CLINICAL ASSESSMENT OF CHILD AND ADOLESCENT BEHAVIOR

CLINICAL ASSESSMENT OF CHILD AND ADOLESCENT BEHAVIOR

H. Booney Vance

Andres J. Pumariega

John Wiley & Sons, Inc

New York • Chichester • Weinheim • Brisbane • Singapore • Toronto

Library of Congress Cataloging-in-Publication Data:
Clinical assessment of child and adolescent behavior / [edited by] H. Booney Vance and Andres J. Pumariega.
    p. cm.
   Includes bibliographical references.
   ISBN 0-471-38046-6 (alk. paper)
   1. Child psychiatry. 2. Adolescent psychiatry. I. Vance, H. Booney,
1941–. II. Pumariega, Andres J.
  RJ499 .C585 2001
  618.92′89—dc21

                                     00-061965

10 9 8 7 6 5 4 3 2

Contents

Preface   xiii

Contributor List   xv

Section I   Processes and Techniques

Chapter 1   The Assessment Process: An Introduction   **3**

Parameters of Assessment   3

Traditional versus New Approaches (Focal Assessment)   4

Exciting Developments   6

Brief Example of Focal Assessment   7

Computer-Assisted Assessment   9

WISC-III Psychological Interpretive Report   10

Summary   15

References   16

Chapter 2   Clinical Assessment of Children and Adolescents: A Place to Begin   **19**

A Brief Review of Psychological Assessment: Past to Present   20

Current and Future Status of Psychological Assessment   26

References   28

Chapter 3   Functional Analysis and Behavioral Assessment of Children and Adolescents   **32**

Introduction   32

History of the Functional Analysis of Behavior   33

Expansion of the Functional Analysis of Behavior   38

Behavioral Assessment of Child and Adolescent Disorders   42

Comprehensive Behavioral Assessment   45

Indirect Behavioral Assessment   61

Behavioral Clinical Case Formulation and Treatment Plan   67

Case Study   68

Current Trends in the Functional Analysis and Assessment of Behavior   76

Special Issues and Populations   78

References   79

Chapter 4   The Mental Status Exam in Child and Adolescent Evaluation   **86**

Definition and Purposes of the MSE   86

Locating the MSE within the Matrix of Child and Adolescent
   Clinical Evaluation   87

Process of the MSE   88

Content of the MSE   89

Age-Related Modifications in the Approach and Technique of the MSE   90

Modifications of the MSE with Special Populations   91

Recording the MSE   93

Case Examples   94

Integration of the MSE and Other Sources of Information in
   Diagnosis and Treatment Planning   96

References   96

Chapter 5   Issues in the Forensic Evaluation of Children and Youth   **98**

Introduction   98

Therapeutic versus Legal Practice Contexts   98

Juveniles and the Law   103

Selected Juvenile Forensic Practice Contexts   104

Conclusion   115

Notes   116

References   116

Chapter 6   The Assessment of Motor Deficits Following Pediatric Brain Injury   **119**

Introduction   119

Epidemiology   119

Neuroanatomical Foundations   120

Neuroanatomy of Motor Functioning   123

Mechanisms of Injury   125

Evaluation of Motor Functioning in Children   126

Motor Impairment Associated with Brain Injury   127

Special Topics   129

Psychological Consequences of Brain Injury   131

Methods of Intervention   132

Case Study   132

Summary   134

References   134

Section II   Disorders of Behaviors, Emotions, and Communications

Chapter 7   Learning Disorders: Real Children, Real Problems   **139**

Introduction   139

Complexity of the Field   140

Definition: What Is a Learning Disability?   140

History   141

The Assessment Process   143

Case Study: Comprehensive Interpretive Psychological Evaluation   148

Additional Issues   155

Medical Factors in Learning Disabilities   158

Approaches to Treatment and Interventions   161

Remediation: Specific Skill Training   161

Summary   163

References   164

Chapter 8   Communicative Disorders   **170**

Rationale for Communication Assessment   170

Developmental Approach   171

Profiles for Impairment   171

Diagnostic Profiles   172

Types of Assessment   174

Case Example   180

Assessment to Treatment   181

Leaders in the Field   181

Summary   182

References   186

Chapter 9   Pervasive Developmental Disorders   **188**

Introduction   188

Autism   189

Asperger's Disorder   192

Changes in Conceptual Considerations   193

Current Definitions of Autism   195

Autism-Related Disorders   199

Assessment   201

Specific Scales for Autism   204

Differential Diagnosis   208

Interventions   210

Controversial and Unorthodox Interventions   219
Summary   224
References   225

Chapter 10   Disruptive Behavior Disorders: Assessment and Intervention   231
Disruptive Behavior Disorders   231
Factors Associated with ODD and CD: Etiology and Correlates   234
Assessment: Diagnosis and Formulation   239
Case Study   243
Interventions   247
Issues and Implications   251
Summary   255
References   256

Chapter 11   Attention-Deficit/Hyperactivity Disorder   263
Introduction   263
Evolution of the Diagnosis of ADHD   264
Treatment Planning   276
Pharmacotherapy   281
Case Examples of the Integration of Assessment and Interventions   288
Outcomes in Adolescence   296
Outcomes in Adulthood   296
References   297

Chapter 12   Eating Disorders: Bulimia and Anorexia Nervosa   307
Introduction and Overview of Eating Disorders   307
Historical Overview   308
Past and Present Leaders in the Field   310
Assessment of Eating Disorders   311
Diagnosis and Formulation   314
Clinical Case Studies   319
Interventions and Rehabilitation   321
Detection and Prevention   323
References   324

Chapter 13   Child Abuse and Psychic Trauma in Children   328
History of Childhood Trauma and Maltreatment   328
History of Legal Protection of Children   330
Definitional Issues   331
Epidemiology of Child Abuse and Childhood Trauma   332
Causes of Child Abuse and Neglect   333

The Impact of Abuse and Psychic Trauma in Childhood 334
Assessment of Child Abuse and Trauma 338
Diagnosis 341
Treatment Interventions for Children Experiencing Severe Traumas 343
Case Examples 348
References 351

Chapter 14 Disorders of Infancy and Early Childhood **358**
Introduction 358
Historical Overview 359
Assessment of Disorders in Infancy and Early Childhood 361
Special Issues in Assessment of At-Risk Populations 368
Diagnosing Disorders in Infancy and Early Childhood 369
Interventions and Rehabilitation: General Comments 377
Interventions and Rehabilitation: Specific Strategies and Approaches 377
Future Directions 380
References 380

Chapter 15 Anxiety Disorders in Children and Adolescents **383**
Introduction 383
Definition 383
Historical Perspective 384
Temperament and Anxiety 385
Behavioral Inhibition 386
Ethological Development 387
Genetic Field Theory 388
Psychological Factors and Anxiety 389
Epidemiology 389
Comorbidity 390
Assessment 390
Clinical Syndromes 398
Course and Outcome 404
Treatment 405
Conclusions 407
References 407

Chapter 16 Childhood Mood Disorders: History, Characteristics, Diagnosis, and Treatment **413**
Introduction 413
Historical Perspective 415
Factors and Changes within Childhood Depression 417

Acute, Chronic, and Masked Childhood Depression   418
Degrees of Depressiveness   419
Depression, Affect, and Mood   419
Childhood Suicide and Depression   420
Depression and Suicidal Threats   421
Depression and Learning Disabilities/ADHD   422
Depression and Aggressive Acting-Out Behaviors   423
Problems and Practices in Diagnosis   423
DSM Criteria Used in Diagnosing Various Mood Disorders   424
MMPI-A Diagnostic Procedures   427
Treatment Considerations   431
Which Therapeutic Intervention Works with Depressed Children?   433
Cognitive-Behavioral Therapy   434
School-Based Interventions   435
Family Therapy   435
Interpersonal Therapy (IPT)   436
Play Therapy   437
Dynamic Psychotherapy   437
Case Studies   439
Summary   442
References   443

Chapter 17   Socially and Emotionally Maladjusted Youth   450
Introduction   450
Historical Overview and Current Trends   451
Clinical Assessment Process: Diagnosis and Treatment   453
Diagnosis and Formulation   457
Clinical Case Study   462
Specific Remedial and Treatment Approaches   464
Psychopharmacology   466
Special Issues   468
References   470

Section III   Special Interventions with Children and Adolescents

**Chapter 18   Psychopharmacological Interventions for Children with
             Challenging Behaviors   475**
Introduction   475
Past and Present Leaders   475

Pharmacological Intervention in Assessment: Its Significance in Relation to
   Diagnosis, Treatment Intervention, and Habitation   476

Formulation and Diagnosis   484

Assessment and Monitoring/Reassessment   486

Specific and Special Issues   487

References   490

Chapter 19   Cultural Competence in Treatment Interventions   494

Rationale for Cultural Competence in Children's Mental Health   494

Concepts of Culture and Impact on Human Behavior   495

Cultural Competence Model   499

Application of Cultural Competence Principles in Clinical Interventions   501

Challenges to the Cultural Competence of Systems of Care   507

References   508

**Chapter 20   Systems of Care for Children and Adolescents with Serious
   Emotional Disturbance   513**

Introduction: The Child with Serious Emotional Disturbance   513

History of Treatment for SED Children   515

Characteristics of the SED Child   517

Assessment of the SED Child   518

The Clinical Model in Systems of Care   520

Clinical Vignettes Illustrating the Wraparound Approach   522

Models of Interagency Collaboration in Systems of Care   523

Accomplishments of Systems of Care Projects   527

Summary   529

References   529

Author Index   533

Subject Index   547

Preface

Clinical Assessment of Child and Adolescent Behavior offers comprehensive coverage of
the most effective approaches to the identification and diagnosis of psychological/psy-
chiatric disorders found in infants, children, and youth plus treatment and intervention
approaches. This book is an interface of school psychology, clinical child psychology,
developmental pediatrics, child and adolescent psychiatry, and child psychopathology
that focuses on psychological disorders found in infants, children and adolescents. It
does not focus on one particular child disorder, or one individual approach to assessing children with challenging behaviors, but offers the student and clinician a wealth of
detailed practical information not only on the clinical assessment of the behavior but
also on applied intervention strategies for each disorder. We believe the chapters offer
an interface between clinical assessment and intervention/treatment approaches, which
most textbooks often treat separately or isolate from each other. For some, keeping up
with the changing nomenclature and progress made in the clinical assessment of children's behavior and treatment approaches has been difficult due to the advances made
within the past five years. We believe this book brings these areas—assessment, treatment, and medication management—together in a systemic manner concurrent with
advances made in the past five years.

Hence, the main objective of *Clinical Assessment of Child and Adolescent Behavior* is
to bring together a group of well-known clinicians to build upon the current knowledge
about identifying and assessing infants, children, and youth with behavior disorders,
developmental problems, and other challenging behavior, and child and adolescent
treatment approaches, including psychopharmacology. This objective is accomplished
by bringing together some of the foremost experts in school psychology, clinical child
psychology, child and adolescent psychiatry, and developmental pediatric to author
chapters that cut across the various complicated issues in the clinical assessment of
children's behavior. Each chapter presents a current consolidated and an integrative description of the assessment process and intervention/treatment approaches for disorders found in infancy, childhood, and adolescence. In addition, each chapter provides
detailed, procedural guidelines for the assessment of these disorders, current descriptions of assessment instruments used in the identification process, detailed case studies,
and an integrated treatment approach, including the use of psychopharmacology
agents in the management of these challenging behaviors.

The consumer of this book is taken through the entire process of identifying and assessing the most common and difficult disorders found in young children and youth.
The organization of each chapter emphasizes the process and procedures for the as-

sessment and treatment for each of the disorders. The book strives to communicate the state of the art in the clinical assessment of child and adolescent behavior and in their treatment approaches. Chief strengths of this book are its

- Balanced coverage of assessment procedures;
- Coverage of issues and disorders not found in other texts, including Forensic Assessment: Eating Disorders, Child Abuse and Psychic Trauma, Mood Disorders, Disorders of Infancy, Psychopharmacological Intervention and Pediatric Brain Injury;
- Enhanced readability through the use of charts and graphs;
- Use of case studies and vignettes for practical application to one's practice; and
- Complete sections on special interventions for children and adolescents.

DESCRIPTION OF SECTIONS

Section I addresses the assessment of children and adolescents, including processes and techniques. Special attention is given to behavior assessment, functional behavior analysis, forensic assessment, and assessment of motor defects following pediatric brain injury. Section II covers specific disorders of behavior, emotions, and communications. Troublesome areas for the clinician such as Autism, Mood Disorders, Eating Disorders, Child Abuse, Disorders of Infancy, and Socially and Maladjusted children and youth are discussed. Section III covers special intervention for children and youth with challenging behaviors such as medication management, cultural competencies in treatment, and systems of intervention for severely emotionally disturbed children and youth.

This book represents an important step in bridging the gap between various disciplines and should lead to improved clinical practices with infants, children, and youth. The book was written with several potential users in mind. It is intended for graduate level courses in assessment, diagnosis, and counseling. It can be used in school psychology, clinical child, developmental pediatric, counseling psychology, and child and adolescent psychiatry courses. The text can be an excellent reference source for clinicians who practice in the public or private domains of health delivery services for children and youth.

This book is the product of the effort of many people. It was truly an honor to work with such outstanding scholars. Each contributor successfully met the challenge of linking the various components of the individual chapters together. For the contributors' hard work, patience, feedback and time, we thank you for your fine work.

We would like to thank the staff of John Wiley & Sons, especially Tracey Belmont for her support, encouragement, and keeping us to the publication schedule. Thank you Tracey! Laura, you deserve a medal! Susan Dodson deserves special recognition for her editing skills.

We are grateful to our families, who have always supported our efforts and demonstrated love and patience. Without our families this book would still be only a topic of discussion. To Sandy and JoAnn, we dedicate this book.

Contributor List

Charles D. Casat, MD
Carolinas Medical Center
Charlotte, North Carolina

Jeanette P. Casat, MS
Charlotte-Mecklenberg Schools
Charlotte, North Carolina

Daniel Castellanos, MD
University of Miami College of Medicine
Miami, Florida

Nancy R. Clanton
University of Alabama
Tuscaloosa, Alabama

Steven P. Cuffe, MD
University of South Carolina
William S. Hal Psychiatric Institute
Columbia, South Carolina

Heather E. Dane
University of Alabama
Tuscaloosa, Alabama

Amor Del Mundo, MD
College of Medicine, East Tennessee
   State University
Johnson City, Tennessee

Mesha Ellis
University of Alabama
Tuscaloosa, Alabama

Gerald B. Fuller, PhD
Director of Psychology
Walden University

R. Andrew Harper, MD
The University of Texas
Horton Medical School
Houston, Texas

Curtis Kauffmann
College of Medicine
East Tennessee State University
Johnson City, Tennessee

Tami V. Leonhardt, PhD
University of South Carolina School of
   Medicine
Columbia, South Carolina

John Lochman, PhD
University of Alabama
Tuscaloosa, Alabama

Thomas N. Magee
University of Alabama
Tuscaloosa, Alabama

Jasjeet Miglani, MD
College of Medicine
University of South Carolina
Columbia, South Carolina

Merry N. Miller, MD
College of Medicine
East Tennessee State University
Johnson City, Tennessee

Ramsey McGowen, PhD
College of Medicine
East Tennessee State University
Johnson City, Tennessee

Freddy Paniagua, PhD
University of Texas Medical Branch
Galveston, Texas

Dustin A. Pardini
University of Alabama
Tuscaloosa, Alabama

Deborah A. Pearson, PhD
University of Texas—Houston Medical
   School
Houston, Texas

Andres J. Pumariega, MD
Quillen College of Medicine
East Tennessee State University
Johnson City, Tennessee

Kenneth M. Rogers, MD
School of Medicine
University of South Carolina
Columbia, South Carolina

Eugenio M. Rothe, MD
University of Miami School of Medicine
Miami, Florida

Eric Roth, PsyD
Quillen College of Medicine
East Tennessee State University
Johnson City, Tennessee

David Sabatino, PhD
East Tennessee State University
Johnson City, Tennessee

Cynthia Santos, MD
The University of Texas
Houston Medical School
Houston, Texas

Thomas Schacht, PsyD
Quillen College of Medicine
East Tennessee State University
Johnson City, Tennessee

Nancy Scherer, PhD
East Tennessee State University
Johnson City, Tennessee

Margaret Shugart, MD
University of South Carolina, William S.
   Hall Psychiatric Institute
Columbia, South Carolina

H. Booney Vance, PhD
Quillen College of Medicine
East Tennessee State University
Johnson City, Tennessee

Nancy Winters, MD
Oregon Health Sciences University
Portland, Oregon

Bonnie G. Webster, MSN, JD
East Tennessee State University
Johnson City, Tennessee

Harry H. Wright, MD, MBA
School of Medicine
University of South Carolina
Columbia, South Carolina

SECTION I

Processes and Techniques

Chapter 1

THE ASSESSMENT PROCESS: AN INTRODUCTION

H. BOONEY VANCE AND ANDRES J. PUMARIEGA

In the referral process the assessment of child or adolescent behavior plays a major role in formulating a diagnosis and treatment/intervention, whether in an outpatient setting, in schools, or in a residential center. Assessment is an interactive student-oriented process. The individual assessment of child or adolescent behavior by a skilled professional is a process that may occur only once in a child's life, when one highly skilled clinician devotes a considerable amount of time (ranging from one to many hours) to that individual. Perhaps the assessment process for a given individual will be a once-in-a-lifetime opportunity for a professional to devote all of his or her skills and knowledge to obtain critical information about a child—information that will be used to answer a number of important questions regarding that child's current and future life, such as mental status, cognitive abilities, presence of emotional/psychiatric disorders, eligibility for remedial/special education programs, placement decisions, and treatment and intervention strategies. The assessment of a child's current performance in different dimensions represents a major challenge to all clinicians who interact with children of all ages and ethnic backgrounds. Cronbach's (1949) definition of a test as a systematic procedure for comparing the behavior of two or more persons still stands as the benchmark of the assessment process.

PARAMETERS OF ASSESSMENT

The last two decades in psychology and psychiatry have seen radical changes in the assessment process and in treatment patterns for children suffering from emotional/behavioral disorders—changes arising from the brief-focus approaches to exciting breakthroughs in psychopharmacology. For instance, medication has reduced the course of depression disorders from months to weeks and has allowed individuals with severe cases of schizophrenia to function productively. These changes have led to a major reorientation toward assessment and treatment; and because of the specificity of the new treatments, the issues of assessment and diagnosis have returned to the center stage. Wetzler and Katz (1989) underscore the importance of understanding how the treatment works to bring recovery from these illnesses. It is necessary to examine in detail the characteristics of the illnesses in order to determine which aspects of behavior, emotions, and cognitions are being affected. To conduct research on the process of treatment/intervention or the mechanisms of treatment, it is necessary to assess and diagnose disorders accurately, to assess the change brought about by the treatment, and to evaluate the outcome.

Traditional psychological assessment of behavior was first introduced over 70 years ago by Herman Rorschach and Henry Murray and was expanded in the 1950s by Rapaport, Gill, and Schafer (1968). That model was appropriate in the 1950s and 1960s for the assessment of problems within the parameters of psychology and psychiatry. Since then, however, numerous changes have affected the assessment procedures: public laws, changing diagnostic systems, new trends in assessment, length of treatment, and the incorporation of children and youth in our theoretical orientations. In addition, we have witnessed a complete change in systems of care, third-party payment, and due process and treatment within a focused time frame, as well as in the language of education, psychology, and psychiatry. For instance, the diagnostic system itself has been revamped (American Psychiatric Association, 1994).

Within the last 15 years, our field has witnessed dramatic growth in managed health care, hospital/school utilization and review committees, quality assurance committees (Individual Treatment Plans, or ITP), and peer-review utilization. These new dimensions, added to the already existing parameters and expectations of assessment of children's behavior, have created an impetus for change. If we as professional clinicians do not change with the times, our procedures, knowledge, and skills will become outdated and anachronistic.

TRADITIONAL VERSUS NEW APPROACHES (FOCAL ASSESSMENT)

Historically and traditionally the standard assessment battery for evaluating children with behavioral difficulties consisted of a projectial instrument (e.g., Children Apperception Test, Draw-a-Person, Bender Gestalt for visual-motor-perceptual difficulties) and a test of cognition (e.g., Wechsler Intelligence Scale for Children—Revised [WISC-R] and Kaufman Assessment Battery for Children [K-ABC]). The aim was to identify or evaluate the child's personality, structure, defenses, ego strengths and boundaries, reality testing, intelligence, mental status, and inner dynamics. Much was based on analytical theory (Weiner, 1983). Traditionally, one of the only self-report instruments available to a clinician was the Minnesota Multiphasic Personality Inventory (MMPI, adult version). Few psychomechanically sound self-report- or behavior-based assessment tools were available to help the child and adolescent school specialist. Regardless of the referral question, the same battery was administered with loyalty.

As the underlying assessment orientation changed and a different climate developed in the fields of education, psychology, and psychiatry, the traditional test battery began to receive criticism. Courts, clinicians, parents, educators, and advocate groups began to raise questions about the usefulness of such a battery in the present day realities; the MMPI did not address the referral questions (Sattler, 1988), and thus their value was questioned.

Clinicians, parents, educators, and physicians were discovering that the traditional assessment strategy used in evaluating child and adolescent behavior was not appropriate to many settings (e.g., school, clinics, residential hospital units). The process was time-consuming, laborious, and of questionable validity, and much of the data obtained from the battery were not used or were even ignored. In practice, in fact, I have seen the psychological assessment results (reports) not included in a child's file until after his or her discharge. What is the value of delaying results in times of rapid discharge? Combined with this, information about a child's developing intropsychic dynamic made the traditional approach grow more vulnerable to criticism. A major concern raised by the consumer was the relevance of the findings in terms of treatment. These traditional assessment instruments are not useless, but this battery was not designed to help choose appropriate treatment modalities or to assist in differential diagnosis, was not developed for children, and is not comparable to the DSM-IV. Further, the influence of ethnic and cultural factors on the development of behavioral/emotional difficulties in children and youth has gained increasing emphasis (Pumariega & Vance, 1999). Cross-cultural assessment issues have given rise to the role of ethnic/cultural factors' influences on the development of behavior/emotional disorders in children and youth. What is the role of one's own cultural biases and values in the assessment process? Could these affect the clinician's use of assessment information? Do our current assessment instruments need new norms for ethnic and cultural minority groups? The benefits of culturally specific tests are rather unclear because the cultural make-up of the United States continues to change, and other intervening variables could affect the results obtained from these instruments.

A More Focused Approach

In recent years there have been several calls for a broader conceptualization of assessment. Such broadening has been noticeable in the use of a focal assessment approach. This approach has contributed greatly in pinpointing psychiatric diagnosis and treatment/interventions. It seems very clear that tools used by assessment specialists and psychologists as recently as 10 years ago are generally different from those used now. Such techniques as computer-based assessment, focal assessment, behavior assessment, structural psychiatric interviews, comprehensive neuropsychological test batteries, and new cognitive batteries are making major contributions in the assessment field. These new assessment procedures have shifted the focus from indirect models to direct acquisition of information and observation. These efforts have bridged the gap between assessment and treatment. There is a distinction between just testing and assessment; assessment is a much broader, thorough concept. Psychologists do not merely *give* tests, but also *perform* assessment, meaning that there are many different ways of evaluating individual differences.

Assessment Schemes

Since the 1960s, a number of comprehensive assessment schemes have been developed (American Psychological Association, 1994; Kamphaus, 1993; Kauffman, 1979; Lazarus, 1973; Sattler, 1988). Sattler's (1988) gold standard test detailed the specifics of his comprehensive model for the assessment of children (see chapters 2 and 3 of his text). Kauffman (1994) provides the interested reader with a seven-step interpretive approach for using the WISC-III. Cautila (1968) describes a three-stage scheme for behavioral assessment at various treatment stages. Kanfer and Saslow (1969) proposed a seven-step model using interviews to organize a patient's complaints into five behavior categories. Their system complemented the existing DSM-II model. Taylor (1983), a behavioral psychiatrist, incorporated the DSM-III conceptual model into an assessment scheme. Wetzler and Katz (1989) elaborate on the multivantaged approach to assessment. Their system consists of eleven state constructs and their associated factors and vantages. According to Wetzler and Katz (1989), these constructs span the area of the psychological functions of affect, activity level, cognition, perception, socialization, and social behavior (p. 19). The American Academy of Child and Adolescent Psychiatrists publishes practice parameters as a guideline for mental health professionals in its official *Journal of Child and Adolescent Psychiatry.* Since 1991, the journal has published 17 practice parameters. The December 1999 issue contained practice parameters for assessment and treatment of individuals with Mental Retardation and comorbid mental conditions, individuals with autism and other Pervasive Developmental Disorders, and children and adolescents who are sexually abusive of others. These supplements to the *Journal of Child and Adolescent Psychiatry* provide clinicians with an excellent conceptual model not only for assessment but also for interventions. They emphasize a shared commitment to a developmental, interdisciplinary collaboration, and a consultation approach with various professionals. Practice parameters, developed by work groups (members of the American Academy of Child and Adolescent Psychiatrists) are strategies or guidelines for patient management based on scientific research, and they describe the generally accepted approaches to assessment and treatment of specific disorders. The parameters are provided as standard care for specific mental disorders or medical procedures.

EXCITING DEVELOPMENTS

Over the last 15 years, two exciting developments have emerged in the field of assessment: behavioral assessment and focal assessment (Bellack and Hensen, 1988). These two approaches were the outgrowth of clinicians' dissatisfaction with the DSM-II and DSM-III, and with the poor relationship between assessment and treatment outcomes. Goldstein and Hersen (1992) attribute the development of behavior assessment and focal assessment to the growing need for precision and accountability, and to the limited relationship between complicated psychological evaluation and eventual treatment. In addition, many clinicians (clinical, child, school) operated as X-ray technicians (Goldstein & Hersen, 1992), using procedures that had a tangential relationship to the diagnostic-behavior descriptors for each clinical group, such as Mental Retardation, learning disorders, mood disorders, Attention-Deficit Hyperactivity Disorder (ADHD), or children with challenging behavior (PDD or severe emotional disturbances). The isolated and extensive psychological evaluation or examination, according to Goldstein and Hersen (1992), "proved to be an empty academic exercise resulting in poetic jargon in the report whose preclinical validity was woefully limited" (p. 9).

Because the behavioral approach to assessment is excellently covered in this book by

Freddy A. Paniagua (Chapter 3), he elaborates on this model. However, within the last decade the field of behavioral assessment has grown dramatically. The behavioral approach to assessment has undergone changes over the past two decades. Nelson and Hayes (1974) indicated that the goal of behavioral assessment was to identify meaningful response units and their controlling variables. Recent research has identified the goal of behavioral assessment as objectively describing discrete human responses that are controlled by environmental events and whose variability is related to a person's environment (specific behaviors and specific environmental events). Behavioral assessment usually provides clients with a description of environmental contexts, of specific behaviors to describe personality constructs, of direct and specific measures of behavior, and of continuous assessment/measurement of ongoing behaviors and outcomes. Emphasis is usually on direct observation, accuracy of observation, and practicality—usefulness, description of behavior, prediction, or what maintains responses and what reduces responses (chances that occur throughout treatment) (Maag, 1999).

The second change, a somewhat different approach to assessment, is focal assessment. Wetzler and Katz (1989) indicated that the roots of focal assessment can be traced back to Galton's day and that focal assessment is not new! Clarkin and Sweeney (1986) suggested that the instruments used in focal assessment serve a different end than do the standard batteries, and that the focal assessment instruments were developed and refined on homogeneous patient populations. In essence they were developed to evaluate outcome variables (treatment). An example is the Conners Scale (Conners, 1990), which was developed for physicians to evaluate the use of medication (stimulants) in treating hyperactive children. These focal assessment instruments are specific to narrower areas of psychopathology (Wetzler & Katz, 1989). Focal assessment instruments cover a wide and diverse range of functioning, such as the Beck Depression Inventory or the Mental Status Exam, to evaluate a patient's mental status. These instruments usually have good normative data, specific rules for scoring, and solid research data for validity purposes. Their research database provides reliable, quantifiable procedures for evaluating behavior. Major advantages of the focal assessment instruments are their focus on efficiency, time saving, cost-effectiveness, and treatment outcome. Consider the use of medication (such as selective serotonin reuptake inhibitors, or SSRIs) to treat depression: A clinician can track clinical changes by administering a weekly serial rating scale. This type of assessment often helps to evaluate effectiveness of treatment modality, to guide treatment planning, and to generate data for research purposes. Focal assessment instruments allow clinicians to be flexible and tailor treatment to clients' needs. Carr (1985), in an excellent review of focal assessment instruments, identified over 100 popular, well-validated tests. Examples of focal assessment instruments and their corresponding measurement domains are provided in Figure 1.1.

BRIEF EXAMPLE OF FOCAL ASSESSMENT

Tom was an 8-year-old elementary school student who had been having serious academic difficulties over the past six months. He was becoming more and more agitated. He was seen as an outpatient at a psychiatric clinic. Tom was administered the

Depression	Hyperactivity/Inattention	Anxiety/Fears	Disruptive/Oppositional	Global
Helplessness Scale	Conners Parent Rating Scale	Social Phobia and Anxiety	Swanson, Nolan, and Pilham Rating Scale	Behavior Assessment System Inventory for Children
Hopelessness Scale	Conners Teaching Rating Scale	Fear Survey for Children	Eyberg Child Behavior Inventory	Child Behavior Checklist
Children Depression Rating Scale	Swanson, Nolan, and Pilham Rating Scale	Revised Children Manifest Anxiety Scale	Sutter-Eyberg Student Behavior Inventory	Devereux Scales of Mental Disorders
Peer Nomination for Depression	Attention Deficit Disorder Evaluation Scale	State-Trait Anxiety Inventory for Children	Devereux Behavior Rating Scale	MMPI-A
Children Depression Inventory	Continuous Performance Tests	Behavioral Avoidance Test	Revised Behavior Problem Checklist	Personality Inventory for Children-R (Youth)
Reynolds Child Depression Scale; also Adolescent Version	Brown Attention Deficit Disorder Scales	Louisville Fear Survey Schedule for Children		Self-Report of Personality
	Attention Deficit/Hyperactivity Test	Fear Survey Schedule		Walker-McConnell Scale
		Feelings, Attitudes, and Behavior Scale		Social Skills Rating System
		Trauma Symptoms Checklist for Children		Child Behavior Checklist
		Behavioral and Emotional Rating Scale		Diagnostic Schedule Interview for Children
				Social Adjustment Inventory for Children

Figure 1.1 Example of Focal Assessment Instruments

Childhood Depression Inventory (Kovacs, 1992), which indicated severe depression. Tom obtained significantly elevated T-scores, a 96 on Negative Mood, 94 on Anhedonia, and 89 on Negative Self-Esteem. His mother and teacher completed the Conners Scale. Results from this scale revealed elevated scores on the Hyperactivity and ADHD Index Scores (T-83 and T-85). Behavior observation during the Diagnostic Interview Schedule for Children (DISC) revealed elevated scores on ADHD, overanxious disorder, and more disorders. Throughout the assessment, Tom was active, often getting out of his seat and turning and twisting in his chair, and he constantly had to be reminded to pay attention. These same behaviors were scored positive on the Conners Scale by his parents and his teachers. In light of these findings, a referral was made to a child psychiatrist. Formulation of findings indicated a child who was depressed and overanxious; ADHD was secondary to depression and overanxiousness. The treatment team decided on a trial dose of Wellbutrin and an aggressive psychoeducational approach with family sessions and individual cognitive behavior therapy.

COMPUTER-ASSISTED ASSESSMENT

Computers and technology have impacted almost every aspect of our society as well as our professions. The availability of computer technology and software engineering has affected the practice of psychological assessment. These effects have influenced test construction, the standardization of new instruments, interactive assessment, continuous-variable assessment, and scoring and interpretation of tests of intelligence and personality. Powerful computers are used today as an adjunct to the assessment process because of their accessibility, affordability, and sophistication, and the emphasis on actuarial-based interpretation of test results.

The first major computer-assisted psychological program began in the early 1960s at the Mayo Clinic in Rochester, Minnesota (Honaker & Fowler, 1990). This system gives a brief interpretation of each of the MMPI scales that were elevated. By the early 1970s there were seven commercial MMPI interpretation services available for clinicians and physicians. Throughout the 1960s, several computerized scoring and interpretation programs were developed for lists such as the Rorschach (Piodrowski, 1964), 16 PF (Elber, 1964, September) and the California Psychological Inventory (Finney, 1966).

The 1970s witnessed a proliferation of more computer applications in psychology, psychiatry, and medicine. The first line testing services became available, led by Johnson and Williams (1980) working at the Veterans Hospital in Salt Lake City (Psychiatric Assessment Unit). According to Honaker and Fowler (1990), there were 320 Psych System owners with more than 700 list terminals in operation by the early 1980s.

The 1980s ushered in powerful, low-cost personal microcomputers, which became accessible to many mental health coaches. Software development for all types of scoring, interpreting, and report writing became available. Many of these systems were developed by individuals or small companies, and only later by the large test publishers. Honaker and Fowler (1990) reported that CompuPsych was one of the first to market microcomputer systems for psychological assessment. Bob Smith, who founded Psychological Assessment Resources (PAR) in 1978, was a leader in marketing software for assessment purposes with a standard microcomputer. Today PAR is perhaps the major leader, developer, and distributor of psychological assessment products. Since the late 1970s, numerous companies have been developed and have contributed to the popularization of computer-assisted assessment. In 1987, Krug reported that there were 72 separate suppliers of over 300 computer-based products with applications in psychological assessment. During this same year, Exner (1987) introduced the assistance of computers in Rorschach interpretations.

WISC-III PSYCHOLOGICAL INTERPRETIVE REPORT

Name: Jacob
Date of Birth: March 19, 1991
Chronological Age: 7 years 7 months
School: ———
Date of Evaluation: November 17, 1998
Grade: First
Examiner: Dr. Vance

Referral Information

Jacob was referred for evaluation by his teacher mainly because of learning problems in school but also due to a possible developmental delay. The main goals of this evaluation were to answer the following questions: Is Jacob in an appropriate classroom setting? Are special education services recommended for Jacob? Are therapeutic interventions advised?

Background Information

Jacob is a Caucasian male, aged 7 years 7 months. The background information presented here about Jacob is based primarily on reports from his teacher but also on his school records and a social history. He lives with his biological parents and is one of two children in his residence. Jacob is the younger child in his family. His family economic status is working class. As a child, his home environment is average—that is, neither impoverished nor enriched. Cultural opportunities at home (e.g., availability of books, family trips to museums) are average, neither inadequate nor excellent. Both Jacob's mother and his father attended some high school.

When she was pregnant with Jacob, his mother reported that she experienced bleeding. Jacob's birth was premature and occurred after a long labor. Following birth, Jacob was placed in an incubator. During early childhood, Jacob was described as difficult. He developed physical skills such as sitting, crawling, and walking at about the same time as most children. His early language development was slow in comparison to that of other children. His early motor development and skills acquisition were about the same as those of his age mates, and his social development was average. His cognitive development (e.g., counting, learning the alphabet) was behind that of others his age.

Jacob went to kindergarten and is now in first grade at a public school. He is reported to enjoy school. Jacob's skill strengths in school are reported to be his ability to please his teacher and to behave correctly. In contrast, his weaknesses are reported to be concentration, organization, and vocabulary, together with verbal expression and understanding concepts.

Appearance and Behavioral Characteristics

Jacob appears the same as his stated age of 7 years. His height is below average for his age, and his weight is average for his build. He has brown eyes, and his hair is blond. At the evaluation, Jacob was dressed appropriately, and his hygiene was good. He appeared pleasant and smiling. He spoke in an age-appropriate manner. Jacob was very willing and compliant when he began the test session. Rapport was easy to establish and maintain.

Jacob displayed good attention during the evaluation; he worked diligently with optimal concentration on the nonverbal tests, which consisted of rapidly copying simple symbols that are associated with shapes, arranging pictures to tell stories, and copying abstract designs with blocks. Jacob showed low risk-taking at times by refusing to guess if unsure of answers on the verbal tests of general information and telling how two concepts are alike. Jacob demonstrated poor expressive language skills while being tested by naming the missing part vaguely or incorrectly or by having to be told "show me where you mean" several times on a test of finding missing parts in pictures, and by giving too much detail or irrelevant information during a test of social comprehension. Jacob demonstrated weak receptive language skills during the evaluation when he didn't seem to understand the wording of some questions on the verbal tests of general information and social understanding. Jacob demonstrated a problem working with numbers when he used "finger writing" to solve some items on a test of arithmetic problem-solving.

The physical environment of the testing session was optimal, and the results of the evaluation are considered valid, though with reservations.

Test Results and Interpretation

Jacob was given the WISC-III, a test that evaluates the present level of intellectual functioning of children and adolescents. He scored in the Low Average range of intelligence (Verbal IQ = 87, Performance IQ = 89, Full Scale IQ = 86), ranking him at about the 18th percentile relative to other 7-year-olds. The chances are very good (about 19 out of 20) that Jacob's true Full Scale IQ falls between 81 and 92. The 2-point difference between his Verbal and Performance IQs is trivial and indicates that he expresses his intelligence equally well when responding verbally to oral questions as when manipulating concrete, nonverbal materials. See Figure 1.2 for the WISC-III results.

The WISC-III contains four indexes. Two are large: Verbal Comprehension (VC), composed of four Verbal subtests; and Perceptual Organization (PO), composed of four Performance subtests. Two are smaller: Freedom from Distractibility (FD), composed of two Verbal subtests; and Processing Speed (PS), composed of two Performance subtests. Jacob earned indexes of 88 on VC (21st percentile), 89 on PO (23rd percentile), 81 on FD (10th percentile), and 93 on PS (32nd percentile).

IQs	IQ Score	Percentile	90% Confidence Interval
VIQ	87	19	82–93
PIQ	89	23	83–97
FFSIQ	86	18	81–92

Factor Indexes	Index Score	Percentile	90% Confidence Interval
VC	88	21	83–95
PO	89	23	83–97
FD	81	10	76–91
PS	93	32	86–102

Verbal	Scaled Score	Percentile
Information	8	25
Similarities	8	25
Arithmetic	7	16
Vocabulary	8	25
Comprehension	7	16
(Digit Span)	6	9

Performance	Scaled Score	Percentile
Picture Completion	7	16
Coding	9	37
Picture Arrangement	9	37
Block Design	9	37
Object Assembly	7	16
(Symbol Search)	8	25

Scaled score profile:

	In	Si	Ar	Vo	Co	DS	PC	Cd	PA	BD	OA	SS
Scaled Score	8	8	7	8	7	6	7	9	9	9	7	8

(Profile axis range 19 to 1)

Figure 1.2 WISC-III Psychometric Summary

Jacob's indexes on the two factors composed only of Verbal subtests (VC and FD) do not differ significantly. That is, he performed about as well on tasks that measure verbal comprehension and expression as he did on tasks that require sequencing and number ability, and that are unusually susceptible to behaviors such as distractibility and anxiety.

Jacob's performance on the FD factor is consistent with his overall performance on the various verbal and nonverbal subtests that constitute the WISC-III. He performed about as well on tasks that measure sequencing and number ability—and that are unusually susceptible to behaviors such as distractibility and anxiety—as would be expected in view of his overall performance on a variety of tasks.

Jacob's indexes on the two factors composed only of Performance subtests (PO and PS) do not differ significantly. He performed about as well on tasks that measure visual/motor coordination and nonverbal reasoning as he did on tasks that require highly speeded paper-and-pencil responding and that are unusually susceptible to behaviors such as low motivation, lack of concentration, and reflectiveness.

Summary

Jacob is a 7-year-old Caucasian male who was referred for evaluation by his teacher because of concerns about learning problems in school. During the evaluation, Jacob displayed good attention. On the WISC-III, Jacob earned a Verbal IQ of 87, a Performance IQ of 89, and a Full Scale IQ of 86. Jacob performed about as well on tests of verbal comprehension and expression as he did on tests of nonverbal thinking and visual-motor coordination. Overall, Jacob performed in the Low Average range of intelligence.

Recommendations

For Jacob's receptive language problems:

1. Be careful that language clarifies, rather than disturbs, learning. Check wording of directions to be sure all basic concepts are within Jacob's working vocabulary.
2. Maintain visual contact with the learner. Use gestures to facilitate oral communication.
3. Speak at a tempo that is slower than usual.
4. Touch Jacob before talking to him.

Jacob has been referred for school learning problems and may require remediation. If so, then the following suggestions may prove beneficial for Jacob:

1. Individualize each area of instruction so that Jacob is taught at the appropriate readiness level for each different skill.
2. Teach to Jacob's tolerance level and avoid pushing beyond. For example, help teachers pinpoint his threshold level and stay at it.
3. Begin new tasks only when you know Jacob is not tired and is "ready" to learn.

4. Employ the following suggestions, which are intended to help strengthen the integration and storage of new learning.

   a. Make use of all available feedback in the remedial setting (for example, the teacher's feedback when Jacob responds to a question or assignment; Jacob's feedback when the teacher confirms or corrects a response; and the internal/external feedback he receives from his own actual and covert response behavior—vocal or motor—and self-corrections in computer instructional materials).

   b. Develop abilities functionally, in natural settings, and avoid contrived or artificial ones. For example, integrate new reading skills by having many easy reading materials for Jacob to "practice" on instead of traditional drills and reviews.

   c. Teach material for which Jacob has a practical need first.

To help a student with a lower IQ like Jacob generalize newly acquired information:

1. Provide set variations of initial learning bits and point out similarities or unity of information.

2. Present the same information in many different ways to create adequate redundancy.

3. Provide generous time allowances for remedial work. Sometimes Jacob does not succeed because he just needs more time on an instructional task.

4. Measure improvement and show the record to Jacob (to prove to him that change is taking place).

5. Employ the following suggestions, which are especially useful for children with multiple areas of deficit.

   a. Remediate prerequisite deficits first (for example, oral language before written language, word recognition before reading comprehension).

   b. Ensure that lessons within each area progress from simple to more complex tasks. This may require preliminary task analyses.

   c. Use minimal steps of increasing difficulty.

   d. If a teacher, allow sufficient time to supervise new learning. Remedial work must be closely monitored until it becomes a work habit.

   e. If a teacher, join Jacob in a cooperative effort to set and attain realistic goals.

   f. Maintain a 90% success rate to avoid negative error learning and feelings of inadequacy.

   g. Get some improvement each session. Don't keep on the same approach if it is not successful.

   h. Work on only one new skill at a time, presenting just a few new stimuli and limiting other variables to a bare minimum. This avoids interference and overloading.

Jacob was reported to have weaknesses in concentration and organization. To improve Jacob's work habits and attention and concentration:

1. Use other pupils in cooperative remedial sessions in addition to individual one-on-one tutoring. Peer tutors will serve as role models for appropriate study techniques and will promote social support at the same time. A side benefit of peer tutors is the encouragement of a spirit of cooperation instead of competition.

2. Select instruction materials that are highly interesting to Jacob. For example, instead of a story in a basal reader, substitute reading the directions of a new game to be played later, or reading instructions about how to put together a model airplane that will be built later.

3. Reinforce Jacob with tangible and intangible rewards when appropriate behavior is demonstrated. Gradually increase the requirements for the reinforcement. For example, classroom privileges, free time, and helping the teacher are tangibles; handshakes, smiles, and praise are intangibles).

4. Write a contract with Jacob that lists expected behaviors and the reinforcements that will follow with each term of the contract that is completed.

5. Structure Jacob's work environment in a way that will promote a reduction of distractions and intervening stimuli.

6. Highlight or circle important information on an assigned work paper that may otherwise be missed. For example, circle the directions, the item numbers to be worked on in math, the main theme in an essay, and so forth.

7. Work on remedial activities when others are working on similar work projects, not during enjoyable activity time.

8. Use learning sets and advanced organizers to enhance motivation for learning by relating previous abilities and knowledge to the present task.

9. Keep lessons very brief for short attention spans. Alternate quiet activities with active ones. Planned interruptions of longer lessons are useful (e.g., have Jacob come to teacher's table after a small task is completed, or get a necessary supply from the shelf when that part of an activity is reached).

10. Manipulate Jacob's sense of space within his learning environment. For example, use partitions, cubicles, screens, quiet corners; remove distracting stimuli by making a window translucent instead of transparent, keeping teacher apparel plain and free from distractions.

SUMMARY

We have provided a brief overview of some of the major areas of psychological assessment and their influence on current practices. There has been a shift from indirect methods to a direct method of gathering information and observing clients. More success has been documented in the last five years of linking our assessment data more closely to treatment outcomes. Roles for psychologists in the area of assessment will be expanding, especially in assessment of medically ill populations, in health psychology, and in behavior medicine. Currently, there is an emphasis on exploring the mind/body dialectic as our measurement instruments become more refined, and this will enable clinicians to identify, treat, and offer suggestions for prevention of stress-related and other psychophysiological disturbances. As Schacht so aptly pointed out, the field of forensic evaluation of children and youth will offer numerous opportunities and challenges for clinicians as more and more clinicians become involved with court cases. This emerging field will require clinicians to upgrade their skills in the forensic practice. Pumariega's paper (Chapter 19, this volume) documents how ethnic variables impact assessment procedures and processes (language, social values, etc.). Rogers (1998) provides an excellent review and offers valuable suggestions to assist psychologists and educational diagnosticians in performing culturally meaningful and technically sound assessment with diverse children and youth. The assessment of a child's behavior will always be a dynamic construct influenced by the individual's age, environment, and culture.

The field of psychological/clinical assessment has expanded rapidly during the last 10 years. New and exciting procedures have been added to the clinician's array of assessment instruments. However, clinical assessment of children's behavior is still dependent on the psychologist's selecting the best possible instrument, whether it be a standardized test, direct observation, or non-norm reference that is firmly rooted in theory and sound psychometric properties (i.e., measuring what it was constructed to do). This may be the most important decision that the clinician makes throughout the assessment process (Vance & Awaad, 1998). The clinical assessment of child and youth behavior requires more than just the ability to select a test, follow the appropriate instructions, and then write a report. Interpersonal and clinical skills are required in addition to a thorough background in assessment and test construction. Interpersonal clinical skills such as report building, accurate observation of behaviors, positive interaction, and interviewing are necessary to be an effective psychologist. The clinical assessment of children behavior is not the mere summation of scores from a test or battery of tests but is a highly complex process that involves the gathering of data from multiple sources and multiple instruments and then extracting diagnostic, meaningful hypotheses regarding the cognitive, social, behavioral, and emotional functioning in a professional and objective manner. It is eminently clear from the chapters in this book that effective, multi-factored assessment of child or youth behavior should be the standard throughout the next decade. As psychology continues to struggle to understand and refine assessment practices, strategic analysis of the *why* of assessment will remain as important as the *how* of assessment. The chapters in this book combine both the why and how as each contributor delineates the purposes of assessing child and youth behavior, matching this to appropriate procedures, and then developing an individualized treatment/intervention plan.

REFERENCES

American Psychiatric Association. (1994). *Diagnostic and statistical manual of mental disorders* (4th ed.). Washington, DC: Author.

Bellack, A. S., & Hensen, M. (1988). Future directions. In A. S. Belleck & M. Hensen, *Behavioral assessment: A practical handbook* (3rd ed., pp. 287–297). Elmsford, NY: Pergamon.

Cautela, J. R. (1968). Behavior therapy and the need for behavior assessment. *Psychotherapy: Theory, Research and Practice, 5,* 175–179.

Clarkin, J., & Sweeney, J. A. (1986). Psychological assessment. In R. Michels et al. (Eds.), *Psychiatry 1* (pp. 241–269). Philadelphia: Sippincott.

Conners, C. K. (1990). *Conners rating scale.* Toronto, Canada. Multi-Health Systems.

Cronbach, L. J. (1949). *Essentials of psychological testing.* New York: Harper & Brothers.

Elber, H. W. (1964, September). Automated personality description with 16 PF data. In R. D. Dregor, *Computer reporting of personality test data.* Symposium of the American Psychological Association, Los Angeles.

Exner, J. E. (1987). Computer assistance in Rorschach interpretation. In J. N. Butcher (Ed.), *Computerized psychological assessment* (pp. 218–235). New York: Basic Books.

Finney, J. C. (1966). Programmed interpretation of the MMPI and CPI. *Archives of General Psychiatry, 15,* 75–81.

Goldstein, G., & Hersen, M. (1992). *Handbook of psychological assessment.* New York: Pergamon.

Honaker, L. M. & Fowler, R. D. (1990). Computer-assisted psychological assessment. In G. Goldstein & M. Hersen (Eds.), *Handbook of psychological assessment* (2nd ed., pp. 521–546). New York: Pergamon.

Johnson, J. H., & Williams, T. A. (1980). Using a line computer technology in a mental health admitting system. In J. B. Sidowski, J. H. Johnson, & T. A. William (Eds.). *Handbook of psychological assessment* (pp. 147–169). New York: Pergamon Press.

Kamphaus, R. (1996). *Clinical assessment of children's intelligence.* Boston: Allyn & Bacon.

Kamphaus, R. W. (1993). *Clinical assessment of children's intelligence.* Boston: Allyn & Bacon.

Kanfer, F. H., & Saslow, G. (1969). Behavioral diagnosis. In C. F. Franks (Ed.), *Behavioral therapy: Appraisal and status* (pp. 148–175). New York: McGraw-Hill.

Katz, M. M. (1989). The multivantaged approach. In S. Wetzler & M. M. Katz (2nd Eds.), *Contemporary approaches to psychological assessment* (pp. 16–42). New York: Brunner/Mazel.

Kauffmann, A. S. (1979). *Intelligence testing with the WISC-R.* New York: Wiley-Interscience.

Kovacs, M. (1992). *Children Depression Inventory.* Toronto, Canada: Multi-Health System.

Krug, S. E. (1987). *Psychware Sourcebook 1987–1988.* Kansas, City, MO: Test Corp. of America.

Lazarus, A. A. (1973). Multimodal behavior therapy: Treating the "basic id." *Journal of Nervous and Mental Disease, 156,* 404–411.

Maag, J. W. (1999). *Behavior management: From theoretical implications in practical applications.* San Diego: Singular Publishing Group, Inc.

Nelson, R. O., & Hayes, S. C. (1974). Some current dimensions on behavioral assessment. *Behavioral Assessment, 1,* 1–6.

Piodrowski, A. Z. (1964). A digital computer administration of inkblot test data. *Psychiatric Quarterly, 38,* 1–26.

Pumariega, A. J., & Vance, B. (1999). School board mental health services. The foundations for system of care for children's mental health. *Psychology in the Schools, 5,* 371–378.

Rapaport, D., Gill, M., & Schafer, R. (1968). *Diagnostic psychological testing* (rev. ed.), R. R. Holt (Ed.). New York: International University Press.

Rogers, M. (1998). Psychoeducational assessment of culturally and linguistically diverse children and youth. In H. B. Vance (Ed.), *Psychological assessment of children: Best practices for school and clinical settings* (pp. 355–384). New York: Wiley.

Sattler, J. M. (1988). *Assessment of children* (3rd ed.). San Diego: Author.

Taylor, C. B. (1983). DSM-III and behavior assessment. *Behavior Assessment, 5,* 5–14.

Vance, H. B., & Awaad, A. (1998). Best practices in assessment of children: Issues and trends. In H. B. Vance (Ed.), *Psychological assessment of children: Best practices for school and clinical settings* (pp. 1–10). New York: Wiley.

Weiner, I. (1983). The future of psychodiagnosis revisited. *Journal of Personality Assessment, 47,* 451–459.

Wetzler, S. (1989). Parameter of psychological assessment. In S. Wetzler & M. M. Katz (Eds.), *Contemporary approaches to psychological assessment* (pp. 3–15). New York: Brunner/Mazel.

Wetzler, S., & Katz, M. M. (Eds.). (1989). *Contemporary approaches to psychological assessment.* New York: Brunner/Mazel.

Chapter 2

CLINICAL ASSESSMENT OF CHILDREN AND ADOLESCENTS: A PLACE TO BEGIN

K. RAMSEY MCGOWEN

Psychological assessment can provide crucial information in formulating a clinical understanding of children and adolescents, although this fact was not always recognized. In the early twentieth century, the psychological status of children and adolescents was often ignored; they were considered incapable of feeling or independent thought. When concerns were acknowledged, children and adolescents were frequently regarded simply as miniature adults, whose problems could be understood in the same terms as those of adults (Ollendick & Hersen, 1993a). There was little understanding of developmental processes, no separate categories in which to classify the different problems experienced by children and adolescents, and poor recognition of the unique interests and concerns of children and adolescents. In fact, the presence of major psychological disorders in children was often disputed, and diagnosis of childhood and adolescent disorders was controversial (Quay & Werry, 1972). In addition, early psychological assessment had limited utility; it focused on identifying the general laws underlying human behavior and the relationship of various physical attributes such as reaction times or physical acuities (French & Hale, 1990). This approach to assessment had little utility in aiding the understanding, diagnosing, or treating of children and adolescents. The applicability of psychological assessment approaches for children and adolescents was certainly disputable under these circumstances.

This state of affairs has changed dramatically for a variety of reasons. During the twentieth century, the recognition and study of developmental processes increased. This has enabled psychologists to better understand normal and abnormal aspects of growth, maturation, learning, intellect, behavior, emotional functioning, and other psychological aspects of development. This exploration has verified the presence of important differences between adults and children and has led to the identification of factors unique to working with children and adolescents. During this same period, approaches to psychological assessment advanced. Assessment approaches have become more sophisticated, and issues from validity to applicability to a wide array of psychological concerns have been addressed. The advances in understanding childhood and adolescence and the advances in psychological assessment have led to a "near universal" psychological assessment of children (Oakland, Gulek, & Glutting, 1996, p. 240).

A BRIEF REVIEW OF PSYCHOLOGICAL ASSESSMENT: PAST TO PRESENT

While a comprehensive history of psychological assessment is beyond the scope of this chapter, a brief review of key developments puts current assessment practices in context. These developments include approaches to the assessment of intelligence, personality, and behavior.

Intellectual Assessment

Many credit the origin of the field of psychological testing to Sir Francis Galton, who, in the mid-1800s, identified important statistical measures (i.e., correlation and regression to the mean) that allowed for the accurate study of mental and other psychological variables. Galton focused primarily on physical and sensory measures that he assumed were related to intelligence (Sattler, 1992). His work had an impact on others who were working in the fledgling field of psychology, including James M. Cattell. Cattell was the first psychologist formally to use the term *mental test,* which appeared in an 1890 publication. Cattell had been an assistant to William Wundt in Germany, where he became interested in studying individual differences—again primarily of physical capacities such as reaction time. He continued his work in this area at Columbia University. The association of Wundt, Galton, and Cattell led to a "cross fertilization of European and American ideas" (French & Hale, 1990, p. 3) and spurred the development of the identifiable field of mental (psychological) assessment. Despite this cross-fertilization, however, approaches to psychological assessment in England, Germany, the United States, and France proceeded with different foci. While English investigators continued focusing on statistical analyses, German investigators moved their emphasis to exploring psychopathology, and American scientists extrapolated. French researchers' methods of testing and analyzing test data related to measuring higher mental functions (Sattler, 1992).

At approximately the same time period that Galton and Cattell were working (late 1800s to early 1900s), Alfred Binet and Theodore Simon were developing methods in France for studying higher mental functions. Although in his early work Binet included some physical measures in attempting to measure mental abilities, he subsequently focused even more on assessing memory, calculation ability, drawing ability, reasoning, and other higher order functions. Binet's and Simon's work culminated in the development of the Binet-Simon Scale, the first widely used test of mental abilities that assessed higher-order thinking and paid attention to standardized administration and normative data. The development of this instrument was precipitated by the French public school system's desire to identify children in need of special academic assistance. The Binet-Simon Scale accomplished this task and evidenced external validity in studies demonstrating that the scale could differentiate students considered by teachers and principals as intelligent from those considered mentally inferior. The Binet-Simon Scale is generally considered the first modern intelligence test (Sattler, 1992). It was imported to the United States and used without significant revision until Terman made extensive additions and revisions to the instrument and undertook major standardization between 1911 and 1926. The instrument subsequently became known as the Stanford-Binet Intelligence Test.

Statistical advances allowed the field of testing to progress. The recognition that physical measures did not correlate well with other measures of mental ability led to the elimination of these sensory and physical measures from tests of mental abilities and cleared the way for theoretical and methodological advances in psychological assessment. Dissatisfaction with the age scale format of the Binet scales led to the development of alternatives in intelligence testing. Most notable were the efforts of David Wechsler, who was prompted by a focus on measuring global intellectual functioning. Wechsler considered intelligence to be the aggregate of mental abilities that allow the individual to "act purposefully, think rationally and deal effectively with the environment" (Sattler, 1992, p. 45). He devised an intelligence test by compiling items from existing measures of intelligence and developing original testing items. The items were organized into eleven subtests that would assess the factors contributing to the global effective intelligence of the individual. Instead of determining a score using the concept of mental age, the Wechsler scale employed measures of deviation from the mean of a standardized sample to determine ranges of intellectual functioning. This was a significant change in the computation of measured intelligence, and the *deviation IQ* method is the approach used by most instruments today. The Wechsler scales were originally designed to assess intelligence in adults but were modified to create intelligence scales for preschool and school-age children. These scales are the Wechsler Preschool and Primary Scale of Intelligence (Wechsler, 1967) and the Wechsler Intelligence Scale for Children—Third Edition (Wechsler, 1991).

Both the Stanford-Binet Scale and the Wechsler scales have been revised throughout the twentieth century to update them, to restandardize and renorm them, and to address issues in measurement and assessment. The most recent revision of the Stanford-Binet Scale (Stanford-Binet Intelligence Scale—Fourth Edition) included a major modification to introduce a point-scale format (Thorndike, Hagen, & Sattler, 1986).

Other intelligence tests have been published, such as the Kaufman Assessment Battery for Children (K-ABC, Kaufman & Kaufman, 1983) and the Kaufman Adolescent and Adult Intelligence Test (KAIT, Kaufman & Kaufman, 1993). Features of the Kaufman scales are their development based on neuropsychological theories of information processing and their focus on identifying the process of mental problem solving. The Kaufman scales have not been universally accepted as primary instruments for intelligence assessment (e.g., Sattler, 1992), but the K-ABC has gained acceptance from a large number of school psychologists (Kemphaus, Kaufman, & Harrison, 1990). Advances in intellectual assessment have also included the development of instruments designed for very young populations (e.g., the Bayley Scales of Infant Development; Bayley, 1969) and instruments with unique features that make them especially suitable for specific populations. Examples of such instruments are the McCarthy Scales of Children's Abilities (McCarthy, 1972) and the Blind Learning Aptitude Test (Newland, 1971). The number of instruments designed to assess intelligence and cognitive functioning has burgeoned in the past three decades. The development of these specialized instruments has added flexibility and scope to psychological assessment, although it has also made it more difficult to stay apace of which instruments are available and their psychometric properties, and therefore to select appropriate instruments for the assessment needs in a specific situation.

Historically, intelligence tests have evidenced outstanding psychometric properties—among the best of all psychological assessment instruments (Meier, 1994). Despite the excellent psychometric properties of intelligence tests, however, concern about their potential misuse is warranted. Not the least of these concerns is that a universally accepted definition of intelligence still eludes psychology. In addition, these instruments frequently have been used for purposes for which they were not intended, and results from these tests have often been ascribed meanings that are not supported (Schlinger & Poling, 1998).

Projective Personality Assessment

In addition to tests designed to measure mental functions, instruments designed to assess personality and other psychological factors in children and adolescents began to be developed in the early twentieth century. Tests in these categories were strongly influenced by the theories of personality and human behavior that dominated the early part of that century. Projective techniques, based on psychoanalytic theory, were among the first instruments to be used in assessment of personality. The Rorschach Inkblot Technique (Rorschach, 1921) and the Thematic Apperception Test (Morgan & Murray, 1935) have been mainstay assessment tools for decades. Interpretive processes for these instruments were originally guided by theoretical tenets, although standardized administration and scoring, along with statistically anchored interpretations, have been developed since the 1970s (Exner, 1974). The problems that haunted early projective assessment in general, such as subjectivity in scoring and the lack of an empirical basis for interpretation, were also issues of concern when these instruments were used with children and adolescents. As advances in projective assessment have accumulated during the past 30 years, however, the reliability and validity of these measures for use with children and adolescents have also improved. Exner's Comprehensive System for Rorschach includes scoring and interpretation information for children 5 to 16 years old (Exner & Weiner, 1982). Proponents of projective testing cite studies (e.g., Parker, Hanson, & Hunsley, 1988) supporting the psychometric soundness of the Rorschach and its utility in differential diagnosis, treatment planning, and assessment of personality characteristics. Meyer and Handler (1997) performed a meta-analysis on the literature related to the Rorschach Prognostic Rating Scale and concluded that there was strong evidence for the Rorschach's predictive validity. The Rorschach is widely used by clinicians and is taught as a core skill in psychological assessment in most graduate programs, but the value of projective techniques is not universally accepted, especially by academics (Weiner, 1997). Exner (1997) identifies the need to relate Rorschach results and interpretations to treatment planning as a key challenge for its future in the field of psychological assessment.

Objective Personality Assessment

Objective measures of personality were also developed in the early twentieth century. One of the earliest of these was developed by Woodworth (1918). He formalized into a paper-and-pencil format the questions previously asked orally of military personnel by psychiatrists. A variety of other measures of traits and personality were developed, but the publication of the Minnesota Multiphasic Personality Inventory (MMPI) (Hathaway & McKinley, 1940) marked the emergence of the first widely accepted criterion-referenced personality assessment instrument. Since its publication, this instrument has been the most widely used measure in clinical settings and has been at the heart of psychological research on personality, diagnosis, treatment planning, and treatment outcome. It was revised and renormed in 1990, and a version for use with adolescents was published in 1992 (Butcher et al., 1992). Designed and normed for 14- to 18-year-olds, the MMPI-A was devised to maintain consistency with the original MMPI, although it is shorter, and many items were changed to simplify wording or to improve relevance to adolescent life (Archer, 1997). In addition to information on the 10 traditional MMPI scales, the MMPI-A provides data on 15 new content scales, 3 supplemental scales, and 4 new validity scales. The new content scales specifically designed for the MMPI-A include Adolescent—Anxiety, Adolescent—Obsessiveness, Adolescent—Depression, Adolescent—Health Concerns, Adolescent—Alienation, Adolescent—Bizarre Mentation, Adolescent—Anger, Adolescent—Cynicism, Adolescent—Conduct Problems, Adolescent—Low Self-Esteem, Adolescent—Low Aspirations, Adolescent—Social Discomfort, Adolescent—Family Problems, Adolescent—School Problems, and Adolescent—Poor Treatment Indicators. This instrument is relatively new and will require an extended period of investigation to determine its utility in a variety of applications. Given the success and widespread acceptance of its parent instrument and the need for sound objective measures of adolescent personality, however, this instrument will likely become a standard measure in adolescent assessment. A body of literature is accumulating on the MMPI-A regarding interpretative practices, research issues, and use with specific populations (Archer, 1997).

Another currently used objective personality inventory designed for assessment of adolescents is the Millon Adolescent Clinical Inventory (MACI; Millon, 1993), a successor to the earlier Millon Adolescent Personality Inventory. This inventory is based on Theodore Millon's theoretical and empirical works, which are directed toward establishing a unified theory and science of personality and psychopathology (Davis, 1999). The MACI is clinically normed and provides a multidimensional assessment. Its scales measure clinical syndromes, personality patterns, and expressed concerns (Romm, Bockian, & Harvey, 1999). The personality styles scales include Introversive, Inhibited, Depressive, Submissive, Dramatizing, Egoistic, Unruly, Forceful, Conforming, Oppositional, Self-Demeaning, and Borderline Tendency. The expressed concerns identified by the MACI are identity confusion, self-devaluation, body disapproval, sexual discomfort, peer insecurity, social insensitivity, and family discord. Clinical indices include eating dysfunctions, academic noncompliance, alcohol predilection, drug proneness, delinquent disposition, impulsivity propensity, anxious feelings, depression affect, and suicidal ideation. The MACI has been well received by clinicians, but published research on the instrument is limited. Davis, Woodward, Goncalves, Meagher, and Millon (1999) state, however, that the MACI fares well when evaluated against criteria for effective assessment instruments and conclude in their description and discussion of the MACI that it is likely to be useful in outcome assessment research with adolescents.

Lachar (1999) recently described a related set of objective personality instruments for school-age children. These include the Personality Inventory for Children—Second Edition (PIC-2), the Personality Inventory for Youth (PIY), and the Student Behavior Survey (SBS). The PIC-2 evaluates information about children from parents; the SBS evaluates it from teachers; and the PIY is a self-report format for children. Lachar reports that these three instruments assess multiple measures of behavior; collect observations from parents, teachers and youth; and provide standardized scores based on contemporary national samples. The PIC-2, PIY, and SBS are designed to assess children from kindergarten through 12th grade. The PIC-2 and PIY provide gender-specific interpretive information related to cognitive impairment, impulsivity and distractibility, delinquency, family dysfunction, reality distortion, somatic concerns, psychological discomfort, social withdrawal, and social skills deficits. The SBS provides information on scales related to academic performance, academic habits, social skills, parent participation, health concerns, emotional distress, unusual behavior, social problems, verbal aggression, physical aggression, behavior problems, Attention Deficit Hyperactivity Disorder, Oppositional Defiant Disorder, and Conduct Disorder.

Behavioral Approaches to Assessment

Behaviorism was also a strong influence in the field of child and adolescent psychology. According to Ollendick and Hersen (1993a), the field of behavioral assessment lagged behind the more general advances in other areas of behavioral intervention for two reasons: the aforementioned lack of attention to normal developmental processes, which impeded the ability to compare specific behaviors to appropriate reference groups; and an overemphasis on operant procedures, which emphasized observable, current, and situation-specific behavior and neglected cognitions, affects, and social systems influences. Wide-ranging behavioral assessment approaches have now been developed and refined, however. These approaches generally involve improved sensitivity to developmental and normative issues, the use of empirically validated procedures, and the use of a variety of procedures to obtain comprehensive pictures of functioning. Systematic behavioral observation, structured and semistructured interviews, questionnaires, self-report inventories, and rating scales that assess a wide variety of behaviors currently help to accomplish effective behavioral assessment (Verhulst, 1995; Ollendick & Hersen, 1993a).

Behavioral observations are a standard part of formal assessment procedures but are rarely studied systematically. Oakland, Gulek, and Glutting (1996) reported on five scales designed to systematically assess test-taking behaviors and indicated that most lack norms and evidence of psychometric soundness. The *Guide to Assessment of Test Session Behavior* (GATSB; Glutting & Oakland, 1993) provides norms and data about reliability and validity and allows behavioral observations to be interpreted in a meaningful way. Behavioral observations can be more reliable than rating scales if the observation is systematic and highly structured (Obrzut & Boliek, 1993). In addition, the limitations of language and reading skills often make structured observations more appropriate for infants, toddlers, and younger children.

Structured and semistructured interviews are also useful assessment techniques. Semistructured interviews provide more structure and control than do standard clinical interviews because they provide guidelines for questioning while still offering some flexibility in interactions with the examinee. Structured interviews use formalized questioning formats that increase precision and accuracy but reduce flexibility in questioning. One commonly used structured interview is the Kiddie-SADS (Schedule for Affective Disorders and Schizophrenia for School Age Children; Puig-Antich & Chambers, 1978), which is designed to assess psychopathology of about 50 symptoms in children ages 6 to 17. The Interview Schedule for Children (Kovacs, 1982) is a semistructured interview for children and their parents designed to assess a wide range of psychopathology. Both these instruments are primarily useful in making diagnoses for clinically referred children. Because of the specificity of the instruments and the extensive training required to use them, their primary utility is in selecting research subjects or in making difficult differential diagnoses (Edelbrock & Costello, 1990). Rating scales of child and adolescent behaviors are numerous. Among the most widely used are the Child Behavior Checklist and related instruments (CBCL; Achenbach, 1999), the Conners Rating Scales–Revised (Conners, 1997), and the Revised Behavior Problem Checklist (Quay & Peterson, 1987).

The CBCL is part of a family of empirically based instruments designed to obtain data on behavioral and emotional problems and competencies, and it includes standardized data obtained from parents and teachers as well as direct observation of the child, including interviews and self-reports. The data is organized in a multiaxial scheme that allows for comprehensive compilation of information. The CBCL and related instruments provide information on eight syndrome scales: Withdrawn, Somatic Complaints, Anxious/Depressed, Social Problems, Thought Problems, Attention Problems, Delinquent Behavior, and Aggressive Behavior. The eight syndrome scales are grouped into two large factors, internalizing and externalizing. The competencies evaluated are organized along the dimensions of activities, social and school. The CBCL and related instruments have been widely used in research, treatment planning and clinical applications, and outcomes assessment (Achenbach, 1999). They are well standardized and have adequate reliability (Sattler, 1992). The Conners scales are designed to identify problem behaviors in children ages 3 to 17. Parent and teacher versions of the rating scales are available. Sattler concludes that these scales have adequate reliability and validity and that the five primary factors provided by the scales are supported by factor analysis. The five primary factors are conduct problems, learning problems, psychosomatic, impulsive-hyperactive, and anxiety. The Conners scales are widely used in clinical and school settings. They are useful in screening, diagnosis, treatment planning, treatment outcome assessment, and research. The Revised Behavior Problem Checklist was devised by factor analysis and rates behaviors along six scales: Conduct Disorder, Socialized Aggression, Attention Problems/Immaturity, Anxiety/Withdrawal, Psychotic Behavior, and Motor Excess.

Another instrument that has been introduced relatively recently is the Behavior Assessment System for Children (BASC; Reynolds & Kamphaus, 1992). This instrument is appropriate for children 4 to 18 years of age. It employs a combination of self-report, rating scales, and structured history elements. The self-report allows children to report on emotions and self-perceptions and allows for the generation of a personality description using the domains of school maladjustment, clinical maladjustment, personal adjustment, and an overall composite score. There are two rating scales, one for teachers and one for parents. The teacher rating scale measures externalizing problems, internalizing problems, school problems, and adaptive skills. The parent rating scale rates similar behavior but omits the behaviors best observed by teachers. The structured history is a detailed structured interview conducted by a clinician who obtains extensive developmental history and background information. Although this structured interview is a part of the BASC instrument, it can also be used alone. Finally, the BASC includes a structured observation form that allows children to be observed and time sampling of behaviors to be recorded. The BASC is a comprehensive assessment instrument that includes multimethod and multidimensional components. Although it is a relatively recent instrument, it shows great promise in providing assessment data about children and adolescents that are grounded in a uniquely broad-based format (Kemphaus, Reynolds, & Hatcher, 1999).

This brief review can provide only an overview of the history of and progress made in psychological assessment over the last century. Certain specialized topics have been omitted entirely. Neuropsychological assessment, assessment of special abilities (e.g., creativity), and assessment of person/environment factors (e.g., stress evaluation or quality of life) have not been reviewed despite the fact that assessment instruments exist for such topics. The instruments cited are key examples, but they certainly do not provide a comprehensive review of current psychological assessment instruments. More detailed information about specific instruments may be found in many other sources (e.g., Maruish, 1999a; Culbertson & Willis, 1993; Ollendick & Hersen, 1993b; Sattler, 1992).

CURRENT AND FUTURE STATUS OF PSYCHOLOGICAL ASSESSMENT

Obviously, the sophistication and application of psychological assessment has grown enormously, and the value of psychological assessment in many venues is evident. Currently, formal psychological assessment is recognized as being more systematic than routine clinical approaches. Formal psychological assessment provides a level of organization, standardization, and precision that is impossible in less systematic approaches to evaluation. Despite vast progress, psychological assessment has not reached a stage of perfection, however. Numerous problems associated with assessment, particularly of children and adolescents, continue to receive attention. Among these are concerns about the appropriateness of psychological instruments for ethnic minority populations. Sattler (1992) has reviewed the arguments both for and against the use of intelligence tests (and, by extension, many other psychological assessment instruments) with ethnic minority populations. Opposition to their use includes arguments that (a) tests have a white, Anglo-Saxon, middle-class bias; (b) national norms are inappropriate for minority populations; (c) ethnic minority children are disadvantaged by poor test-taking skills; (d) test results are negatively influenced by impaired examiner/examinee rapport and examiner expectations for poorer performance by these populations; and (e) test results are used to place ethnic minority children in inferior special education classrooms. Sattler extensively discusses data relating to each of these concerns and concludes that intelligence tests are generally not biased; that national norms are important, although pluralistic norms may have some utility; that the extent of the influence of minority children's poorer test-taking skills is not clear; that rapport problems and negative expectancies have not been confirmed; and that there is insufficient data to support arguments that placements in special education classrooms are harmful. Sattler also discusses issues related to testing ethnic minority children, such as poverty, and cautions that these factors may be shared factors among ethnic minority populations that influence outcomes. The issue of possible test bias and the need to be cognizant of differences in test appropriateness in certain populations will likely continue to be an issue in psychological assessment.

Others have pointed out certain chronic controversies in psychological measurement (Meier, 1994). Individually and in combination, these controversies have posed problems in psychological assessment in the past and continue to do so for measures currently in use or under development. The variability caused by such factors as motivation (e.g., fatigue or boredom), affective influences (e.g., test anxiety), dissimulation and malingering, response sets (e.g., social desirability responding), and response styles (e.g., acquiescence) can distort assessment and interpretation. These factors require specific attention and must be addressed on a number of fronts, notably through rigorous training in appropriate administration and assessment technique as well as through rigorous test design. Another potential problem in accurate psychological assessment of children and adolescents is that children and adolescents are "works in progress" and change rapidly. There have been great advances in recognizing and understanding developmental processes. However, there is no comprehensive model of development that places all aspects of psychological assessment in appropriate context (Yule, 1993). Developmental processes that can influence assessment in children include variations in attention span, motivation, and cooperation with the testing process; variability in exhibiting appropriate test-taking behavior; separation-individuation processes that result in periods when fears or oppositional behaviors are normal; and the emergence at different age periods of physical, cognitive, and affective skills. Also, children and adolescents are vulnerable to the influences of their environment. They may carry the distress of their parents or demonstrate behavior problems that are precipitated not so much by child psychopathology as by problems in the living environment (Culbertson & Willis, 1993). Finally, psychological assessment is not a simple undertaking. It requires a comprehensive and careful approach that starts with a review of referral information. It includes consideration of the function and influence of relevant adults in the child's life, of observation in various settings, and of selection and administration of tests appropriate to the referral question and to the child's age-related, physical, and language proficiencies, among others. Psychological assessment also requires careful interpretation of data, the formulation of hypotheses related to the data, and the development of intervention strategies supported by the conclusions (Sattler, 1992). This sequence is challenging and time-consuming, and it is not always followed when psychological assessment occurs in the real world.

All these concerns deserve attention when the use of psychological assessment is considered. Despite these potential problems, however, there are a number of sound reasons to employ psychological testing. Lachar (1999) points out that assessment can be especially useful with children and adolescents, who are unlikely to refer themselves and may be noncompliant with the requests of significant adults in their lives. Therefore, children and adolescents may not clearly present the nature or scope of their problems in less structured formats; they may not have the academic, cognitive, or motivational status to complete self-report inventories and may not have the verbal abilities to respond accurately to clinical interviews. Also, the use of multisource psychological assessment strategies can overcome the divergent pictures of child and adolescent functioning that emerge when only single sources of information (e.g., child, parent, or teacher) are questioned. Maruish (1999b) comprehensively reviewed the current status of psychological assessment in treatment planning and outcomes assessment. He concluded that the future for psychological assessment is bright, despite the recent constraints imposed by managed care on health care practices, which have led others to conclude that assessment is a dying professional endeavor. Maruish reached this conclusion based on the potential contributions of assessment in providing an empirical basis for diagnostic and treatment decisions that can make treatment more cost-effective. Maruish argued that assessment can be a force for accurate clinical decision making and a treatment technique itself (by identifying, organizing, and discussing problems during results feedback sessions), and that it can be used for effective treatment monitoring and outcome determination, which will make treatment more accountable and precise. Beutler, Goodrich, Fisher, and Williams (1999) provided a similarly positive picture regarding the future of assessment. They heralded the empirical advantages of psychological assessment over unstandardized clinical methods but added that assessment practices must become more tailored, brief, practical, and treatment-centered to be meaningful in current and future clinical practice. In particular, they reviewed the literature about seven factors related to treatment outcome and argued that psychological assessment can provide systematic information about these factors that will predict treatment outcome and differential response to available treatments by individual patients. These seven factors are the degree of functional impairment, subjective distress, problem complexity, readiness for/stage of change, potential to resist therapeutic influences, social support, and coping styles. This ability—to predict differential responses to treatments and treatment outcomes—is highly valuable in promoting cost-effective and successful care. If further work supports the ability of assessment to provide such predictions, the future of psychological assessment, though different from the omnibus assessments of the past, will be secure.

The evolution of psychological assessment over the past century has resulted in a much improved field. Although problems in measurement and application must be taken seriously and assessment must be undertaken with utmost professional rigor and integrity, there is ample evidence that psychological assessment can enhance clinical practice. A multitude of instruments exists for a wide range of psychological concerns and behaviors. These can be used for screening, differential diagnosis, treatment planning, treatment monitoring, and treatment outcome purposes; and their appropriate use can enhance provision of service. Tying assessment results and interpretations to treatment interventions and outcome ultimately closes the circle of psychological intervention and makes both assessment and treatment more relevant and effective.

REFERENCES

Achenbach, T. M. (1999). The Child Behavior Checklist and related instruments. In M. E. Maruish (Ed.), *The use of psychological testing for treatment planning and outcomes assessment* (2nd ed., pp. 429–466). Mahwah, NJ: Erlbaum.

Archer, R. P. (1997). Future directions for the MMPI-A: Research and clinical issues. *Journal of Personality Assessment, 68,* 95–109.

Bayley, N. (1969). *Bayley Scales of Infant Development: Birth to two years.* San Antonio, TX: Psychological Corp.

Beutler, L. E., Goodrich, G., Fisher, D., & Williams, O. B. (1999). Use of psychological tests/instruments for treatment planning. In M. E. Maruish (Ed.), *The use of psychological testing for treatment planning and outcome assessment* (2nd ed., pp. 81–113). Mahwah, NJ: Erlbaum.

Butcher, J. N., Williams, C. L., Graham, J. R., Archer, R. P., Tellegen, A., Ben-Porath, Y. S., & Kaemmer, B. (1992). *MMPI-A (Minnesota Multiphasic Personality Inventory—Adolescent): Manual for administration, scoring and interpretation.* Minneapolis: University of Minnesota Press.

Conners, C. R. (1997). *Conners Ratings Scales—Revised technical manual.* North Tonawanda, NY: Multi-Health Systems.

Culbertson, J. L., & Willis, D. J. (Eds.). (1993). *Testing young children: A reference guide for developmental, psychoeducational, and psychological assessments.* Austin, TX: Pro-Ed.

Culbertson, J. L., & Willis, D. J. (1993). Introduction to testing young children. In J. L. Culbertson & D. J. Willis (Eds.), *Testing young children: A reference guide for developmental, psychoeducational, and psychological assessments* (pp. 1–10). Austin, TX: Pro-Ed.

Davis, R. D. (1999). Millon: Essentials of his science, theory, classification, assessment and therapy. *Journal of Personality Assessment, 72,* 330–352.

Davis, R. D., Woodward, M., Goncalves, A., Meagher, S. E., & Millon, T. (1999). Studying outcome in adolescents: The Millon Adolescent Clinical Inventory and Millon Adolescent Personality Inventory. In M. E. Maurish (Ed.), *The use of psychological testing for treatment planning and outcomes assessment* (2nd ed., pp. 381–397). Mahwah, NJ: Erlbaum.

Edelbrock, C., & Costello, A. J. (1990). Structured interviews for children and adolescents. In G. Goldstein & M. Hersen (Eds.), *Handbook of psychological assessment* (2nd ed., pp. 308–323). New York: Pergamon.

Exner, J. E. (1974). *The Rorschach: A comprehensive system.* New York: Wiley.

Exner, J. E. (1997). The future of the Rorschach in personality assessment. *Journal of Personality Assessment, 68,* 37–46.

Exner, J. E., & Weiner, I. B. (1982). *The Rorschach: A comprehensive system: Vol. 3. Assessment of children and adolescents.* New York: Wiley.

French, J. L., & Hale, R. L. (1990). The history of the development of psychological and educational testing. In C. R. Reynolds & R. W. Kamphaus (Eds.), *Handbook of psychological and educational assessment of children* (pp. 3–28). New York: Guilford.

Glutting, J., & Oakland, T. (1993). *Guide to the assessment of test session behavior.* San Antonio, TX: Psychological Corp.

Hathaway, S. R., & McKinley, J. C. (1940). A multiphasic personality inventory schedule (Minnesota): Construction of the schedule. *Journal of Psychology, 10,* 249–254.

Kaufman, A. S., & Kaufman, N. L. (1983). *Interpretive manual for the Kaufman Assessment Battery for Children.* Circle Pines, MN: American Guidance Services.

Kaufman, A. S., & Kaufman, N. L. (1993). *Manual for the Kaufman Adolescent and Adult Intelligence Test.* Circle Pines, MN: American Guidance Services.

Kemphaus, R. W., Kaufman, A. S., & Harrison, P. L. (1990). Clinical assessment practice with the Kaufman Assessment Battery for Children (K-ABC). In C. R. Reynolds & R. W. Kemphaus (Eds.), *Handbook of psychological and educational assessment of children* (pp. 259–276). New York: Guilford Press.

Kemphaus, R. W., Reynolds, C. R., & Hatcher, N. M. (1999). Treatment planning and evaluation with the BASC: The Behavior Assessment System for Children. In M. E. Maruish

(Ed.), *The use of psychological testing for treatment planning and outcome assessment* (2nd ed., pp. 563–597). Mahwah, NJ: Erlbaum.

Kovacs, M. (1982). The Interview Schedule for Children (ISC). Unpublished interview schedule. Pittsburgh: Department of Psychiatry, University of Pittsburgh.

Lachar, D. (1999). Personality Inventory for Children, 2nd edition, Personality Inventory of Youth, and Student Behavior Survey. In M. E. Maruish (Ed.), *The use of psychological testing for treatment planning and outcomes assessment* (2nd ed., pp. 399–427). Mahwah, NJ: Erlbaum.

Maruish, M. E. (1999a). *The use of psychological testing in treatment planning and outcomes assessment* (2nd ed.). Mahwah, NJ: Erlbaum.

Maruish, M. E. (1999b). Introduction. In M. E. Maruish (Ed.), *The use of psychological testing in treatment planning and outcome assessment* (2nd ed., pp. 1–40). Mahwah, NJ: Erlbaum.

McCarthy, D. A. (1972). *Manual for the McCarthy Scales of Children's Abilities.* San Antonio, TX: Psychological Corp.

Meier, S. T. (1994). *The chronic crisis in psychological measurement and assessment: A historical survey.* San Diego: Academic.

Meyer, G. J., & Handler, L. (1997). The ability of the Rorschach to predict subsequent outcome: A meta-analysis of the Rorschach Prognostic Rating Scale. *Journal of Personality Assessment, 69,* 1–38.

Millon, T. (1993). *The Millon Adolescent Clinical Inventory manual.* Minneapolis, MN: NCS.

Morgan, C., & Murray, H. A. (1935). A method for investigating phantasies: The Thematic Apperception Test. *Archives of Neurological Psychiatry, 34,* 289–306.

Newland, T. E. (1971). *The Blind Learning Aptitude Test.* Champaign: University of Illinois Press.

Oakland, T., Gulek, C., & Glutting, J. (1996). Children's test-taking behaviors: A review of literature, case study, and research on Turkish children. *European Journal of Psychological Assessment, 12,* 240–246.

Obrzut, J. E., & Boliek, C. A. (1993). Assessment of the child with social and emotional disorders. In J. L. Culbertson & D. J. Willis (Eds.), *Testing young children: A reference guide for developmental, psychoeducational, and psychological assessments* (pp. 345–382). Austin, TX: Pro-Ed.

Ollendick, T. H., & Hersen, M. (1993a). Child and adolescent behavioral assessment. In H. Ollendick & M. Hersen (Eds.), *Handbook of child and adolescent assessment* (pp. 3–14). Boston: Allyn & Bacon.

Ollendick, T. H., & Hersen, M. (Eds). (1993b). *Handbook of child and adolescent assessment.* Boston: Allyn & Bacon.

Parker, K. C. H., Hanson, R. K., & Hunsley, J. (1988). MMPI, Rorschach, and WAIS: A meta-analytic comparison of reliability, stability, and validity. *Psychological Bulletin, 103,* 367–373.

Puig-Antich, J., & Chambers, W. (1978). *The Schedule for Affective Disorders and Schizophrenia for school-aged children.* Unpublished interview schedule, New York State Psychiatric Institute. New York, NY.

Quay, H. C., & Peterson, D. R. (1983). *Interim manual for the Revised Behavior Problem Checklist.* Coral Gables, FL: University of Miami Press.

Quay, H. C., & Werry, J. S. (1972). *Psychopathological disorders of childhood.* New York: Wiley.

Reynolds, C. R., & Kamphaus, R. W. (1992). *Behavior Assessment System for Children.* Circle Pines, MN: American Guidance Service.

Romm, S., Bockian, N., & Harvey, M. (1999). Factor-based prototypes of the Millon Adolescent Clinical Inventory in adolescents referred for residential treatment. *Journal of Personality Assessment, 72,* 125–143.

Rorschach, H. (1921). *Psychodiagnostick.* Bern: Bircher.

Sattler, J. M. (1992). *Assessment of children* (3rd ed.). San Diego: Author.

Schlinger, H. D., & Poling, A. (1998). *Introduction to scientific psychology.* New York: Plenum.

Thorndike, R. L., Hagen, E. P., & Sattler, J. M. (1986). *Stanford-Binet Intelligence Scale* (4th ed.). Chicago: Riverside.

Verhulst, F. C. (1995). Recent developments in assessment and diagnosis of child psychopathology. *European Journal of Psychological Assessment, 11,* 203–212.

Wechsler, D. (1967). *Manual for the Wechsler Preschool and Primary Scale of Intelligence.* San Antonio, TX: Psychological Corp.

Wechsler, D. (1991). *Manual for the Wechsler Intelligence Scale for Children* (3rd ed.). San Antonio, TX: Psychological Corp.

Weiner, I. B. (1997). Current status of the Rorschach Inkblot Method. *Journal of Personality Assessment, 68,* 5–19.

Woodworth, R. S. (1918). *Personal Data Sheet.* Chicago: Stoelting.

Yule, W. (1993). Developmental considerations in child assessment. In H. Ollendick & M. Hersen (Eds.), *Handbook of child and adolescent assessment* (pp. 15–25). Boston: Allyn & Bacon.

Chapter 3

FUNCTIONAL ANALYSIS AND BEHAVIORAL ASSESSMENT OF CHILDREN AND ADOLESCENTS

FREDDY A. PANIAGUA

INTRODUCTION

The questions, "Why do children and adolescents develop mental disorders?," "Which measurement strategies are available to assess these disorders?," and "Which experimental approach should be used to evaluate the effects of treatment in the management of these disorders?" could be answered in many ways. The reason for these many ways to answer such questions is that sciences involved in the analysis of behavior (both private and overt behaviors; more details of this difference discussed later) are multiparadigmatic in nature (Kuhn, 1970; Paniagua, 1991; Paniagua & Baer, 1981). In general, Kuhn defines a paradigm in terms of the "entire constellation of beliefs, values, techniques, and so on shared by the members of a given [scientific] community" (1970, p. 175). A paradigm, then, governs the scientific behavior of a given group of practitioners, including their answering the above questions.

This chapter provides a summary of scientific behaviors of two groups of practitioners who share many of the assumptions of the paradigms of applied behavior analysis and behavior therapy in their efforts to answer the above questions. These groups are know as *behavior analysts* and *behavior therapists* depending on whether the group emphasizes only environmental variables in the explanation and measurement of behavior (the behavior analysts) or emphasizes both environmental and organismic variables (the behavior therapists). A detailed explanation of this distinction can be found in Paniagua and Baer (1981).

The generic term *behavioral psychologists* is often used to refer to these two groups, because the majority of these practitioners are psychologists trained in departments of psychology with emphasis on the behavioral model and not on other approaches in the analysis and assessment of human behavior, including, for example, the psychoanalytic and humanistic models (Kazdin, 1978).

The term *functional analysis* is generally used to name the process involved in the explanation of why people behave in the way they do, including both normal (e.g., social play in children) and abnormal (e.g., physical aggression during social play) behavior. The term *behavioral assessment* is often used to name the process of measuring variables in a functional analysis of behavior, as well as the experimental approach used to demonstrate functional relationships between behavioral changes (i.e., dependent variables) and interventions or treatments (i.e., independent variables). This second element of behavioral assessment is termed *functional assessment* (see Haynes & O'Brien, 2000, p. 42). The first portion of this chapter is a summary of the process involved in a functional analysis of behavior. The second part deals with the process of behavioral assessment in diagnosis and treatment, with emphasis on child and adolescent disorders. Clinical cases will illustrate the applicability of this type of assessment in the present context.

HISTORY OF THE FUNCTIONAL ANALYSIS OF BEHAVIOR

The question, "Why do children and adolescents develop mental disorders?" cannot be answered experimentally using children and adolescents as research subjects. Behavioral psychologists, however, claim that children and adolescents learn such disorders through a functional *relationship* among antecedent events (i.e., receiving a "failing grade" in school), the behavior under consideration (e.g., symptoms suggesting depression), and its consequence (e.g., symptoms of depression followed by social attention, thus increasing the occurrence of such symptoms over time). To demonstrate this relationship experimentally, it would be necessary to expose one group of children to the independent variable (e.g., a difficult school task) and keep a second group from it. In addition, parents in the first group would be instructed to provide social attention (or social reinforcement, in technical terms) contingent upon symptoms of depression in those children who did not pass the test. Institutional Review Boards (IRBs), which deal with human subject consents, however, would consider this type of experiment unethical.

If that question cannot be answered empirically using children as research subjects, where are the empirical data to support indirectly the explanation of normal and abnormal behavior in terms of that type of functional relationship? As noted by Haynes and O'Brien (2000) and Wilson and O'Leary (1980), the answer to this question could be traced to the work of experimental psychologists such as R. E. Guthrie, C. Hull, J. Watson, and B. F. Skinner (see Bower & Hilgard, 1981, for a review of contributions made by these experimental psychologists). The most widely accepted answer to that question, however, is in the special branch of experimental psychology Skinner termed the *Experimental Analysis of Behavior* (EAB). Skinner is credited with the development of this particular field (Catania, 1984), which he also termed *operant conditioning* because he was interested in the study of behaviors that "change or operate on the environment" (Ferster & Parrott, 1968) instead of the type of responses termed "reflexes" in the Pavlovian conditioning paradigm (Catania, 1984).

Skinner conducted many experiments using pigeons and white rats as experimental subjects and showed that these organisms could learn *new* behaviors and maintain them over time through the experimental manipulation of antecedents and consequences in a chamber he specifically designed to conduct his experiments (Ferster & Skinner, 1957; Skinner, 1938; Skinner, 1961). This chamber is known as the Skinner box. For example, Skinner showed that in order for his rats to learn to press a lever (a new behavior), he would have to gradually reinforce (with food) responses that led to the final (target) behavior (lever pressing). This procedure, in which only responses approximating the target behavior (e.g., approaching the lever, sniffing at the lever, touching the lever) are reinforced, is termed "shaping" (Catania, 1984). This procedure is based on the process of *differential reinforcement,* in which only responses leading to the target behavior are reinforced. In this experiment, responses that are not part of this chain of responses (e.g., running inside the Skinner box rather than approaching the lever) would be considered maladaptive because they would not lead to the target (final) behavior. Therefore, in his experiments Skinner placed these maladaptive responses under extinction (i.e., food was not delivered contingent upon responses that did not lead to the chain of responses needed to achieve the experimental goal, in this case lever pressing).

In another set of experiments, Skinner (1938, 1961) introduced an experimental manipulation in which the rat would have to press the lever in the presence of a particular stimulus (e.g., a green light projected inside the Skinner box) in order to receive the reinforcer (food). In these experiments, if the rat pressed the lever when the green light was off, the behavior was not reinforced. In this specific case, a rat's lever pressing would be considered maladaptive because they lead to extinction rather than reinforcement. In these experiments, the stimulus (green light) that follows the target behavior is called an antecedent event, and in this particular experimental procedure this antecedent event is also termed *discriminative stimulus* because its sets "the occasion on which responses [e.g., lever presses] have consequences" (Catania, 1984). (A different type of antecedent events, namely, establishing operations, is discussed in the section Current Trends in the Functional Analysis and Assessment of Behavior.)

Concurrent with the above experiments, Skinner also showed that the *programming* of the reinforcer was also a critical variable to consider if one expects to maintain behavioral changes over time in the absence of reinforcement (Catania, 1984). Skinner found that if lever presses are reinforced continuously or regularly (i.e., each level press leads to reinforcer or food in the Skinner box), the organism would stop pressing the lever almost immediately after the reinforcer is not delivered contingent upon the target behavior (i.e., the extinction procedure). Skinner then changed the programming of the reinforcer (i.e., the schedule of reinforcement in technical terms), and created a condition in which the reinforcer was delivered *intermittently.* In this experimental manipulation, the reinforcer (food) followed some lever presses whereas other (similar) responses were not and this resulted in the maintenance of lever presses for a longer period. Many schedules of reinforcement were investigated by Skinner and his students (e.g., Catania, 1984; Ferster & Skinner, 1957), but the overall finding was that behaviors that are reinforced intermittently (i.e., the organism would find it difficult to predict when the reinforcer would follow the behavior) would persist for a longer period in the absence of reinforcement, in comparison with behaviors reinforced regularly or continuously (which tend to stop as soon as the reinforcer is not available). Therefore, to create a new behavior the organism would be reinforced regularly; once the behavior has been established it could be maintained for a extended period in the absence of reinforcement in those cases when the reinforcer is scheduled intermittently (Skinner, 1961). The adaptive behavior (lever pressing) in the above experiments was maintained through this particular change in the schedule reinforcement.

In Skinner's experiments (see Skinner, 1961), lever presses were followed by food (the reinforcer), and the frequency of these responses increased over time. This process in establishing a behavior and maintaining it over time is called *positive reinforcement* (Catania, 1984). Skinner considered a different process in establishing and maintaining the target behavior, which he termed *negative reinforcement.* This second process is the experimental analysis of escaping and *avoiding* in the operant paradigm. Skinner created a condition in which the rat would have to press the lever to terminate an electric shock in the Skinner box. After several trials, the rat learned that pressing the lever as soon as the shock was presented could terminate or remove this aversive event from the chamber. In this situation, the removal or termination of the shock *is* the reinforcer that follows lever presses. The target behavior (lever presses) is called *escaping,* because it terminates an aversive event; and the operation or process involved in this manipulation is termed *negative reinforcement.*

Skinner also showed that his rats did not have to wait to receive the shock in order to press the lever (and terminate the shock). In this case, a discriminative stimulus (e.g., the green light) was presented seconds before the shock was introduced. The rat quickly learned that lever presses could postpone the shock. Skinner termed *avoidance* the behavior (e.g., lever press) that prevented the delivery of the shock, and the same process of negative reinforcement was involved. That is, the adaptive behavior (lever press), was negatively reinforced (its frequency increased over time) because it led to the absence of the shock.

Therefore, Skinner showed that the adaptive behavior (lever press) could be learned and maintained either through positive reinforcement (behavior followed by food), or by the removal of an aversive event (behavior followed by the termination of the electric shock, called escaping), or by preventing the occurrence of aversive stimulus (avoidance) by responding (e.g., lever presses) in the presence of an antecedent event.

In 1953 Skinner published *Science and Human Behavior,* in which he extrapolated his findings to the analysis of adaptive and maladaptive behaviors among humans. This book does not summarize Skinner's empirical data, but shows only how these data could be used to explain why people behave the way they do (both in terms of normal and abnormal behavior). In the specific case of a functional analysis of abnormal behavior, one of Skinner's students, Charles B. Ferster, published a paper (Ferster, 1965) in which he employed the Skinnerian operant paradigm to argue that what is known as deviant, maladaptive, inappropriate, or disruptive behaviors are determined by environmental stimuli (i.e., functional relationships similar to those described above), and not by underlying illness or intrapsychic conflicts. These and other theoretical extrapolations of Skinner's empirical findings to the analysis of human behavior were crucial in teaching behavioral psychologists how to apply such findings in the explanation of adaptive and maladaptive behaviors among people.

The first set of experiments provided behavioral psychologists with the first clue concerning the explanation of maladaptive or abnormal behaviors among people and their maintenance over time without the need to replicate similar experiments with human subjects. That is, just as the rats in the experiments conducted by Skinner and his associates learned adaptive and maladaptive behaviors through functional relationships involving only behavior and its consequences, people also would learn similar behaviors when exposed to similar behavior/consequence relationships in the social environment.

For example, in terms of the Skinnerian paradigm, a child would learn behaviors characteristic of Oppositional Defiant Disorder (*Diagnostic and Statistical Manual of Mental Disorders—4th Edition,* American Psychiatry Association, 1994) in those cases in which parents reinforce these behaviors with "attention" (i.e., a social reinforcer); psychotic verbalizations are learned through the same mechanism of positive reinforcement (e.g., social reinforcement contingent upon verbalizations involving delusions and hallucinations).

The second set of experiments introduced a more complex functional relationship, in which antecedents (e.g., discriminative stimuli) served as the occasion or the opportunity for the emission of adaptive behaviors (e.g., lever presses) resulting in reinforcement and maladaptive behaviors (e.g., running around the Skinner box) leading to extinction (i.e., absence of reinforcement). The hypothetical case of the depressed adolescent is an example of the extrapolation of Skinner's experimental findings (Skinner, 1961), in which failing grades would serve as the occasion for the emission of symptoms of depression followed by social attention from parents, thus increasing the probability of these symptoms in the future. Another example is self-injurious behavior (SIB) among children with mental retardation and associated disabilities. In general, according to behavioral psychologists, SIB is in itself an *automatic reinforcer* because the behaviors involved in SIB (e.g., self-stimulation, scratching body parts) increase the probability that such behaviors would be repeated. Certain antecedent events could also set the occasion for the occurrence of SIB. Miltenberger (1998) provided the following example: "If an individual engages in self-injury and a particular staff member typically reinforces the behavior with attention, that staff is [a discriminative stimulus] for the self-injury, and the behavior will be more likely to occur in the presence of that staff person" (p. 49).

In the extrapolation of findings from the third set of experiments (i.e., escaping and avoiding situations), behavior psychologists argue that children and adolescents can learn maladaptive behaviors through the same process of negative reinforcement described above (Haynes & O'Brien, 2000; Barkley, 1990; Wilson & O'Leary, 1980). For example, children who are nagged, isolated in a room, teased, or ridiculed in the classroom would display oppositional responses (e.g., refusal to complete schoolwork) and physical aggression toward teachers and peers to escape these aversive events. These children, however, do not need to experience these events; they could avoid such aversive events by displaying maladaptive behaviors as soon as they enter the school setting, prompting the school principle to contact parents to remove the child from school because of his or her oppositional behaviors and aggressive acts prior to the beginning of the school session on a given day. Additional examples of the applicability of this process of negative reinforcement among children and adolescents can be found in Bucher and Lovaas (1968) and Sulzer-Azaroff and Mayer (1977).

Skinner's experimental approach was initially named operant conditioning to differentiate it from the Pavlovian conditioning (Catania, 1984; Skinner, 1938). In 1957, however, Skinner published a paper titled "The Experimental Analysis of Behavior," in which he summarized his major empirical contributions in the area of experimental psychology (Skinner, 1957a). Many Skinnerian (experimental) psychologists adopted this title (rather than operant conditioning) to name this new branch of experimental psychology (Catania, 1984). During earlier replication of Skinner's findings, however, experimental psychologists contributing with new studies could not publish their findings in current experimental journals because their paradigmatic approach to the analysis of behavior did not correspond with "the traditional scientific strategy of the statistical analysis of group data" (Wilson & O'Leary, 1980, p. 12) and did not emphasize the formulation of hypotheses, but focused instead on direct observation of behavior and its changes through experimental manipulations of antecedent/behavior/consequence functional relationships. One year after the publication of Skinner's 1957 paper, these experimental psychologists found a solution to this difficulty by creating a new journal called *Journal of the Experimental (JEAB)*, devoted exclusively to the empirical analysis of these functional relationships with emphasis on overt (observable) behavior as the "only acceptable subject of scientific investigation" (Wilson & O'Leary, 1980, p. 11).

The applicability of Skinner's experimental findings in the functional analysis and assessment of adaptive and maladaptive behaviors among people resulted in a new field called *Applied Behavior Analysis* or *Behavior Modification*. Among early demonstrations of this field in the management of maladaptive behaviors are the studies by Ayllon and Michael (1959), Brady and Lind (1961), Fuller (1949), and Williams (1959). Several of these early applications were published in the *JEAB* (e.g., Ayllon & Michael, 1959), but at that time the *JEAB* was exclusively devoted to basic research with minimal interest in publishing applied research illustrating the applications of the Skinnerian paradigm in analysis of human behavior, particularly in the case of understanding and managing maladaptive behaviors among people. This constituted the first obstacle that behavior analysts encountered in their struggle to publish their findings in peer-reviewed journals.

The second obstacle was similar to the one confronted by Skinner and his associates that led to the formation of *JEAB;* that is, applied studies submitted by behavioral analysts were also systematically rejected by journals that published only applied research emphasizing hypothesis testing and complex statistical procedures in the analysis of the significance of results in statistical terms. Behavioral analysts were interested in the direct observation of behavior, measurable (rather than inferred) behavioral changes, and evaluation of these changes using a different set of experimental designs known as *single-subject designs* or *intrasubject replication designs* as opposed to the standard designs (e.g., between-group designs) favored by editors and reviewers in journals emphasizing group data and hypothesis testing (Beck, Andrasick, & Arena, 1984; Kazdin, 1980). Behavioral analysts found two ways to quickly publish their findings without the need to send their studies to such journals. First, leader behavioral psychologists served as editors of textbooks publishing chapters written by other behavioral psychologists. Examples of these edited books included *Research in Behavior Modification: New Developments and Implications* (Krasner & Ullman, 1965) and *Operant Procedures in Remedial Speech and Language Training* (Sloane & Macaulay, 1968). Second, in 1968 behavioral analysts also created their own journal which they named the *Journal of Applied Behavior Analysis (JABA)* devoted exclusively to the functional analysis of observable behavior in terms of behavioral laws discovered by Skinner and his associates (e.g., Ferster & Skinner, 1957; Catania, 1984). The first volume of *JABA* included papers by prominent behavioral psychologists illustrating the applications of the functional analysis methodology (e.g., Ayllon & Azrin, 1968; Bijou, Paterson, & Ault, 1968; Hall, Lund, and Jackson, 1968; Risley, 1968).

In the first volume of JABA, Donald M. Baer, Montrose Wolf, and Todd R. Risley (among the most influential leaders in this field) published a paper in which they provided the criteria a study should have in order to be considered within the framework of the applied behavior analysis or functional analysis of behavior represented in JABA. Baer, Wolf, and Risley (1968) wrote that "the study must be *applied, behavioral,* and *analytic;* in addition, it should be *technological, conceptually systematic,* and *effective,* and it should display some generality" (p. 92, italics in the text). Table 3.1 shows the characteristics of these dimensions with examples.

EXPANSION OF THE FUNCTIONAL ANALYSIS OF BEHAVIOR

Earlier applications of the operant paradigm in the development of adaptive behaviors and control of maladaptive or problematic behaviors emphasized the so-called ABC model, in which the only critical elements in a functional analysis of a given behavior was the identification of the antecedent (A) event leading to behavioral (B) probability as a result of consequences (C) contingent upon behavior. In this model, what the organism was thinking, imagining, processing, believing, or feeling was not of importance in explaining why the organism was behaving in a certain way. In 1963, Skinner published a paper in which he summarized the main assumption of his radical behaviorism (Skinner, 1963). Briefly, Skinner argued that private or subjective experiences were real (i.e., thinking is another way of behaving, but mentally), but he added that they did not play a role in the regulation of behavior. Mental events are real entities, but the problem is not the reality of these entities but their use in the explanation of why people behave in the way they do. That is, the issue is not the mental, but *mentalism,* which is the use of private events to explain human behavior (Paniagua, 1987a; Skinner, 1963). Therefore, early applied studies conducted by behavior analysts (particularly those published in *JABA*) consistently ignored cognitive processes (private events) because they cannot be directly observed and reliably measured. A group of applied researchers, however, departed from this tradition and adopted "a broader approach that emphasizes the importance of cognitive factors in the treatment of complex clinical disorders" (Wilson & O'Leary, 1980, p. 26). This group constitutes the behavior therapists (Paniagua & Baer, 1981).

Behavior therapists and behavior analysts share many of the exemplars of the experimental analysis of behavior or operant conditioning. Behavior therapists, however, propose that a functional analysis of human behavior cannot be achieved without considering the explanatory role of private events (e.g., cognitions, affective processes) in that analysis. That is, not only are these subjective experiences of private events within the organism (O) real (in agreement with behavioral analysis) but they also can be critical in the explanation of why people behave in the way they do. This led to the AOBC model in which antecedent events (A; e.g., school failure) lead to cognitive processes (O; e.g., negative thoughts) preceding both the overt behavior (B; e.g., decrease in social activities suggesting "depression") and its consequences (C; e.g., attention contingent upon symptoms of depression). Early demonstrations of this expansion of the

Table 3.1   Dimensions of Applied Behavior Analysis

Applied:	Emphasis on solutions to social problems rather than confirmation of theories. *Example:* Investigating procedures to decrease aggressive acts in children instead of an evolutionary analysis of aggression (Barrash, 1977).
Behavioral:	Emphasis on observable behaviors and reliable measurement of behaviors. *Example:* Children are "oppositional" not because they have a negative attitude or lack of interest in the presence of teachers' instructions but because they do not stop "pushing" others and refuse to "sit down" five seconds after teachers' instructions to perform the appropriate behavior (e.g., sitting). At least two trained observers should *directly* measure these observable behaviors; teachers' and parents' verbal reports, and children's self-report of behavioral changes are indirect measures, which are not as reliable as direct behavioral observations.
Analytic:	Traditional approaches in the evaluation of treatment effects (e.g., statistical test of grouped data, clinical interviews, rating scales) are too inferential and unreliable. Reliable demonstration of experimental control of a given behavior during the introduction of a given treatment can only be achieved with the programming of baseline observations upon target behavior followed by the intervention in an intrasubject-replication design format (e.g., reversal designs, multiple-baseline designs, etc.). *Example:* The frequency of "out-of-seat" is noted during 10 baseline sessions; in sessions 11 through 20, a token program is introduced in which tokens are contingent upon "in-seat" behavior and exchanged for tangible reinforcers (e.g., small toys); the intervention is removed across 10 consecutive sessions (a return to baseline), and it is reintroduced for an additional 10 sessions. This intrasubject-replication design is called *reversal design* (Kazdin, 1980).
Technological:	A given behavioral procedure (e.g., token programs, time-out from positive reinforcement, overcorrection) should be described in such a way that other practitioners would be able to replicate the same procedure to produce similar behavioral changes, giving only a general reading of that description. Techniques such as play therapy and individual psychotherapy are not "technological" because they can be used in many different ways depending on who is applying these techniques. *Example:* Each 30 seconds, deliver one token contingent upon "in-seat" behavior; do not deliver the token if "in-seat" does not correspond with the operational definition both observers are using to record this behavior; at the end of the session (a total of ten 30-second intervals, or five minutes), exchange tokens for tangible reinforcers according to the following format: 5 tokens = extra 5 minutes recess and 10 tokens = access to 20 minutes in the game room.
Conceptual:	Procedures must be based on a comprehensive theory about behavior. For behavioral psychologists this comprehensive theory is the operant paradigm. Freud's theory about behavior is also comprehensive, but its exemplars (Kuhn, 1970; Paniagua & Baer, 1981) are not useful in an experimental analysis of behavior, which does not deal with the analysis of behavior in terms of struggles among the id, ego, and superego, but with functional relationships among antecedents, behavior, and consequence. The applied, behavioral, analytic, and technological dimensions should be conceptualized in terms of the exemplars of the operant paradigms.

(continued)

Table 3.1   Continued

Example: The "mental" is not what is crucial in the analysis of "mental retardation" but the fact that children often display behavioral deficits (e.g., low frequency of self-care skills) and "behavioral excess" (e.g., physical aggression, self-injury behavior). The mental is not a social event of importance, but what the child is actually doing (or not doing); the mental cannot be directly measured because it is an unobservable (or invented) event; but one can directly observe and measure how many times a "mentally retarded" child dresses without assistance from the staff, for example; and the technological approach to these deficits and excesses in behavioral terms should also be conceptualized in terms of the exemplars of the operant paradigm. For example, overcorrection procedures would be more effective than time-out (TO) from positive reinforcement in the management of these children because overcorrection teaches these children adaptive behaviors, whereas TO only suppresses maladaptive behaviors temporarily.

Effective: Behavioral procedures must produce "large enough effects for practical value" (Baer et al., 1968, p. 96). The main criterion is not whether the procedure resulted in significant changes during treatment, relative to baseline observations, but the social validity of these changes (Wolf, 1978).

Example: During the introduction of the token program (above example), the child under treatment displays "in-seat" behavior 50% of the total number of intervals during which the behavior is recorded, relative to percentages below 10 during baseline. Similar results are replicated in the reversal design. Are these results socially important? The answer is no because teachers would expect children to display that behavior for more than five minutes (see example). Therefore, in this context the token program would not be effective because it is not socially valid. Parents with a child diagnosed with Elective Mutism would be perceived as very significant minor increases in the child's verbal communication with the therapist; minimal reduction in self-injury behavior among autistic children would also be seen as socially significant by parents and staff. The first case for the social validity of behavioral changes deals with people's (e.g., teachers) expectancy of what should be the norm in the frequency and duration of behavior; the second case deals with the approximation of this normality assumption in the clinical setting considering the low frequency of behavior (e.g., mutism) or its severity (e.g., self-injury).

Generality: Behavioral changes noted during the introduction of behavioral interventions should be generalized beyond the setting (e.g., clinic) and people (e.g., therapists, staff) in which these interventions were initially programmed. These changes should also continue over time (i.e., maintained after the intervention has been removed).

Example: If "in-seat" behavior is also noted in classrooms other than that in which the token program was initially programmed, one would say that this behavior was generalized across different settings (classrooms) and teachers; observing the same behavior daily is a case of maintenance of behavior over time.

functional analysis of behavior include the work of Albert Bandura, Aaron T. Beck, Joseph Cautela, Albert Ellis, and Joseph Wolpe (Paniagua & Baer, 1981).

According to Bandura (1969, 1996) people can learn maladaptive (and adaptive) behaviors only by observing others (the models or antecedent events) performing these behaviors in the absence of direct reinforcement of overt behavior (e.g., attention contingent upon aggressive act). In Bandura's social learning theory of behavior, people's ability to display three cognitive processes (attention, retention, and production) and one motivational process (including external incentives, vicarious incentives, and self-incentives) is what permits people to learn adaptive and maladaptive behaviors (see Bandura, 1996, Figure 1, p. 330). According to Beck (1976), maladaptive behaviors are the result of faulty patterns of thinking or negative cognitions in the presence of antecedent events. For example, an adolescent would develop symptoms suggesting depression because he or she engages in self-derogation and self-blaming in the presence of the antecedent event (e.g., failing in school).

Cautela (1973) argued that functional relationships among antecedents, behavior, and consequences can be imagined by the client during the treatment of maladaptive behaviors. Cautela's approach is called *covert conditioning* (Cautela & Kearney, 1986; Paniagua, 1993), which included a series of covert techniques clinicians can use to modify maladaptive behaviors including covert reinforcement, covert extinction, and covert modeling. According to Ellis (1977), maladaptive behaviors are not exclusively determined by environmental events, but by people's irrational beliefs, thoughts, and other distorted cognitions about that environment. For example, an adolescent would develop symptoms suggesting depression in those cases in which he or she experiences difficulties with school performance on a given test, and develop a cognitive distortion of this situation by believing that one must be thoroughly competent, intelligent, and achieving in this and similar situations.

Wolpe (1973) also emphasized private events or subjective experience in the functional analysis of behavior. Wolpe argued that *underlying* anxiety responses (i.e., anxiety states within the organism) are the causal agent of *overt* anxiety disorders (e.g., the case of specific phobia). For example, Wolpe pointed out that people develop overt anxiety responses (i.e., observable responses suggesting anxiety) because an antecedent event (e.g., harmless snake) causes a perceptual (i.e., perception of the event) response leading to an underlying response for anxiety "either immediately (i.e., perceptual response followed by the underlying anxiety) or through the intermediary of the conditioned concept 'danger'" (p. 25); that is, perceptual response leads to "danger," which leads to underlying anxiety. This underlying anxiety is then manifested overtly; it becomes "public."

Five textbooks with many examples of early applications of the AOBC model alone or in combination with the ABC (behavioral analytic) model are (1) *Handbook of Behavior Modification and Behavior Therapy* (Leitenberg, 1976); (2) *The Practice of Behavior Therapy* (Wolpe, 1973); (3) *Learning Foundations of Behavior Therapy* (Kanfer & Phillips, 1970); (4) *Principles of Behavior Therapy* (Wilson & O'Leary, 1980); and (5) *Principles of Behavior Modification* (Bandura, 1969). Examples of journals with a tradition in publishing conceptual and empirical studies in which the role of private or subjective experiences are emphasized in a functional analysis of behavior include *Be-

havior Modification, Behavior Therapy, Behaviour Research and Therapy, and *Journal of Behavior Therapy and Experimental Psychiatry.*

Even though some behavior analysts still maintain that adaptive and maladaptive behaviors are a function of antecedent/behavior/consequences relationships *without the need to appeal to mediating process* (see the special issue of *JABA,* Vol. 27, 1994, pp. 385–418), the current trend among many behavioral psychologists (behavior analysts and behavior therapists) is to emphasize the AOBC model in the analysis of behavior. Some behavior analysts deny the role of private events (e.g., images, thought processes) in the functional analysis of behavior "not because such [private events] do not exist but because they are out of the reach of their methods" (Skinner, 1963, p. 953). Other behavioral psychologists, however, have taken a different approach by arguing that such methods are, indeed, available but that they are not part of the exemplars (Kuhn, 1970; Paniagua & Baer, 1981) of the operant paradigm (Wilson & O'Leary, 1980).

BEHAVIORAL ASSESSMENT OF CHILD AND ADOLESCENT DISORDERS

Functional Analysis versus Behavioral Assessment

The question, "Why do children and adolescents develop mental disorders?" is the domain of a *functional analysis* of behavior (Durand, 1993). For example, a child might display oppositional responses (e.g., refusal to complete schoolwork) in the classroom to escape from events this child perceives as aversive (i.e., completion of math problems, reading, etc.). A functional analysis would involve a systematic introduction and removal of these events and an introduction and removal of "positive" events (e.g., allowing the child to engage in self-selected activities such as reading comic books, drawing, or talking to other students). In both conditions (negative versus positive trials), the child would be instructed to engage or not to engage in certain tasks, and oppositional responses would be assessed across each condition. If oppositional responses are noted only during the aversive condition and not during the positive condition, the assumption is that a process of negative reinforcement is involved in the development and maintenance of such responses in the classroom.

Another example of a functional analysis of behavior is the answer to the question, "Why do children diagnosed with mental retardation or autism display self-injurious behaviors?" This question was answered by Carr, Newsom, and Binkoff (1976) with an 8-year-old boy named Tim, and their findings led to many other publications by prominent applied researchers, including the work of Brian A. Iwata, who is considered the most influential researcher in the functional analysis and treatment of self-injurious behaviors among children with pervasive developmental disorders (e.g., Iwata, Dorsey, Slifer, Bauman, & Richman, 1982; Iwata, Pace, Kalsher, Cowdery, & Cataldo, 1990).

Carr et al. (1976) placed Tim in a "free time" and a "tact" condition in which *demands* from teachers requesting Tim to fulfill certain tasks (e.g., "Point to the door") were not scheduled. During the free time condition, Tim was allowed to roam freely about the classroom, lie down, and engage in activities in which no demands were scheduled. During the "tact" condition, the teacher approached Tim, mentioned Tim's name, looked Tim in the eye, and presented a *tact* (a special type of verbal behavior; Paniagua, 1985a, 1987a; Skinner, 1957b) regarding what Tim was doing (e.g., "The grass is green"). These conditions were repeated several times in an intrasubject replication design format, and the results showed significant increases in the level of self-destructive behaviors during the "demand" condition, relative to extremely low frequency of these behaviors during either the free time or tact condition. This functional analysis of Tim's self-destructive behaviors showed that the antecedent event leading to these maladaptive behaviors was related to teachers' demands and not to the other two conditions.

The question, "What is the frequency or the rate of responding of a behavior in a given condition, and which experimental approach should be used to demonstrate functional relationships between dependent (target behavior) and independent (e.g., antecedents, treatment modalities) variables?" is the domain of a behavioral assessment. For example, Carr et al. (1976) recorded "hits per minute" during each condition and found that this rate of responding was between zero and two per minute during free time and tact conditions, and about 80 per minute during the demand condition; the results were analyzed in reversal (intra-subject replication) design (described in the next section).

The History of Behavioral Assessment: Techniques and Instruments

During the initial applications of the Skinnerian paradigm (e.g., *JABA*, Vol. 1, 1968), most assessment techniques of adaptive and maladaptive behaviors were considered by many behavioral psychologists (particularly behavior analysts) inferential, speculative, invalid, and unreliable, including children's self-reports, parents' reports of children's emotional difficulties, and use of projective tests. Behavioral psychologists took a different approach: the selection of valid and reliable measures of behavior with no room for inferential analysis and a strong emphasis on *direct* observation of observable behavior under consideration. This emphasis on observable behavior and use of valid and reliable measurement strategies is the essential feature of the behavioral dimension in Table 3.1 (Baer et al., 1968), which has its root in the Experimental Analysis of Behavior (Skinner, 1957a).

In the cited experiments illustrating the history of the functional analysis of behavior, the *rate* of responding (e.g., number of lever presses per seconds, minutes, etc.) constituted the main dependent variable Skinner elected to investigate. Skinner measured the rate of responding with an instrument called a cumulative recorder (see Catania, 1984, p. 60; Skinner, 1961, p. 85), which includes a roller with paper and a pen (similar to the lie-detector machine). Each time the rat pressed the lever in the Skinner box, the pen moved a fixed distance across the paper. At the end of the session, Skinner reviewed the cumulative curve displayed on top of that roll of paper to determine the exact number of responses (lever presses) his rats displayed per minute. In Skinner's experiments (and those published in the *JEAB* by his followers), the behavior under study is, indeed, observable (i.e., one can observe that the rat is actually pressing the lever); and one can say that the cumulative curve clearly indicates that this behavior is occurring at a given rate (e.g., 40 responses per minute) without the need of speculation or inferential reasoning (which is the problem with indirect measurement of behaviors such as children's self-record of their own behavior in the absence of direct or independent observations of similar behaviors by trained observers).

Skinner, however, wrote that "in choosing rate of responding as a basic datum and in recording this conveniently in a cumulative curve, we make important temporal aspects of behavior visible. . . . We use such curves as we use a microscope, X-ray camera, or telescope" (Skinner, 1961, p. 93, italics in the original). What Skinner is really saying is that the concept of response rate was an *abstract* or *unobservable* event until he used an instrument (the cumulative recorder) that allowed him and other experimental psychologists to "see" that event and the patterns of acceleration and deceleration produced by a distinctive schedule of reinforcement. Paniagua and Baer (1981) called the rate of responding an *instrumentally proximal event* because it is within the class of events whose reality must be inferred by looking at the outputs of instruments such as the cumulative recorder (for rate of responding), EEG (for neurological electrical circuits in the brain), and the sphygmomanometer (for the assessment of blood pressure).

In Skinner's operant paradigm, the dependent variable is not lever presses (i.e., observing the rat pressing the lever in the Skinner box) but the *rate of responding* (this is the "basic datum" in the experimental analysis of behavior developed by Skinner and used in all studies published in the *JEAB*). The rate of responding, however, cannot be observed directly. It has to be inferred with the assistance of the cumulative recorder, which displays a cumulative curve of that rate (e.g., 40 lever presses per minute). This explains why Skinner wrote that "the [the cumulative recorder] revealed things in the rate of responding, and in changes in that rate, which would certainly otherwise have been missed" (Skinner, 1961, p. 85).

Therefore, although the root of behavioral assessment in applied or clinical research is associated with the measurement of observable behavior in Skinner's research program (e.g., observing a rat pressing a lever) the basic datum resulting from such observation is not visible except with the aid of mechanical instruments or trained (human) observers who apply specific behavioral assessment techniques to make such a basic datum observable. For example, when trained observers record the frequency of a given maladaptive behavior (e.g., physical aggression in the classroom), display this observation on a graph, and conclude (by reading the results displayed on that graph) that the mean rate of aggression decreased from 10 responses per minute to zero responses per minute during treatment, relative to baseline observations, this conclusion is a case of a *statistical guess* (Paniagua, 1990a). In this example, inferences about changes in the rate of aggression are made by analyzing the data points between baseline and treatment phases. The behavior under study was directly observed (e.g., a child hitting other children in the classroom), but the basic datum resulting from this observation (rate of aggression) is not visible until the data are plotted on a graph.

The main point in the above analysis is that a behavioral assessment strategy in the measurement of adaptive and maladaptive behaviors not only includes direct observation of observable target behaviors by trained observers but also deals with a great deal of indirect interpretation of the basic datum resulting from that observation. This probably explains why recent trends in behavioral assessment show an emphasis on both traditional assessment strategies (e.g., the so-called indirect measures such as self-reports and rating scales) and direct observation in the setting where the target behavior actually occurs (e.g., Goldstein & Hersen, 1999; Haynes & O'Brien, 2000; Hersen & Bellack, 1998; Mash & Terdal, 1997; Milternberger, 1998). For a behavioral assessment of child and adolescent disorders to be comprehensive, many behavioral psychologists (behavior analysts and behavior therapists) maintain that both direct and indirect measurement of behavioral changes should be emphasized (e.g., Haynes & O'Brien, 2000; Miltenberger, 1998). In addition, in many clinical situations, a behavioral assessment with emphasis only on *direct* observation in the natural environment would not be feasible or ethical. This is the measurement problem of sexual dysfunctions, marital sexual encounters, and obsessive thoughts, to mention only some examples.

COMPREHENSIVE BEHAVIORAL ASSESSMENT

Following are examples of how *comprehensive behavioral assessment* could assist clinicians in the evaluation and diagnosis of behavior disorders in children and adolescents, as well as in the valuation of desirable (i.e., socially expected) behavioral changes resulting from the programming of behavioral interventions. A given behavioral assessment would be comprehensive in terms of an emphasis on three basic components: (a) direct measures of behavior; (b) indirect measures of behavior; and (c) the programming of these measures using multiple methods of measurement, multiple informants, multiple occasions, and multiple settings (Haynes & O'Brien, 2000; Miltenberger, 1998). For example, children diagnosed with Attention-Deficit Hyperactivity Disorder (ADHD; DSM-IV) should be assessed with unstructured clinical interviews using DSM-IV criteria or structured clinical interviews using instruments listed in Table 4, direct behavioral measures (see Table 3), rating scales (e.g., the Child Behavior Checklist, see Table 4), and vigilance and sustained attention tests (see Table 4). Multiple informants would include parents, children, teachers, and staff members. These multiple methods of measurement should be scheduled at different times during the day, on different days (i.e., multiple occasions), and in multiple settings (i.e., home, school, clinics). Box 3.1 summaries these three components.

Direct Behavioral Assessment

Selection of Target Behavior

In general, the frequency, intensity (severity), and duration are three measures used by behavioral psychologists to select the target (observable) behavior in a behavioral treatment plan. For example, the target behavior is selected because it must be decreased (not totally eliminated) in a given setting. This is the case of "out-of-seat" behavior in which children are expected to move from their seat but not at a very high frequency within a given observational period (Paniagua, 1992). Another example is compulsion in a child with diagnosis of Obsessive Compulsive Disorder (DSM-IV; Barrios & Hartmann, 1988), in which repetitive behaviors (e.g., hand washing) are seen as maladaptive because their frequency is beyond that expected by the community (i.e., repetitive hand washing is a good social behavior, except when its high frequency prevents the individual from fulfilling other expected social activities).

Box 3.1   Components in a Comprehensive Measurement of Behavior

---

A. **Direct Behavioral Measures**
   1. Selection of Target Behavior
   2. Behavioral Definition of Target Behavior
   3. Measurement of Target Behaviors by Independent Observers
B. **Indirect Behavioral Measures**
   4. Unstructured Clinical Interview
   5. Structured Clinical Interview
   6. Selection of Intellectual Development Tests
   7. Selection of Social Development Tests
   8. Selection of Language Development Tests
   9. Selection of Achievement Tests
   10. Selection of Parent/Child Relationship Measures
   11. Selection of Rating Scales
   12. Selection of Neuropsychological Tests
C. **Programming of Above Measures**
   1. Multiple Methods of Assessment (e.g., direct observations, rating scales)
   2. Multiple Informants (e.g., children, parents, teachers, staff members)
   3. Multiple Occasions (e.g., different times of the day, different days)
   4. Multiple Settings (e.g., school, home, clinics)

In another instance, the behavior has to be not only decreased but also totally eliminated in a given context. This is the case of physical aggression, in which the frequency and the severity of the behavior make it impossible to tolerate or accept in that context (Paniagua & Black, 1990). If out-of-seat behavior occurs at least two times during a 30-minute observational period, this frequency would not be of clinical significance for intervention. On the other hand, two instances of physical aggression in the classroom by a child diagnosed with Conduct Disorder (DSM-IV) would be a clinically significant problem requiring immediate intervention.

Other behaviors are selected for direct observation and intervention because their frequency is too low. What makes the behavior maladaptive is not the behavior per se but its extremely low frequency. For example, children with diagnosis of Elective Mutism (DSM-IV) "elect" not to talk to people outside the range of their immediate family (e.g., parents). In the classroom, this mutism is often considered abnormal or maladaptive because the child's verbalization in this setting is significantly low across teachers and peers (Paniagua & Saeed, 1988). Another example includes low frequency of behaviors suggesting childhood depression (Kazdin, 1988), including substantial reduction in the frequency of talking, playing with others, participating in group activities, and other social activities with a frequency below the expected frequency in a given context.

In other cases, a behavior is selected not because it has a high or a low frequency, but because its duration is either too high or very low. For example, the length of time a child takes to complete a set of math problems would be seen by teacher as too long if it prevents the child from completing additional tasks in the classroom. A child diagnosed with ADHD would display attention in the presence of a given task, but this attention would be too short, which could lead to significant errors during the performance of the task (i.e., fast responses might lead to errors because the child does not spend enough time attending to important features in such a task; see Barkley, 1990, p. 331). In the first example, the goal of the treatment plan would be to decrease the duration of the behavior; the inverse goal would be established in the second example.

In addition to the frequency, severity, and duration parameters in the selection of observable behaviors, the absence of the behavior could also be the problem. In this case, what constitutes a problem behavior is the fact that the behavior is not present in a given context. This is the strategy used by behavioral psychologists employing the technique of differential reinforcement of other behavior (DRO) in the management of maladaptive behaviors. For example, in the case of behavioral treatment plans designed to reduce the frequency of self-stimulation in mentally retarded children, the absence of head weaving, body-rocking, and other instances of self-stimulatory behaviors is the target (overt) behavior, which leads to reinforcement in a DRO condition (e.g., Paniagua, Braverman, & Capriotti, 1986).

A special case in the selection of the target observable behaviors involves those situations in which two observable behaviors must occur but the intervention is programmed not upon these behaviors but on the relationship between them. For example, in the field of verbal/nonverbal correspondence training (Paniagua, 1990b), the reinforcer is contingent upon a relationship between the subject's verbalization of a future behavior (e.g., "I'll complete 10 math problems") and the actual fulfillment of the corresponding (nonverbal) behavior. In this example, three target behaviors are recorded: Behavior 1, verbal behavior (i.e., a report about either past or future behavior); Behavior 2, the nonverbal (reported) behavior; and Behavior 3, the relationship between these two behaviors. It should be noted that the third behavior is inferred by directly observing Behaviors 1 and 2 (i.e., overt verbal and corresponding nonverbal behaviors). This inferential feature in verbal/nonverbal correspondence training is what makes this selection of the target behavior a special case in direct behavioral assessment of behaviors. That is, direct behavioral assessment is programmed upon two observable behaviors (verbal report and its corresponding nonverbal behavior), but the behavioral intervention is contingent upon an inferred relationship (correspondence) between two observable behaviors, i.e., Behavior 1 and Behavior 2 (e.g., Paniagua, 1987b; Paniagua & Baer, 1982; Risley & Hart, 1968; Rogers-Warren & Baer, 1976).

Behavioral Definition of Target Behavior

Behavioral psychologists are interested in the assessment of most psychiatric diagnoses listed in the DSM-IV. These professionals, however, do not target the diagnosis per se (e.g., ADHD, Conduct Disorder, Oppositional Defiant Disorder, Pervasive Developmental Disorders) but specific behaviors leading to the application of such diagnostic categories (Wilson & O'Leary, 1980). For example, behavioral interventions are not programmed to treat ADHD but to manage specific behavior children with this diagnosis often display. In this case, two critical target behaviors are inattention to task materials and overactivity (e.g., Paniagua, 1987b; Paniagua, Pumariega, & Black, 1988). These are examples of two classes of behaviors in the management of children with ADHD. Specific responses within each class must be identified and a behavioral definition applied to such responses from which the level of the class of behavior under consideration is inferred.

Table 3.2   Behavioral Definition of Target Behavior in Direct Behavioral Assessment

Class of Behavior	Response	Definition
Conduct Problem	Aggressiveness	Kicking, hitting, pushing others (Paniagua, 1992).
Helping Behavior	Bathroom Cleaning	Wash the toilet bowl and mop the floors daily.
	Kitchen Cleaning	Scour the sink after each meal, sweep and mop the floor (Paniagua, 1985b).
	Living Room Cleaning	Dust and vacuum the floor daily (Paniagua, 1985b).
Inattention	Off-Task Behavior	Eyes not oriented toward task materials for at least 15-second duration during any 30-second record intervals.
	Activity Change	Physical contact with a new toy or task materials. New is defined as any toy, group of toys, or materials that the child is not engaged with at the start of the interval (e.g., Paniagua et al., 1988).
Overactive	Grid-Marked Changes	Crossing a gridline under own power; both feet must be completely in new quadrant to be scored as "grid changes."
	Out-of-Seat Behavior	Any situation where normal seating surface of neither buttocks is applied to the child's chair (e.g., Paniagua et al., 1988).
Pica	Mouthing Objects	Holding nonedible objects (or fingers) to the lips or tongue, or placing nonedible objects in the mouth (e.g., Finney, Russo, & Cataldo, 1982; Paniagua et al., 1986).
Self-Stimulation	Head Weaving	Moving head from side to side in a figure-eight pattern.
	Body-Rocking	Moving the trunk at the hips rhythmically back and forth or from side to side (e.g., Paniagua et al., 1986).

Table 3.2 shows examples of behavioral definitions of target behaviors in terms of the present analysis. For example, inattention includes two specific responses: off-task behavior and activity change, which are operationally defined to permit two or more observers to record these responses with a certain degree of accuracy and agreement. For example, if the child does not make physical contact with a new toy at the start of a given interval of observation, the response is not considered an example of inattention to task materials, which is inferred from the absence of activity change in that definition. In this example, a behavioral intervention would be programmed to decrease off-task behavior and overactivity; and if the treatment actually reduces these responses over time, the management of two important elements in the diagnosis of ADHD is said to be controlled (i.e., inattention and hyperactivity). A similar conclusion could be reached when analyzing additional examples in Table 3.2.

The Measurement of Target Behavior

In the area of direct behavioral assessment, only behaviors that can be observed (not inferred) by at least two independent are emphasized. The selected measure must be valid and reliable. In the exemplars (Kuhn, 1970; Paniagua & Baer, 1981) of behavioral psychologists, a given measurement system is valid if it is *"appropriate* to the variable that it is to measure" (Sulzer-Azaroff & Mayer, 1977, p. 50; emphasis added). For example, the use of the permanent product recording system is not a valid (appropriate) measure for the assessment of self-stimulatory behaviors (see Table 3.2 for specific examples) because the observer cannot measure the "trace" of such behaviors after it has occurred. This measure (permanent product), however, would be a valid measure in the assessment of children with diagnosis of Encopresis and/or Enuresis (DSM-IV). An example of a valid measurement of self-stimulatory behaviors is the partial-interval time-sampling recording system described below (Paniagua et al., 1986).

In the present context, a given measurement system is reliable if it is consistent in terms of the level of agreement derived from at least two independent observers. Sulzer-Azaroff and Mayer (1977) summarized behavior analysts' interpretation of what exactly a "reliable" measure is in the following terms:

> Behavior analysts must demonstrate that their recording systems are reliable. One way is to try simultaneous recording by *two independent observers.* There must be close *agreement between the two,* demonstrating that the behavior under observation is being measured in the same way [by both observers]. If a *high percentage* of agreement is not obtained, any recorded change in observed behavior by a single observer may reflect a change in observing and recording responses, rather than in the observed behavior itself. (p. 52; emphasis added)

The selection of the formula used to determine the reliability between two observers depends on the measures employed (see below for examples of computation of the inter-observers reliability in this context).

Table 3.3 shows a summary of common recording techniques used in the measurement of observable behaviors. In the case of the frequency, it is recommended when the number of behaviors under observation is relatively low (e.g., from one to three) and each behavior has a clear beginning and end. For example, number of math problems completed, failure to complete given task, and refusal to stop getting up from a chair in the classroom could be recorded at the same time on the same data sheet, and they would be easy to assess because observers would know when they begin and end.

In many clinical situations, the goal of treatment is to either reduce or increase the length of time (duration) during which the target behavior occurs. For example, a child would be oppositional in the sense that he or she takes a long time to complete schoolwork. In this case, a measure of the duration of the target behavior should be considered within the context of the task the child is expected to complete within a reasonable time period. For example, a teacher would determine that the completion of reading should take no more than 10 minutes, whereas the completion of math problems would take 30 minutes. Children who are instructed to follow these expected durations of target behavior and fail to follow the instructions (e.g., taking one hour instead of 30 min-

Table 3.3   Recording Techniques in the Assessment of Observable Behavior

	Frequency	Example
Description	Measures how many times the behavior occurs across a given time period.	Number of times a child with diagnoses of Conduct Disorder and Oppositional Defiant Disorder hits other children in the classroom, does not complete classroom work, and refuses to follow teachers' instruction to stop getting-up from a chair without permission from teachers.
Appropriateness	Low frequency behavior; with small number of behaviors observed at the same time.	

	Duration	Example
Description	Measures the length of time a behavior occurs.	Length of time to complete school work; number of minutes in-seat behavior occurs.
Appropriateness	Measures behavior with a clear beginning and end.	

	Permanent Product	Example
Description	Measures the "trace" of behavior.	Number of times feces are noted in inappropriate places—encopresis (e.g., bed); number of times urine is noted in inappropriate places—enuresis (e.g., bed, clothes); number of math problems are completed correctly; number of times the kitchen is cleaned after each meal.
Appropriateness	Assesses behavior which can be recorded after it has occurred in the absence of direct observation.	

Interval Recording System

	Momentary Time Sampling	Example
Description	The behavior is recorded at the end of the interval.	In five 10-sec intervals, self-stimulation is recorded only if it occurs right after one of 10-sec interval.
Appropriateness	Measures behaviors that tend to persist for a long time.	

	Partial Interval Time Sampling	Example
Description	The behavior is recorded if it occurs at least once within the interval.	In five 10-sec intervals, inattention is recorded if it occurs anywhere within a given 10-sec interval.
Appropriateness	Measures behaviors that tend not to last for a long time but which sometimes occur within the observational interval.	

Table 3.3   Continued

	Whole Interval Time Sampling	Example
Description	The behavior is recorded only if it occurs across the entire observational interval.	In five 10-sec intervals, on-task behavior is recorded only if it occurs across the entire interval (e.g., 10 sec) without interruption.
Appropriateness	Measures behaviors that are required to continue until verbal (e.g., "It is time to stop working on this test") or nonverbal (e.g., the ringing bell in school) stimuli are introduced to indicate the termination of the behavior in a given context (e.g., on-task behavior in the classroom).	

	Direct Self-Monitoring	Example
Description	The child is instructed to record his/her own behavior within a given time period. For practical reasons, the frequency of behavior is generally selected because it would be difficult for the child to use more complex measures (e.g., interval recording systems).	In the classroom, the teacher instructs a child to check on a data sheet whether or not "study behavior" occurred during the last five minutes, and independent observers record the same behavior.
Appropriateness	Recommended in settings where multiple subjects are included in direct observation of target behaviors (e.g., "study behavior" in a classroom with 10 children or more); could be used as a treatment modality in itself (e.g., self-recording of increments in "study behavior" might result in future occurrence of similar behavior over time).	

utes to complete the set of math problems) would display oppositional behaviors because they do not meet the expected duration for the completion of a given task. Inversely, if the child completes the task in a short time period (i.e., below the expected duration of the behavior as established by school rules), the child would be considered inattentive or hyperactive because he or she is not taking enough time to complete the task without making errors.

Because of practical reasons, limitation in the number of people available to record behaviors or the nature of the behavior under observation the *permanent product* recording system might be the best alternative measure. For example, it would be impractical to wait until children diagnosed with Encopresis or Enuresis (DSM-IV) display instances of these disorders in a given setting (e.g., inpatient treatment, school, home, etc.). Observers, however, could check the environment in which these disorders occur (e.g., bed, pants, underwear, etc.) and record the traces of incidents of Encopresis and Enuresis. Similarly, busy teachers might not have the time to continuously record each task completed by students, but the teacher could collect materials and record whether or not a given student completed the task. In the case of children diagnosed with Feeding Disorder of Infancy or Childhood (DSM-IV) observers would wait until the mealtime period is completed (e.g., lunch) and would record the number and type of foods the child ate.

In the assessment of behaviors that are not clearly discrete (i.e., having unclear beginning and end) or behaviors that tend to last for a long time, the selection of one of the interval recording systems (Table 3.3) would be the measurement of choice. Examples of behaviors with unclear beginning and end include self-stimulation, self-injury, disruptive noise, and shouting. In general, it would be very difficult to record either the frequency or duration of such maladaptive behaviors. Examples of behaviors that often last for a long time include (i.e., might be observed at least every 10 seconds across twenty 30-second intervals, or a total of 10 minutes of observation) on-task behavior (attention to task materials), eating, and playing in the school playground. In general, all interval-recording systems include steps in Box 3.2.

In general, the goal of the treatment plan determines which specific interval recording system should be used (Powell, Martindale, & Kulp, 1975). For example, if teachers expect children to display on-task behavior (e.g., completion of math problems, reading, etc.) until they are instructed to stop the behavior (see Table 3.3), the *whole-interval recording system* would be used, because in this case the behavior must occur throughout the interval to be recorded. If only a sampling of intervals is required for the assessment of on-task behavior, the *partial interval time sampling* is recommended in which the

---

Box 3.2   Steps in Interval Recording Systems

1. Select a block of time, such as 10 minutes per session.
2. Divide this block of time into shorter intervals (e.g., 30 seconds per interval). In this example, a total of 10 minutes (per session) is divided into twenty 30-second intervals for recording (see Paniagua, 1987b).
3. Within each interval (e.g., 30 seconds) the occurrence versus nonoccurrence of the behavior is recorded.

occurrence and nonoccurrence of the behavior is recorded only once within each interval (i.e., the behavior must occur any time within the interval to be recorded).

If the treatment plan does not require the behavior to be present (in the case of increasing behavior) or absent (in the case of decreasing behavior) within the interval but only at the moment the interval ends, the *momentary time sampling recording* system would be used (i.e., the behavior must occur at the end of the interval to be recorded). For example, self-stimulatory behaviors might occur many times within the interval (e.g., within each 10-second interval in a block of 5 minutes), but such behaviors would be recorded only if they are observed at the end of the interval. A review of earlier applications of recording systems listed in Table 3.3 can be found in Kazdin and Straw (1976) and Sulzer-Azaroff and Mayer (1977).

Another observational method used by behavioral psychologists is self-monitoring. This measure could be either direct or indirect, depending on the nature of the behavior being observed and the context in which that observation is scheduled. For example, instructing a client to record the frequency of "premature ejaculation" when engaging in sexual relationships with his wife at home would be a case of indirect self-monitoring of behavior. Instructing a child to record the frequency of "study behavior" (e.g., on-task behavior) in the classroom and then matching this self-monitoring with observations conducted by independent observers in the same setting would be an example of direct self-monitoring of behavior. In the second case, the objectivity of self-monitoring is validated with direct observations by two independent observers. Two earlier applications of this direct self-monitoring of target behaviors can be found in Broden, Hall, and Mitts (1971) and Glynn, Thomas, and Shee (1973). It should be noted that self-monitoring in itself could function as a behavioral intervention in the treatment plan. For example, in the study by Broden et al. (1971) the percentage of study behavior increased significantly during the self-recording phase, relative to lower percentages of the same behavior during the baseline phase. This finding suggests that observations of one's own behavioral (socially expected) changes could be reinforcing in itself (i.e., self-awareness of such changes might lead to future behavioral changes; see Broden et al., 1971, pp. 197–98). Boxes 3.3 through 3.6 show examples of methods to assess the reliability of these measures.

Box 3.3   Frequency

Computation of Reliability

Method A: Smaller frequency/higher frequency × 100. For example, Observer 1 records 10 instances of physical aggression, and Observer 2 records 12. The reliability is 83% (or 10/12 × 100 = 83%).

Method B: Agreements/agreements + disagreements × 100. For example, Observers 1 and 2 record physical aggression across three time blocks (e.g., 9:00am, 10:00am, and 11:00am).

	Block 1	Block 2	Block 3	Reliability
Observer 1	10	20	15	
Observer 2	10	10	15	A/A + D = 25/25 + 10 = 71%
Agreement	10	10	15	
Disagreement	0	10	0	

Box 3.4   Duration

Computation of Reliability

Duration/Longer Duration × 100. For example, Observer 1 records "working on math problems" across 20 consecutive minutes in the classroom; Observe 2 records 21 minutes. The reliability is 20/21 = 95%.

Box 3.5   Permanent Product

Computation of Reliability

Agreements/Agreements + Disagreements × 100. For example, Observers 1 and 2 record bed-wetting (Enuresis):

Monday	Tuesday	Wednesday	Thursday	Friday	Reliability
Observe 1	Yes	Yes	Yes	Yes	
Observer 2	Yes	No	Yes	Yes	A/A + D = 3/3 + 1 = 75%
Agreement	1	0	1	1	
Disagreement	0	1	0	0	

The above reliability indexes ranged from 65% to 95%. The question is, "Which reliability result is the best?" The answer: All are acceptable. The first volume of the *Journal of Applied Behavior Analysis,* published in 1968, not only introduced examples of what exactly a functional analysis of behavior should be, which specific direct measures to use, and what types of experimental designs would be needed to demonstrate the effects of the treatment with a minimal amount of inferences and speculations from the clinician (Baer et al., 1968); that volume also provided examples of which levels of reliability indexes would be acceptable in future development of the field. In that volume, reliability indexes ranged from 65% to 100% (e.g., Bijou et al., 1968; Hall et al., 1968; Walker & Buckley, 1968; Zelberger, Sampen, & Sloane, 1968). In subsequent years, these conventional indexes of reliability continued to be reported in *JABA,* and in some studies even reliability indexes below 65% were accepted. For example, in the study by Kennedy and Haring (1993), several reliability indexes ranged from 50% to 100%.

These indexes of reliability are calculated across individual sessions, and sessions with 50% reliability would, of course, be less reliable than sessions with 100% reliability (see Sulzer-Azaroff & Mayer, 1977, p. 52). Regardless of how low or high that range is, studies conducted by behavioral psychologists included all sessions in the analysis of results. The reason for this is that behavioral psychologists generally report that range as well as the overall mean interobserver agreement reliability, which is always higher than the lower reliability index in a range of scores. For example, in the study by Kennedy and Haring (1993), examples of overall mean reliability (with ranges from 50% to 100%) include 92% and 97%. Sessions with 50% reliability, however, were also included in the results. Let's suppose that two observers record inattention across five consecutive sessions (using any of the measures in Table 3.3). The reliability results are Session 1, 50%; Session 2, 100%; Session 3, 100%; Session 4, 100%; and Session 5,

---

Box 3.6   Interval Recording Systems

Calculation of Reliability

Agreements/Agreements + Disagreements × 100. For example, inattention to task materials in the classroom is observed across 10 consecutive minutes during five baseline sessions (one session per day). Each 10 minutes is divided into twenty 30-second intervals for recording using one of the interval recording formats described above (e.g., partial interval time sampling method):

	Intervals																				
	1	2	3	4	5	6	7	8	9	10	11	12	13	14	15	16	17	18	19	20	Total
Observer 1	x	x	x	x	n	x	x	x	x	n	n	n	x	n	x	x	x	n	x	x	20
Observer 2	x	x	x	n	x	x	n	n	x	x	x	n	x	n	x	x	x	x	x	x	20
Agreement	1	1	1	0	0	1	0	0	1	0	0	1	1	1	1	1	1	0	1	1	13
Disagreement	0	0	0	1	1	0	1	1	0	1	1	0	0	0	0	0	0	1	0	0	7

Reliability = A/A + D = 13/13 + 20 = 65%

xx = Agree
nx = disagree

100%. The reliability scores range from 50% to 100%, but the overall mean reliability is 83%. Sessions 1 and 3, however, would be part of the data analysis even though these scores were not as reliable as sessions with 100% reliability.

The practice of including sessions with low reliability indexes in the analysis of results is not unique to behavioral psychologists publishing in JABA. For example, in the study by Paniagua et al. (1986) published in the *American Journal of Mental Deficiency,* the overall reliability index was 78% for self-stimulation and was 83% for Pica. The range of these scores, however, was 55% to 88% and 33% to 100%, for self-stimulatory behaviors and Pica, respectively. All sessions were included in the data analysis regardless of how low or high their respective reliability indices were. Other examples can be found in studies published in *Behavior Modification, Behavior Therapy,* and the *Journal of Behavior Therapy and Experimental Psychiatry,* to mention only a few of the journals in which most behavioral psychologists publish their work.

The Reliability and Validity of Indirect versus Direct Measures of Behavior

Many behavioral psychologists, particularly those who restrict their scientific behaviors to the functional analysis and assessment of behavior in terms of Skinner's operant paradigm, point to two major disadvantages of indirect behavioral assessment (Baer et al., 1968; Miltenberger, 1998): (1) This type of assessment is often based on people's recall of past events, and this recall might be inaccurate because of biases, memory problems, or lack of direct contact with the events being reported; (2) in addition, results obtained through an indirect assessment of behavior might be interpreted in many different ways because of the "equivocal reliability and validity of data" (Miltenberger, 1998, p. 55) derived from indirect assessment such as people's self-report of their public behavior (e.g., children's self-report of behavioral changes in school) or private experiences (e.g., children's self-report of obsessive thoughts), and from rating scales such as, for example, the Conners Rating Scales and the Child Behavior Checklist (Barkley, 1988).

To deal with the above two disadvantages effectively, many behavioral psychologists propose direct behavioral assessment of observable behavior and the use of assessment strategies that are reliable and valid. As just noted, although a direct behavioral assessment emphasizes observing what exactly an individual is doing in a given context (e.g., children playing with other children versus children hitting other children in the playground), a great deal of indirect interpretation of the basic datum also results from that observation when cumulative results are plotted on graphs, for example. To demonstrate why the second proposal (i.e., the use of reliable and valid assessment strategies) might not be logistical (in methodological terms), it is necessary to point to a distinction between the ways the terms *reliability* and *validity* are used by many behavioral psychologists versus the use of similar terms in the field of test construction, that is, the area devoted to the development of psychometric tests, rating scales, or psychological tests (Anastasi, 1988).

It should be noted that in the field of inferential statistical analyses or hypothesis testing with emphasis on group comparisons designs, the results of an experiment would be *internally valid* if (a) a null hypothesis is rejected when it should have been accepted—Type I error, (b) a false null hypothesis is not rejected—Type II error, and (c) the wrong experiment was conducted—Type III error. The experiment would be *externally valid* if its result can be generalized outside the context in which they were initially obtained—for example, Treatment A substantially decreases inattention and overactivity among preschool children treated in Setting A, but this treatment is not effective in treating a different group of children in Setting B. In this example, the experiment might be internally valid, but it is not externally valid (see Smith and Sechrest, 1995, pp. 567–570). In addition, an experiment might not be externally valid because it is not clinically significant; that is, it does not resolve social problems despite the statistical significance of the findings. This issue involves the *social validity* of the experiment or the *opinion* of the community regarding the relevance of experimental findings in the solution of social problems (see Wolf, 1978). In the present chapter, the term validity is discussed in the context of either direct or indirect measures in Tables 3.3 and 3.4.

As just noted, in the direct behavioral assessment, the appropriateness of the measurement strategy (e.g., permanent product versus interval recording systems) is what defines the measurement as valid in a given context of measurement. In the area of test construction, the validity of a measurement system "refers to many aspects of its use and definition, but the central feature is the *correlation* of the test with some other behavior of interest, such as performance in college or jobs" (Green, 1992, p. 182; emphasis added). Examples of validity methods in the development and use of psychometric tests (e.g., projective tests, self-report inventories, rating scales, intelligence tests, etc.) include (Anastasi, 1988; Green, 1992): content validity, criterion-related validity or predictive validity, construct validity, concurrent validity, and discriminant validity. In the case of the content validity of the test, the question is "Is the content [i.e., items, questions, etc.] of the test relevant to the characteristic being measured?" (Hammond, 1995, p. 208). For example, the Conners Rating Scales and the Child Behavior Checklist (CBCL; Barkley, 1988) include items relevant to behaviors considered by clinicians, teachers, and parents as examples of impulsivity-hyperactivity, conduct problems, learning problems, and anxiety. The content of these rating scales cannot be used to assess, for example, the IQ of children experiencing these disorders; the Wechsler Intelligence Scale for Children—Revised (WISC-R) includes items relevant to the assessment of general intelligence among children (Golden, 1990).

The question, "Does the test predict later behavior?" (Hammond, 1995, p. 209) is the domain of *criterion-related* or *predictive validity*. For example, the predictive validity of the Conners Rating Scales and the CBCL would be assessed in those cases when scores on these tests are correlated with teachers' reports about emotional disorders among children who initially took such tests (Achenbach & Elderbrock, 1983; Barkley, 1988); similarly scores below two standard deviations on the WISC-R (in which the mean is 100 and the standard deviation is 15) would predict behaviors characteristic of mental retardation in children assessed with the Vineland Adaptive Behavior Scales (mean = 100; standard deviation = 15), which provides an assessment of mental retardation across four observable domains (communication, daily living skills, socialization, and motor skills) as well as a measure of maladaptive behaviors in such children (Anastasi, 1988).

In the field of test construction, the question, "What is the underlined concept, dimension, and trait this test measures?" (see Sechrest, 1984, p. 41) deals with the *construct validity* of the test. For example, the 90-item Eysenck Personality Questionnaire measures four traits: extroversion, neuroticism, psychoticism, and response bias (Hammond, 1995); rating scales such as the Conners Scales measure "learning problem," "anxiety," "psychosomatic," "impulsive-hyperactive," among others (Barkley, 1988); the Beck Depression Inventory measures "depression" (Sechrest, 1984), and so on. The question, "Do the results of this test correlate with ratings from a different test measuring the same event or construct?" is the domain of *concurrent validity* (also termed convergent validity; see Sechrest, 1984, pp. 41–42). For example, the Conners Rating Scales correlate significantly with ratings from the CBCL, Werry-Weiss-Peters Activity Scales, and the Behavior Problem Checklist (Barkley, 1988, p. 118). Finally, the question "Can this test discriminate between normal and abnormal situations or between two different disorders?" deals with the *discriminant validity* of the test. For example, the Conners Rating Scales and the CBCL have been used to separate (discriminate) hyperactive children from nonhyperactive children, depressed from nondepressed children, and clinic-referred from nonferred children (Barkley, 1988).

In the area of direct behavior assessment the term *reliability* is not associated with the event being measured but with the level of agreement between two or more observers. Therefore, the measure (e.g., frequency, duration, and permanent product) would be reliable if at least two observers are consistent in their observations of the behavior under consideration. In the field of test construction, however, reliability "refers to the consistency of scores obtained by the same persons when reexamined with the same test on different occasions, or with different sets of equivalent items, or under other variable examining conditions" (Anastasi, 1988, p. 109). In this application of the concept, a test is reliable if its score can be repeated and is stable over time (Green, 1992). Therefore, the application of this concept in the area of test construction has nothing to do with the level of agreement between two observers recording the target (observable) behavior with a given direct behavioral assessment strategy (e.g., frequency). Examples of three common reliability coefficients in the area of test construction include (Anastasi, 1988) *test-retest reliability* (repetition of the same test on a second occasion), *parallel forms reliability* (two forms of the same test, Form A and Form B, are constructed, and a person is tested with Form A on the first occasion, and with the equivalent Form B on the second; the correlation between scores in Form A and Form B provide an index of the reliability coefficient of the test); and *internal consistency reliability* or *alpha* (the intercorrelation of individual items on the test). Behavioral psychologists who emphasize a combination of direct and indirect assessments of target behavior (e.g., Conners Scales, CBCL, rating scales, the Schedule of Affective Disorders and Schizophrenia, Diagnostic Interview Schedule for Children, etc.) generally use psychometric tests that are reliable in terms of one or more of the above methods (see Rutter, Tuma and Lann, 1988, for a summary of such methods across widely used tests).

The assumption that indirect assessment of target behavior is not useful because of its equivocal reliability and validity appears logical only when these concepts are interpreted in terms of the exemplars (Kuhn, 1970) of the applied behavior analysis. When such concepts are interpreted in terms of the exemplars of the field of test construction (e.g., Anastasi, 1988; Green, 1992), the reliability and validity of indirect measures of behavior (e.g., rating scales) become evident and unquestionable. The use of valid and reliable direct measures is, of course, a critical issue in a direct behavioral assessment of target behavior: The measure should be appropriate, or valid, in the assessment of a given observable, and a certain level of agreement between at least two observers should be achieved. It is important to recognize, however, that this usage of such concepts is only one example of the many ways in which similar concepts are used (e.g., in the field of test construction) in the assessment of adaptive and maladaptive behaviors.

Functional Assessment of Behavioral Changes

As noted earlier, this is the second element in the area of behavioral assessment, and it also constitutes the *analytic* domain in Table 3.1 (Baer et al., 1968). The goal of a functional assessment is the selection of the most appropriate experimental design to demonstrate that behavioral changes (i.e., changes in the dependent variable) are the result of the intervention or treatment (independent variable), rather than the result of variables unrelated to the goal of the treatment plan (see Haynes & O'Brien, 2000, p. 42, for alternative definitions of functional assessment). In this particular context, intra-subject replication (or single-case or Skinnerian) designs are used (e.g., Hersen & Barlow, 1976; Kazdin, 1980), rather than traditional group comparison designs (Beck et al., 1984; Kazdin). Many variants of intrasubject replication design exist (see Hersen & Barlow), but the most common variants include reversal designs, multiple-baseline designs, and changing-criterion designs. A brief summary of each of these designs is provided below; a more extensive description of such designs can be found in Hersen and Barlow, Kazdin, and Vollmer and Camp (1998).

The *reversal design* is the classic single-case or intrasubject replication design (Hersen & Barlow, 1976). In this design, the target behavior is recorded during a period termed baseline (A) in the absence of the behavioral intervention; the intervention is programmed across several sessions (B); and a return to baseline (A) is again programmed. An earlier application of the ABA reversal design is the study by Hall et al. (1968; incidentally, this is the first study in the series of studies published in the first volume of the *JABA*). In this study, children's study behavior (e.g., orientation toward the appropriate task in the classroom) was recorded across a five-day consecutive baseline period (A); social reinforcement was programmed contingent on study behavior (B) across nine consecutive days; and this interval was removed (a return to A) from day 17 through day 21. The results showed that study behavior dramatically increased during the social reinforcement condition, relative to baseline observations. In the same study, social reinforcement (B) was again programmed after the second baseline, and a follow-up assessment followed this repetition of Phase B (i.e., observations of behavior in the absence of treatment). This illustrates one of the many variants of the ABA reversal design, and an ABAB design (with a maintenance phase). Other variants of the ABA reversal design can be found in Hersen and Barlow. The study by Hall et al. (1968) also illustrates the importance of a return to treatment (after the second baseline) for ethical reasons (i.e., if the treatment is effective in controlling a maladaptive behavior, e.g., lack of "study behavior," the treatment plan should not end in a baseline—ABA—but in a repetition of the treatment—ABAB). Figure 3.2 (for Cases 1 and 2) shows another example of the reversal design.

In multiple-baseline designs (MBD), the effect of behavioral interventions is assessed at different points in time following a baseline period. In these designs, the intervention does not need to be removed or withdrawn (e.g., ABA designs) to demonstrate experimental control of dependent variables (i.e., treatments). The MBD can take different formats, but (a) in each format the target behavior is recorded across two or more baselines (e.g., Classroom 1 and Classroom 2); (b) the intervention is programmed after observations have been completed in the first baseline period (e.g., in Classroom 1); (c) observation of target behavior continue in the second baseline period (e.g., Classroom 2); and (d) at a given point or session in the design the intervention is also programmed after the completion of the second baseline observations (e.g., in Classroom 2). This example illustrates the MBD across settings (e.g., Classroom 1 and Classroom 2; see Case 8, Figure 3.6). The same experimental format is used in the MBD across subjects or groups (e.g., baseline observations scheduled with Subject 1 or Group 1 and Subject 2 or Group 2, and then the programming of the intervention with both subjects/groups but at different points in time following baseline observations; see Cases 3 and 4, Figure 3.3, and Cases 5 and 6, Figure 3.4); and the MBD across behaviors (e.g., similar format to the MBD across settings and subjects/groups, but with emphasis on the programming of the intervention sequentially on two or more behaviors; see Case 7, Figure 3.5).

Paniagua (1990c) introduced a new variant of the MBD termed the MBD *across exemplars.* The logic of the MBD across exemplars takes "into account the possibility that the component of what appears to be one behavior class, the 'exemplars' of that class, could in certain circumstances serve as the baseline of an MBD across behaviors: the experimental treatment could be applied sequentially to these exemplars" (Paniagua, 1990c, p. 178). For example, "play behavior" could include two exemplars: crayon and bead play; meat and fruit consumption could be the exemplars for "eating" behavior, and the exemplars for "conversational skills" could include subject's questions and the subject's interjection. Figure 3.1 shows a general description of the general format in this new variant of the MBD (see Paniagua, 1990c, p. 180, for examples of studies in which this variant of the MBD was used).

In the case of the changing-criterion design, the target behavior is initially observed

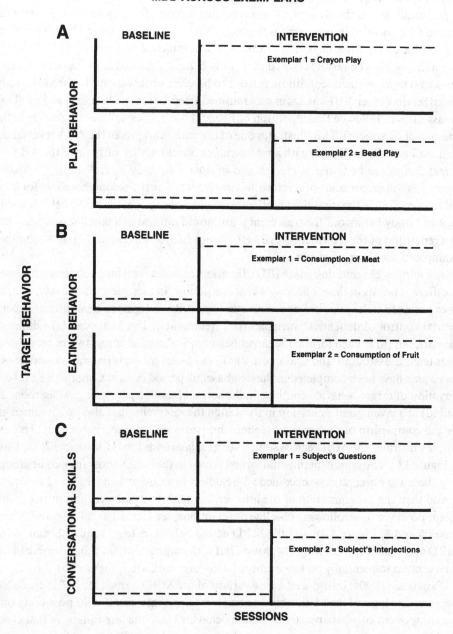

Figure 3.1   Format of the MBD

Note: In A, the target behavior (play behavior) is divided into two exemplars (crayon and bead play). In B, eating behavior is measured across the exemplars "consumption of meat" and "consumption of fruit"; in C, the subject's questions and interjection are the two exemplars for "conversational skills." In each case, the intervention is introduced sequentially across exemplars.

Source: Paniagua (1990), pp. 177–188.

during a baseline period. If the goal of the intervention is to increase the frequency of the behavior gradually over time (i.e., shaping) from the baseline sessions to treatment sessions, specific criteria (i.e., at what level that frequency should be prior to the delivery of the consequence) are established during the programming of the intervention. For example, if a child only completes two math problems correctly during baseline, during the intervention phase (treatment) social praise and tokens will be delivered contingent upon meeting the following criteria for the occurrence of the target behavior (completion of math problems correctly): Criterion 1 = 2 problems, Criterion 2 = 3 problems, Criterion 3 = 5 problems, and so on, until the child is able to complete the maximum number of math problems expected by the teacher in the classroom. Case 9, Figure 3.7, shows an example of this design in those cases when the goal of the intervention is to increase the frequency of behavior (Paniagua & Saeed, 1987). If the goal of the intervention is to decrease the frequency of behavior, an inverse direction (from high to low levels) in criterion levels is selected. This is the case of the programming of the reinforcer contingent upon gradual decreases in weight levels (Favell, 1977), and gradual reduction of instances of inattention and overactivity in children diagnosed with ADHD (e.g., Paniagua, 1987b; see also Cases 1 and 2, 3 and 4, and 7, Figures 3.2, 3.3, and 3.5, respective).

INDIRECT BEHAVIORAL ASSESSMENT

Factors Justifying the Use of Indirect Measures

As noted, many behavioral psychologists (behavior therapists, in particular) emphasize a combination of direct and indirect assessments of target behavior (Miltenberger, 1998). In general, four factors led to the appreciation of the use of indirect measures of behavior among behavioral psychologists. First, it is either unethical, impractical, or impossible to measure the target behavior with recording systems listed in Table 3.3. For example, many clients would not permit the use of direct observational methods to assess sexual dysfunctions (e.g., Sexual Aversion Disorder, Premature Ejaculation, and paraphilias such as Exhibitionism, Fetishism, and Pedophilia; APA, 1994). In this case, behavioral psychologists would emphasize self-report and indirect self-monitoring measures (Schumancher & Lloyd, 1976). Similarly, symptoms of anxiety disorders in children and antecedent events leading to such symptoms may be difficult to assess directly. For example, it would be impossible to create a condition in which symptoms suggesting Separation Anxiety Disorder (APA, 1994) could be assessed in the presence of antecedent events such as the death of parents or being alone. That is, a child would self-report that he or she feels afraid that parents could be killed in an accident or that they would be alone at home for a extended period of time; but it would be unethical (i.e., forcing the child to stay alone at home) to show that such events are the actual cause of such symptoms. A better strategy would be use a self-report instrument such as the Fear Survey Schedule for Children (Ollendick, 1983, 1984; Scherer & Nakamura, 1968). Another example is the assessment of Anorexia Nervosa and Bulimia Nervosa (APA, 1994), in which structured clinical interviews, self-report questionnaires, and indirect self-monitoring are more practical than direct behavioral assessment methods (Wilson & Pike, 1993).

Second, indirect measures of target behaviors are essential in conducting a preliminary assessment of such behaviors in a cost-effective way prior to the programming of direct behavioral observation strategies (Mash & Terdal, 1988). For example, during the clinical interview parents often bring their children to mental health clinics and report behaviors they consider problematic in their children. As noted by Ollendick and Meador (1984), parents' reports during the (unstructured) clinical interview are an "indispensable part of assessment" (p. 355). In addition, Edelbrock and Costello (1988) rightly pointed out that the clinical interview (e.g., use of *DSM* criteria) should be followed by a structured psychiatric interview to enhance the collection of reliable and valid information during the interviewing process (e.g., the programming of the Schedule for Affective Disorders and Schizophrenia for Children or the Diagnostic Interview for Children and Adolescents).

Third, prominent behavioral psychologists such as Barkley (1990), Kazdin (1988), Ollendick and Meador (1984), and Wilson and O'Leary (1980) have emphasized the fact that indirect measures of behavior are reliable and valid methods, but in the context of the test construction approach (Anastasi, 1988) as opposed to the interpretation of reliable and valid measures in terms of the methodology used by behavioral psychologists identified with the operant paradigm.

Fourth, the use of direct behavioral assessment strategies picked up in the mid-1970s and 1980s (Haynes & O'Brien, 2000). During these periods, prominent behavioral psychologists edited textbooks illustrating the utility of both direct and indirect measures of behavior. Examples of these early textbooks include *Behavioral Assessment: A Practical Handbook* (Hersen & Bellack, 1976), *Behavioral Assessment of Childhood Disorders* (Mash & Terdal, 1988), and *Handbook of Psychological Assessment* (Goldstein & Hersen, 1984). For example, Ollendick and Meador (1984) and Haynes (1984) titled their chapters "Behavioral Assessment of Children" and "Behavioral Assessment of Adults," respectively, and each chapter includes an emphasis on both direct and indirect measures of adaptive and maladaptive behaviors. The successful acceptance of these textbooks by behavioral and nonbehavioral psychologists led to subsequent editions (Goldstein & Hersen, 1999; Hersen & Bellack, 1998; Mash & Terdal, 1997). Future generations of behavioral psychologists (including the author of this chapter) followed a similar trend in their efforts to develop a comprehensive assessment of behavior by emphasizing both direct and indirect measurement strategies in the functional analysis of behavior, behavioral assessment of behavior, and functional assessment of behavioral changes (see Miltenberger, 1998).

As noted by Mash and Terdal (1988), direct behavioral assessment of adaptive and maladaptive behaviors among children and adolescents (as well as adults) represented a "break from traditional psychometric test approaches" (p. 50). These authors, however, correctly added that despite that break the use of these approaches should be "a common practice among both behavioral and nonbehavioral clinicians" (Mash & Terdal, 1988, p. 50; see also Haynes & O'Brien, 2000, p. 16).

Selection of Indirect Measures

Table 3.4 includes examples of indirect measures that behavioral psychologists often use to enhance direct behavioral assessment of many of the psychiatric or emotional difficulties described in the DSM-IV (APA, 1994). Discussion related to the reliability

Table 3.4 Examples of Indirect Measures of Target Behavior in Behavioral Assessment

Measure	Description
Unstructured Clinical Interview	
Diagnostic and Statistical Manual of Mental Disorders (DSM-IV)	Provide a preliminary assessment of disorders self-reported by the child or parents (APA, 1994); a mental status exam is also conducted (Siassi, 1984).
Structured Clinical Interview	
Behavioral Screening Questionnaire	Identifies preschool-age children with emotional disorders (Richman & Graham, 1971).
Child Screening Inventory	Identifies children aged 6–18 with emotional disorders (Langner et al., 1976).
Diagnostic Interview for Children	Assesses a wide range of emotional disorders in children and adolescents aged 6 and older (Herjanic & Reich, 1982).
Kiddie-SADS: Schedule for Affective Disorder and Schizophrenia	Assesses a wide range of emotional disorders, children aged 6–17 (Puig-Antich & Chambers, 1978).
Interview Schedule for Children	Emphasize current symptoms related to depression (Kovacs, 1985).
The Functional Assessment Interview	Assesses distal antecedent events (e.g., sleep pattern, eating routines, daily activities) and proximal antecedent events immediately related to the target behavior, e.g., time of day, settings, and people that might be functionally related to the target behavior (Miltenberger, 1998; O'Neill et al., 1997).
Intellectual Development Tests	
Bayley Scale of Infant Development	Assess the developmental status of infants age two months and 2½ years and mentally retarded children (Black & Matula, 2000).
Cattell Culture Fair Intelligence Tests	For children ages four to adulthood and retarded. Emphasis on relationships among figures and shapes to help minimize the effect of language and educational levels on performance (Anastasi, 1988).
Hiskey-Nebraska Test of Learning Aptitude	Recommended for deaf and hearing-impaired children ages three to 16 and mentally retarded (Goldman et al., 1983).
Kaufman Assessment Battery	Recommended for children ages 2½ to 12½ years. Does not emphasize innate abilities, but what the child has learned in the past (Goldman et al., 1983).
McCarthy Scales of Children's Abilities	Recommended with children ages 2½ and 8½ years. This test provides an overall development of children (Anastasi, 1988).
Raven's Progressive Matrices	This test is recommended with children 5 years old and older, with adults, with mentally retarded children and adults, and with immigrants and individuals with language deficiency (Anastasi, 1988).
Stanford-Binet Intelligence Scale	Assesses general intelligence in children, adolescents, and adults. This test (and the Wechsler scales) is generally used to assess the levels of mental retardation in the DSM-IV. The mean of this test is 100, and its standard deviation (SD) is 16. Individual scores 2 SD below the mean = mild retardation; 5 SD below the mean = profound mental retardation (Anastasi, 1988).

(continued)

Table 3.4   Continued

Measure	Description
Test of Nonverbal Intelligence	Recommended to measure intellectual functioning in a non-verbal format (requiring no listening, speaking, reading, or writing by the individual being examined). Designed for children with mental retardation, language and/or hearing-impaired individuals (Anastasi, 1988; Goldman et al., 1983).
Wechsler Intelligence Scale for Children	Recommended with children $6\frac{1}{2}$ through $16\frac{1}{2}$ years old; generally used to determine levels of mental retardation in the DSM-IV; mean = 100, SD = 15; 2 SD below the mean = "mild retardation" (or $100 - 30 = 70$; 30 derived from 15×2 SD = 30); 5 SD below that mean = "profound mental retardation" (or $100 - 75 = IQ$ of 25; 75 derived from 15×5 SD = 75) (Anastasi, 1988).
Wechsler Preschool and Primary Intelligence	Used with children 4 to $6\frac{1}{2}$ years; mean = 100, SD = 15. Can be used to assess levels of mental retardation in the DSM-IV (Anastasi, 1988).

Social Development Tests

The American Association on Mental Deficiency Adaptive Behavior Scale	Assesses adaptive functioning of impaired individuals, particularly mentally retarded persons, three to 12 years old. This scale emphasizes the assessment of behaviors the individual needs to cope with the demands in the social and natural environment (e.g., language, self-care skills, social skills). Classifying people with mental retardation only on the basis of IQ performance on a intelligence test could lead to an underestimation of the individual's ability (Goldman et al., 1983).
The Vineland Social Maturity Scale	This is a widely used test to assess many adaptive skills in individuals ranging in ages from under one month to 25 years, across four domains: communication, daily living, socialization, and motor skills. The maladaptive behaviors that could interfere with adaptive functioning in these domains are also recorded. The mean of this test (for each domain and all domains together in a "adaptive behavior composite score") is 100 with 15 SD. Thus, two standard deviations below the mean of this test on the adaptive behavior composite scale (i.e., $100 - 30 = 70$) would suggest deficit in adaptive skills leading to a diagnosis of mild mental retardation. For the diagnosis of profound mental retardation, a score between 20 and 25 will be needed (or 5 SD below the mean of that test). If an intelligence test (e.g., the Wechsler scales) used with children previously tested with the Vineland scale are tested with an intelligence test and their IQ scores correlated with the above scores, one would conclude that the Vineland is a valid test in the assessment of the levels of mental retardation among children (see Anastasi, 1988, p. 289).

Table 3.4   Continued

Measure	Description

Language Development Tests

Peabody Picture Vocabulary Test	Covers the age range 2 years 6 months to 18 years; assesses an individual's hearing or receptive vocabulary, and can be used as a predictor of school success. Provides a quick measure (approximately 15 minutes) of a child's language development, particularly with cerebral-palsied and deaf children (Goldman et al., 1983).
The Illinois Test of Psycholinguistic Abilities	For children age 2 to 10 years; assesses disabilities in critical domains of learning (auditory-vocal, visual-motor, receptive and expressive language). This test is widely used in the design of language programs for children in need of remedial education (Goldman et al., 1983).

Achievement Tests

Metropolitan Achievement Tests	Recommended with children in grades K–12. It assesses a child's academic achievement in reading, vocabulary, mathematics, computation, language, and spelling (Anastasi, 1988; Fox & Zinkin, 1984; Goldman et al., 1983).
Wide Range Achievement Test	Measures word recognition and pronunciation, writing, spelling, and arithmetic computation (Goldman et al., 1983).

Parent-Child Relationship Measures

Child Report of Parental Behavior Inventory	Assesses children's perception of their parents with emphasis on acceptance versus rejection, psychological autonomy versus psychological control, and firm control versus lax control (Jacob & Tennebaum, 1988).
Parent-Adolescent Communication Scale	Assesses children's and parents' perception regarding their communication among themselves (Jacob & Tennenbaum, 1988).

Rating Scales and Self-Report Questionnaires

Conners Rating Scales	Parents' and teachers' rating of emotional disorders in children aged 3–17 (Barkley, 1988; Conners, 1973).
Child Behavior Checklist	Parents' and teachers' rating of emotional disorders in children aged 6 to 16 ½ (Achenbach & Edelbrock, 1983; Barkley, 1988).
Children's Depression Inventory	Assesses symptoms of depression based on the Beck Depression Inventory (Ollendick & Meador, 1984).
Eating Disorder Inventory	Assesses symptoms for anorexia and bulimia nervosa (Wilson & Pike, 1993).
Fear Survey Schedule	Assesses fear of physical injury/personal loss and fear of natural or supernatural events in children aged 4–18; completed by parents, teachers, or children (Barkley, 1988; Miller et al., 1971).
Fear Survey Schedule for Children	Used by younger and middle-aged children during self-report of specific fears (e.g., dark places, riding in a car, being punished by parents) integrated across five factors (e.g., fear of failure, the unknown, death) (Ollendick, 1983).

(continued)

Table 3.4   Continued

Measure	Description
Home Situations Questionnaire	Assesses where at home (setting) the child is displaying the target behavior, as opposed to what type of problem the child is having (Barkley & Edelbrock, 1987).
Louisville Behavior Checklist	Assesses academic disability and a wide range of emotional disorders (Barkley, 1988; Miller, 1984).
School Behavior Checklist	Emphasis on teachers' rating of emotional disorders in children aged 3–13 (Barkley, 1988; Miller, 1981).
School Situations Questionnaire	Assesses where in school (setting) the child is displaying the target behavior, as opposed to what type of problem the child is having (Barkley & Edelbrock, 1987).
Self-Control Rating Scale	Assesses deficit in self-control in children aged 8–11 as perceived by teachers and parents (Barkley, 1988; Kendall et al., 1981).
Werry-Weiss-Peters Activity Rating Scale	Emphasis on children's level of activity across specific settings (e.g., play, television, meal time); children aged 2–9 (Barkley, 1988).
Viligance and Sustained Attention Tests	
Continuous Performance Tests	Assesses sustained attention and impulse control in children with ADHD; provides an indirect measures of self-control skills (Barkley, 1990).
Matching Familiar Figures Test	Assesses impulse control in normal and disturbed children and adolescents; provides an indirect measure of self-control skills (Barkley, 1990; Kagan, 1966).

and validity of these measures can be found in Anastasi (1988); Barkley (1988); Edelbrock and Costello (1984, 1988); Goldman, Stein, and Guerry (1983); and Mash and Terdal (1988, 1997). With the exception of the unstructured clinical interview, which is indispensable in the assessment of adaptive and maladaptive behaviors (Ollendick & Meador, 1984), the selection of additional measures in Table 3.4 depends on the nature of the behavioral problem being measured. For example, intellectual, social, and language development tests would be particularly useful during the assessment of children with DSM-IV diagnoses of Mental Retardation and Pervasive Developmental Disorders; language development and achievement tests should be emphasized during the assessment of children with diagnosis of ADHD or Learning Disorders (APA, 1994). Parent-child measures, structured clinical interviews, rating scales, and self-report questionnaires would greatly enhance direct behavioral assessment of other psychiatric disorders usually first diagnosed in infancy, childhood, or adolescence (e.g., Conduct Disorder, Oppositional Defiant Disorder, Selective Mutism, etc.), as well as other disorders such as, for example, Major Depression and Anxiety Disorders (APA, 1994). Neuropsychological tests would help in the assessment of visual-spatial, construction, somatosensory, and motor problems among children experiencing developmental disabilities (Taylor, Fletcher, & Satz, 1984). Finally, it should be noted that in the specific case of the unstructured clinical interview it is important to include the mental status exam because difficulties in thought processes, orientation, insight and judgement, perception and other elements in this exam (Siassi, 1984) could provide critical information (e.g., the probability of suicidal behavior in children and adolescents with Major Depression) that direct observation would not reveal.

BEHAVIORAL CLINICAL CASE FORMULATION AND TREATMENT PLAN

In general, the goal of a clinical case formulation is to provide guidelines to clinicians with respect to their choice of specific variables considered to be of social significance in the treatment plan, including the selection of target behaviors, interventions, measurement strategies, and the experimental manipulation in the evaluation of treatment effects. In the specific case of the practice of behavioral psychologists, examples of models guiding a behavioral clinical case formulation include the problem-solving, cognitive-behavioral, and the functional analytic models (Haynes & O'Brien, 2000). A summary of selected components of a behavioral clinical case formulation using elements from each of these models follows.

Selected Components of a Behavioral Clinical Case Formulation

Make a list of problems. Include overt behaviors and the client's beliefs leading to behavior problems. For example, a child may be diagnosed with Oppositional Defiant Disorder (ODD) and believe that "external" forces (e.g., parents' demands) are causing this problem.

Determine which problem or set of problems would be initially intervened or treated. Use findings derived from multiple assessment methods (e.g., direct observations and rating scales) and informants (e.g., clients, parents, teachers) to make this decision.

Determine the most feasible intervention. Children with internalizing disorders (e.g., anxiety, depression) would respond better to techniques in which cognitive processes are emphasized (e.g., covert modeling, covert reinforcement, rational-emotive therapy); in the case of children with externalizing disorders (e.g., ODD, ADHD, Conduct Disorder), techniques that emphasize external manipulations of events (e.g., token programs, timeout from positive reinforcement) would be recommended in the treatment plan.

Rank the order of behavioral problems. Problem behaviors that have an immediate effect on the client's life or upon social, occupational, and family areas should be placed first in the list of problems for intervention. For example, in the case of child with diagnoses of Major Depression and a Reading Disorder (APA, 1994), the first problem should have priority in the treatment plan.

Determine antecedent events leading to identified problem behaviors. Examples of antecedent events that have been shown to trigger maladaptive behaviors include situational events such as complexity of school tasks and multiple instructions to perform multiple behaviors leading to oppositional responses; demands leading to self-injurious behaviors in children with Pervasive Developmental Disorder; and physiological conditions such as sleep deprivation leading to fatigue, resulting in refusal to go to school the following day.

Determine the consequence of problem behaviors. Many childhood and adolescent disorders are the product of either positive reinforcement (e.g., social attention contingent on oppositional responses would increase the probability of occurrence of such responses in the future) or negative reinforcement (e.g., aggression to escape from an aversive event). When the consequences of maladaptive behaviors are identified, the treatment should emphasize a change in the consequences leading to behaviors. For example, if a functional analysis suggests that physical aggression in the classroom allows a child to escape from this setting (i.e., the process of negative reinforcement), physical aggression should be followed not by the removal of the child from the classroom (the consequence) but by creating a condition in which the child would be positively reinforced (e.g., a token program) for staying in the classroom (which is an indirect way to manage aggression in this case).

Conduct a functional assessment of behavioral changes. In the treatment plan, schedule direct behavioral observations on a continuous basis (e.g., one session of 10-minute duration daily in the classroom) across several sessions. The programming of indirect measures would depend on the nature of the problem and the measure selected. For example, direct observations of inattention and impulsivity in children diagnosed with ADHD would be scheduled daily in combination with vigilance and sustained attention tests (e.g., the Matching Familiar Figures test; Kagan, 1966). Rating scales and self-report questionnaires (e.g., Conners Scales, Children's Depression Inventory) would be scheduled once during the baseline and treatment phase.

Consider the social validity of behavioral changes. Parents, teachers, and other social agents are not concerned about behavioral changes displayed on graphs or summarized using statistical techniques (e.g., percentages of attention or parents' instructions followed by a child); they want to know whether findings derived from the treatment plan could be generalized and maintained outside the clinic. Parents' and teachers' satisfaction with the intervention should emphasize not whether they agree with behavioral changes in the clinic (i.e., effective treatment of the child's problem behaviors) but whether they could see these changes in the natural environment (e.g., school, home, etc.).

CASE STUDY

The following cases show examples of a combination of direct and indirect assessments of target behaviors, as well as example of intrasubject replication designs in the functional assessment of behavioral changes. A detailed description of behavioral interventions and procedures can be found in the original publication.

Cases 1 and 2

The participants included two girls diagnosed with ADHD (Paniagua & Black, 1992). Prior to participation, both subjects received this diagnosis on the basic of an unstructured clinical interview conducted by child psychiatry residents using the ADHD criteria in the DSM-III-R (1987; the study was conducted prior to the release of the DSM-IV). Examples of selection criteria included age between 6 and 12 (Case 1 = 8 years old, Case 2 = 6 years old); IQ greater than 70 on the Wechsler Intelligence Scale for Children-Revised (Case 1 = 90, Case 2 = 75; see Table 3.4); cutoff mean factor score of at least 1.5 on the Abbreviated Conners Teacher Rating Scale (ACTRS; both subjects scored about 2.5 on this scale, suggesting a great deal of ADHD); and a history of ADHD according to parents' reports.

The aim of these cases was to decrease behaviors considered as examples of ADHD by programming the reinforcer contingent upon the verbal behavior about the inhibition of these (nonverbal) behaviors and the actual decrease of such behaviors using the verbal-nonverbal correspondence training method (Paniagua, 1990b). The target nonverbal behaviors include inattention (eyes not oriented toward task materials, teachers, or trainer for at least a 15-second duration during any 30-second recording interval); overactivity (any situation where the normal sitting surface of neither buttock was applied to the child's seat, i.e., out-of-seat behavior, or moving hands, legs, torso, head without apparent purpose, i.e., fidgeting); noise (clapping hands, tapping pencils, or any other nonverbal noise); and academic performance (arithmetic and spelling problems completed correctly during the observations scheduled for the recording of inattention, overactivity, and noise). The verbal behavior include self-reports about the inhibition of past (nonverbal) behavior (i.e., inattention) in the forms of "I sat in my chair," "I paid attention to my tasks," or "I did not clap my hands" in response to specific questions from the therapist (e.g., "Did you sit still in your chair?"). Answers such as "I don't know," "I don't remember," and "probably" were not considered verbal reports of past nonverbal behavior in this study.

Nonverbal behaviors were recorded with the partial time-sampling recording system, during which a total of 10 minutes per session was divided into 20 30-second intervals for recording. Verbal reports were recorded verbatim on a data sheet during a verbalization period of approximately 5 minutes. The formula: number of intervals of agreement/number of intervals of disagreement + agreement × 100 was used to determine the reliability of observations by two independent observers. The reliability of recording corresponding verbal reports (i.e., reports matching the nonverbal behaviors) and academic performance was 100% in each case. The overall reliability across observations of nonverbal behaviors (inattention, overactivity, and noise) ranged from 40% to 100%, and mean (overall) reliability ranged from 93% to 100%.

A combination of ABABC reversal design and changing-criterion design was used with both subjects. During Phase A, baseline observations were scheduled. In Phase B, Case 1 received an intervention termed *Reinforcement of Do-Report Correspondence* (Paniagua, 1990b, 1998a; also known as Reinforcement of Corresponding Reports; Paniagua, 1987b), in which only reports matching the actual inhibition (in terms of certain criterion levels, e.g., Criterion 1 = 40% of intervals with no inattention or overactivity responses) of maladaptive behaviors were reinforced with small toys, stickers, and so forth (see Paniagua, 1990b); and Case 2 observed Case 1 (observational learning process in Bandura's theory of behavior, e.g., Bandura, 1969) performing the expected (adaptive) nonverbal behaviors *and* Case 1's self-reports of such behaviors. After several sessions in Phase B, baseline observations were repeated (Phase A) with both sub-

Treatment Room

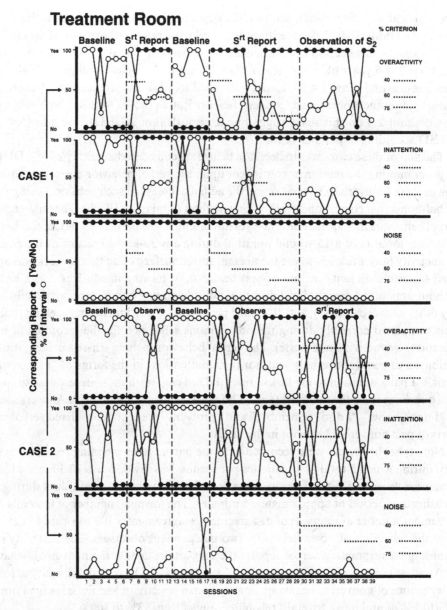

Figure 3.2   Daily Percentages of Intervals

Note: Daily percentages of intervals for overactivity, inattention, and noise and occurrence (Yes) versus nonoccurrence (No) of corresponding reports during baseline, reinforcement of report-do correspondence, and observational learning for Cases 1 and 2.

Source: Paniagua and Black (1992), pp. 1–19.

jects, which were followed by the repetition of Phase B. In the last phase of the design (C), the interventions were reversed: Case 2 received the Reinforcement of Do-Report Correspondence technique, whereas Case 1 observed Case 2. Figure 3.2 shows the format for this combination of intrasubject replication designs, in which substantial behavioral changes (i.e., a functional assessment of behavioral changes) occurred during Phases B and C, relative to baseline observations. In addition, the percentage of intervals in which maladaptive behaviors did not occur gradually increased across sessions as a result of the delivery of reinforcers contingent upon the child's meeting of such criteria in a changing-criterion design format. Children's academic performance also increased during the intervention, relative to baseline (see Paniagua & Black, 1992, p. 11 and p. 14, Figures 3.3 and 3.4, respectively).

Cases 3 and 4

Two boys, 10 (Case 3) and 9 (Case 4) years old, participated in this case (Paniagua, 1987b). Each subject was diagnosed with ADHD by a child psychiatrist during an unstructured clinical interview using criteria in the DSM-III-R (1987). Their IQ was also assessed with the WISC-R (Case 3 = 89, and Case 4 = 87). An indirect assessment of ADHD with the ACTRS was also conducted. Target behaviors similar to those described in Case 1 were selected, as well as the same recording system and behavioral intervention (i.e., Reinforcement of Corresponding Reports). Reliability between observers was calculated using the same formula as in Cases 1 and 2 (mean for Case 3 = 81 and 90 in the classroom and treatment room, respectively; for Case 4 = 91 and 92 in the classroom and treatment room, respectively).

In this case, a functional assessment of behavior changes was conducted with the multiple baseline design across subjects in combination with the changing-criterion design. For purpose of illustration, only results involving attentional problems are showed in Figure 3.3. In general, the intervention dramatically decreased inattention (in this case, off-task behavior and overactivity as defined in Table 3.2), relative to baseline observations. In addition, subjects fulfilled the pre-established criterion level for the inhibition of the corresponding nonverbal behavior leading to a matching (verbal-nonverbal correspondence) between the child's verbalization to inhibit inattention and the actual inhibition of inattention during the introduction of the behavioral intervention. Results in Figure 3.3 also correlated with results on the ACTRS. During baseline, the ACTRS scores were Case 3 = 3.0, Case 4 = 3.0 (maximum score, suggesting severe symptoms for ADHD). During the intervention, these scores decreased dramatically (Case 3 = 0.9, Case = 1.0). Figure 3.3 also show that treatment effects were maintained during a follow-up phase in the treatment room, and generalized (bottom section of Figure 3.3) in the classroom (where subjects continued under direct behavioral observations in the absence of treatment).

Cases 5 and 6

Subjects include 6 boys ranging in ages from 15 to 17 years (Paniagua, 1985b), who were residents of a group home for adolescents with emotional problems (e.g., antisocial behaviors, oppositional behaviors). Among target behaviors, helping behavior was a critical behavior to establish and maintain among these adolescents. Examples of this behavior included bathroom cleaning (wash the toilet bowl and mop the floor daily), living and dining room cleaning (dust the furniture and vacuum or sweep the floor daily), kitchen cleaning (scour the sink after each meal, sweep and mop the floor), and trash removal (put the day's trash in the garage and later place the trash accumulated during the weekend in a container on the sidewalk). The permanent product recording

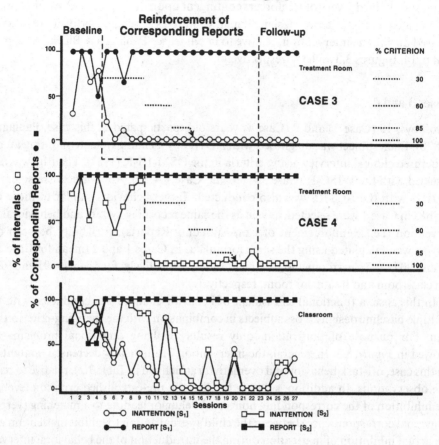

Figure 3.3   Daily Percentages of Inattention

Note: Daily percentages of inattention and corresponding reports during baseline, reinforcement of corresponding report, follow-up, and generalization (classroom) for Cases 3 and 4.

Source: Paniagua (1987), pp. 1–23.

system was used to assess instances of helping behavior. The mean interobserver agreement of recording helping behavior was 100% (using the formula described previously). Subjects were divided into two groups (Case 5 and Case 6) of three subjects each, and the intervention described in Cases 1 and 2 was programmed in a multiple baseline design across groups. Figure 3.4 shows that baseline subjects' reports about their engagement in helping behaviors did not correspond with subjects' actual participation in such behaviors. During the programming of the intervention (reinforcement of correspondence or corresponding reports), a clear match between reports and their corresponding nonverbal (reported) behaviors was noted. These results were maintained in a 6-day follow-up phase. This case also shows that although Skinnerian designs were initially used with single subjects (as opposed to the traditional group designs) resulting in the generic names "single case experimental designs" (e.g., Hersen & Barlow, 1976), the logic and format of these designs also applied when results represent group data (e.g., Figure 3.4).

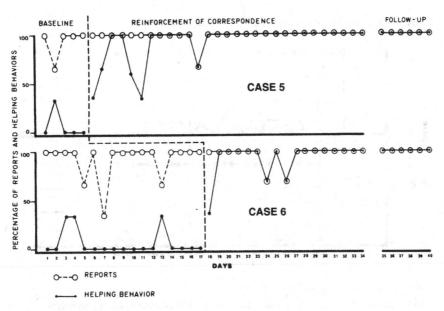

Figure 3.4   Daily Percentages of Reports

Note: Daily percentages of reports and helping behaviors during baseline, reinforcement of correspondence, and follow-up conditions, for Cases 5 (Group 1) and 6 (Group 2).

Source: Paniagua (1985), pp. 237–244.

Case 7

The subject was a boy aged 7 years (Paniagua, 1987b). This case included procedures similar to those described in Cases 3 and 4 during the definition of target nonverbal (e.g., inattention) and verbal (e.g., "I'll sit in my chair") behaviors and the measurement of such behaviors. The intervention, however, included a variant of verbal-nonverbal correspondence training techniques (Paniagua, 1990b, 1998a), namely *Reinforcement Set-Up on Promises* (i.e., a report about future behaviors), in which the reinforcer was initially presented contingent upon a promise to display the nonverbal (promised) behavior (e.g., a promise about the inhibition of instances of overactivity and inattention) and was later available contingent on the correspondence between the verbal behavior (i.e., a promise) and its corresponding nonverbal behavior. This case illustrates a functional assessment of behavioral changes with the multiple baseline design across behaviors in combination with the changing-criterion design. In baseline (Figure 3.5), the percentage of intervals of both overactivity and inattention were above 50% during the introduction of the treatment. When the first behavior was intervened across specific criterion levels (e.g., Criterion 1 = 30% of intervals for the delivery of the reinforcer), it decreased substantially across 20 consecutive sessions; similar results are noted when the intervention was used with the second behavior (inattention). Again, indirect measures of ADHD using the ACTRS showed dramatic decreases in the overall scores in this scale from baseline (score = 1.6) to treatment (score = 0.9).

Case 8

This case (Paniagua et al., 1986) involved a 4-year-old girl diagnosed with profound mental retardation. The Bayley Scales of Infant Development (see Table 3.4) were used

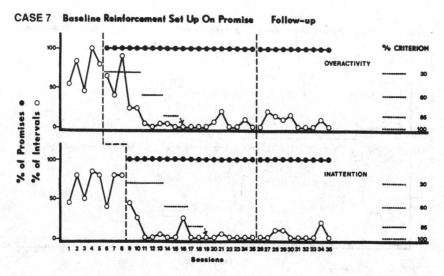

Figure 3.5   Daily Percentages of Overactivity

Note: Daily percentages of overactivity, inattention, and promises during baseline, reinforcement of set-up on promises, and follow-up for Case 7.

Source: Paniagua (1987), pp. 1–23.

to assess her IQ (which was below 20). Medical records and parents' reports during an unstructured clinical interview indicated two significant maladaptive behaviors: self-stimulatory behaviors and Pica. Self-stimulation consisted of head weaving (moving head from side to side in a figure-eight pattern), body rocking (moving the trunk at the hips rhythmically back and forth or from side to side), finger/hand flapping, (placing one or both hands/fingers in front of her face and vigorously moving the fingers/hands back and forth), and body rubbing (hands repetitively rubbing any body part such as face, eyes, mouth, arms, ears, hair). Pica involved mouthing objects (either holding nonedible objects or fingers in contact with the mouth, touching these objects/fingers to the lips or tongue, or placing nonedible objects in the mouth).

A 10-second partial-interval-sampling method was used. Two observers watched the subject (in an inpatient and outpatient clinic for handicapped children) for the entire interval and recorded any occurrence of self-stimulation or Pica in the interval. In the inpatient setting, data were collected four times per day during 5-minute sessions. Similar observations were scheduled in the outpatient setting (after the child was discharged from the clinic). Reliability between observers was assessed by dividing the number of interval of agreement by the number of intervals of agreement and disagreement and multiplying by 100 to yield a percentage. The mean interobserver agreement in the inpatient setting was 80% (range = 33% to 100%) and 78% (55% to 88%) for pica and self-stimulation, respectively; in the outpatient setting the reliability for these percentages was 93% (80% to 100%) for Pica, and 95% for self-stimulation (85% to 100%).

A treatment package was employed, consisting of differential reinforcement of other behavior (DRO), verbal reprimand (e.g., "No!" contingent on maladaptive behaviors), and overcorrection techniques (Foxx & Azrin, 1973). A functional assessment of behavioral changes was conducted with the programming of the intervention in a

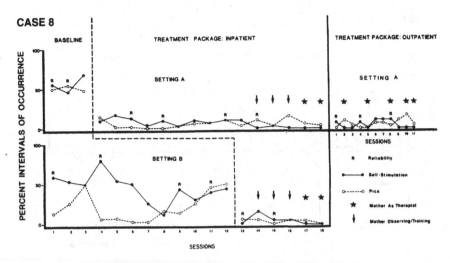

Figure 3.6 Daily Percentages of Occurrence

Note: Daily percentages of occurrence of pica and self-stimulation across baseline and treatment sessions for Case 8.

Source: Paniagua, Braverman, and Capriotti (1986), pp. 550–557.

multiple baseline design across settings: Setting A = a treatment room, and Setting B = a playroom. In Figure 3.6, baseline observations were conducted in Setting A and B. In session 4, the intervention was introduced in Setting A and baseline observations continued in Setting B; in session 13, the same intervention was scheduled in both settings. The results show substantial decreases in target behaviors only when the intervention was introduced.

Case 9

The participant was an 11-year-old girl with normal social and academic functioning who was admitted for assessment and treatment of Elective Mutism (Paniagua & Saeed, 1987). Her IQ was 101 on the Test of Nonverbal Intelligence (see Table 3.4). No abnormalities in hearing or language comprehension were noted. One of the selected behaviors for intervention included productive labeling (naming the content of a given picture card within 30 seconds, e.g., saying "cat" in the presence of the corresponding picture). During baseline and treatment sessions, two observers recorded whether the child fulfilled a particular criterion level and the number (frequency) of productive labeling responses (see Figure 3.7) occurred. The mean interobserver reliability of recording productive labeling was 99% (range = 90% to 100%). The treatment for the establishment of productive labeling included verbal instructions, imitative (modeling) procedures, praise, and response cost (removal of tokens contingent upon the absence of productive labeling responses).

This case illustrates a functional assessment in which the evaluation of the intervention is conducted with the changing-criterion design alone. In this case, praise and tokens were available contingent upon meeting a given criterion for productive labeling responses (e.g., Criterion 1 = naming one experimental picture card across seven consecutive sessions). Once the child met this criterion, the next criterion was introduced

CASE 9

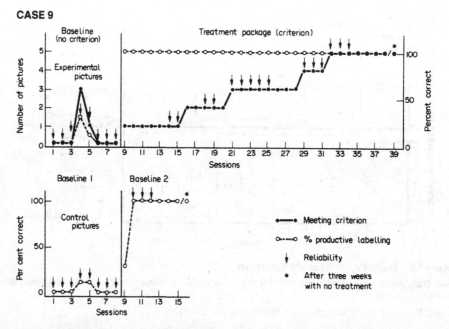

Figure 3.7   Number of Productive Labeling Responses

Note: Number of productive labeling responses and criterion levels (left-hand, top section) and percentages of productive labeling of experimental (right-hand, top section) and control (bottom section) picture cards for Case 9.

Source: Paniagua and Saeed (1987), pp. 259–267.

(e.g., naming two picture cards across a given number of sessions). Figure 3.7 shows that the behavioral intervention was effective in terms of gradually increasing the percentage of productive labeling responses over time (i.e., across criterion levels). In session 38, the child was stricken with chicken pox, and all interventions stopped for 3 weeks. At the end of this period, the treatment package was again introduced in session 39 (marked with the asterisk) and the child fulfilled the criterion level (after three weeks without intervention). Baselines 1 and 2 (bottom portion of Figure 3.7) show the child's performance during the introduction of control pictures in the absence of interventions. In Baseline 1, the percentage of productive labeling responses in the presence of these pictures was almost zero; during Baseline 2 (when the intervention was programmed with the experimental pictures), that percentage increased dramatically. The child's performance during Baseline 2 shows the generalization of treatment effects (i.e., productive labeling responses in the presence of control pictures that were not targeted during the intervention).

CURRENT TRENDS IN THE FUNCTIONAL ANALYSIS AND ASSESSMENT OF BEHAVIOR

Despite the increasing number of behavioral analysts and behavior therapists emphasizing direct and indirect measures of problem behaviors (Haynes & O'Brien, 2000), substantial differences still exist regarding the application of this combinatory measurement approach across current behavioral journals. For example, journals such as *Behavior Modification* (e.g., 1999, Vol. 23, No. 1–4), *Behavior Therapy* (e.g., 1996, Vol. 27, No. 1), and *Journal of Behavior Therapy and Experimental Psychiatry* (e.g., 1996, Vol. 27, No. 4) continue with a tradition of emphasizing direct and indirect behavioral assessment strategies (e.g., Tables 3.3 and 3.4), whereas the *Journal of Applied Behavior Analysis* (e.g., 1999, Vol. 32, No. 1–3) continues emphasizing direct measures of the type listed in Table 3.3 across studies, with the exception of studies (e.g., Durand, 1999; Graff & Libby, 1999) involving children with diagnosis of Mental Retardation and Pervasive Developmental Disorders (APA, 1994) in which indirect measures of symptoms (see Table 3.4) are required (and in some cases enforced) regardless of the theoretical or paradigmatic orientation of the clinician. For example, it would be clinically unacceptable to conclude that a child is mentally retarded only with the use of direct measure of observable behaviors; assessments of significant deficit in intellectual functioning (e.g., measured with the WISC-R; see Table 3.4) and deficits in adaptive behaviors (e.g., measured with the Bayley Scales of Infant Development; see Table 3.4) are also required (and demanded by the American Association of Mental Deficiency; Hamilton & Matson, 1992).

In general, no significant advancements are currently noted in the area of behavioral assessment strategies with emphasis on direct measure of behavior and a functional assessment of behavioral changes (Haynes & O'Brien, 2000). For example, measurement techniques shown in Table 3.3 and intrasubject replication design formats (e.g., ABA reversal and multiple baseline designs) continue in use without significant variations across studies published in the journals just mentioned in the last 10 years (e.g., Vollmer & Camp, 1998). One exception is the variant of the MBD (across exemplars) proposed by Paniagua (1990c).

The functional analysis of behavior with emphasis on antecedent events is an area with significant advancements in the clinical and research practice of behavioral psychologists (e.g., see the special issue of *JABA* on functional analysis approaches to behavioral assessment and treatment, 1994, Vol. 27, No. 2, and Lindberg, Iwata, & Kahng, 1999). As noted earlier, an example of antecedent events is termed a *discriminative stimulus,* which serves as the occasion or the opportunity for the occurrence of a target behavior (Catania, 1984; Miltenberger, 1998). This point was illustrated previously with the functional analysis of self-injurious behaviors in terms of their occurrence in the presence of a staff member serving as a discriminative stimulus for self-injury because of a history in that staff's social attention contingent upon self-injurious behaviors (Miltenberger, 1998). In the same example, if self-injurious behaviors previously maintained with attention do not receive (are deprived of) attention (e.g., from staff members) "over a long period, attention becomes a more powerful reinforcer, and self-injury is more likely to occur" (Miltenberger, 1988, p. 49). In this case, deprivation of attention not only increases the power of the reinforcer (i.e., attention) but also makes the discriminative stimulus (i.e., the presence of that staff member) more effective in terms of providing the opportunity for the emission of more rapid (i.e., shorter duration between the presence of the staff and the emission of these maladaptive behaviors) and severe (e.g., increases in bleeding, number of injuries, etc.) self-injurious behaviors. This deprivation of attention is an example of another kind of antecedent event known as establishing operations. Other examples of establishing operations include "eating salt," which makes "looking" at a restaurant and water a more powerful reinforcer and discriminative stimulus, respectively, for the behavior of "drinking" water; and "sleep deprivation" which could make prior aversive classroom tasks even more aversive, the discriminative stimulus (e.g., a classroom) more effective, and the probability of avoiding related behaviors (e.g., physical aggression in the classroom) even more probable (Miltenberger, 1998). As noted by Miltenberger (1998), in these examples establishing operations (e.g., deprivation of attention) are the "motivation" for the target behavior, and discriminative stimuli (e.g., staff members) are the "opportunity" for such behavior.

The term establishing operations in the functional analysis of antecedent events leading to adaptive and maladaptive behaviors was initially used in 1950 by two prominent experimental psychologists in the Skinnerian tradition (Keller & Schoenfeld, 1950). Jack Michael, a leading behavioral analyst, is credited with the introduction of the utility of this term in applied research (Michael, 1982, 1993). Currently, an emphasis on establishing operations as critical antecedent events in a functional analysis of behaviors constitutes a major research activity among behavioral psychologists, particularly behavior analysts. An extensive review of the function of establishing operations in the functional analysis of a wide range of problem behaviors (e.g., self-injury, self-stimulation, aggression, and oppositional responses) can be found in McGill (1999).

SPECIAL ISSUES AND POPULATIONS

A distinctive feature of studies published in behavioral journals (e.g., *Behavior Modification, Behavior Therapy, JABA*) is the exclusion of cultural and ethnic variables in the descriptions of the sample. Typical examples of the description of the client's characteristics in these journals resemble the following formats: "Thirty-two children were involved in the three experiments, 19 males and 13 females, in age from 3 yr, two months, to 5 yr, six months" (Rogers-Warren & Baer, 1976, p. 337), or, "The 4 participants in this study were Mike and Walter, age 9; Steve, age 11; and Roy, age 14" (MacDuff, Krantz, & McClannahan, 1993, p. 90). In these formats, readers do not know if subjects in the study included only Anglo-American, African American, American Indian, Asian, or Hispanic children, or combinations of racial groups in the sample (e.g., Anglo-American and African American children). In addition, ethnic variables such as level of acculturation, belief systems, and immigrant status are also missed in that format.

The underlined assumption is that cultural variables are not needed in the present context, because in the behavioral model functional, assessment, and treatment techniques are based on laws of behavior that can be generalized across people regardless of cultural and ethnic differences. This underlined assumption might be partially correct in the case of treatment (behavioral) techniques. For example, treatment based on the "behavioral model" (e.g., token programs, problem-solving, cognitive-behavioral, social skills training techniques) are often recommended not only with Anglo-American children and adolescents, but also among the other culturally diverse clients mentioned above (Paniagua, 1998b). For example, social skills training has been recommended in treatment plans targeting African American clients who lack "assertive responses" (see Paniagua, 1998b, p. 35). This technique, however, might not be appropriate with many Hispanic children and adolescents raised under the cultural values of *machismo* and *marianismo* (Paniagua, 1998b; pp. 40–41). For example, teaching an adolescent to be "assertive" with the assistance of social skills training would be seen as a sign of "lack of respect" toward the expected authority of the father by Hispanic families who believes in the phenomenon of *machismo* (Comas-Diaz & Duncan, 1985).

In addition, the cross-cultural literature indicates that racial and ethnic variables might, indeed, impact on the development of problem behaviors and measurement of such problems (Dana, 1993; Cuellar & Paniagua, 2000; Paniagua, 1998b; see also Chapter 19 in this volume). For example, a cultural antecedent event (and more likely an establishing operation) in immigrant children diagnosed with Conduct Disorder would be their prior exposure to aggressive behaviors in countries where such behaviors are expected to survive in such countries (see the DSM-IV, p. 88; Paniagua, 1998b, p. 128). Another cultural antecedent event is the case of immigrant children unfamiliar or uncomfortable with the new language (e.g., Asian and Hispanic immigrant children into the United States) who elect not to talk to strangers but only to family members (i.e., the case of Elective Mutism). Hispanic adolescents with diagnosis of Major Depression might be experiencing difficulties with different levels of acculturation between them and their parents, and this difference in acculturation levels might serve as a cultural antecedent event leading to symptoms of depression (see Paniagua, 1998b, p. 46). Additional discussion involving the impact of cultural variables in a functional analysis of maladaptive behaviors and its measurement can be found in Forehand and Kotchick (1996). In future applied research dealing with the functional analysis of behavior and its measurement, for issues involving cultural variables within (e.g., only African American clients) or between (e.g., Anglo-American vs. African American children) clients, the potential impact of cultural antecedent events (e.g., acculturation, client's belief system) should be considered to avoid misclassifications of culturally diverse children and adolescents with problem behaviors or psychiatric disorders.

REFERENCES

Achenbach, T. M., & Edelbrock, C. (1983). *Manual for the Child Behavior Checklist.* Burlington: Department of Psychiatry, University of Vermont.

American Psychiatric Association. (1994). *Diagnostic and statistical manual of mental disorders* (4th ed.). Washington, DC: Author.

Anastasi, A. (1988). *Psychological testing* (6th ed.). New York: Macmillan.

Ayllon, T., & Michael, J. (1959). The psychiatric nurse as a behavioral engineer. *Journal of the Experimental Analysis of Behavior, 2,* 323–334.

Ayllon, T., & Azrin, N. H. (1968). Reinforcer sampling: A technique for increasing the behavior of mental patients. *Journal of Applied Behavior Analysis, 1,* 13–20.

Baer, D. M., Wolf, M. M., & Risley, T. R. (1968). Some current dimensions of applied behavior analysis. *Journal of Applied Behavior Analysis, 1,* 91–97.

Bandura, A. (1969). *Principles of behavior modification.* New York: Holt, Rinehart & Winston.

Bandura, A. (1996). Ontological and epistemological terrains revised. *Journal of Behavior Therapy and Experimental Psychiatry, 27,* 323–345.

Barkley, R. A. (1988). Child behavior rating scales and checklists. In M. Rutter, A. H. Tuma, & I. S. Lann (Ed.), *Assessment and diagnosis in child psychopathology* (pp. 113–155). New York: Guilford Press.

Barkley, R. A. (1990). *Attention Deficit Hyperactivity Disorder.* New York: Guilford Press.

Barkley, R. A., & Edelbrock, C. S. (1987). Assessing situational variation in children's behavior problems: The Home and School Situations Questionnaires. In R. Prinz (Ed.), *Advances in behavioral assessment of children and families* (pp. 157–176). Greenwich, CT: JAI.

Barrios, B. A., & Hartmann, D. P. (1988). Fears and anxiety. In E. J. Mash & L. G. Terdal (Eds.), *Behavioral assessment of childhood disorders* (pp. 196–262). New York: Guilford Press.

Barrash, D. P. (1977). *Sociobiology and behavior.* New York: Elsevier.

Beck, A. T. (1976). *Cognitive therapy and the emotional disorders.* New York: International University Press.

Beck, J. G., Andrasick, F., & Arena, J. G. (1984). Group comparison designs. In A. S. Bellack & M. Hersen (Eds.), *Research methods in clinical psychology* (pp. 100–138). New York: Pergamon Press.

Bijou, S. W., Paterson, R. F., & Ault, M. H. (1968). A method to integrate descriptive and experimental field studies at the level of data and empirical concepts. *Journal of Applied Behavior Analysis, 1,* 175–191.

Black, M. M., & Matula, K. (2000). *Essentials of Bayley Scales of Infant Development-II Assessment.* New York: Wiley.

Bower, G. H., & Hilgard, E. R. (1981). *Theories of learning* (5th ed.). Englewood Cliffs, NJ: Prentice-Hall.

Brady, J. P., & Lind, D. L. (1961). Experimental analysis of hysterical blindness: Operant conditioning techniques. *Archives of General Psychiatry, 4,* 331–339.

Broden, M., Hall, R. V., & Mitts, B. (1971). The effect of self-recording on the classroom behavior of two eighth-grade students. *Journal of Applied Behavior Analysis, 4,* 191–199.

Bucher, B., & Lovaas, O. I. (1968). Use of aversive stimulation in behavior modification. In M. R. Jones (Ed.), *Miami symposium on the prediction of behavior 1967: Aversive stimulation* (pp. 77–145). Coral Gables, FL: University of Miami Press.

Catania, A. C. (1984). *Learning* (2nd ed.). Englewood Cliffs, NJ: Prentice-Hall.

Carr, E. G., Newsom, C. D., & Binkoff, J. A. (1976). Stimulus control of self-destructive behavior in a psychotic child. *Journal of Abnormal Child Psychology, 4,* 139–153.

Comas-Diaz, L., & Duncan, J. W. (1985). The cultural context: A factor in assertiveness training with mainland Puerto Rican women. *Psychology of Women Quarterly, 9,* 463–476.

Cautela, J. R. (1973). Covert processes and behavior modification. *Journal of Nervous and Mental Disease, 157,* 27–36.

Cautela, J. R., & Kearney, A. J. (1986). *The covert conditioning handbook.* New York: Springer.

Conners, C. K. (1973). Rating scales for use in drug studies with children. *Psychopharmacology Bulletin* (Special issue; Pharmacotherapy with Children), 24–84.

Cuellar, I., & Paniagua, F. A. (2000). *Handbook of multi-cultural mental health: Assessment and treatment of diverse populations.* New York: Academic Press.

Dana, R. H. (1993). *Multicultural assessment perspectives for professional psychology.* Boston: Allyn & Bacon.

Durand, V. M. (1993). Functional assessment and functional analysis. In M. D. Smith (Ed.), *Behavior modification for exceptional children and youth* (pp. 38–60). Boston: Androver Medical.

Durand, V. M. (1999). Functional communication training using assistive devices: Recruiting natural communities of reinforcement. *Journal of Applied Behavior Analysis, 32,* 247–267.

Edelbrock, C., & Costello, A. (1984). Structured psychiatric interviews for children and adolescents. In G. Goldstein & M. Hersen (Eds.), *Handbook of psychological assessment* (pp. 276–304). New York: Pergamon Press.

Edelbrock, C., & Costello, A. (1988). Structured psychiatric interviews for children. In M. Rutter, A. H. Tuma, & I. S. Lann (Eds.), *Assessment and diagnosis in child psychopathology* (pp. 87–112). New York: Guilford Press.

Ellis, A. (1977). Rational-emotive therapy: Research data that support the clinical and personality hypotheses of RET and other models of cognitive-behavior therapy. *Counseling Psychologist, 7,* 2–42.

Favell, J. (1977). *The power of positive reinforcement.* Springfield, IL: Thomas.

Ferster, C. B. (1965). Classification of behavioral pathology. In L. Krasner & L. P. Ullmann (Eds.), *Research in behavior modification* (pp. 6–26). New York: Holt, Rinehart & Winston.

Ferster, C. B., & Parrott, M. C. (1968). *Behavior principles.* New York: Meredith Corp.

Ferster, C. B., & Skinner, B. F. (1957). *Schedule of reinforcement.* New York: Appleton-Century-Crofts.

Finney, J. W., Russo, D. C., & Cataldo, M. F. (1982). Reduction of pica in young children with lead poisoning. *Journal of Pediatric Psychology, 7,* 197–207.

Forehand, R., & Kotchick, B. A. (1996). Cultural diversity: A wake-up call for parent training. *Behavior Therapy, 27,* 187–206.

Fox, L. H., & Zinkin, B. (1984). Achievement tests. In G. Goldstein & M. Hersen (Eds.), *Handbook of psychological assessment* (pp. 119–131). New York: Pergamon Press.

Foxx, R. M., & Azrin, N. H. (1973). The elimination of autistic self-stimulatory behavior by overcorrecting. *Journal of Applied Behavior Analysis, 6,* 1–14.

Fuller, P. R. (1949). Operant conditioning of a vegetative human organism. *American Journal of Psychology, 62,* 587–590.

Glynn, E. I., Thomas, J. D., & Shee, S. M. (1973). Behavioral self-control of on-task behavior in an elementary classroom. *Journal of Applied Behavior Analysis, 6,* 105–113.

Golden, C. J. (1990). *Clinical interpretation of objective psychological tests* (2nd ed.). Needham, MA: Allyn & Bacon.

Goldman, J., Stein, C. L., & Guerry, S. (1983). *Psychological methods of child assessment.* New York: Brunner/Mazel.

Goldstein, G., & Hersen, M. (Eds.) (1984). *Handbook of psychological assessment.* New York: Pergamon Press.

Goldstein, G., & Hersen, M. (Eds.) (1999). *Handbook of psychological assessment* (3rd ed.). New York: Pergamon Press.

Graff, R. B., & Libby, M. E. (1999). A comparison of presession and within-session reinforcement choice. *Journal of Applied Behavior Analysis, 32,* 161–173.

Green, B. F. (1992). A primer of testing. In A. E. Kazdin (Ed.), *Methodological issues and strategies in clinical research* (pp. 173–192). Washington, DC: APA.

Hall, R. V., Lund, D., & Jackson, D. (1968). Effects of teacher attention on study behavior. *Journal of Applied Behavior Analysis, 1,* 1–12.

Hamilton, M., & Matson, J. J. (1992). Mental retardation. In S. M. Turner, K. S. Calhoun, & H. E. Adams (Eds.), *Handbook of clinical behavior therapy* (pp. 317–326). New York: Wiley.

Hammond, S. (1995). Using psychometric tests. In G. M. Breakwell, S. Hammond, & C. Fife-Schaw (Eds.), *Research methods in psychology* (pp. 194–212). Thousand Oaks, CA: Sage.

Haynes, S. N. (1984). Behavioral assessment of adults. In G. Goldstein & M. Hersen (Eds.), *Handbook of psychological assessment* (pp. 369–401). New York: Pergamon Press.

Haynes, S., & O'Brien, W. (2000). *Principles of behavioral assessment.* Norwell, MA: Kluwer Academic/Plenum.

Herjanic, B., & Rich, W. (1982). Development of a structured psychiatric interview for children: Agreement between children and parent on individual symptoms. *Journal of Abnormal Child Psychology, 10,* 173–189.

Hersen, M., & Bellack, A. S. (Eds.). (1976). *Behavioral assessment: A practical handbook.* New York: Pergamon Press.

Hersen, M., & Bellack, A. S. (Eds.). (1998). *Behavioral assessment: A practical handbook* (4th ed.). New York: Pergamon Press.

Hersen, M., & Barlow, D. H. (1976). *Single case experimental designs.* New York: Pergamon Press.

Iwata, B. A., Dorsey, M. F., Slifer, K. J., Bauman, K. E., & Richman, G. S. (1982). Toward a functional analysis of self-injury. *Analysis and Intervention in Developmental Disabilities, 2,* 3–20.

Iwata, B. A., Pace, G. M., Kalsher, M. K., Cowdery, G. E., & Cataldo, M. F. (1990). Experimental analysis and extinction of self-injurious escape behavior. *Journal of Applied Behavior Analysis, 23,* 11–27.

Jacob, T., & Tennenbaum, D. L. (1988). Family assessment methods. In M. Rutter, A. H. Tuma, & I. S. Lann (Eds.), *Assessment and diagnosis in child psychopathology* (pp. 196–231). New York: Guilford Press.

Kanfer, F. H., & Phillips, J. S. (1970). *Learning foundations of behavior therapy.* New York: Wiley.

Kazdin, A. E. (1978). *History of behavior modification.* Baltimore, MD: University Park Press.

Kazdin, A. E. (1980). *Research design in clinical psychology.* New York: Harper & Row.

Kazdin, A. E. (1988). Childhood depression. In E. J. Mash & L. G. Terdal (Eds.), *Behavioral assessment of childhood disorders* (pp. 157–195). New York: Guilford Press.

Kazdin, A. E., & Straw, M. (1976). Assessment of behavior of the mentally retarded. In M. Hersen & A. S. Bellack (Eds.), *Behavioral assessment: A practical handbook* (pp. 337–368). New York: Pergamon Press.

Kagan, J. (1966). Reflection-impulsivity: The generality and dynamics of conceptual tempo. *Journal of Abnormal Psychology, 71,* 17–24.

Keller, F. S., & Schoenfeld, W. N. (1950). *Principles of psychology.* New York: Appleton-Century-Crofts.

Kendall, P. C., Zupan, B. A., & Braswell, L. (1981). Self-control in children: Further analyses of the Self-Control Rating Scale. *Behavior Therapy, 12,* 667–681.

Kennedy, C. H., & Haring, T. G. (1993). Teaching choice making during social interactions to students with profound multiple disabilities. *Journal of Applied Behavior Analysis, 26,* 63–76.

Kovacs, M. (1985). ISC (The Interview Schedule for Children). *Psychopharmacology Bulletin, 21,* 991–994.

Krasner, L., & Ullmann, L. P. (Eds.). (1965). *Research in behavior modification: New developments and implications.* New York: Holt, Rinehart & Winston.

Kuhn, T. S. (1970). *The structure of scientific revolutions* (2nd ed.). Chicago: University of Chicago Press.

Langner, T., Gersten, J., McCarthy, E. D., Eisenberger, J. G., Greene, E. L., Herson, J. H., & Jameson, J. D. (1976). A screening inventory for assessing psychiatric impairment in children aged 6–18. *Journal of Consulting and Clinical Psychology, 44,* 286–296.

Leitenberg, H. (Ed.). (1976). *Handbook of behavior modification and behavior therapy.* Englewood Cliffs, NJ: Prentice-Hall.

Lindberg, J. S., Iwata, B. A., & Kahng, S. W. (1999). On the relation between object manipulation and stereotypic self-injurious behavior. *Journal of Applied Behavior Analysis, 32,* 51–62.

Mash, E. J., & Terdal, L. G. (1988). Behavioral assessment of child and family disturbance. In E. J. Mash & L. G. Terdal (Eds.), *Behavioral assessment of childhood disorders* (pp. 3–65). New York: Guilford Press.

Mash, E. J., & Terdal, L. G. (1997). *Assessment of childhood disorders* (3rd ed.). New York: Guilford Press.

McDuff, G. S., Krantz, P. J., & McClannahan, L. E. (1993). Teaching children with autism to use photographic activity schedules: Maintenance and generalization of complex behavior. *Journal of Applied Behavior Analysis, 26,* 89–97.

McGill, P. (1999). Establishing operations: Implications for the assessment, treatment, and prevention of problem behavior. *Journal of Applied Behavior Analysis, 32,* 393–418.

Michael, J. (1982). Distinguishing between discriminative and motivational functions of stimuli. *Journal of the Experimental Analysis of Behavior, 37,* 149–155.

Michael, J. (1993). Establishing operations. *Behavior Analyst, 16,* 191–206.

Miller, L. C. (1981). *School Behavior Checklist Manual.* Los Angeles, CA: Western Psychological Services.

Miller, L. C. (1984). *Louisville Behavior Checklist Manual.* Los Angeles, CA: Western Psychological Services.

Miller, L. C., Barrett, C. L., Hampe, E., & Nobel, H. (1971). Factor structure of childhood fears. *Journal of Consulting and Clinical Psychology, 39,* 264–268.

Miltenberger, R. G. (1998). Methods for assessing antecedent influences on challenging behaviors. In J. K. Luiselli & M. J. Cameron (Eds.), *Antecedent control: Innovative approaches to behavioral support* (pp. 47–65). Baltimore, MD: Brookes.

Ollendick, T. H. (1983). Reliability and validity of the Revised-Fear Survey Schedule for Children (FSSC-R). *Behaviour Research and Therapy, 21,* 685–692.

Ollendick, T. H., & Meador, A. E. (1984). Behavioral assessment of children. In G. Goldstein & M. Hersen (Eds.), *Handbook of psychological assessment* (pp. 351–368). New York: Pergamon Press.

O'Neill, R. E., Horner, R. H., Albin, R. W., Sprague, J. R., Storey, K., & Newton, J. S. (1997). *Functional assessment and program development for problem behavior: A practical handbook.* Pacific Grove, CA: Brooks/Cole.

Paniagua, F. A. (1985a). The relational definition of reinforcement: Comment on circularity. *Psychological Record, 35,* 193–202.

Paniagua, F. A. (1985b). Development of self-care skills and helping behaviors of adolescents in a group home through correspondence training. *Journal of Behavior Therapy and Experimental Psychiatry, 16,* 237–244.

Paniagua, F. A. (1987a). "Knowing" the world within the skin: A remark on Skinner's behavioral theory of knowledge. *Psychological Reports, 61,* 741–742.

Paniagua, F. A. (1987b). Management of hyperactive children through correspondence training procedures: A preliminary study. *Behavioral Residential Treatment, 2,* 1–23.

Paniagua, F. A. (1990a). Skinner's senses of "guessing." *New Ideas in Psychology, 8,* 73–79.

Paniagua, F. A. (1990b). A procedural analysis of correspondence training procedures. *The Behavior Analyst, 13,* 107–119.

Paniagua, F. A. (1990c). The multiple baseline design across exemplars. *Behavioral Residential Treatment, 15,* 177–188.

Paniagua, F. A. (1991). Kuhn's paradigmatic view of psychology and Skinner's theory of behavior. *Theoretical and Philosophical Psychology, 11,* 122–125.

Paniagua, F. A. (1992). Verbal-nonverbal correspondence training with ADHD children. *Behavior Modification, 16,* 226–252.

Paniagua, F. A. (1993). Anomalies in covert conditioning. *Psychological Reports, 73,* 323–327.

Paniagua, F. A. (1998a). Correspondence training and verbal mediation. In J. K. Luiselli & M. J. Cameron (Eds.), *Antecedent control: Innovative approaches to behavioral support* (pp. 223–242). Baltimore, MD: Brookes.

Paniagua, F. A. (1998b). *Assessing and treating culturally diverse clients: A practical guide.* Thousand Oaks, CA: Sage.

Paniagua, F. A., & Baer, D. M. (1981). A procedural analysis of the symbolic forms of behavior therapy. *Behaviorism, 9,* 171–205.

Paniagua, F. A., & Baer, D. M. (1982). The analysis of correspondence training as chain reinforceable at any point. *Child Development, 53,* 786–798.

Paniagua, F. A., & Black, S. A. (1990). Management and prevention of hyperactivity and conduct disorders in 8–10 year old boys through correspondence training procedures. *Child and Family Behavior Therapy, 12,* 23–56.

Paniagua, F. A., & Black, S. A. (1992). Correspondence training and observational learning in the management of hyperactive children: A preliminary study. *Child & Family Behavior Therapy, 14,* 1–19.

Paniagua, F. A., Braverman, C., & Capriotti, R. M. (1986). Use of a treatment package in the management of a profoundly mentally retarded girl's pica and self-stimulation. *American Journal of Mental Deficiency, 90,* 550–557.

Paniagua, F. A., Pumariega, A. J., & Black, S. A. (1988). Clinical effects of correspondence training in the management of hyperactive children. *Behavioral Residential Treatment, 3,* 19–40.

Paniagua, F. A., & Saeed, M. A. (1988). Labeling and functional language in a case of psychological mutism. *Journal of Behavior Therapy and Experimental Psychiatry, 18,* 259–267.

Powell, J., Martindale, A., & Kulp, S. (1975). An evaluation of time-sampling measures of behavior. *Journal of Applied Behavior Analysis, 8,* 463–469.

Puig-Antich, J., Blau, S., Marx, N., Greenhill, L. I., & Hambers, W. (1978). Prepubertal major depressive disorders: A pilot study. *Journal of the American Academic of Child and Adolescent Psychiatry, 17,* 695–707.

Richman, N., & Graham, P. (1971). A behavioural screening questionnaire for use with three-year-old children: Preliminary findings. *Journal of Child Psychology and Psychiatry, 12,* 5–33.

Risley, T. R. (1968). The effects and side effects of punishing the autistic behaviors of a deviant child. *Journal of Applied Behavior Analysis, 1,* 21–34.

Risley, T. R., & Hart, B. (1968). Developing correspondence between the non-verbal and verbal behavior of preschool children. *Journal of Applied Behavior Analysis, 1,* 267–281.

Rogers-Warren, A., & Baer, D. M. (1976). Correspondence between saying and doing: Teaching children to share and praise. *Journal of Applied Behavior Analysis, 9,* 335–354.

Rutter, M., Tuma, A. H., & Lann, I. S. (Eds.). (1988). *Assessment and diagnosis in child psychopathology.* New York: Guilford Press.

Sechrest, L. (1984). Reliability and validity. In A. S. Bellack & M. Hersen (Eds.), *Research methods in clinical psychology* (pp. 24–54). New York: Pergamon Press.

Scherer, W. M., & Nakamura, C. Y. (1968). A fear survey schedule for children (FSS-FC): A factor analytic comparison with manifested anxiety (CMAS). *Behaviour Research and Therapy, 6,* 173–182.

Schumacher, S., & Lloyd, C. W. (1976). Assessment of sexual dysfunction. In M. Hersen & A. S. Bellack (Eds.), *Behavioral assessment: A practical handbook* (4th ed., pp. 419–435). New York: Pergamon Press.

Siassi, I. (1984). Psychiatric interview and mental status examination. In G. Goldstein & M. Hersen (Eds.), *Handbook of psychological assessment* (pp. 259–275). New York: Pergamon Press.

Skinner, B. F. (1938). *The behavior of organisms.* New York: Appleton-Century-Crofts.

Skinner, B. F. (1953). *Science and human behavior.* New York: Macmillan.

Skinner, B. F. (1957a). The experimental analysis of behavior. *American Scientist, 45,* 343–371.

Skinner, B. F. (1957b). *Verbal behavior.* New York: Appleton-Century-Crofts.

Skinner, B. F. (1961). *Cumulative record* (2nd ed.). New York: Appleton-Century-Crofts.

Skinner, B. F. (1963). Behaviorism at fifty. *Science, 140,* 950–958.

Sloane, H. N., & Macaulay, B. D. (1968). *Operant procedures in remedial speech and language training.* New York: Houghton Mifflin.

Smith, B., & Sechrest, L. (1995). Treatment of attitude × treatment interactions. In A. E. Kazdin (Ed.), *Methodological issues and strategies in clinical research* (pp. 557–584). Washington, DC: APA.

Sulzer-Azaroff, B., & Mayer, G. R. (1977). *Applied behavior analysis procedures with children and youth.* New York: Holt, Rinehart & Winston.

Taylor, H. G., Fletcher, J. M., & Saltz, P. (1984). Neuropsychological assessment of children. In G. Goldstein & M. Hersen (Eds.), *Handbook of psychological assessment* (pp. 211–234). New York: Pergamon Press.

Vollmer, T. R., & Camp, C. M. V. (1998). Experimental designs to evaluate antecedent control. In J. K. Luiselli & M. J. Cameron (Eds.), *Antecedent control: Innovative approaches to behavioral support* (pp. 87–100). Baltimore, MD: Brooks.

Walker, H. M., & Buckley, N. K. (1968). The use of positive reinforcement in conditioning attending behavior. *Journal of Applied Behavior Analysis, 1,* pp. 245–250.

Williams, C. D. (1959). The elimination of tantrum behavior by extinction procedures. *Journal of Abnormal Social Psychology, 59,* 269.

Wilson, G. T., & O'Leary, K. D. (1980). *Principles of behavior therapy.* Englewood Cliffs, NJ: Prentice-Hall.

Wilson, G. T., & Pike, K. M. (1993). Eating disorders. In D. H. Harlow (Ed.), *Clinical handbook of psychological disorders: A step-by-step treatment manual* (pp. 278–317). New York: Guilford Press.

Wolf, M. M. (1978). Social validity: The case for subjective measurement, or how behavior analysis is finding its heart. *Journal of Applied Behavior Analysis, 11,* 203–214.

Wolpe, J. (1973). *The practice of behavior therapy.* New York: Pergamon.

Zelberger, J., Sampen, S. E., & Sloane, H. N. (1968). Modification of a child's problem behavior in the home with the mother as therapist. *Journal of Applied Behavior Analysis, 1,* 47–53.

Chapter 4

THE MENTAL STATUS EXAM IN CHILD AND ADOLESCENT EVALUATION

CHARLES D. CASAT AND DEBORAH A. PEARSON

The Mental Status Exam (MSE) occupies an important and unique place in the clinical evaluation of children and adolescents and contributes significantly to the information base available to the clinician for making decisions regarding diagnosis and treatment planning. Its use spans evaluation of children and adolescents in pediatrics and family practice, as well as in mental health–related disciplines such as psychiatric social work, marriage and family counseling, psychology, and psychiatry. Thus, skill and experience in the performance and integration of findings from the MSE are fundamental to good practice with these populations. As with any other skill, use of the MSE requires a set of processes and procedures. This chapter will engage in a discussion of these premises and techniques for clinical employment of the MSE.

DEFINITION AND PURPOSES OF THE MSE

The MS Exam is a systematic interview assessment template for evaluating a patient's current functioning in domains of orientation, motor activity, mood and affects, emotional control, thought content, speech, phenomena of special senses, perception, cognitive functioning, reasoning, apperception, insight, social judgement, and social relatedness. Effective employment of the MSE template requires a thorough understanding of its elements and the information that each adds to the understanding of the patient's current functioning. The emphasis on the term *template* reflects the idea that although all the elements included therein must necessarily be accounted for to achieve completeness, in practice the template is for the reference of the examiner, and not, with the exception of the recording of the MSE, a recipe to be followed rotely and without deviation within the interview. In fact, the skillful clinician will learn to weave extensive parts of the MSE into the general interview with the child, adolescent, or family unobtrusively, without resorting to discontinuity in the process of the interview, and often following the leads of the patient as the natural narrative of current concerns unfolds. As pointed out by Lewis (1996), "The child or adolescent acts as a whole and in the context of a given environment, and his or her present behavior is always continuous with past behavior" (p. 4).

The purposes of the MSE are (a) to gain a systematic, cross-sectional view of a patient's emotional, behavioral, cognitive, and social strengths, as well as capabilities, deficiencies, and deviations from age- and situation-appropriate expectations; (b) to add these observational and verbal response findings to the larger process of information gathering for purposes of establishing diagnoses and developing a treatment plan that addresses psychological, behavioral, cognitive, and social needs; and (c) to establish a baseline of current functioning to be used for future comparison for determining response to interventions. The MSE has often been likened to the physical exam in office medical evaluations, and indeed, the MSE should be included as a part of the physical exam as well.

LOCATING THE MSE WITHIN THE MATRIX OF CHILD AND ADOLESCENT CLINICAL EVALUATION

Good clinical practice requires a *multitrait, multimodality, multi-informant approach* to gain the best available picture of a child or adolescent's functioning, strengths, deficits, and needs. For thoroughness, the evaluation should include standard information sources and procedures, as outlined in Table 4.1.

Table 4.1   Elements of the Child and Adolescent Office Evaluation

1. The Parent Interview
   Reasons for seeking consultation at this time
   Description of symptoms, duration, and impairment
   History of past intervention attempts, including psychosocial approaches and medications
   Developmental history
   Parenting style and discipline attitudes
   Medical history
   Family history of medical, psychiatric, and substance-abuse disorders
   Current family situation and possible family stressors

2. School Information
   Verbal reports of behavior, classroom organization, peer relations, and academic progress
   Results of individual and standardized academic achievement testing
   Results and recommendations from other evaluations: speech and language, occupational therapy, Individuals with Disabilities Education Act (IDEA), or Section 504

3. Symptom and Behavioral Rating Scales and Personality Inventories

4. The Interview with the Child or Adolescent
   Perceptions of his or her reasons for the evaluation and current problem areas
   View and perceptions of his or her relations with parents, siblings, and other family members, peers, teachers, and other adults
   Personal experience, including potential or real traumas
   Psychological concerns and attitudes
   Assessment of the child or adolescent's ability to identify emotions and affects
   Assessment of the child or adolescent's capacity for self-monitoring and self-regulation

It is important to understand the unique addition the MSE makes to the overall available information. For effectiveness, the clinician must discipline him- or herself always to record the findings of the MSE in a standard fashion, using the template as a guide. This permits reference to the MSE when weighing different diagnostic possibilities, and when constructing a clinical intervention plan.

PROCESS OF THE MSE

The MSE is part of a category of social interactions seen generally as an information-eliciting interview undertaken for purposes of receiving advice, opinion, and alternatives for resolution of concerns and problems, set in an expert/client relationship. This relationship is both reciprocal and limited. Close attention must be paid to the climate and process of this relationship if it is to be effective, and therefore successful. Crucial to the success of the endeavor is the development of a rapport and a trust that allows for divulging and exploring sometimes painful revelations and concerns. The clinician must have a strong awareness of the sense of vulnerability of family experiences in the interview, tinged as they often are with denial, defensiveness, and resentment. To ease past these tendencies that the family brings to the situation, the clinician must be able to establish an atmosphere of trust, acceptance, and respect for the family, by conveying through attentiveness, good eye contact, and a friendly, nonjudgmental manner, an interest and willingness to be of help. Communication should be facilitated through these means, together with anticipatory statements, clarifications, and explorations of the family members' statements. Questions should be short and open-ended, whenever possible, and should be free of jargon or phrases that might be confusing to the interviewees. Questions should be formulated to avoid embarrassing or offending the family. Appropriate and expanded replies should be encouraged, circumventing the "uh-huh/uh-uh" variety of response that conveys minimal information to the interviewer. The clinician must also have continuously in mind the separation between *accepting* and *endorsing* the interviewee's communications (Sattler, 1998). The former conveys that the clinician acknowledges the patient's or family's point of view, whereas the latter means the clinician is in agreement with the patient's perspective. Effectiveness as an expert advisor may mean at times that the clinician accepts the patient's perspective, but that does not necessarily constitute embracing the point of view, and forgetting that this view may require reassessment and modification for more successful future outcomes.

At times during the interview, it may be useful or necessary to reflect emotions or content. Doing this skillfully allows the patient to experience the emotion; may ease the further discussion of painful thoughts, concerns, or experiences; and conveys that the interviewer is attentive (Sattler, 1998). Such technique facilitates identifying and uncovering material that is pertinent to the consultation and is helpful in developing trust and rapport. As noted previously, many of the MSE template items may be garnered from the general interview, or may be blended into the general flow of the interview to minimize patient guardedness. Those that cannot be, such as arithmetic and assessment of recall, among others, can be introduced as low-key games to lighten up an otherwise heavy, anxiety-arousing exploration of symptoms and functioning.

CONTENT OF THE MSE

Returning to the idea of the MSE as having a template for included items, the clinician must become conversant with the meanings and potential significance of each of the MSE items and categories. The template used by the individual clinician must be both inclusive and concise, if it is to have feasibility and individual clinical utility. With experience, each clinician will settle upon both a process and a content for eliciting the MSE that is suitable to that clinician's style, yet comprehensive enough to surpass the threshold for good clinical practice.

The following represents one approach to a MSE template that is informative and sufficiently inclusive to meet the standards of good clinical practice. Again, *flexibility* is the watchword in obtaining the needed information, while *consistency* is required during the recording of the MSE for maximizing the utility of this important element in the clinical interview.

1. General appearance (dress, grooming, nutritional state, presence of physical stigmata, unusual head size, evidences of bruising, manner of relating)
2. Motor status (overactive, tremor, restless, mannerisms, retardation of movement, catatonia)
3. Activity level, organization
4. Facial expression
5. Language
   a. Communicative
   b. Idiosyncratic (nonfunctional, odd syntax, odd pronomial usage)
6. Speech
   a. Rate (rapid, slow, mute, latency to response)
   b. Rhythm (fluid, stuttering, sing-song)
   c. Volume (quiet, loud)
   d. Coherence
   e. Logicality and goal-directedness (flight of ideas, drift of ideas, loss of logical association)
   f. Blocking
   g. Circumstantiality (unnecessary overinclusiveness, but finally achieves the point)
   h. Perseveration (inability to move from one topic to another in timely manner; returns frequently to previous theme)
7. Mood (happy, sad, anxious, detached; a pervasive emotional climate)
8. Affect (cheerful, elated, aloof, detached, irritable, negative, withholding, sullen, resentful, sarcastic, angry)
   a. Intensity
   b. Flattened or blunted
9. Suicidal or homicidal thoughts, impulses, intent
   a. Directed toward self
   b. Directed toward others
   c. Presence of a plan or method

10. Thought content
    a. Preoccupations
    b. Morbid
    c. Ideas of reference
    d. Delusions
        i) Mood congruent
        ii) Mood incongruent
        iii) Persecutory
        iv) Grandiose
        v) Of being controlled
        vi) Self-depreciatory, self-worthlessness
        vii) Somatic
    e. Hallucinations
        i) Simple versus complex
        ii) Command
        iii) Visual
        iv) Auditory
        v) Tactile
        vi) Olfactory
    f. Depersonalization
    g. Feelings of unreality
    h. Obsessions and compulsions
11. Orientation and awareness
    a. Self
    b. Place
    c. Time
    d. Situation
12. Memory
    a. Remote memory (past experiences)
    b. Recent memory
    c. Immediate memory
    d. Recall
13. Cognitive functioning
    a. General information
    b. Calculations
    c. Abstract reasoning
14. Insight and judgment
15. Adaptive capacities and positive attributes
16. Self-esteem

AGE-RELATED MODIFICATIONS IN THE APPROACH AND TECHNIQUE OF THE MSE

With younger children, especially preschoolers with developmentally imposed limitations in social skills and separation in a strange environment, it is probably best to interview in the presence of the parent or guardian, at least initially. Gentle attempts may be made at separating the child from the parent; but if this is met with resistance, interviewing with the parent in the room will probably be more effective and will not jeopardize future work. However, a good deal can be learned about the child's ability to tolerate separation by attempting a separation. Use of simple language and ideas are vital when working with the young child, as is a knowledge and understanding of the generally acceptable developmental norms for age. These general principals have recently been applied to the assessment of mental status in infants and toddlers (Benham, 2000). In this Infant-Toddler MSE, an observer documents the domain of behaviors displayed by infants and young children in the context of their relationship with their caregivers.

Elementary school–aged children (ages 5–11), especially those who have attained first-grade status, are generally able to tolerate separation, and more serious attempts should be made to separate the child and interview the child alone. Although the goal is to engage the child verbally, the availability of a limited set of play materials to ease anxiety and facilitate conversation may be appropriate, especially for the younger or more reticent, slow-to-warm-up individuals. This information about the characteristic style of relating is important. Children who have experienced out-of-home placements, on the other hand, may be inappropriately engaging, without the expected respect for boundaries with strangers. Older elementary school children will have less reticence and are increasingly capable of verbal expression and meaningful elaboration of concerns. All, however, will have some developmental incapability in giving an accurate historical account of their past. It is important to interview these children separately. Issues of confidentiality will begin to arise among the older members of this age range.

Middle school and high school students will be noted to be less spontaneous and more guarded in their responses. The clinician must work hard to appear interested, attentive, accepting, and nonjudgmental. There is often a suspicion about the confidentiality of the material that is inquired about, and this issue must be dealt with in a frank and active manner. One strategy is to have an initial meeting with adolescents and family members together, then to see the parent individually, and, lastly, to see the adolescent alone. This allows the clinician to observe the family interaction and style of relating, to hear the parental concerns in the presence of the adolescent, to hear further from the parent the adolescent's history and the history of the present difficulties, and to outline the diagnostic and treatment-planning process. Lastly, the adolescent has an opportunity to be heard without parental prompting or censure. A great deal of the time spent with the adolescent is given over to the development of trust and communication, as these qualities are difficult to develop in this age group and in an adolescent culture that relies on other adolescents for information and values.

MODIFICATIONS OF THE MSE WITH SPECIAL POPULATIONS

In addition to its adaptability to young children, the MSE can also be adapted for use with individuals from special populations, such as those with Mental Retardation (MR) and other Developmental Disorders (DD). Specific adaptations of the MSE for adolescents and adults with Mental Retardation include the Folstein Mini-Mental State Exam (Folstein, Folstein, & McHugh, 1975), the Test for Severe Impairment (a downward extension of the Folstein; Albert & Cohen, 1992), and the New York State Institute Adapted Mental Status Exam (Wisniewski & Hill, 1985). All of these forms of the MSE employ simplified items assessing appearance, orientation, motor performance, language, memory, conceptualization, general knowledge, and emotional state. Such instruments are used to assess current mental status and to document declines in functioning over time, for example, tracking the course of dementia in adults with Down syndrome (Burt et al., 1999; Cosgrave et al., 1998; Devenny, Wisniewski, & Silverman, 1993).

In addition to these standardized instruments, less formal versions of the MSE are frequently used to assess mental status in children and adolescents with developmental disabilities such as MR and Pervasive Developmental Disorders (PDDs). When working with these special populations, it is important to present items that are appropriate for the individual's estimated mental age and communication abilities. For instance, it might be appropriate to substitute recognition for recall in some situations; for example, if a child or adolescent cannot identify the city they are in, a multiple-choice format can be used (e.g., "Are you in Houston? Seattle? Chicago?"). Other appropriate modifications include reducing the number of items to be recalled in the memory section, and gauging expectations for vocabulary and syntax to the individual's estimated mental age and educational level. As with any MSE, it is appropriate to gather information using a semistructured interview format.

In addition to adapting items to cognitive and language ability, special care must be taken to identify specific behaviors often associated with MR/DD, and with specific subgroups within MR/DD. Such behaviors include immature posture (i.e., resembling that of a much younger child), self-injurious and self-stimulatory behaviors, and body rocking and other repetitive movements (stereotypies). Abnormalities of speech are often present, including misarticulation, and oddities in tone and volume (especially in children with autism/PDD). Abnormalities in general appearance often seen in children with autism/PDD include poor eye contact and significant restriction in the range of facial expressions. Even verbal children with autism/PDD tend to exhibit very concrete language and often use stereotyped utterances, pronominal reversals, and neologisms or other idiosyncratic language. These children will also make far less use of communicative gestures (e.g., pointing, nodding, headshaking) during the interview, as compared to everyday school-age children. Specific abnormalities in the motor skills of children and adolescents with autism/PDD include repetitive hand and finger movements, such as finger flicking, and unusual sensory interests (e.g., smelling objects in the office). A person with Rett syndrome will manifest unusual midline hand movements such as hand wringing. Children with autism/PDD manifest significantly less social relatedness during an MSE than do children with other forms of MR/DD, such as Down syndrome. Indeed, children with Down syndrome are often noted to exhibit relatively good social-relatedness and engagement in the interview process. Children with Williams syndrome are often very loquacious during an interview, although the actual content of their speech is often sparse. In contrast, children with Fragile X syndrome are often very hard to engage in an interview, due to social aversion and limited language abilities. It is imperative that the interviewer be familiar with the behavioral repertoire of various subgroups of MR/DD, in order to avoid misinterpreting behaviors manifested during the interview process.

In general, items elicited in traditional MSEs are most often administered to older and higher functioning children and adolescents with MR/DD. In contrast, for lower functioning children and adolescents, it is sometimes very difficult to distinguish communication disorders from thought disorders on the basis of standard MSE-type questions. For this reason, the clinical assessment of younger and lower functioning individuals will rely more heavily upon observation as opposed to direct questioning. Because it is crucial that these observations be interpreted objectively within the context of a child's typical everyday function, these assessments also rely heavily upon caretaker reports (Nezu, Nezu, & Gill-Weiss, 1992). It has been our experience that a particularly helpful adjunct to the MSE with children and adolescents with MR/DD is an adaptive behavior instrument, such as the Vineland Adaptive Behavior Scales (Sparrow, Balla, & Ciccetti, 1984), which assesses everyday living skills, including communication and socialization.

Other valuable sources of adjunctive information include parent and teacher questionnaires. As Aman (1991) has noted, standard behavior rating scales such as the Conners Parent and Teacher Rating Scales (Conners, 1997) and the Child Behavior Checklist (Achenbach, 1991) are appropriate for children with mild to moderate mental retardation because the domains of behavior seen in these children are often similar to those seen in children without mental retardation (i.e., the children on whom most standard rating instruments are normed). However, use of these psychometric instruments (which are normed for the general child and adolescent population) becomes increasingly suspect as the level of cognitive ability diminishes because the domains of behavior displayed in these lower functioning individuals are often divergent from higher functioning individuals. For this latter group, helpful adjuncts to the MSE would be rating scales developed specifically to assess the domains of behaviors often seen in children and adolescents with mental retardation. Examples of such instruments include the Aberrant Behavior Checklist (Aman, Singh, Stewart, & Field, 1985), the Nisonger Child Behavior Rating Form (Aman, Tasse, Rojahn, & Hammer, 1996), and the Reiss Scales for Children's Dual Diagnosis (Reiss & Valenti-Hein, 1990, 1994).

Finally, in order to interpret the findings obtained during the MSE appropriately, it is very important to obtain copies of previous clinical and educational assessments (e.g., school testing and previous psychological/psychiatric evaluations). Such information provides the foundation for current functional abilities and allows inferences to be made regarding developmental progression or regression.

RECORDING THE MSE

The taking of notes during an interview is a mixed bag. On the one hand, note-taking improves recall, and therefore accuracy. On the other hand, if not done discretely, it may interfere with the development of rapport and raise anxiety or suspiciousness. This latter is especially important when dealing with adolescents. If the clinician elects to take notes, there should be a brief but clear discussion about the purposes of note-taking, and, again, a discussion of confidentiality. There is often the need for defining the limits of confidentiality, which include breaking that confidentiality when issues of the personal safety of the adolescent, or others arise.

The MSE should routinely be recorded as soon as possible after termination of the interview to guarantee accuracy and detail of recall. Whether dictated or completed on a standard form, the MSE should not deviate from the MSE template of the clinician, and should adhere to standards of good clinical practice for completeness. Personal discipline in exercising good and timely recording habits is required and expected, both for clinical and medical/legal purposes. If dictated, transcribed interviews and MSEs should be read through for accuracy and corrected soon after their return, and before being placed in the patient's chart. Requirements about the protection and retention of records must be adhered to.

CASE EXAMPLES

Case Study: MSE for a Child with ADHD and Comorbid Oppositional Defiant Disorder

Raydonn was a 9-year-old African American male referred for evaluation by his school guidance counselor. (For more information regarding his history, please see Chapter 11 in this volume.) He appeared for the interview accompanied by his mother, who at first sat in on the interview. He appeared as a clean, well-groomed, casually dressed African American male who was quite large for his age. There were no notable abnormalities of posture or gait. No evidence was seen of tics, tremors, or mannerisms. While seated, he was observed to be restless, fidgety, and easily distractible. Initially, he had poor eye contact, was difficult to engage, and offered little in the way of spontaneous information or conversation. He appeared notably irritable and resistant in responses to comments and urgings on the part of the mother. This negative style became more pronounced when the examiner inquired about his adjustment with his mother, teacher, peers, and siblings. When the mother was asked to wait outside, so that the examiner could talk privately with Raydonn, the boy pulled his legs onto the seat of the chair and sat in a defensive, slightly turned-away position, with his arms crossed on his chest. Only gradually did he unfold himself and become minimally more positive toward the examiner. He continued to be distracted by objects on the examiner's desktop, and to appear fidgety.

Raydonn's language was communicative, with no idiosyncrasies noted. His speech was moderate in rate, rhythm, and volume. Content was logical, coherent, and goal-directed, if somewhat sparse. Mood was one of mild anxiety, and affect was sullen and defiant, especially initially. This anxiety and sullenness decreased with time as the patient warmed up slightly to the examiner. Raydonn denied suicidal or homocidal thoughts, impulses, or intents. Thought content was normal for a boy Raydonn's age, with no notable morbid preoccupations, ideas of reference, excessive somatic concerns, or delusional content. Raydonn denied auditory or visual hallucinatory experiences.

Raydonn was alert and oriented to self, place, time, and the nature of the interview proceedings. Remote memory, as tested by events from his last birthday, was intact, as was memory for recent events. Immediate memory and recall were intact, as tested by repeating back the names of three objects. In his cognitive functioning, general information was adequate for his age. Calculations, as tested by simple addition and subtraction problems, were appropriate to age and grade level. Reasoning was concrete, which was age-appropriate.

The patient's insight was limited. He did not (or would not) see that his style was obstructive and that it added to his woes, and he tended to externalize responsibility for his temper outbursts at peers and his mother, indicating that he was misunderstood both by his teacher and his mother. Raydonn's judgment was poor, even for his age.

Regarding positive attributes, Raydonn appeared intelligent and responsive to praise. His self-esteem appeared tenuous, and he seemed on the watch for evidence of a lack of regard on the part of the examiner.

Case Study: An Adapted MSE in an Adolescent with Mental Retardation and ADHD

Jeffrey S. was brought to the outpatient child psychiatry clinic by his parents. (For more information regarding his history, please see Chapter 11 in this volume.) He separated very easily from his parents to begin the interview. Jeff was a 14-year-old boy with a history of Mental Retardation (IQ = 56) and Attention-Deficit Hyperactivity Disorder (ADHD) who was tall for his age and had a slender build. He was well-groomed and casually (but neatly) dressed, and appeared his stated age. No abnormalities of gait, posture, tics, tremors, or body rocking were noted. He showed no evidence of tactile or auditory defensiveness. He displayed no unusual habits or mannerisms, self-injurious behaviors, or self-stimulatory behaviors. Throughout the interview, Jeff was very active physically, fidgeting in his seat, and also getting up and moving about the interview room. Despite this movement, he was engaged with his interviewer, made good eye contact, was very cooperative, and smiled frequently. His mood was euthymic.

Jeff was very talkative throughout the interview. His syntax and vocabulary were estimated to be on the first- to second-grade level. He could follow multistep commands ("Pick up the red paper, fold it, and put it on the table"). His tone and volume were normal, and there was no evidence of pronoun reversals, perseveration, or echolalia. A slight stutter was noted, and he had some disarticulation (in particular, "r" and "f" sounds; Jeff is receiving speech therapy through his special education placement at school). Although he was frequently distracted by sounds outside the interview room (e.g., high heels clicking in the hallway) or even objects within it (e.g., holiday decorations), the clinician could easily reorient Jeff to the interview by saying his name. In all of his responses, Jeff was goal-directed and coherent. His thought content was mood-congruent, and he denied having suicidal or homicidal thoughts.

Regarding orientation, Jeff knew his name, age, the month and day of his birth (but not the year), and that he was living at home with his parents. With regard to place, Jeff knew that he was "downtown" but could not be more specific. He did indicate that he was on the second floor of the building. Jeff was able to say that it was "morning" but could not identify the time (even though there was an analog clock in the room). He knew that it was "winter" and that it was "December" but could not identify the exact date (it should be noted that school was out of session when this evaluation was performed; Jeff's parents indicated on the Vineland that he is aware of the date only when he is in school and has seen it on the blackboard all day).

Cognitive functioning appeared to be consistent with his estimated mental age (approximately 7–8 years old). He was able to identify colors and was able to name body parts and common objects (wristwatch, pencil). He did not know who the current president was, nor any previous presidents. Jeff was able to do simple rote arithmetic ($3 - 1 = 2$) but could not do simple word problems verbally ("If you have eight books and lose three, how many do you have left?"). He used his fingers to compute written arithmetic problems ($6 + 3 = 9$) but could not do written problems involving two-digit numbers

(18 – 11 = ?). Jeff could print all the letters in the alphabet proficiently but had considerable difficulty doing cursive writing. He had a mature pencil grip and was right-handed.

Regarding memory, Jeff's long-term ("What did you do on vacation last summer?") and short term ("What did you get for Christmas?") memory skills were intact. He could not identify where he had been born. Jeff was able to repeat three objects immediately, and to recall them after five and ten minutes.

Insight and judgment were congruent for his estimated mental age. Jeff exhibited appropriate social judgment when asked what he would do if he saw a fire in a public building. He was not able to explain what was meant by the saying, "A bird in hand is worth two in the bush." However, Jeff displayed some insight into his difficulty keeping friends ("I talk too much"). Some evidence of low self-esteem was noted; for example, he expressed concern that he was not as smart as others, or as well-liked. Jeff also said that he thought his sister was mad at him a lot, but that he did not know why. It was noted that Jeff often started answering questions before the interviewer had finished asking them, this observation was consistent with parent and teacher behavior rating scales (Conners, Aberrant Behavior Checklist) noting significant problems with impulsivity.

INTEGRATION OF THE MSE AND OTHER SOURCES OF INFORMATION IN DIAGNOSIS AND TREATMENT PLANNING

The MSE represents a systematic, cross-sectional view of a patient's emotional, behavioral, cognitive, and social strengths, as well as his or her capabilities, deficiencies, and deviations from age- and situation-appropriate expectations, and provides a baseline of current functioning for future reference regarding the effects of intervention. A structure (template) is provided to the clinician for the MSE for completeness. However, rather than beginning at the top and going straight through, the skillful clinician will weave extensive parts of the MSE into the general interview with the child, adolescent, or family unobtrusively, without resorting to discontinuity in the process of the interview.

The MSE is one element in a multitrait, multimodality, multi-informant approach to gain the best available picture of a child or adolescent's functioning, strengths, deficits, and needs. When organized with information from other sources, the total data can be arranged in the form of symptom complexes to establish diagnosis and comorbid conditions. Equally, information about individual capabilities and styles of functioning can provide direction about treatment approaches. Together, the information should convey "how and why" (Lewis, 1996) a child or adolescent functions the way he or she does by integrating organic, environmental, and individual psychological factors to render a complete picture, and suggesting to the clinician an integrated approach to meeting the needs of the individual and family.

REFERENCES

Achenbach, T. M. (1991). *Manual for the Child Behavior Checklist/4-188 and 1991 Profile.* Burlington: University of Vermont Department of Psychiatry.

Albert, M., & Cohen, C. (1992). The Test for Severe Impairment. An instrument for the assessment of patients with severe cognitive dysfunction. *Journal of the American Geriatric Society, 40,* 449–453.

Aman, M. G., Singh, N. N., Stewart, A. W., & Field, C. J. (1985). Psychometric characteristics of the Aberrant Behavior Checklist. *American Journal of Mental Deficiency, 89,* 492–502.

Aman, M. G., Tasse, M. J., Rojahn, J., & Hammer, D. (1996). The Nisonger CBRF. A Child Behavior Rating Form for children with developmental disabilities. *Research in Developmental Disabilities, 17,* 41–57.

Aman, M. G., & Turbolt, S. H. (1991). Prediction of clinical response in children taking methylpharidate. *Journal of Autism Developmental Disorders, 21,* 211–228.

Benham, A. L. (2000). The observation and assessment of young children including use of the Infant-Toddler Mental Status Exam. In C. H. Zeanah, Jr. (Ed.), *Handbook of infant mental health* (2nd ed., pp. 249–265). New York: Guilford Press.

Burt, D. B., Pearson, P., Lesser, J., Lewis, K. R., Cummings, E., Chen, Y. W., Loveland, K. A., Primeaux, S., & Cleveland, L. (1999). Use of the Mini-Mental State Examination for assessing dementia in adults with Mental Retardation. Presented at the 123rd Annual Meeting of the American Association on Mental Retardation, May 1999, New Orleans.

Conners, C. K. (1997). *Conners' Rating Scales—Revised, Technical Manual.* North Tonawanda, NY: Multi-Health Systems.

Cosgrave, M. P., McCarron, M., Anderson, M., Tyriell, J., Gill, M., & Lawlor, B. A. (1998). Cognitive decline in Down syndrome: A validity/reliability study of the Test for Severe Impairment. *American Journal on Mental Retardation, 103,* 193–197.

Devenny, D. A., Wisniewski, K. E., & Silverman, W. P. (1993). Dementia of the Alzheimer's type among high-functioning adults with Down's syndrome: Individual profiles of performance. In B. Corain, K. Iqbal, M. Nicolini, B. Winblad, K. Wisniewski, & P. Zatta (Eds.), *Alzheimer's disease: Advances in clinical and basic research* (pp. 47–53). New York: Wiley.

Folstein, M. F., Folstein, S. E., & McHugh, P. R. (1975). "Mini-Mental State": A practical method for grading the cognitive state of patients for the clinician. *Journal of Psychiatric Research, 12,* 189–198.

Lewis, M. (1996). Psychiatric assessment of infants, children and adolescents. In M. Lewis (Ed.), *Child and adolescent psychiatry: A comprehensive textbook* (2nd ed., pp. 440–457). Baltimore: Williams & Wilkens.

Lord, C., Rutter, M., & Le Couteur, A. (1994). Autism Diagnostic Interview, Revised. A revised version of a diagnostic interview for caregivers of individuals with possible pervasive developmental disorders. *Journal of Autism and Developmental Disorders, 24,* 659–685.

Nezu, C. M., Nezu, A. M., & Gill-Weiss, M. J. (1992). *Psychopathology in persons with Mental Retardation. Clinical guidelines for assessment and treatment.* Champaign, IL: Research Press.

Reiss, S., & Valenti-Hein, D. (1990). *Reiss Scales for Children's Dual Diagnosis.* Chicago: International Diagnostic Systems.

Reiss, S., & Valenti-Hein, D. (1994). Development of a psychopathology rating scale for children with mental retardation. *Journal of Consulting & Clinical Psychology, 62,* 28–33.

Sattler, J. M. (1998). *Clinical and forensic interviewing of children and families: Guidelines for the mental health, education, pediatric, and child maltreatment fields.* San Diego: Author.

Sparrow, S., Balla, D., & Ciccetti, D. (1984). *Vineland Adaptive Behavior Scales.* Circle Pines, MN: American Guidance Service.

Wisniewski, K., & Hill, A. L. (1985). Clinical aspects of dementia in Mental Retardation and developmental disabilities. In M. Janicki & K. Wisniewski (Eds.), *Aging and developmental disabilities: Issues and approaches* (pp. 195–210). Baltimore: Brookes.

Chapter 5

ISSUES IN THE FORENSIC EVALUATION OF CHILDREN AND YOUTH

THOMAS E. SCHACHT

INTRODUCTION

This chapter presents an overview of forensic practice for mental health professionals working with children and adolescents. The primary goals of the chapter are to introduce general distinctions and boundaries between clinical and forensic practice and to familiarize the reader with issues from selected major areas of specialized forensic practice with this population. This chapter will not address legal issues integral to ordinary clinical practice, such as rights to informed consent, involuntary treatment, malpractice risk management, liability associated with managed care, confidentiality and its limits, and so on. The reader interested in these subjects may profitably consult general texts on legal issues in clinical practice, such as Appelbaum and Gutheil (1991), Schetky and Benedek (1992), and Simon (1987).

THERAPEUTIC VERSUS LEGAL PRACTICE CONTEXTS

Most services provided by health professionals occur in a therapeutic context. Such therapeutic services are typically provided at the request of the patient (or guardian) for diagnosis of impairment, relief of suffering, or improvement of functioning. The corresponding professional duties of the practitioner revolve around maintenance of a therapeutic alliance guided by core principles related to the welfare of the patient, including efforts to avoid activities that may cause harm.

In contrast, a forensic assessment is conducted to assist a trier-of-fact (a judge or jury or both) in resolving a legally disputed issue. The forensic examiner's duties are primarily to the court, rather than to the individual being examined, and revolve around providing relevant and accurate information that will help the court adjudicate the legal matter at hand. If a therapeutic encounter results in distress or harm to a patient, this is generally regarded as an unfortunate outcome. In contrast, a successful forensic examination may be distressing or even harmful to the individual evaluated precisely because the examination is successful in assisting the trier-of-fact. For example, a forensic examination may discover evidence that contradicts an individual's legal position or that indicates the individual has not been accurate in his or her claims. Although legal action is sometimes undertaken in the belief that it will prove therapeutic and empowering, forensic examiners are fully cognizant of the inherent potential for litigation to be traumatic. Recent seminal analyses by Greenberg and Shuman (1997) and Strasburger, Gutheil, and Brodsky (1997) cogently argue that a therapeutic role is incompatible with providing professional services to the legal system. Any mental health professional venturing into the forensic arena should be intimately familiar with these role differences as well as with relevant forensic practice guidelines and specialized ethics codes promulgated by various professional organizations.[1]

Who Is the Client?

In a therapeutic relationship, the individual being evaluated and treated is the client or patient, and all services are provided for his or her benefit. In a forensic evaluation context, the court or referring attorney is the client; there is no treatment agenda (except for the possible exception of emergency interventions); and services are provided for the benefit of the court. In a forensic evaluation there is no doctor/patient relationship, and the subject of a forensic evaluation is an *examinee* or *evaluee* rather than a *patient* or *client.*

What Rules Govern Privacy of the Information Generated?

In a therapeutic relationship, the governing principle is the therapist/patient privilege. Except for specific circumstances that create a duty to report (such as child abuse), therapists can generally offer their clients reasonable assurances about the uses to which information will be put, as well as a high degree of confidence in the privacy of information. In contrast, the governing privacy principles in a forensic relationship are attorney/client privilege, attorney work-product doctrine, and (in some cases) the power of a court to seal a record. Forensic evaluators can make no promises about how information will be used once it is introduced into the legal process. For this reason, prior to commencing an examination, forensic examiners must be prepared to inform examinees and their legal counsel of the intended uses of the information and of the potential lack of privilege for information that is introduced into a legal proceeding.

What Is the Structure of the Professional Relationship?

A therapeutic relationship is rarely adversarial. Consistent with the goals of forming a therapeutic alliance and helping the client, a therapeutic relationship typically requires a supportive, accepting, and empathic stance and may often be relatively unstructured; the structure may even be substantially under the control of the patient. Therapists may often suspend critical judgment in order to promote the therapeutic alliance. In contrast, the truth-seeking goals of a forensic evaluator typically result in a more neutral, detached, and objective stance, and procedures are relatively structured and directed by the evaluator. A forensic examination is explicitly evaluative, demands critical judgment, and may include adversarial elements.

In psychotherapeutic relationships, the entire clinical process may be conceptualized more as a search for meaning than as a search for facts. This distinction has been widely recognized as the difference between narrative truth and historical truth (Spence, 1982). A psychotherapist may actively and tactically suspend disbelief in order to enter the patient's inner reality and personal mythology empathically. Although helping the patient reach a more objective self-understanding is a goal of psychotherapy, improvements in insight are not generally subjected to the validation necessary for meeting legal standards of proof. Furthermore, psychotherapeutic work often occurs in an atmosphere of ambiguity and possibility, rather than the "reasonable degree of clinical or medical certainty" that is required for expert testimony.

Of course, not all therapeutic activities focus more on the patient's subjective reality than on historical accuracy. For example, in a diagnostic context, professionals may rely on somewhat objectifiable diagnostics procedures. However, even in this role, therapeutic professionals typically obtain most or all of their information directly from the patient and generally engage in little scrutiny for the accuracy of information provided by the patient. Most often it is presumed that information provided by the patient is accurate because the patient is seeking relief of suffering, and giving inaccurate information would interfere with this goal.

What Information and Evaluation Techniques Are Used?

In a forensic context, the type of traditional diagnosis conducted for purposes of health care may be irrelevant. Thus, forensic professionals focus in some contexts on criteria that illuminate the relationship between psychological factors and specialized legal concepts (such as cause-and-effect relationships necessary for establishing legal liability, various types of competency, or factors related to the determination of criminal responsibility). Forensic evaluators may use specialized instruments or procedures that have little application to therapeutic contexts, such as Grisso's (1998) Instruments for Assessment of Understanding of Miranda Rights, or Rogers, Bagby, and Dickens (1992) Structured Interview of Reported Symptoms. Forensic assessment may employ laboratory testing of breath, urine, blood, or hair samples to evaluate the accuracy of reported substance abuse and compliance with prescribed medical regimens (Rogers & Kelly, 1997). Interview techniques employed in forensic evaluation are often highly structured, directive, and probing, with many questions aimed toward illuminating specific legal standards or issues (Rogers, 1995). Forensic examinations may be observed by third parties or may be electronically recorded for independent analysis by opposing experts. This forensic approach contrasts markedly with confidential, nondirective, patient-centered clinical interviews designed to foster a therapeutic alliance. Furthermore, forensic evaluators typically scrutinize information for evidence of its accuracy and generally obtain collateral information from clinical and nonclinical records and third-party interviews.

Forensic assessment procedures address not only the content of information but also its accuracy and completeness. Children have historically been viewed as less reliable informants than adults. This general belief is supported by observations of developmental limitations in the capacity to appreciate the nature and value of truth-telling, particularly in very young children and also by developmental limitations in capacity for self-observation and description.

Little is known empirically about the general accuracy of childrens' accounts of their own psychological symptoms and functioning. Further complicating any search for a gold standard of diagnostic accuracy is the commonly encountered poor agreement between the reports of children, their parents, and teachers (cf. the meta-analysis of 119 studies by Achenbach, McConaughy, & Howell, 1987).

It is clear that children are capable of effective dissimulation and that these skills are acquired at an early age. For example, Lewis (1993) conducted a series of studies in which child subjects were instructed to stay in a room and not to look at a toy. Subsequently, the children were asked if they had peeked. Using subjects from ages 2½ to 6, the researchers were unable to identify any differences in verbal or nonverbal behavior that reliably distinguished truth-tellers from liars. Indeed, adults were unable to detect liars at any age beyond chance levels when the children were questioned with simple closed-ended inquiries.

Whereas Lewis's research indicates that the lies told by very young children tend to take the form of simple denial or misleading affirmation, older children and adolescents are more likely to offer elaborated prevarications (Bussey, 1992) that require more complex skills of role playing and impression management. Oldershaw and Bagby (1997) note that this developmental shift has important implications for interviewing children. Specifically, to the extent that interviewers ask open-ended questions that do not lend themselves to "yes" or "no" responses, younger children should have greater difficulty in crafting elaborate lies, and their deceptions should be more readily detectable.

It is also important for evaluators to recognize that children's motivations for deception may also reflect developmental factors. Compared to adults, whose motives may be more concretely linked to overt goals such as attaining compensation or avoiding prosecution, children may be more likely to respond to emotionally-based motives such as protection of the family or an attachment relationship, a desire for attention and approval, a desire to "fit in" socially, or a desire to reduce family conflict by avoiding certain topics or by following family rules about disclosure or meeting the expectations of adults. Children may be more likely to respond defensively during assessments in the presence of certain background factors (Oldershaw & Bagby, 1997), such as being raised in a highly religious family; having a mother who works outside the home; or being raised in family environments notable for rejection, inconsistent discipline, parental manipulativeness and dishonesty, and pressure to perform. Interviewing principles likely to improve the accuracy and completeness of reports by children include the following:

- Making sure the child has a clear, understandable, and nonthreatening rationale for his or her participation in an assessment interview;
- Using developmentally appropriate vocabulary in the interview;
- Asking for descriptions of behavior in specific situations rather than asking for generalizations, abstractions, or labels;
- Avoiding subtle or overt social reinforcement for particular answers or content;
- Avoiding leading or closed-ended questions in favor of open-ended inquiry;
- Avoiding questions that evoke defensiveness, such as asking *why;* asking, "What don't you like about X?" instead of "Why don't you like X?"

What Is Done in Court?

Courts recognize two major types of witnesses: fact witnesses and expert witnesses. In general, therapists should limit themselves to service as fact witnesses, whereas forensic evaluators inevitably function as expert witnesses. The distinction between a fact witness and an expert witness does not rest on whether a witness happens to be an expert in some field, but on the type of testimony the witness will offer. A fact witness is generally limited to observations they have personally made, such as observations of a patient in therapy, and to immediate conclusions that flow directly from those observations, such as diagnosis, response to treatment, and prognosis. Fact witnesses may be compelled to testify by issuance of a subpoena, subject to restrictions associated with rules of privilege.

In contrast, expert witnesses are paid consultants and are generally not subject to being compelled to testify by subpoenas. An expert witness may draw conclusions based on reports or data generated by others, including professional and scientific literature, and may offer testimony in the form of opinions and inferences (rather than just observations), including opinions expressed in response to hypothetical questions. Under some circumstances, experts may be asked to state an opinion directly on the ultimate issue that is before the court, such as "Was this person able to understand his/her Miranda rights at the time he/she signed the waiver form?" In some situations, ultimate issue testimony is illegal; and, even when it is allowable, many experts refrain from speaking to ultimate issues on the grounds that such testimony invades the duties of the trier-of-fact. Thus, in response to the foregoing question about Miranda rights, experts might limit their opinions to statements that can be made with a reasonable degree of clinical certainty about psychological capacities that are relevant to the court's decision-making. Experts may also be required to conform their testimony to requirements for scientific soundness, general acceptance within the field, and so forth (cf. *Daubert v. Merrell-Dow Pharmaceuticals,* 1993).

As the foregoing analysis should clarify, the differences between clinical and forensic roles are substantial. Failure to respect these differences jeopardizes not only the integrity of the professional services, but also legal rights of involved parties. It is extremely difficult, if not impossible, for a mental health professional ethically to engage in both a therapeutic and a forensic relationship with the same individual. The conflict between therapeutic and forensic roles ultimately threatens the fundamental purpose of forensic services, which is to provide objective and accurate information to the court. Due to concerns about the negative implications of performing dual therapeutic and forensic functions in relation to the same client, professional organizations have adopted formal practice guidelines and ethics statements that discourage conflicting dual professional roles with patient/litigants, for example:

A treating psychiatrist should generally avoid agreeing to be an expert witness or to perform an evaluation of his patient for legal purposes because a forensic evaluation usually requires that other people be interviewed and testimony may adversely affect the therapeutic relationship. (American Academy of Psychiatry and the Law, 1989)

In most circumstances, psychologists avoid performing multiple and potentially conflicting roles in forensic matters. (American Psychological Association, 1992)

Psychologists generally avoid conducting a child custody evaluation in a case in which the psychologist served in a therapeutic role for the child or his or her immediate family. . . . In addition, during the course of a child custody evaluation, a psychologist does not accept any of the involved participants in the evaluation as a therapy client. Therapeutic contact with the child or involved participants following a child custody evaluation is undertaken with caution. . . . A psychologist asked to testify regarding a therapy client who is involved in a child custody case is aware of the limitations and possible biases inherent in such a role and the possible impact on the ongoing therapeutic relationship. Although the court may require the psychologist to testify as a fact witness regarding factual information he or she became aware of in a professional relationship with a client, that psychologist should decline the role of an expert witness who gives a professional opinion regarding custody and visitation issues" (American Psychological Association, 1994).

JUVENILES AND THE LAW

For scientists and health professionals, childhood and adolescence are formative periods whose boundaries are best described as empirically supported continua rather than as discrete categories bounded sharply by chronological age. In contrast, the timetables and sequences of biological and psychological development are reduced under the law to a matter of convention, subject to revision at any time by legislative action or judicial interpretation. Legal conventions often implement arbitrary distinctions that have no counterpart in scientific views of human development. For example, the U.S. Supreme Court has held that the Constitution does not prohibit subjecting persons aged 16 to capital punishment (*Stanford v. Kentucky*, 1989), but the court declared that persons under this age are insufficiently mature to receive this ultimate penalty (*Thompson v. Oklahoma*, 1988).

Full adult legal empowerment ("majority") is a legal status that depends primarily on chronological age, not on determination of any particular mental or physical attributes. Solely because of their age, the law gives children a special status of legal disability, also referred to as minority. Between roughly A.D. 1600 and 1800, this meant that children were legally regarded as the property of their parents, without significant independent rights. Subsequent legal developments over the next two centuries established a benevolent and protective legal function ensuring that children have certain enforceable legal rights. As embodied in the doctrine of *parens patriae,* the state came to be seen as owing a protective duty to citizens with legal disabilities, a group that by definition includes children.

Legal disability differs from the concept of disability typically understood by health professionals. No particular health infirmity is required for legal disability. Rather, this term refers to limitations in an individual's status under the law. Children are legally disabled because, as compared to adults, their rights, duties, and liabilities under the law are restricted. The law presumes that children need protection from themselves and others and that society needs to be protected from any dangers that may flow from childrens' immaturity. Thus, under typical legal circumstances, minors may own property but not manage it; minors may unilaterally void contracts that would be binding on an adult; and very young children (typically under seven) are presumed incapable of the negligence required for some types of liability. Young children are likewise presumed incapable of forming the necessary mental state for commission of a crime, but at the same time minors may be held responsible for conduct, such as curfew violation, that would not be a crime if committed by an adult (so-called "status offenses").

Consistent with the international age of majority expressed in Article I of the United Nations Convention on the Rights of the Child, the age of majority in most states has been fixed by law at 18 for purposes of entering into contracts, marriage without parental consent, military service, and voting. The age for other purposes (receiving a license to drive an automobile, purchasing alcohol or tobacco, consenting to sexual activity, consenting to or refusing health care) may be set differently in different states. There is a poorly defined concept known as the *mature minor,* which may be employed by courts on a case-by-case basis, particularly when a minor may seek a court's permission to be declared emancipated. A court's finding of sufficient maturity to grant a petition for emancipation severs the parents' legal right to control their child's earnings and services and terminates the parents' obligation to provide support. However, emancipation per se is not a shortcut to legal majority and does not affect other legal disabilities of a minor.

The fact that minors' rights, duties, and liabilities are legally limited does not diminish the legal system's interest in minors; nor does it necessarily simplify the task of courts and attorneys called upon to respond to legal situations involving minors. Rather, the special status of minors calls upon correspondingly specialized legal settings (such as family court and juvenile court) and specialized legal procedures (such as hearings to determine the fitness of a juvenile to be tried as an adult for violent criminal acts).

SELECTED JUVENILE FORENSIC PRACTICE CONTEXTS

Education

In 1954, the Supreme Court reviewed the issue of racial segregation of schools and established that "education is a right which must be made available to all on equal terms" (*Brown v. Board of Education,* 1954). Nearly two decades passed, however, before federal legislation was first passed to extend this basic constitutional protection to handicapped children as well as racial minorities (e.g., Sec. 504 of the Rehabilitation Act of 1973, Education for all Handicapped Children Act of 1975, and the Individuals with Disabilities Education Act [IDEA] of 1991 and subsequent amendments). These statutes require school systems to provide all handicapped children with an evaluation that leads to an individualized education plan for a free and appropriate public education. Disabilities specifically identified in the IDEA include mental retardation, visual and hearing impairment, speech and language impairment, specific learning disability, serious emotional disturbance, autism, traumatic brain injury, and orthopedic impairment. Special education and related services must be reasonably calculated to provide educational benefit in the least restrictive environment. The law gives children and their parents or guardians specific enforceable legal rights, whose scope is continually evolving both through amendments to the law and by court interpretation of the meaning and boundaries of statutory language (Schacht & Hanson, 1999).

Unfortunately, the educational entitlement created by the IDEA did not come from Congress fully funded. School systems thus face a perverse incentive to identify disabled children as nondisabled because of the potentially large costs associated with providing special education and related services. The somewhat vague terms of the federal law were designed to allow varied implementation by the states. However, this same vagueness may also be used to skirt the spirit of the law and may give rise to litigation when a family and school system cannot agree on a program to meet a child's educational needs. Forensic evaluation services are frequently required in such cases. Either party or the court on its own may seek expert consultation regarding determination of key facts, including:

- Determination of whether a condition is present that meets the legal definitions of handicapped or disabled. While clinicians may regard either suffering or functional impairment as sufficient to diagnose a mental disorder, the IDEA emphasizes functional impairment in the educational setting as the sine qua non of eligibility for special services. Furthermore, certain causes of inabilities to learn, such as mere social maladjustment, do not qualify a child for special services. For these reasons, the mere presence of a DSM-IV diagnosis will not satisfy the legal definition of disability. Forensic evaluation of intelligence; language and communication skills; perceptual abilities; academic achievement; and behavioral, interpersonal and emotional deficits must all be geared toward identifying the legal relevance of functioning in each domain to the juvenile's capacity to learn and benefit from education.

- Determination of the extent to which conduct problems are causally related to a covered disability, such as serious emotional disturbance (in which case purely disciplinary options may be restricted and therapeutic options may be required).

- Determination of the type of special educational interventions necessary to help the child compensate for his/her disability.

- Determination of whether and which type of specific related services are necessary to allow the child to benefit from the educational program. Related services cannot involve treatment by a physician and must typically be supportive services provided during school hours that enable the child to benefit from education.

- Determination of the least restrictive environment in which appropriate educational services may be delivered, including specific evaluation of prospects for delivering educational services in a mainstreamed environment. It is important for evaluators to remember that least restrictive environment is not a clinical concept, but a legal term that expresses a judgment posed by a particular intervention program or educational environment about the degree of intrusion into civil rights and liberty interests.

Mental health evaluations conducted under the IDEA are one element in a multidisciplinary proceeding for the creation of an Individual Education Plan (IEP). The law prohibits use of any single evaluation procedure as the sole criterion for determining an appropriate education program (for example, an IQ test may not be the sole criterion determining class placement). As with all forensic evaluations, reliability may be enhanced by surveying multiple sources of information. Thus, in addition to direct clinical evaluation of a child, an evaluator should consult school and clinical records; examine samples of student work; make classroom observations; and interview parents, teachers, other clinicians, and child-care personnel. Including trial interventions in a longitudinal evaluation process can be very helpful. Psychological tests should be chosen carefully to insure that they will past legal muster. This generally requires selection of instruments that are clearly relevant to the disability in question and are well standardized and appropriately normed for the population to which the child belongs.

The law is very particular about distinguishing between clinically and scientifically undefined categories such as serious emotional disturbance versus social maladjustment. For this reason forensic evaluators in educational contexts should become intimately familiar with the jargon employed in the law and should incorporate exact legal terminology in their reports. The meanings of the legal terms should be operationalized by reference to the specific clinical findings that were judged to support the use of a particular legal category.

Divorce and Child Custody

Involvement in child custody proceedings is the most volatile area of child forensic practice. Expert testimony from mental health professionals is common in litigated divorces and in child custody disputes between unmarried parents. Formal custody determination usually occurs only in the most conflicted circumstances, such as when the parties are utterly unable to negotiate their family relationships and effectively abandon family decision-making to a group of hopefully well-meaning strangers in a courtroom. Testifying experts are bound to make at least one party unhappy, and may achieve this result with both sides. Consequently, it is not uncommon for dissatisfied marital litigants to shift their aim from the ex-spouse to the expert. Published data on ethics complaints indicate that involvement with child custody poses a significant professional risk. In the most recent 10-year period for which statistics have been compiled by the American Psychological Association Ethics Committee (1988–1998), child custody disputes have been the single most common context for complaints of inappropriate professional practice.[2] One proposed defense against this threat is the extension of judicial immunity to the expert.[3] However, even judicial immunity does not halt administrative proceedings resulting from complaints to professional ethics committees and state licensing bodies. Furthermore, there is no immunity for experts who are not court appointed, such as treatment experts who step outside their clinical role to participate in a client's divorce. Treating clinicians should never attempt to play the roles of independent custody evaluators and should not make recommendations about the proper disposition of a child in a custody dispute. To ignore this principle is to invite immeasurable legal woe.

Forensic clinicians should carefully structure their involvement in custody cases. At a minimum, the evaluation should be conducted under the auspices of a court order that sets forth the scope and ground rules of the evaluation. Ideally the evaluator should draw major guidance from empirical literature (cf. Galatzer-Levy & Kraus, 1999) and from professional organizations that have published guidelines for professional involvement in child custody and child abuse cases (see Note 1).

Of course, merely working under a court order and following general guidelines does not ensure that the resulting evaluation will be focused, relevant, affordable, and respectful of a family's right to be spared unnecessary intrusion and psychological trauma in the process of revealing intimate details of family life in a courtroom. Unfortunately, useless or harmful evaluation outcomes occur with distressing frequency, in part because many courts order a custody evaluation as if this constituted a standard procedure, whose scope, direction, level of effort, and relevance to the proceedings at hand may be taken for granted, and because many professionals are correspondingly willing to provide a one-size-fits-all form of evaluation.

Evaluators can improve the usefulness of their custody evaluations to courts if they structure their work in a two-phase procedure. In the first, or *scoping,* phase, the expert conducts a preliminary reconnaissance to determine which issues are likely to be the key issues for a particular family. It is critical that the expert retain control over this scoping process, in order to avoid corruption of the entire subsequent evaluation process by legal gerrymandering. Based on this scoping evaluation, a preliminary report is presented to the parties and the court for the limited purpose of identifying the likely agenda for a full custody evaluation. It is possible that the clarification achieved by a scoping evaluation will permit a family to proceed into some form of alternative dispute resolution, such as mediation. If not, then the second phase of a custody evaluation, based on the results of the scoping evaluation, may be performed in a manner that increases the likelihood of producing a product that makes efficient use of the family's resources and is maximally relevant to the needs of the court and the parties.

Professionals wishing to work regularly in the area of child custody should consider establishing a multidisciplinary team. The expertise and balance embodied in such a team should allow an improved execution of the various incarnations of the *best interests of the child* standard.[4] A best interests standard is laudable in principle but is often so vague in execution that it opens the door to error, bias, or frank abuse of discretion. An evaluation team may be better able than a single individual to resist the idiosyncratic personalized reactions that may be evoked by outrageous and provocative behavior on the part of litigating spouses. A team should also be better able to define the desired scope of a best interests evaluation in a particular case, allowing more efficient targeting of evaluation efforts to relevant, as opposed to peripheral, issues.

There is a common belief that false child-abuse allegations may be raised in custody disputes as part of an effort by one parent to gain leverage over the opposing spouse or to undermine the child's relationship with the other parent (Gardner, 1987). This belief is supported, in part, by observations that in cases of suspected abuse, there is a high frequency of custody dispute (Green, 1986). However, the fact that custody disputes occur in cases of sexual abuse does not mean that the sexual abuse allegations were caused by the custody dispute. A recent empirical study of a large sample of consecutive family court cases for an entire year suggests that the base rate incidence of alleged sexual abuse may be as low as 2% of contested custody cases and less than 1% of all family court cases (McIntosh & Prinz, 1993). However, these statistics do not speak to the correlated issues of how frequently allegations may be false or of how often this issue may be raised and settled informally, resulting in the issue's never being litigated or appearing in court documents.

Unfortunately, some courts expect mental health professionals not only to determine the impact of documented abuse, but also to overcome problems posed by absent or equivocal evidence and to determine whether or to what extent abuse allegations are true. However, psychological evaluation to determine whether alleged abuse occurred is a treacherous enterprise even under the best of circumstances. Psychological evaluation was never designed or intended to replace criminal investigation. Improper psychological evaluation may cause children to make statements that are biased or distorted, or that are even outright false memories. Improper evaluation techniques may fuel the modern equivalent of witch trials, in which even denials of abuse become reframed as evidence that abuse has actually occurred but has been so traumatic that the child must deny it in order to cope psychologically.

Ideally, suspected abuse victims are interviewed once, not repeatedly. The interview situation should be nonthreatening and devoid of any elements of pressure or coercion. Leading questions, praise for "correct" answers, and suggestive props such as anatomically correct dolls should be avoided. Ceci and Bruck (1995) and Perry and Wrightsman (1991) provide comprehensive analyses of the empirical literature related to children as witnesses and supporting various "do's and don'ts" of abuse evaluation.

Most mental health professionals are aware of the existence of child-abuse reporting laws, some version of which has been enacted in all states. Every state now requires the reporting of suspected child abuse, although professional knowledge and compliance with these laws is inconsistent. One study of a large sample of psychologists found that "protecting the child" was rated more highly than "upholding the law" as a determinant of whether to make a report of suspected abuse (Kalichman & Brosig, 1993). These professionals may confuse the professional duty to testify in accordance with the best interests of the child, which does not authorize breach of confidentiality, with the legal duty to report suspected abuse. Some professionals, caught up in the throes of a high-conflict divorce situation, appear to forget that reporting laws typically provide immunity from liability only for disclosures that are made under limited circumstances specified by the statute (such as reports made directly to police, human service authorities, juvenile courts, etc.). Unauthorized testimony in a divorce action, even when given in response to allegations of abuse or neglect, is not covered by immunity provisions of reporting statutes, which generally apply only to reports made to designated authorities. Thus, a recent New Jersey case found a psychologist liable for damages to a former patient, whom she had counseled along with her husband for five years prior to a divorce, after the psychologist testified against the mother in a custody hearing, believing that her testimony was permissible because it was intended to foster the best interests of the child (*Runyon v. Smith*, 1999).

Delinquency/Criminal Court

The idea of a special court for juveniles is relatively modern. It was not until 1899 that Illinois implemented the first Juvenile Court Act in the United States. In theory, a special court for juveniles expresses a state's desire to act in the role of parent rather than policeman. Accordingly, juvenile court proceedings are confidential and are characterized as civil rather than criminal. Theoretically, a primary goal of juvenile court is to organize resources for education, treatment, and rehabilitation in accord with the best interests of the child. The therapeutic orientation of juvenile court contrasts sharply with the primary goals of the adult correctional system, which are protection of society, deterrence of future crime, rehabilitation, and punitive retribution. The language of the juvenile court is euphemized consistent with its special mission. Thus: *arrested* becomes *taken into custody; trial* becomes *hearing; crime* becomes *delinquency; conviction* becomes *adjudication; sentence* becomes *disposition;* and *prison* becomes *reformatory* or *training school.*

Of course, the paternalistic, rehabilitative approach of the juvenile court has not been without its own price. In the name of judicial flexibility, juveniles were historically deprived of the basic rights and protections afforded to adults in criminal proceedings. Juvenile matters were routinely handled without requirements for notice, without hearings, without rights to counsel or to discover evidence or to confront or summon witnesses, and without rights to appeal. Juveniles could be confined to institutions for much longer periods than adults who had committed similar offenses. This situation did not change materially until the mid-1960s, when a series of landmark Supreme Court cases criticized juvenile justice as its worst as "kangaroo court" (cf. *In re Gault* 387 U.S. 1, 1967) and began awarding basic due process rights to minors. Rights presently afforded to juveniles include the following:

- Notice of charges
- Representation by counsel
- Privilege against self-incrimination
- Formal hearing, similar to a trial
- Access to records, evidence, and witnesses, and the right to confront witnesses
- Proof beyond a reasonable doubt (in delinquency proceedings)
- Protection from double jeopardy
- Limited rights of appeal

Major adult rights still not enjoyed by juveniles include:

- Jury trial
- Freedom from warrantless searches on school property, provided there is "reasonable suspicion"
- Freedom from preventive detention if deemed potentially dangerous
- Freedom from prosecution for "status" offenses (acts that would not be prosecuted but for the juvenile status of the individual, such as truancy, running away, curfew violation, habitual disobedience, etc.)

Waiver of Rights

In *Miranda v. Arizona* (1966) the U.S. Supreme Court established the principle that, to be used as evidence at trial, statements made by suspects in the custody of police should be made with knowledge of the Constitutional rights to avoid self-incrimination and to be represented by counsel. To implement the court's decision, police departments established procedures for informing suspects of these rights and for obtaining a waiver of the rights from suspects who wished to make a statement despite their right to refrain. Following standard procedure for waiver of any rights, any such waiver must be made in a "knowing," "intelligent," and "voluntary" manner. Subsequent Supreme Court cases (*Kent v. U.S.,* 1966; *In re Gault,* 1967) made it clear that the Miranda requirements extended to juveniles as well as adults. Juveniles as a group appear to be at elevated risk for impairments in the capacity to waive rights knowingly, intelligently, and voluntarily. Although the court did not find that the mere fact of being a juvenile automatically invalidated a waiver of rights, it did recognize a need for case-by-case scrutiny of the totality of the circumstances, including features of the situation in which the statement was given and characteristics of the juvenile that might affect his or her capacity to understand and apply the Miranda warnings. Grisso (1981) conducted an empirical study of how well juveniles understand Miranda warnings. His results indicated that as compared to criminal adults matched for IQ, adolescents have greater difficulty understanding the warnings and their significance. The risk of impaired understanding increased in the presence of cognitive deficits and as age decreased.

Expert evaluation of a juvenile's capacity to waiver Miranda rights begins, as with virtually all forensic evaluations, with a review of records and interviews of collateral sources. Documents that may be of value include school records (including academic and school psychological evaluations); medical and mental health records; previous juvenile offense records, including indications of prior experience with interrogation and rights waivers; and the police investigative report, including copies of whatever statement the juvenile made. If the statement was recorded, the examiner should review the recording. The evaluator should obtain a copy of the exact Miranda waiver form that was used with the juvenile. It may be useful to subject the form to a reading-level analysis to compare to the measured reading level of the juvenile. It may also be useful to have the juvenile read the form aloud, and to make a verbatim recording of his or her performance, including all errors. Collateral interviews may be very useful. Potential resources for collateral interviews include parents, teachers, and the arresting and interrogating officers.

The evaluator must develop a detailed understanding of the juvenile's general level of functioning, particularly regarding capacity to process verbal material. It is also critical to uncover the specific situational pressures that may have operated at the time of the interrogation and rights waiver. This effort may benefit from investigation into factors such as:

- Circumstances in the days prior to the arrest
- Circumstances of the arrest itself, including transportation to the police station and detention prior to questioning
- The physical and interpersonal circumstances of the interrogation itself, including communications with others (such as parents), prior to making a rights waiver
- Behavioral observations of the interrogation process, including specifics of how the Miranda rights were presented and how the waiver was obtained

Direct evaluation of the juvenile generally follows record reviews and collateral interviews. In addition to the usual dimensions of a clinical interview, the evaluator should emphasize any past experiences with the legal system and should obtain a detailed description of the current legal situation, including descriptions of the arrest and the interrogation. Psychological testing may be useful to objectify clinical estimates of general levels of intellectual and academic functioning, as well as to evaluate the presence of emotional disturbances that could affect reasoning or decision-making. Specialized validity-indicating instruments can be important in addressing issues of exaggeration or malingering of deficits with adults, but very few of these instruments have been validated for use with children and adolescents. Standardized measurements of functional abilities to waive Miranda rights can be very informative and can be conducted with Grisso's (1998) *Instruments for Assessing Understanding and Appreciation of Miranda Rights.* These four instruments were developed under the auspices of the National Institute of Mental Health in a study that compared responses of 431 male youths in juvenile detention facilities, evaluated within a few days of arrest, with responses of 203 male adults living in halfway houses as part of a postprison community reentry program. The instruments assess comprehension of Miranda rights through separate procedures designed to tap:

• Capacity to paraphrase and explain the Miranda rights
• Capacity to discriminate correct from incorrect information about the rights
• Knowledge of typical vocabulary employed in Miranda warnings
• Comprehension of the function of the Miranda rights (distinguishing, for example, between mere superficial awareness of the right to an attorney and meaningful knowledge of the advocacy and help an attorney can offer)

Waiver to Adult Criminal Court

Balancing the movement toward expanding the rights of juveniles is an opposing concern with law and order and community safety. A relative emphasis on law and order stems in part from a public perception that the juvenile court's presumption of rehabilitation is too costly for society because it fails to control dangerous juvenile felons. One marker of the level of public hysteria with regard to juvenile crime may be found in a study of attitudes toward capital punishment by Crosby, Britner, Jodl, and Portwood (1995), who reported that 60% of a sample of 250 persons rotating off jury duty would vote to execute a 10-year-old defendant convicted of robbery and murder. In response to such public concerns, the federal government and many states have made it much easier to bypass juvenile court and treat young offenders as adults. The legal procedure by which juveniles may be adjudicated as adults is known as *transfer* or *waiver* to adult court. Waiver is an extremely serious matter, as it may carry lifetime exclusion from further jurisdiction of the juvenile court and may expose the juvenile to virtually the full range of adult punishments, with the general exception of the death penalty.

The specific requirements for waiver vary across jurisdictions, so practitioners must become familiar with the law in their particular locale. Although all but three states provide a mechanism for judicial waiver by juvenile courts, about three quarters of the states have statutes that make waiver automatic when the alleged offense is sufficiently serious, and about 20% of states allow prosecutors the discretion to bypass juvenile court and file charges directly in adult court (Torbet, Gable, Hurst, Montgomery, Szymanski, & Thomas, 1996).

Although the specific legal criteria and procedures for juvenile waiver vary from state to state, most jurisdictions follow a prototypic decision-making process. First, the court must determine the status of a set of threshold conditions, such as age, level of offense, history of prior offenses, and probable cause that the currently alleged offense was committed by the defendant. Once the threshold conditions have been met, establishing potential eligibility for waiver, the court then attends to specific legal standards that govern the ultimate decision.

Mental health expertise may be relevant in determining a number of the factors that a juvenile court may consider in deciding whether to transfer a juvenile to adult court. In the absence of some threshold demonstration of likely mental impairment, there is no universal legal requirement for routine mental evaluation in waiver cases. When evaluation is deemed necessary, relevant questions may include:

- What psychosocial characteristics are relevant to commission of the offense? Is there a mental disease or defect? What are the important environmental factors?

- What types of change are necessary in the juvenile and/or the environment?

- What is the nature of past intervention efforts, if any, as well as intervention response?

- Is the juvenile committable to an institution for the mentally ill or mentally retarded?

- What factors affect prospects for rehabilitation by use of relevant procedures, services, and facilities currently or reasonably available to the court?

- What factors affect the risk of further criminal behavior (risk assessment)?

- What factors and security measures may affect the likelihood that a program of structured supervision (probation) will be successful?

Under its *parens patriae* powers, a juvenile court may appoint a mental health expert on its own motion (*sua sponte*). It is critical for an expert to determine, at the outset, the scope of the requested examination and whether he or she has been appointed to serve one side (defense/prosecution) or to serve as the court's own expert. Once the scope of an evaluation has been determined, experts should be careful to respect its boundaries. For example, if the court asks only for a determination of whether an individual is mentally retarded, an expert should not evaluate or opine about unrelated issues such as future dangerousness or state of mind at the time of the alleged offense. Defense attorneys may be justifiably leery of mental evaluations ordered by the court and may oppose them, fearing that the expert will simply undertake a fishing expedition that will benefit the prosecution. Although it is typical for court rules to restrict use of statements made during a waiver proceeding in a subsequent adult prosecution, some attorneys may nonetheless advise their clients not to answer certain questions.

For similar reasons, some attorneys may demand that they or their own expert be present at an evaluation. While such arrangements are intrusive by clinical standards, the U.S. Supreme Court has clearly held that forensic mental examinations require adequate notice to defense counsel describing the evaluation and its intended scope and purpose. Examining a defendant without these steps, even with a court order, may violate the Constitution's 6th Amendment right to counsel (similar to the police interrogating a represented suspect without an attorney present). Offering to videotape an examination may be an acceptable substitute for the potentially intrusive presence of a live observer.

Some jurisdictions have rules that prohibit examiners from discussing details of the alleged offense in a waiver examination. Failure or inability to inquire about the offense may sometimes be unfortunate for the youth, because a detailed understanding of the offense and its surrounding motivations may provide an important element of the foundation for an opinion regarding future risk. When prohibited from discussing details of the offense directly, an examiner may be forced to rely on alternative sources of information, including past history of similar offenses and reports of third parties who are familiar with the defendant or are witnesses to the alleged offense.

In most jurisdictions, the legal standards that guide a waiver decision are expressed in terms of factors related to the overlapping issues of *amenability to rehabilitation* and *dangerousness*. Successful rehabilitation is that which is likely to produce a substantial reduction in the risk of recidivism or future harm. Rehabilitation amenability decisions are inextricably linked to time contexts, because a juvenile may be subject to the court's jurisdiction only until he or she reaches majority. Other considerations potentially relevant to judgments about amenability to rehabilitation include the following.

- Individuals who are satisfied with themselves and who view their behaviors as justified are unlikely to work hard at personal change. The examiner should look for ego-dystonic attitudes toward offending behavior. It is important to distinguish public displays of remorse (which may be emotionally shallow) from more mutative but perhaps private experiences of shame and guilt.

- Most psychosocial rehabilitation relies to a significant extent on the formation of a therapeutic alliance. The capacity to enter into a helping relationship is a valuable asset in this endeavor. The examiner should look for interpersonal history demonstrating some capacity for trusting attachment with an adult and some concern about the appraisals of others that would lead to a desire to engage in socially approved behavior in order to receive adult approval. Sometimes, the history of offending behavior may itself provide evidence of desire for attachment, when the behavior appears to reflect a dysfunctional mode of coping with a frustrated desire for acceptance.

- Behavioral patterns that have an early life onset and a chronic generalized course are more difficult to change than are patterns that begin later and represent acute reactions to particular circumstances. The examiner should attempt to characterize the rehabilitation behavioral targets in relation to these dimensions.

- System factors, including both clinical resources and availability of family and community support, may be critical elements in determining amenability to rehabilitation. Amenability to rehabilitation is typically interpreted in the context of rehabilitation resources realistically available to the court. Even if clinically appropriate, recommendations for services that are nonexistent or financially infeasible may carry little weight in the court's eyes. For example, a juvenile whose condition requires psychotropic medication may be a poor candidate for rehabilitation in a system that lacks adequate capacity to provide outpatient psychiatric services.

Dangerousness may refer not only to the risk of recidivism in the community, but also to such issues as the potential for harm to other youths or staff in juvenile detention or rehabilitation facilities; the likelihood of attempts to escape; or the question of whether rehabilitation efforts have reduced the risk of future harm. Such questions are obviously important, but courts may sometimes ask experts to make predictions of dangerousness over impossibly long intervals and without any guarantees of recommended rehabilitation that is integral to the risk estimate.

It is likely that the same methodological caveats that apply to estimating dangerousness in adults should apply to juveniles. That is, efficient and accurate prediction of violent behavior is difficult in general because of the low population base-rate of violent behavior and because of the important role of unpredictable life circumstances that may trigger violence. However, as compared to adult populations, risk assessment of future dangerousness with adolescents has very little empirical foundation. There are no psychological tests that specifically assess the risk of future violence among juveniles. Direct application of specific methods for estimating violence risk with adult offenders is unsubstantiated in juveniles. Indeed, any method for assessing risk with juveniles must consider the life span developmental differences between adolescent-limited offending and lifelong-persistent offending (Moffitt, 1993) and the fact that most adolescents discontinue their delinquent behavior as they approach adulthood (Gottfredson & Hirschi, 1990). As summarized by Quinsey, Harris, Rice, and Cormier (1998), "If one examines the number of male offenders convicted each year as a function of their age, the curve looks like a testosterone output curve, rising steeply with puberty and declining gracefully after young adulthood" (p. 193).

Grisso (1998) usefully outlines the major considerations that should inform an assessment of risk factors potentially relevant to estimating future dangerousness:

1. The evaluation must consider the characteristics of the juvenile in the present and likely future social contexts that the youth will encounter. The predictive value of individual characteristics considered outside social context factors may be markedly reduced. In some cases, the most accurate risk estimate will be expressed in different opinions about the degree of risk for different situations and time frames.

2. The evaluator should recognize the limitations of prediction and offer risk estimates rather than predictions. A risk estimate is a comparison of the juvenile in question to some reference population. For example, whereas a prediction might state, "This youth will reoffend given an opportunity," a risk estimate might state, "Relative to the average juvenile who comes before this court facing similar charges, the degree of risk for recidivism under conditions of unsupervised probation is above average."

3. Specific factors potentially associated with risk of future harm to others include:
   a. Past violent behavior (including chronicity, frequency, recency, context, and severity);

   b. Substance abuse;
   c. Peer and community influences;
   d. Commitment to school and level of academic achievement;
   e. Family stability, quality of attachment to parents, domestic conflict and aggression, and family modeling of substance abuse or antisocial behavior;
   f. Quality of social stressors and social supports, including opportunity to reoffend and access to weapons or other means to reoffend;
   g. Psychological characteristics including personality traits (such as anger, impulsivity, and impaired capacity for empathy) and mental disorders, such as severe affective disorders, Attention-Deficit Hyperactivity Disorder, psychoses, trauma-spectrum disorders, and brain syndromes; and
   h. Expected residential situation (e.g., secure facility vs. community).

The evaluation should specifically identify each factor deemed relevant to increased or decreased risk. The examiner should be prepared to explain why the factor is relevant, how the data on each factor were obtained in this particular case, and what reasoning was employed to combine the factors into an overall assessment of risk.

CONCLUSION

The difference between forensic and clinical roles was well distilled by Strasburger, Gutheil, and Brodsky (1997):

> At a time when forensic experts have been held liable for negligence in evaluation, the therapist who attempts to combine the roles of treating clinician and forensic evaluator embarks upon especially treacherous waters. Even a clinician who testifies as a fact witness may find this seemingly unambiguous role compromised . . . [and] a therapist whose factual testimony displeases the patient may later be charged with negligence for having failed to carry out the investigative tasks of a forensic expert. . . . The clinician who does testify as a fact witness should rigorously maintain role boundaries by declining to perform the functions of an expert witness, such as reviewing the reports or depositions of other witnesses. . . . A therapist who is asked to give expert testimony about a patient can respond. . . . with a disclaimer such as this: "Having observed the patient only from the vantage point of a treating clinician, I have no objective basis for rendering an expert opinion, with a reasonable degree of medical certainty, on a legal as opposed to a clinical question." (p. 454)

This chapter should make clear that forensic services by health professionals differ drastically from services provided for therapeutic reasons, and that therapeutic and legal practice contexts are fundamentally incompatible. Readers who desire more in-depth forensic knowledge should consult major texts such as Melton, Petrila, Poythress, and Slobogin (1997) or Nurcombe and Partlett (1994) as well as specialized journals such as *Law and Human Behavior,* the *Bulletin of the American Academy of Psychiatry and the Law,* the *International Journal of Law and Psychiatry, Behavioral Science and the Law,* and the *Mental and Physical Disability Law Reporter.* Development of specialized professional skills can be fostered via formal training programs and continuing education and supervision as may be found under the auspices of major professional organizations, such as the American Academy of Psychiatry and the Law and the American Academy of Forensic Psychology.

NOTES

1. American Academy of Psychiatry and the Law (1991), *Ethical Guidelines for the Practice of Forensic Psychiatry;* Bloomfield, CT: AAPL. Committee on Ethical Guidelines for Forensic Psychologists (1991), Specialty guidelines for forensic psychologists; *Law and Human Behavior, 15,* 655–665. American Academy of Child and Adolescent Psychiatry (1997), Summary of practice parameters for child custody evaluations, *Journal of the American Academy of Child and Adolescent Psychiatry, 36*(12), 1784–1787. American Academy of Child and Adolescent Psychiatry (1997), Practice parameters for the forensic evaluation of children and adolescents who may have been physically or sexually abused, *Journal of the American Academy of Child and Adolescent Psychiatry, 36,* 423–442. American Psychological Association (1994), Guidelines for child custody evaluations in divorce proceedings, *American Psychologist, 49*(7), 677–680. American Psychological Association Committee on Professional Practice and Standards (1998), *Guidelines for psychological evaluations in child protection matters;* Washington, DC: American Psychological Association. Association of Family and Conciliation Courts (1994), Model Standards of Practice for Child Custody Evaluation, *Family and Conciliation Courts Review, 32,* 504. American Academy of Matrimonial Lawyers, *AAML Standards of Conduct in Family Law Litigation,* available at http://www.aaml.org/boundsof.htm.

2. Yearly statistical reports of the APA Ethics Committee are published in the annual archival issue of *American Psychologist,* usually in July or August. Each report includes a table that among other facts enumerates the numbers of cases arising in the context of custody disputes.

3. For example, see *Howard v. Drapkin,* 271 Cal. Rptr. 893, 222 Cal. App. 3d 843 (Cal. App. 2 Dist. 1990) and *Lavit v. Superior Court of the State of Arizona,* 1-CA-5A920015, Ariz. Ct. App.

4. "In all actions concerning children, whether undertaken by public or private social welfare institutions, courts of law, administrative authorities or legislative bodies, the best interests of the child shall be a primary consideration" (Article 3, United Nations Convention on the Rights of the Child, 1989).

REFERENCES

Achenbach, T. M., McConaughy, S. H., & Howell, C. T. (1987). Child/adolescent behavioral and emotional problems: Implications of cross-informant correlations for situational specificity. *Psychological Bulletin, 101,* 213–232.

American Academy of Psychiatry and the Law. (1989). Ethical guidelines for the practice of forensic psychiatry. In *Membership directory of the American Academy of Psychiatry and the Law* (pp. x–xiii). Bloomfield, CT: Author.

American Psychological Association. (1992). Ethical principles of psychologists and code of conduct. *American Psychologist, 47,* 1597–1611.

American Psychological Association. (1994). Guidelines for child custody evaluations in divorce proceedings. *American Psychologist, 49,* 677–680.

Appelbaum, P. S., & Gutheil, T. G. (1991). *Clinical handbook of psychiatry and the law* (2nd ed.). Baltimore: Williams & Wilkins.

Brown v. Board of Education, 347 U.S. 483 (1954).

Brown v. Board of Education, 349 U.S. 294 (1955).

Bussey, K. (1992). Children's lying and truthfulness: Implications for children's testimony. In S. J. Ceci, M. D. Leichtman, & M. E. Putnick (Eds.), *Cognitive and social factors in early deception* (pp. 89–109). Hillsdale, NJ: Erlbaum.

Ceci, S. J., & Bruck, M. (1995). Jeopardy in the courtroom: A scientific analysis of children's testimony. Washington, DC: APA.

Crosby, C. A., Britner, P. A., Jodl, K. M., & Portwood, S. G. (1995). The juvenile death penalty and the Eighth Amendment: An empirical investigation of societal consensus and proportionality. *Law and Human Behavior, 19*(3), 245–261.

Daubert v. Merrell-Dow Pharmaceuticals, 113 S. Ct. 2786 (1993).

Galatzer-Levy, R., & Kraus, L. (1999). *The scientific basis of child custody decisions.* New York: Wiley.

Gardner, R. (1987). *The parental alienation syndrome and the differentiation between fabricated and genuine child sex abuse.* Trenton, NJ: Creative Therapeutics.

Gottfredson, M., & Hirschi, T. (1990). *A general theory of crime.* Stanford, CA: Stanford University Press.

Green, A. (1986). True and false allegations of sexual abuse in child custody disputes. *Journal of the American Academy of Child Psychiatry, 25,* 449–456.

Greenberg, S. A., & Shuman, D. W. (1997). Irreconcilable conflict between therapeutic and forensic roles. *Professional Psychology: Research and Practice, 28*(1), 50–57.

Grisso, T. (1981). *Juveniles' waiver of rights: Legal and psychological competence.* New York: Plenum.

Grisso, T. (1998). *Forensic evaluation of juveniles.* Sarasota, FL: Professional Resource Exchange Press.

Grisso, T. (1998). *Instruments for assessing understanding and appreciation of Miranda rights.* Sarasota, FL: Professional Resource Exchange Press.

Kalichman, S., & Brosig, C. (1993). Practicing psychologists' interpretations of and compliance with child abuse reporting laws. *Law and Human Behavior, 17*(1), 83–93.

Kent v. U.S., 383 U.S. 541 (1966).

Lewis, M. (1993). The development of deception. In M. Lewis & C. Saarni (Eds.), *Lying and deception in everyday life* (pp. 90–105). New York: Guilford Press.

McIntosh, J., & Prinz, R. (1993). The incidence of alleged sexual abuse in 603 family court cases. *Law and Human Behavior, 17*(1), 95–101.

Melton, G. B., Petrila, J., Poythress, N. G., & Slobogin, C. (1997). *Psychological evaluations for the courts: A handbook for mental health professionals and lawyers* (2nd ed.). New York: Guilford Press.

Miranda v. Arizona, 384 U.S. 436 (1966).

Moffitt, T. E. (1993). Adolescence-limited and life-course-persistent antisocial behavior: A developmental taxonomy. *Psychological Review, 100,* 674–701.

Nurcombe, B., & Partlett, D. F. (1994). *Child mental health and the law.* New York: Free Press.

Oldershaw, L., & Bagby, R. M. (1997). Children and deception. In R. Rogers (Ed.), *Clinical assessment of malingering and deception* (2nd ed., pp. 153–166). New York: Guilford Press.

Perry, N. W., & Wrightsman, L. S. (1991). *The child witness: Legal issues and dilemmas.* Newbury Park, CA: Sage.

Quinsey, V. L., Harris, G. T., Rice, M. E., & Cormier, C. A. (1998). *Violent offenders: Appraising and managing risk.* Washington, DC: PA.

Rogers, R. (1995). *Diagnostic and structured interviewing: A handbook for psychologists.* Odessa, FL: Psychological Assessment Resources.

Rogers, R., Bagby, R. M., & Dickens, S. E. (1992). *Structured interview of reported symptoms: Professional manual.* Odessa, FL: Psychological Assessment Resources.

Rogers, R., & Kelly, K. S. (1997). Denial and misreporting of substance abuse. In R. Rogers (Ed.), *Clinical assessment of malingering and deception* (2nd ed., pp. 108–129). New York: Guilford Press.

Runyon v. Smith, A-1533-97T1, NJ Ct. App., 1999.

Schacht, T. E., & Hanson, G. (1999). The evolving legal climate for school mental health services under the Individuals with Disabilities Education Act. *Psychology in the Schools, 36*(5), 415–426.

Schetky, D. H., & Benedek, E. P. (1992). *Clinical handbook of child psychiatry and the law.* Baltimore: Williams & Wilkins.

Simon, R. I. (1987). *Clinical psychiatry and the law.* Washington, DC: American Psychiatric Press.

Spence, D. P. (1982). *Narrative truth and historical truth: Meaning and interpretation in psychoanalysis.* New York: Norton.

Stanford v. Kentucky, 492 U.S. 361 (1989).

Strasburger, L. H., Gutheil, T. G., & Brodsky, A. (1997). On wearing two hats: Role conflict in serving as both psychotherapist and expert witness. *American Journal of Psychiatry, 154*(4), 448–456.

Thompson v. Oklahoma, 487 U.S. 815 (1988).

Torbet, P., Gable, R., Hurst, H., Montgomery, I., Szymanski, L., & Thomas D. (1996). *State responses to serious and violent juvenile crime.* Washington, DC: Office of Juvenile Justice and Delinquency Prevention.

Chapter 6

THE ASSESSMENT OF MOTOR DEFICITS FOLLOWING PEDIATRIC BRAIN INJURY

R. ERIC ROTH

INTRODUCTION

The incidence of pediatric traumatic brain injury is significant and results in emotional and financial costs to the patient, the family, and society. Appropriately, the research literature is replete with studies that attend neuropsychological consequences of pediatric brain injury, including deficits in memory, behavioral dysregulation, and impaired academic performance. However, relative to these areas of study, research concerning motor sequelae has received little attention. As a result, this chapter will provide a structured review with regard to epidemiology, mechanisms of injury, methods of motor assessment, and current neuropsychological research.

EPIDEMIOLOGY

In testimony provided to the United States Senate Committee on Labor and Human Resources in 1998, former Surgeon General C. Everett Koop reported that one in four children under the age of 14 would be injured to the degree that formal medical attention would be warranted. On a yearly basis this translates to more than 14 million children. According to data compiled by the Center for Disease Control (1990), injury causes approximately 40% of fatalities of children ages 1 to 4 and 70% in children and adolescents ages 5 to 19. Rouse and Eichelberger (1992) report that more than 460,000 to 600,000 children not fatally injured will require hospitalization. Of these children, an estimated 100,000 to 120,000 will be permanently disabled (Center for Disease Control, 1995; Rouse & Eichelberger, 1992).

Between birth and age 19, head injury occurs at a rate of approximately 219 per 100,000 per year (Kraus, Rock, & Hemyari, 1990). However, causes of traumatic brain injury in the majority of cases varies significantly by age. The cause of traumatic brain injury in 56% of cases of children less than 1 year old is assault (Kraus et al.). This figure drops to 5% in children ages 1 to 4. More specific scrutiny of the data, however, suggests that assault accounts for 90% of the most serious brain injuries in this age group. For children ages 5 and older, injuries as a result of motor vehicle accidents and accidents associated with sporting or recreation are the most common causes of death and head injury (Tibbs, Haines, & Parent, 1998). The statistics, which clarify the frequency of motor deficits as a function of brain injuries versus musculoskeletal injuries, are unclear.

NEUROANATOMICAL FOUNDATIONS

A thorough review of neuroanatomy is clearly beyond the need or scope of this chapter. However, to better understand the mechanisms that result in patterns of neuropsychological deficits, it is necessary to have a working understanding of the brain. This section will broadly review the organization of the cerebral cortex, subcortex, protective central nervous system membranes, and cerebral vascularization. Although the spinal cord plays an obvious role in motor output, this chapter focuses more narrowly on the impact of injury to motor areas of the brain itself.

Development and Cellular Structures

From a period just following conception, development of the brain begins. During the earliest stages, cell proliferation and differentiation begin to develop from a rudimentary neural tube. The basic building block of the brain is the *neuron*. Neurons are filamentous units that serve to conduct bioelectrical information throughout the nervous system. Although neurons are developed in various shapes, sizes, and lengths based on their purpose, they consist of four primary components. The *dendrite* is a branching root-like structure that receives input from other neurons. The *cell body* collects information and conducts that information down the *axon*, a fiber that projects toward other neurons in the nervous system. At the end of neurons lies the axon terminal, the site from which various neurotransmitters are released to transmit a signal or message to the receptor sites on contiguous dendrites and cell bodies. Among the cell bodies are *glial cells*, which provide a range of functions including structural support, insulation, and clean up and production of cerebral spinal fluid. Coating the axonal projections in *myelin*, a fatty substance that provides insulation and improves conduction between cells. The adult brain weighs about 3 pounds and may be composed of 10 billion (Beaumont, 1988) to 1 trillion (Young, 1985) cells.

Cortical Organization

The maturing brain (Figure 6.1) is composed of an upper layer or mantle called the *cortex*. On visual examination the cortex appears as a highly convoluted mantle of gray matter. The deep fissures observable on the surface are referred to as a *sulci*, while the observable folds are *gyri*. These landmarks denote the various cortical areas or lobes.

The cortex is the most complex and highly organized aspect of the brain. Although the cortex comprises approximately 80% of total brain volume, it is only 1.5 to 3 mm thick (Kolb & Wishaw, 1990, p. 15). It is composed of four primary lobes. The *frontal lobe* comprises approximately one third of the cortical mass. It extends from the frontal pole to the central sulcus. The more anterior areas of the lobe are typically considered

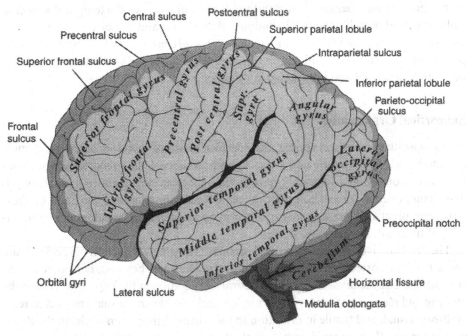

Figure 6.1   Lateral Surface of the Brain

to be involved in mental processes such as planning, organizing, and inhibiting response. The posterior portion of the frontal lobe, which is bounded by the central sulcus, is referred to as the *precentral gyrus* or *primary motor area*. In this area all parts of the body are represented in terms of motor homunculus. This area will be discussed more in depth later.

The *parietal lobes* are located in mirror fashion in both of the cerebral hemispheres. The boundaries are commonly considered the central sulcus anteriorly, the parieto-occipital sulcus posteriorly, and the preoccipital notch inferiorly. The dominant and nondominant hemispheres of the parietal lobes differ significantly in function. The dominant lobe, most often the left hemisphere, has general responsibilities for complex neuropsychological functions such as writing, arithmetic, and praxis, or the ability to carry out sequential tasks correctly. The nondominant parietal lobe is broadly responsible for neuropsychological functions including facial recognition, constructional praxis (i.e., the ability to copy designs or construct multidimensional objects), visuo-perceptual abilities, and the ability to be aware of one's strengths and weaknesses. The most important function of the parietal lobe for the purpose of this chapter concerns sensory/perceptual abilities. The postcentral gyrus or primary somesthetic area lies just posterior of the central sulcus. As with the primary motor area, all parts of the body are represented in terms of a sensory homunculus. Although impairments in sensation are not a focus of this chapter, the integration of sensory and motor abilities in daily functional motor activities is clear.

The *temporal lobes* are represented bilaterally and are located inferior to the lateral sulcus and anterior to the preoccipital notch. The dominant hemisphere of the temporal lobe regulates expression and comprehension of speech. It is also associated with verbal learning and memory. The nondominant hemisphere of the temporal lobe controls aspects of speech processes including volume, tone, and prosody. It is also viewed as regulating nonverbal learning and memory. The *occipital lobe* of the brain lies most posteriorly. Visuosensory information is provided along the visual tracts and is believed to be analyzed and interpreted in this area.

Subcortical Organization

Lying beneath the cortical mantle are complex series of interconnected areas most commonly referred to as the *subcortex*. As with the cortex, the subcortex is not a continuous or homogeneous organ. Typically the subcortex is thought to have three primary components: forebrain, midbrain, and hindbrain (Figure 6.2). Each of these structures plays a vital role in motor functioning and tends to be vulnerable to the effects of traumatic brain injury.

The *forebrain* is comprised of several sections. The greatest portion of the forebrain consists of the cortex itself. The remaining structures are, however, considered to be subcortical. The *thalamus* is a primary neural relay station in the brain, involved in the sending and receiving of sensory information. Relay nuclei in the thalamus act to relay auditory, visual, and tactile information to the cortex. Association nuclei in the thalamus are indirectly connected with frontal and parietal association cortices. The *hypothalamus* is primarily responsible for regulation of homeostatic functions and control over the autonomic nervous system. It also receives olfactory information and projects information to the reticular formation. Several relay nuclei are collectively referred to as the *basal ganglia*. Broadly, this portion of the subcortex is responsible for complex motor integration and planning. Toward this end two of the nuclei, the *putamen* and *caudate nucleus*, receive topographically organized input from the cerebral cortex, and subsequently project this input forward to the *globus pallidus*. From the globus pallidus information is sent to the thalamus and to nuclei in the brain stem. The *limbic system* is a set of structures that are the substrate of emotional functioning and memory.

The *midbrain* has two primary divisions: the tectum and tegmentum. Together these structures form the roof and floor of the cerebral aqueduct. Throughout the midbrain are a series of nuclei including the red nucleus and the substantial nigra. The red nu-

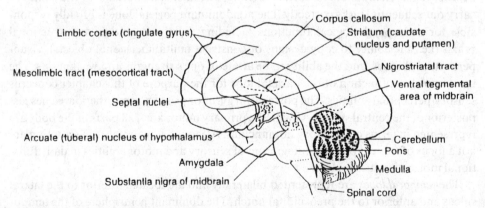

Figure 6.2   Medical View through the Center of the Brain

cleus receives afferent projections from the cerebellum and sends efferent projections to the spinal cord. The substantial nigra has connections to and from the basal ganglia, previously noted to be involved in motor integration and planning.

The third portion of the subcortex, the *hindbrain,* plays a prominent role in motor functions. A portion of the *pons* houses three major fiber tracts, which interconnect with the cerebellum and the cerebral cortex. The *cerebellum,* like the cerebral cortex, has two fundamentally parallel hemispheres and is composed of three phylogenetically differentiated lobes. Together, the cerebellar lobes impact gait coordination, muscle and postural tone, and integration of complex voluntary movements. The *medulla* is the most caudal aspect of the hindbrain and is an extension of the spinal cord. Through the medulla runs a complex set of fiber tracts connecting the cortex, subcortex, and spinal cord.

Protecting the Brain

The brain as a whole sits suspended in the cranial vault surrounded by cerebral spinal fluid. Three protective membranes encapsulate the brain, the dura, arachnoid, and pia mater. The *dura* itself is composed of two thin layers. An outer or periosteal layer has many blood vessels and nerves and adheres to the cranium. The inner layer is referred to as the meninges. The *pia mater* is the innermost layer and closely follows the contours of the sulci and gyri. Existing between the dura and pia mater is the *arachnoid* layer. Unlike the pia mater, the arachnoid layer does not follow the convolutions of the cerebral cortex. The area between the arachnoid membrane and the pia mater is called the subarachnoid space. This area is filled with cerebral spinal fluid and serves to absorb the shock and movement of the brain within the cranial vault. The size of this space varies by area of the brain. Over the convexities of the cerebral cortex the space is rather small, but areas around the hindbrain contain significantly larger spaces.

Vascularization

Blood is supplied to the brain via the internal carotid artery, which rapidly branches into the anterior, middle, and posterior cerebral arteries. Each of these arteries in turn has multiple branches, which vascularize the brain. Overall the brain requires nearly one quart of oxygen-rich blood per minute to maintain normal functioning. Once the blood has been depleted of its oxygen and additional nutrients, it is directed into venous structures, many of which run through the subdural space and back toward the lungs.

NEUROANATOMY OF MOTOR FUNCTIONING

Motor tracts, or pathways, begin in the precentral gyrus. This area is topographically organized and can be mapped into motor (and sensory) homunculi (Figure 6.3). The homunculi yield distorted representations of the human body. The distortions reveal the disproportionate amount of motor cortex associated with the face and hands, the areas associated with the most complex motor movement.

From the precentral gyrus the projections are complex, and an extensive explanation

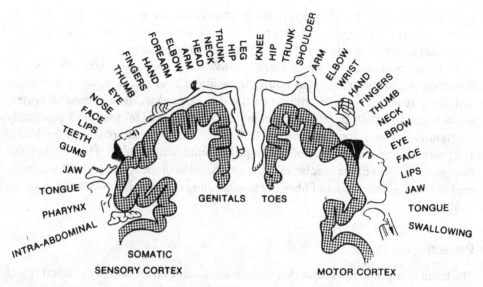

Figure 6.3   Functional Locations on Sensory and Motor Strips

is beyond the needs or goals of this chapter. However, it is important to understand that there are parallel but interactive systems providing gross, fine, and postural motor controls. Projections from the cerebral cortex may be directly connected to the basal ganglia, cerebellum, thalamus, brain stem, or spinal cord. The vast projections among the basal ganglia, thalamus, cerebellum, and spinal cord serve to produce a rapid series of movements that allow us to carry out any number of simultaneous and vastly complex motor behaviors. Such complexities of motor movement are, of course, not present at the time of birth. Twitchell (1965) provided a description of the longitudinal development of motor development in the grasp response in infants. Twitchell noted that motor movement advanced through a sequence of observable developmental stages. Prior to birth the infant's movements comprise all aspects of the body simultaneously (whole body movements). Following birth is the development of the grasp reflex. Shortly thereafter the infant demonstrates the ability to move its arm in a scooping motion. It appears that this type of motor behavior does not occur until around 1 month of age. Between the ages of 1 month and about 4 months the infant will begin to develop a whole grasp response in which all parts of the hand simultaneously attempt to hold an object that comes into contact with the hand. From 3 to 4 months and upwards to 11 months of age the infant begins to orient the reach and grasp response if there has been stimulation to that hand. Between 8 and 11 months a pincer grasp develops and represents the development of a well-integrated fine motor behavior that increasingly integrates sensoriperceptual information to improve precision.

This progression of motor skills does not occur by chance. It appears that the progression of motor behaviors has a strong but not absolute relationship to the progression of myelination in the brain. Work by Yakovlev and LeCours (1967; see also Spreen, Tupper, Risser, Tuokko, & Edgell) correlates the degree of myelination and specific developmental behaviors. At birth motor roots are heavily myelinated and sensory roots and cerebellar tracts are only moderately myelinated. Subsequently, reflex actions are observed, and integrated postural controls and movement are not. By 6 months the infant can grasp with either hand, can roll over, and may be able to support his body weight if standing with assistance. These behaviors are correlated with highly myelinated ascending fibers from the spinal cord, cerebellar tracts, and only a moderately myelinated corpus callosum and primary motor tracts. In contrast, a 5-year-old's motor system is well myelinated with the exception of the corpus callosum.

MECHANISMS OF INJURY

Many of the early theories of head injury were based on the general concepts of coup and contre coup effects. That is, the area of direct impact (coup) and the area of the brain opposite the impact (contre coup) were considered to be the areas most likely to sustain damage. In the eighteenth century this general brain injury paradigm was understood in terms of the vibration theory (Pudenz & Sheldon, 1946). This theory suggested that vibrations began at the point of impact and moved across the brain, creating damage at the contre coup site. Russell's (1932) displacement theory was similar but indicated that damage at the contre coup site was caused by a vacuum-like effect as the brain was pulled away from the skull.

More recent research indicates that strong rotational forces contribute to various aspects of brain injury. Holbourn (1943, 1944) theorized that rotational acceleration produces a shearing and straining of brain tissue as one layer of brain substance slides against another, especially along the cortical-subcortical boundary. Similarly, injury occurs as the brain slides against the inner surface of the skull. Research with a variety of animal and gelatin models (Pudenz & Sheldon, 1946; Ommaya, Boretoz, & Beile, 1969) lends support the Holbourn's work.

The mechanisms that create the actual damage to the brain can be broadly classified as *mechanical injury* and *neurochemical injury*. The two main mechanical phenomena occur secondary to contact (i.e., friction) and inertial loading (i.e., acceleration) forces. Contact injury refers to situations in which the cortex is damaged against the bony aspects of the interior of the skull. As previously noted, the aspects of the skull in the vicinity of the orbital frontal and temporal poles (e.g., lesser wing of the sphenoid) have rough protuberances that can easily damage the cortex when contact occurs. Coup injuries, and to a lesser degree contre coup injuries, can result in hemorrhages and resulting hematomas (Bigler, 1988). A subarachnoid hemorrhage is the most common pathologic consequence of head trauma found at autopsy (Lezak, 1995). The subarachnoid space becomes larger at different points around the brain and forms subarachnoid cisterns. Within many of these cisterns are arteries supplying blood to the brain. When blood fills these cisterns it acts as an irritant on the arteries, which can subsequently result in occlusion of the vessels and loss of necessary blood flow. Epidural and subdural hemorrhages can result in the development of hematoma, which can produce space-occupying lesions. Such lesions can lead to focal neurological deficits or diffuse injury caused by a mass effect resulting in the shifting or compression of the brain tissues. Although epidural hemorrhages are more commonly associated with skull fractures, subdural hemorrhages tend to occur secondary to tearing of the bridging vessels.

There are several mechanical effects related to the influence of accelerative forces

(Katz, 1992). Strain deformations occur due to tensile forces. Neural tissue is, in effect, stretched until it tears. Acceleration forces can also result in compression and destruction of brain tissue. And finally, shearing effects occur when one layer of tissue slides against another. Any of these processes can result in diffuse axonal injury (DAI) or more focal contusions.

A second mechanism of injury is neurochemical injury. Cerebral blood flow is the primary agent of metabolism in the brain (Bigler, 1988; Katz, 1992). Oxygen and blood sugars, among others, are delivered via the cerebral arteries while the cerebral veins remove toxins. Ischemia, a loss of blood flow to the brain, therefore results in both an interrupted delivery of requisite oxygen and the accumulation of toxic by-products (Bigler). Jennett and Teasdale (1981) note that significant neuronal dysfunction can occur within seconds as metabolic energy (primarily oxygen) is interrupted. Studies (Barclay, Zemcov, Richert, & Blass, 1985; Jennett & Teasdale) indicate that more than 91% of all patients sustaining traumatic brain injury continue to have reduced blood flow resulting in a chronic head injury syndrome.

It is relatively unlikely that closed head injury will result in only mechanical or metabolic injury. In general both types of injuries will be present, though one may be primarily mechanical injuries with secondary metabolic effects. For example, rotational acceleration forces on the brain cause injury secondary to mechanical shearing of neural tissue, but can also result in tearing and subsequent bleeding in cortical arteries (Katz, 1992), reducing necessary blood flow or potentially causing mass effects from pooled blood. Research by Povlishock and Coburn (1989) indicates that this process also occurs at a cellular level. This study reports that there are delayed autodestructive processes that, within hours to days after even a mild head injury, lead to axonal stretching and the formation of retraction balls. The swelling and stretching of the cells results in abnormal axonal transport and eventually complete rupture of the cells.

EVALUATION OF MOTOR FUNCTIONING IN CHILDREN

Systematic neuropsychological evaluation of pediatric motor functions can be traced back to Ralph Reitan's (1969) Reitan-Indiana Test Battery for Children ages 5 to 8 and the Halstead-Reitan Neuropsychological Test Battery for Children ages 9 to 14 (Reitan & Davidson, 1974). Standard aspects of motor evaluation for both batteries include the Grip Strength Test and Finger Tapping Test. In the former the child is directed to squeeze a hand dynamometer with both the dominant and nondominant hands for several trials to maximize reliability. The Grip Strength Test yields information regarding hand strength. In the Finger Tapping Test the child is asked to use his or her index finger to tap a counter device over several trials. Both the dominant and nondominant hands are tested to provide a measure of fine motor speed and dexterity. The Marching Test is added to the Reitan-Indiana Battery. On this test children are asked to touch a series of connected circles rapidly. Overall the Marching Test is viewed as a measure of upper extremity motor functions and coordination. As part of a larger battery of tests, these tests yield valuable information about lateralization and localization of neuropsychological deficits. Individually they provide important information about gross motor strength and fine motor functioning.

The Bayley Scales of Infant Development (Bayley, 1969) also utilize a battery approach to the evaluation of cognitive and motor delays in children up to 30 months of age. The battery was developed to detect the presence of underlying cognitive or motor deficits in children with risk factors for dysfunction. The motor scale evaluates domains including crawling, sitting, walking, and grasping. Examiners utilize standard stimuli to elicit specific motor or cognitive behaviors. Though the Bayley was developed to identify underlying disabilities in children, there have been efforts (Mayo, 1991) to use it to measure the outcomes of physical therapy in children with cerebral palsy.

A more recent contribution to the neuropsychological evaluation of motor impairments is the NEPSY (Korkman, Kirk, & Kemp, 1998), a comprehensive developmental neuropsychological battery for children ages 3 to 12. Within the sensorimotor domain, children are evaluated for fine motor speed and ability to imitate hand positions and to carry out a series of rhythmic motor movements. Sensori perceptual abilities and visuomotor abilities are also evaluated. The NEPSY was validated on a small group of children with moderate and severe traumatic brain injury. Significant deficits were found for the sensorimotor domain as a whole and more specifically on measures of finger tapping speed and visuomotor integration. Overall, the NEPSY has good reliability and validity and demonstrates some promise in evaluating neuropsychological functions in children, including motor abilities.

At this time one of the most comprehensive batteries for assessing motor functions in children is the Bruininks-Oseretsky Test of Motor Proficiency (BOTMP; Bruininks, 1978). The test is individually administered and targets children ages 4.5 to 14.5 years. The test consists of 46 items divided into eight subtests: Running Speed and Agility, Balance, Bilateral Coordination, Strength, Upper-Limb Coordination, Response Speed, Visual-Motor Control, and Upper-Limb Speed and Dexterity. A complete battery yields Gross Motor Composite, Fine Motor Composite, and Battery Composite scores. Composite scores are expressed as normalized standard scores with a mean of 50 and standard deviation of 10. Reliability and validity are good, and the battery has been successfully utilized in evaluation of children with traumatic brain injury.

In addition to the above tests, many other tests include tests of motor functions as a portion of a larger neuropsychological battery. Examples include the Luria-Nebraska Neuropsychological Battery—Childrens Revision (Golden, 1986) and the McCarthy Scales of Children's Abilities (McCarthy, 1972). Other batteries have a more focused evaluation of motor abilities. The System of Multicultural Pluralistic Assessment (Mercer & Lewis, 1978) utilizes developmentally appropriate motor tasks to evaluate a range of motor abilities in children ages 5 to 12. The Alberta Infant Motor Scale (Piper & Darah, 1994) is an observational assessment scale developed to evaluate gross motor maturation in children 18 months old or younger. Although it appears to have good reliability and validity in detecting abnormal functioning, there appears to be little evidence of its validity for ongoing evaluation and treatment planning (Ketelaar & Vermeer, 1998).

MOTOR IMPAIRMENT ASSOCIATED WITH BRAIN INJURY

Despite the prevalence of brain injury and the associated cost and emotional turmoil, there has been relatively little interest in evaluating motor performance deficits in children, and even less in infants and toddlers. Relatively early studies (Levin & Eisenberg, 1979; Gagnon, Forget, Sullivan, & Friedman, 1998) strongly supported the notion that children experience motor deficits even after mild head injury. Nevertheless, complaints of motor symptoms are frequently attributed to psychological factors without additional examination of subtle but real motor impairments (McCordie, 1988). This section will attempt to review the limited but most current literature pertaining to issues of impact of injury severity and age of onset.

Ewing-Cobbs and colleagues (Ewing-Cobbs, Miner, Fletcher, & Levin, 1989) sought to evaluate the effects of closed head injury (CHI) on intellectual, language, and motor functioning in infants and toddlers. Their study evaluated 21 children ages 4 months to 5 years. Subjects were initially evaluated at approximately 30 days following the injury and again an average of 8 months later. Potential subjects who had a history of neuropsychological disorders, developmental delays, abuse, or penetrating head injuries, or who were non-English speakers, were excluded from the study. The youngest subjects (ages 4–42 months) were evaluated with the Bayley Motor Scale, and older children (ages 42–72 months) were examined with the McCarthy Motor Scale. Results of the study support a positive correlation between injury severity and motor performance deficits. Children categorized as having severe CHIs were more severely impaired on motor measures than children categorized as having mild to moderate CHIs. Comparison of the baseline evaluation with the follow-up exam indicates that the rate of recovery is equal for children with mild to moderate injuries and those with severe injuries. However, children with severe injuries continue to demonstrate statistically significant impairments at the time of the follow-up evaluation, whereas children in the mild to moderate category are generally functioning within a normal developmental range.

Advancing this work further, Jaffe headed a research team (Jaffe et al., 1993) that looked at 94 children with varying degrees of brain injury shortly after presentation to an emergency room and then again one year later. Factors including low premorbid intelligence, psychiatric history, prior traumatic brain injury, history of physical abuse, and prior motor impairments were controlled for well. Subjects were matched with children of similar age, premorbid achievement, and behavior, as well as similar family demographic variables. Jaffe's team evaluated a wide range of cognitive abilities as well as motor performance. The measures of motor ability showed a significant association of change across the year. However, at the follow-up they found no correlation between injury severity and performance on four of their motor task variables, coding, name writing, finger tapping speed, and grip strength. In contrast, there was a significant correlation with the parent-reported measures of functional, fine, and gross motor skills.

Seventy-two of the original children were evaluated 3 years after the injury (Fay, Jaffe, Polissar, Liao, Rivera, & Martin, 1994). The authors noted that parent reports from the Woodcock Johnson Scale of Independent Behavior continue to demonstrate a relationship between both fine and gross motor skills and injury severity. Although there was no correlation between injury severity and performance on measures of fine motor speed as evaluated by the Finger Tapping Test at 1 year, there was a significant correlation at the 3 year follow-up. Explanations for such differences are not clear and may be a statistical artifact more so than a functional impairment. No correlations were found for severity of injury and gross motor ability.

Prior studies tend to indicate a consistent relationship between severity of injury and degree of impairments found on motor testing. Parental reports appear to suggest functional, fine, and gross motor impairments, and standardized evaluation tends to suggest a presence of statistically significant fine motor impairments and gross motor abilities comparable to matched cohorts. The pattern of results supports the presence of residual impairments though methods of measurement may not have been adequately sensitive. Measurements of fine motor speed and hand strength are sensitive to lesions in the motor cortex but may not be sensitive to significant but subtle deficits in motor integration. In a study by Chaplin, Deitz, and Jaffe (1993), 14 children with histories of traumatic brain injury and a loss of consciousness of at least 24 hours were evaluated with the BOTMP. The evaluation was completed at least 16 months after injury (range 16 to 49 months) and was compared to a cohort group. Children in the normal group performed within normal limits on both the Fine and Gross Motor Composites. Children with TBI performed significantly worse on measures comprising the Gross Motor Composite, but there was no significant difference between the TBI group and the normal group for the Fine Motor Composite. In an analysis of BOTMP subtests, significant differences were observed on four subtests from the Gross Motor Composite and one from the Fine Motor Composite. The common factor among the subtests is response speed.

Gagnon and colleagues (Gagnon, Forget, Sullivan, & Friedman, 1998) also utilized the BOTMP to evaluate motor deficits following pediatric traumatic brain injury. Twenty-eight children between the ages 5 to 15 were evaluated 13 to 18 days following a mild TBI. More than 40% of the children with a mild TBI demonstrated below average performance on three of the eight motor domains evaluated by the BOTMP. Subjects performed within this range on tasks of running speed and agility, response speed, and balance. In her discussion of the results, Gagnon underscores the fact that only three of the subjects performed more than 2 standard deviations below the mean, and no child performed more than 3 standard deviations below the mean. Overall, children with a mild TBI have a trend toward motor performance deficits on speeded tasks and balance, although only 7 to 11% of the sample was considered to have a statistically clear performance deficit. Upon closer examination of the data the authors suggested that factors including performance speed, reaction time, and deficits in balance account for the core motor deficits observed on the BOTMP. Observations of balance deficits are significant. One balance test directs children to stand on one foot and close their eyes. The authors believed deficits on this single item contributed to systematically lower test scores. The test intentionally targets both proprioceptive and vestibular components of this motor control, underscoring the integrative nature of motor impairments.

SPECIAL TOPICS

Skull Fractures and Open Head Injuries

As was previously noted, there has been limited research regarding the relationships between traumatic brain injury and subsequent motor impairments in a pediatric population. The literature that is available largely utilizes subjects with closed head injuries. Subsequently, the available research regarding motor deficits and skull fractures or open head injuries is all the more limited.

Tibbs, Haines, and Parent (1998) note that a child's age plays a significant role in the type of skull fractures that may occur. In infants, the open areas (fontanelles) are areas where the brain has limited protection and is most vulnerable. However, the skull is less rigid, and skull fractures tend to be less common in infants. As children mature the skull becomes more thick and rigid. Consequently, as children get older they are increasingly likely to experience true fractures. In an examination of 530 cases of pediatric head injury, Ersahin, Mutluer, Mirzai, and Palali (1996) found that depressed skull fractures were present in 7 to 10% of all cases of pediatric head injury and that depressed skull fractures accounted for 15 to 25% of skull fractures in children. Both linear and depressed skull fractures are typically associated with blunt head trauma incurred from falls, motor vehicle accidents, assault, or falling or thrown objects.

The type of neuropsychological deficits and the severity of that deficit is primarily related to the location of the insult and the degree to which the skull is depressed. The severity of the deficits is associated with the degree to which the fracture tears the protective membranes, involves focal damage to brain parenchyma, and disrupts metabolic processes. In cases where there are focal depressed skull fractures in the absence of diffuse axonal injury, motor impairments will most commonly be associated within trauma to the area of the calvarium immediately over the precentral gyrus (primary motor area). Fractures that occur to the base of the skull are typically associated with severe trauma in which a broad range of neuropsychological deficits may be present. In such cases it may be difficult to determine the degree to which motor deficits are a result of the fracture or diffuse axonal injury that can accompany severe trauma.

Child Abuse

Injury inflicted in the form of child abuse accounts for a significant percentage of cases of traumatic brain injury, especially for children younger than 5 years old. In a comprehensive study, Ewing-Cobbs et al. (1998) evaluated 40 children ages 4 weeks to 6 years admitted for either inflicted or noninflicted brain injury. The results demonstrated that children with inflicted injuries had extensive signs of preexisting brain injury, evidenced by cerebral atrophy, ex vacuo ventriculomegaly, subdural hematoma, and a higher rate of seizures. In contrast, the presence of epidural hematomas and shear injuries was found only in children with noninflicted brain trauma, as was the presence of internal organ injuries. Intraparenchymal hemorrhage, edema, infarction, cranial nerve injury, hemiparesis, and skull fractures were found with similar frequency in children with both inflicted and noninflicted injuries, thus limiting diagnostic specificity.

Ratings of motor ability were achieved with the Bayley Scales of Infant Development—Second Edition (Bayley, 1993) for the youngest children and with the McCarthy Scales of Children's Abilities motor scales (McCarthy, 1972) for children 43 to 71 months of age. Approximately 25% of both inflicted and noninflicted TBI samples were within the deficient range. These results tend to suggest that motor deficits are found around the time of injury, though with equal frequency in inflicted and noninflicted brain injury.

What is not clear is the degree to which such motor deficits maintain themselves over time. This study provides indications that there are both significant similarities and differences regarding the mechanisms of injury in inflicted and noninflicted injury. However, it is not known whether the motor deficits seen in both groups are a function of the common frequency of injury secondary to shear and infarction, or differentially caused by epidural versus subdural injuries.

Sports Injuries

Sports injuries in general and, more specifically, brain injuries from sports activities have garnered an increasing amount of research interest. In a study of 23,566 high school athletes (Powell & Barber-Foss, 1999) mild TBI was found in 1,219 (5.5%) of the cases reviewed. Of these, football accounted for 63.4% of cases, wrestling 10.5%, girls' soccer 6.2%, boys' soccer 5.7%, girls' basketball 5.2%, boys' basketball 4.2%, softball 2.1%, baseball 2.1%, field hockey 1.1%, and volleyball 0.50%. Based on these figures, the authors predicted that nearly 63,000 mild TBIs from sports activities occur yearly. In the vast majority of more current studies (Ferguson, Mittenberg, Barone, & Schneider, 1999; Harmon, 1999; Powell & Barber-Foss, 1999; Daniel, Olesniewicz, Reeves, Bleiberg, Thatcher, & Salazar, 1999; Roberts, Brust, & Leonard, 1999), concussions or mild diffuse cognitive deficits are the focus. Efforts to find well-constructed studies or reviews regarding motor deficits following sports-related brain injuries in children were not successful.

Interpolation of the available data suggests that motor impairments as a function of sports-related injuries are not common. Powell and Barber-Foss (1999) revealed only 6 cases of subdural hematoma and intracranial injury related to football accidents. These types of injuries clearly have a higher rate of motor deficits than does simple concussion. Nevertheless, more specific research regarding motor deficits following sports-related traumatic brain injury is an area in need of study.

PSYCHOLOGICAL CONSEQUENCES OF BRAIN INJURY

Depending on the type and severity of pediatric brain injury (i.e., focal contusion vs. diffuse axonal injury), the sequelae can be quite varied. Lehr (1990) noted that there are three general patterns of presentation. First, there may be acute deficits that resolve with no residual impairments. Second, there may be gradual resolution of the acute impairments with notable static deficits remaining across the lifespan. Finally, initial impairments may appear insignificant and later become more prominent as environmental demands increase in complexity. The types of deficits may be present as cognitive impairments, including declines in intellect, memory functions, and higher-order problem solving (Dalby & Obrzut, 1991), and as behavioral disruption (Dalby & Obrzut, 1991; Bergland & Thomas, 1991).

The consequences of brain injury can result in more specific psychological effects as well. Bergland and Thomas (1991) evaluated adolescents' emotional reactions to brain injury. They note that adolescent awareness of their cognitive, emotional, behavioral, and physical impairments results in feeling different and apart from others. The degree to which underlying physical limitations, overt physical differences (e.g., scarring, hemiplegia, use of a wheelchair), behavioral disturbance, and cognitive impairments may impact development of self and self-esteem is unclear.

METHODS OF INTERVENTION

Although treatment of emotional and cognitive sequelae of pediatric brain injury clearly falls to the expertise of the psychologist and neuropsychologist, treatment of motor impairments typically goes to other disciplines, including physical therapy and occupational therapy. Where musculoskeletal impairments are noted, the physical therapist may develop a program of treatment including positioning, joint mobilization, prolonged static stretching, serial castings, and electrical stimulation (Blaskey and Jennings, 1999). The authors recommend that higher level goals be based on prior level of functional ability and the interests of the child. Methods of therapy utilize activities in which functional abilities are the focus. Ambulation and more complex motor integration activities should be practiced in activities known to the child, including various aspects of play and functional routines found at home or school.

The psychologist's role will be directed at patient and family education, issues of compliance with treatment or environmental demands, behavior management, family counseling and psychotherapy with the child, and staff training. Such interventions are sculpted to meet the needs of the patient and family and are highly dependent on patient-family resources (e.g., level of education, opportunity to be involved with daily therapy processes, number of caregivers, stability of the family unit, etc.) and patient variables (e.g., age/developmental level, cognitive abilities, severity of behavioral disturbance, and personal interests/goals).

CASE STUDY

The patient, KL, is a female, aged 9 years 4 months, who was involved in a motor vehicle accident. According to available police records and the report of parents, her mother was traveling at approximately 45 mph when she swerved to avoid an animal running across the road; her car left the pavement and struck large tree. KL was initially restrained in the rear passenger-side seat. However, in the minutes before the accident she had removed her seatbelt to adjust her clothing. As a result of the impact, KL was thrown against the windshield. KL and her mother were found unconscious at the scene by residents of the area who had witnessed the accident. Emergency medical technicians were contacted and found KL breathing but unconscious. She was transported to the local trauma center, where she regained consciousness approximately 45 minutes after the accident (her mother had regained consciousness before the EMT's arrival). Computed tomography of the brain suggested multiple areas of small punctate hemorrhages and a focal small left fronto-temporal subdural hematoma. There was no indication of a midline shift. Although KL had suffered multiple abrasions and a laceration to the right frontal area, there were no significant orthopedic injuries. Gross motor testing was evaluated and considered intact. The patient was admitted and followed in the hospital for five days. During this time the subdural hematoma resolved without surgical intervention. Mental status testing suggested grossly intact cognition prior to discharge.

Following discharge the patient and her family chose to pursue a two-week period of home-bound schooling followed by a gradual reintroduction to school over a period of two weeks. Approximately three weeks after her full-time return to school, the parents met with teachers who reported that KL's thinking continued to be mildly slowed, and that her ability to recall new information was noticeably decreased compared to baseline. As an aside, the teacher also reported that KL was less effective in playground athletics and seemed to fall more often.

Based on teachers' input, KL was referred for a neuropsychological evaluation. Although she was given a comprehensive battery of tests, only the results of motor testing will be reviewed here. KL was seen for evaluation approximately 16 weeks following the accident. As a component of that exam she was administered the BOTMP. Her Gross Motor Composite Score was 73, representing performance at the 54th percentile. The Fine Motor Composite was 55, reflecting performance at the 69th percentile. Her overall Battery Composite was 54, representing motor abilities at the 66th percentile. Closer examination of subtest scores indicates that she was functioning in the High range for Bilateral Coordination and Strength, the Above Average range for Upper-Limb Speed and Dexterity, and the Average range for Response Speed and Visual-Motor Control. Examination of her performance for Running Speed and Agility reveals Below Average ability (6–11th percentile) while her score for Balance is within the Low range (less than 4th percentile).

Focused intervention was conducted by both physical therapy and neuropsychology departments. KL was seen for several sessions to improve balance and motor speed. Significant training was conducted with the patient and family to ensure good carry-over of home-based interventions. KL's mother reported significant guilt with regard to the accident and KL's injuries. Beginning with the acute stages of hospitalization, her parenting approach had become more passive. As an apparent result, KL had become more attention-seeking and was initially allowed to forgo normal household chores and school assignments while getting more focused attention than before the accident. KL's father expressed frustration over a lack of unified parenting approach. He believed it was beginning to cause an atypical amount of stress in the marriage. KL's parents were seen for eight counseling sessions toward the goal of increasing their knowledge of head injury as well as improving their communication and efficacy in parenting matters. Both were active participants and were able to effect changes in their parenting approach in just a few meetings.

KL was seen for a routine follow-up at 1 year after the injury. Her parents indicated that her cognitive skills were better and that her grades were at premorbid levels across the board. Consistent feedback from the teacher appeared to indicate a gradual resolution of the motor deficits. Repeat assessment with the BOTMP revealed average or better performance across all subtests with the exception of Balance. KL continued to score near the upper limits of the Below Average range in this area. At 18 months, KL's pediatrician requested another follow-up although no overt symptoms were present. At this follow-up KL scored in the Average or better range in all motor domains.

SUMMARY

Each year several hundred thousand children experience a traumatic brain injury. In the youngest of these children, abuse appears to be the primary agent of injury; in older children, accidents, especially with motor vehicles, play a more primary role. Over the years the research has clearly established that mechanisms of injury result in a high rate of focal injury to the developing frontal and temporal lobes in addition to the presence of diffuse axonal injury. Neuropsychologically, these children have higher rates of impaired memory and learning, behavioral difficulties, and academic problems. In the past decade there has been some increased focus on the rates and severity of motor deficits following brain injury. At this time the results seem to suggest that motor deficits are observed with all levels of severity and that recovery of motor deficits occurs at an equal rate across severity levels. Evidence also appears to suggest that gross motor disturbance after a substantial period of time, even with severe brain injury, is not significant. The validity and reliability of these findings, however, require further investigation. The instruments traditionally utilized by neuropsychologists may not sufficiently capture the dynamic quality of motor speed, coordination, and balance. It will be important for future investigation to implement longitudinal or cross-sectional models in conjunction with a comprehensive standardized motor battery.

REFERENCES

Barclay, L., Zemcov, A., Richert, W., & Blass, J. P. (1985). Cerebral blood flow decrements in chronic head injury syndrome. *Biological Psychiatry, 20,* 146–157.

Bayley, N. (1969). *Bayley Scales of Infant Development.* New York: Psychological Corp.

Bayley, N. (1993). *Bayley Scales of Infant Development* (2nd ed.). San Antonio, TX: Psychological Corp.

Beaumont, J. G. (1988). *Understanding neuropsychology.* Oxford, England: Basil Blackwell.

Bergland, M. M., & Thomas, K. R. (1991). Psychosocial issues following severe head injury in adolescence: Individual and family perceptions. *Rehabilitation Counseling Bulletin, 35,* 5–22.

Bigler, E. D. (1988). *Diagnostic clinical neuropsychology* (rev. ed.). Austin: University of Texas Press.

Blaskey, J., & Jennings, M. C. (1999). Traumatic brain injury. In S. K. Campbell (Ed.), *Decision making in pediatric neurologic physical therapy* (pp. 84–139). Philadelphia: Livingstone.

Bruininks, R. H. (1978). *Bruininks-Osteretsky Test of Motor Proficiency.* Circle Pines, MN: American Guidance Service.

Center for Disease Control, Center for Environmental Health and Injury Control, Division of Injury Control (1995). Childhood injuries in the United States. *American Journal of the Diseases of Children, 144,* 627–646.

Chaplin, D., Deitz, J., & Jaffe, K. M. (1993). Motor performance in children after traumatic brain injury. *Archives of Physical Medicine and Rehabilitation, 74,* 161–164.

Dalby, P. R., & Obrzut, J. E. (1991). Epidemiologic characteristics of closed-head injured children and adolescents: A review. *Developmental Neuropsychology, 7,* 35–68.

Daniel, J. C., Olesniewicz, M. H., Reeves, D. L., Tam, D., Bleiberg, J., Thatcher, R., & Salazar, A. (1999). Repeated measures of cognitive processing efficiency in adolescent athletes: Implications for monitoring recovery from concussion. *Neuropsychiatry, Neuropsychology and Behavioral Neurology, 12,* 167–169.

Ersahin, Y., Mutluer, S., Mirzai, H., & Palali, I. (1996). Pediatric depressed skull fractures: Analysis of 530 cases. *Child's Nervous System, 12,* 323–331.

Ewing-Cobbs, L., Kramer, L., Prasad, M., Canales, D. N., Louis, P. T., Fletcher, J. M., Vollero, H., Landry, S. H., & Cheung, K. (1998). Neuroimaging, physical and developmental findings after inflected and noninflicted traumatic brain injury in young children. *Pediatrics, 102,* 300–307.

Ewing-Cobbs, L., Miner, M. E., Fletcher, J. M., & Levin, H. S. (1989). Intellectual, motor and language sequelae following closed head injury in infants and preschoolers. *Journal of Pediatric Psychology, 14,* 531–547.

Fay, G. C., Jaffe, K. M., Polissar, N. L., Liao, S., Rivara, J. B., & Martin, K. M. (1994). Outcome of pediatric traumatic brain injury at three years: A cohort study. *Archives of Physical Medicine and Rehabilitation, 75,* 733–741.

Ferguson, R. J., Mittenberg, W., Barone, D. F., & Schneider, B. (1999). Postconcussion syndrome following sports-related head injury: Expectation as etiology. *Neuropsychology, 13,* 582–589.

Gagnon, I., Forget, R., Sullivan, J. S., & Friedman, D. (1998). Motor performance following a traumatic brain injury in children: An exploratory study. *Brain Injury, 12,* 843–853.

Golden, C. J. (1986). *Manual for the Luria-Nebraska Neuropsychological Battery: Childrens Revision.* Los Angeles: WPS.

Hahn, Y. S., Raimondi, A. J., McLone, D. G., & Yamanouchi, Y. (1983). Traumatic mechanisms of head injury in child abuse. *Childs Brain, 10,* 229–241.

Harmon, K. G. (1999). Assessment and management of concussion in sports. *American Family Physician, 60,* 887–894.

Holbourn, A. H. S. (1943). Mechanics of the head injury. *The Lancet, 2,* 438–441.

Holbourn, A. H. S. (1944). The mechanics of trauma with special reference to herniation of cerebral tissue. *Journal of Neurosurgery, 1,* 190–200.

Jaffe, K. M., Fay, G. C., Polissar, N. L., Martin, K. M., Shurtleff, H. A., Rivara, J. B., & Winn, H. R. (1993). Severity of pediatric traumatic brain injury and neurobehavioral recovery at one year: A cohort study. *Archives of Physical Medicine and Rehabilitation, 74,* 587–595.

Jennett, B., & Teasdale (1981). *Management of head injuries.* Philadelphia: Davis.

Katz, D. I. (1992). Neuropathology and neurobehavioral recovery from closed head injury. *Journal of Head Trauma Rehabilitation, 7*(2), 1–15.

Ketelaar, M., & Vermeer, A. (1998). Functional motor abilities of children with cerebral palsy: A systematic literature review of assessment measures. *Clinical Rehabilitation, 12,* 369–380.

Kolb, B., & Wishaw, I. Q. (1990). *Fundamentals of human neuropsychology* (3rd ed.). New York: W. H. Freeman and Co.

Korkman, M., Kirk, U., & Kemp, S. (1998). *NEPSY: A Developmental Neuropsychological Assessment.* San Antonio: Psychological Corp.

Korn, N. (1998). Testimony of C. Everett Koop to United States Senate Committee on Labor and Human Resources. Washington, DC: National Safe Kids Campaign.

Kraus, J. F., Rock, A., & Hemyari, P. (1990). Brain injuries among infants, children, adolescents, and young adults. *American Journal of Diseases of Children, 144,* 684–691.

Lehr, E. (1990). *Psychological management of traumatic brain injuries in children and adolescents.* Rockville, MD: Aspen.

Levin, H. S., & Eisenberg, H. M. (1979). Neuropsychological outcome of closed head injury in children and adolescents. *Child's Brain, 5,* 281–292.

Lezak, M. D. (1995). *Neuropsychological assessment* (3rd ed.). New York: Oxford University Press.

Mayo, N. E. (1991). The effect of physical therapy for children with motor delay and cerebral palsy: A randomized clinical trial. *American Journal of Physical Medicine and Rehabilitation, 70,* 258–267.

McCarthy, D. (1972). *McCarthy Scales of Children's Abilities.* New York: Psychological Corp.

McCordie, W. R. (1988). Twenty-year follow up of the prevailing opinion on posttraumatic or postconcussional syndrome. *Clinical Neuropsychologist, 2,* 198–212.

Mercer, J. R., & Lewis, J. F. (1978). *System of Multicultural Pluralistic Assessment.* New York: Psychological Corp.

National Center for Injury Prevention and Control, Centers for Disease Control & Prevention. (1997). *U.S. injury mortality statistics: Unintentional and adverse-event-related* (E800–E949). Washington, DC.

National Center for Injury Prevention and Control, Centers for Disease Control & Prevention. (1998). *Leading causes of death. United States, 1995.* Washington, DC.

Ommaya, A. K., Boretos, J. W., & Beile, E. E. (1969). The lexan calvarium: An improved method for direct observation of the brain. *Journal of Neurosurgery, 30,* 25–29.

Piper, M. C., & Darrah, J. (1994). *Motor assessment of the developing infant.* Philadelphia: Saunders.

Povlishock, J. T., & Coburn, T. H. (1989). Morphopathological changes associated with mild head injury. In H. S. Levin, H. M. Eisenberg, & A. L. Benton (Eds.), *Mild head injury.* New York: Oxford Press.

Powell, J. W., & Barber-Foss, K. D. (1999). Traumatic brain injury in high school athletes. *Journal of the American Medical Association, 282,* 958–963.

Pudenz, R. H., & Sheldon, C. H. (1946). The lucite calvarium: A method for direct observation of the brain: II. Cranial trauma and brain movement. *Journal of Neurosurgery, 3,* 487–505.

Reitan, R. M. (1969). *Manual for the administration of neuropsychological test batteries for adults and children.* Indianapolis: Author.

Reitan, R. M., & Davidson, L. A. (Eds.). (1974). *Clinical neuropsychology. Current status and applications.* Washington, DC: Winston.

Roberts, W. O., Brust, J. D., & Leonard, B. (1999). Youth ice hockey tournament injuries: Rates and patterns compared to season play. *Medical Science and Sports Exercise, 31,* 46–51.

Rouse, T. M., & Eichelberger, M. R. (1992). Trends in pediatric trauma management. *Surgical Clinics of North America, 72*(6), 1347–1364.

Russell, W. R. (1932). Cerebral involvement in head injury. *Brain, 55,* 549–603.

Spreen, O., Tupper, D., Risser, A., Tuokko, H., & Edgell, D. (1984). *Human developmental neuropsychology.* New York: Oxford University Press.

Tibbs, R. E., Haines, D. E., & Parent, A. D. (1998). The child as a projectile. *The Anatomical Record, 253,* 167–175.

Twitchell, T. E. (1965). The automatic grasping response of infants. *Neuropsychologia, 3,* 247–259.

Yakolev, P. E., & LeCours, A. R. (1967). The myelogenic cycles of regional maturation of the brain. In A. Minkowski (Ed.), *Regional development of the brain in early life.* Oxford: Blackwell.

Young, J. Z. (1985). What's in a brain? In C. W. Coen (Ed.), *Functions of the brain.* Oxford, England: Clarendon Press.

SECTION II

Disorders of Behaviors, Emotions, and Communications

Chapter 7 —————————————————————————

LEARNING DISORDERS: REAL CHILDREN, REAL PROBLEMS

H. BOONEY VANCE AND RAMSEY McGOWEN

INTRODUCTION

This chapter acquaints you with the difficult process of diagnosing the learning disabled student. The contents will provide you with information on the history of the field, learning authorities, various definitions, assessment procedures used to diagnose a learning problem, case examples, and the medical aspects of learning disabilities. Special problems such as morbid condition will be discussed. The case study and other information in this chapter reflect real-world situations to which professionals have had to respond. The field of study of learning disabilities/disorders is relatively new and poses great challenges to clinicians, teachers, parents, and individuals themselves. The types of problems presented by the student with learning disorders are very frustrating for the student, parents, teachers, and other professionals.

Bobby finished his first year in school with below-average grades; when he got to the second grade, he began to experience problems with his school work and in his behavior. He could not recognize words, reversed letters, had "sloppy handwriting," and could not understand the stories that he read. Bobby enjoys math and does OK in arithmetic. Bobby's parents don't understand his problems in school, because they see that he studies hard each night for at least an hour. Bobby is often teased by his peers.

Bobby is a real person who needs help. He is one of the estimated millions of students with a learning disorder (LD). Forty percent of all children identified as handicapped are learning disabled (Algozzine & Ysseldyke, 1987). Bobby is the unusual student who has difficulty in some facet of academic or behavior functioning that is not related to any other handicapping condition. Often students like Bobby perform acceptably well in certain academic areas but very low in others. Children like Bobby represent a real challenge to the clinician in terms of accurate diagnosis; pinpointing areas of strengths and weaknesses; ruling out comorbid conditions; investigating the neuropsychological aspects of LD; and developing a report comprising the information that teachers, parents, and professionals can use to develop an appropriate intervention/treatment program. Complicating this are various types of assessment reports such as eligibility, psychoeducational, neuropsychological, clinical, educational/curriculum-based, and clinical. This assessment information comes from multiple informants (sources) and from the results obtained by individuals on multitest instruments.

COMPLEXITY OF THE FIELD

Why is the field of LD so complex? There are several reasons for its complexity. One of the primary reasons is definitions. Since the term LD was introduced in 1962 (Kirk, 1988), there have been numerous definitions posed for LD from different perspectives. The definitions also vary widely from one state to another. Professionals in the field of LD come from widely diverse backgrounds (psychiatry, education, medicine, language development, optometry, neurology, psychology, audiology). Many of these professionals work independently of each other. The interaction between definitions of LD and social policy (funding patterns and who receives services) is another reason for the field's complexity (Algozzine & Ysseldyke, 1987). Currently there are major efforts to identify relevant subgroups of the LD populations (subtyping research); these also add to the complexity. Numerous treatment approaches are used with children and youth identified as learning disabled. Many of these programs, such as visual perception learning, movigenic curricula, motor skills approaches, and neurological organization approaches, are supported by conclusive research. With any relatively young field, 37 years of age, there will continue to be complex issues facing the parents of learning disabled children and professionals who work in the assessment and service delivery areas. A major challenge to this field of study is to find a working definition of LDs that is generally acceptable (Beitchman & Young, 1997).

DEFINITION: WHAT IS A LEARNING DISABILITY?

Hammill (1990) reviewed various definitions of LD and found similarities among the definitions. Hammill pointed out that there is increasing agreement among professionals on the definitions of LD. According to Hammill, the National Joint Committee on Learning Disabilities (NJCLD) definition is the most widely accepted in the field.

> Learning disabilities is a general term that refers to a heterogeneous group of disorders manifested by significant difficulties in the acquisitions and use of listening, speaking, reading, writing, reasoning, or mathematical abilities. These disorders are intrinsic to the individual presumed to be due to central nervous system dysfunction, and may occur across the life span. Problems in self-regulatory behaviors, social perception and social interaction may exist with learning disabilities but do not by themselves constitute a learning disability. Although learning disabilities may occur concomitantly with other handicapping conditions (for example, sensory impairment, mental retardation, serious emotional disturbances) or with extrinsic influences (such as cultural differences, insufficient or inappropriate instruction), they are not the results of those conditions or influences. (NJCLD, 1988, p. 1)

Although this definition appears straightforward, serious conceptual and pragmatic-problems exist, such as the identification of the discrepancy, what constitutes a discrepancy, and what constitutes "serious." Added to this are the varying guidelines that exist from state to state. Depending on the definition and formula used to determine a discrepancy and the variations of individual school districts' approaches to identifying LD students, each of the above variables will identify a somewhat different group of children as LD (Reynolds, 1984).

Learning disabilities are usually diagnosed when a student's achievement on individually administered, standardized tests in basic areas of achievement is significantly below that expected for age, schooling, and level of intelligence. The term LD is used to represent a syndrome of academic difficulties that interfere with a student's ability to acquire academic skills. In addition to the above criteria for an LD, the *Diagnostic and Statistical Manual of Mental Disorders—Fourth Edition* (American Psychiatric Association, 1994) recognizes three major diagnostic categories of LD: mathematics, written expression, and reading disorders. According to the *DSM-IV,* the estimates of students with an LD range from 2 to 10%. Approximately 5% of all students in public schools in the United States are diagnosed as having an LD.

Developmental dyslexia is often defined as a severe difficulty in learning to read. According to Kamphaus (1993), dyslexia is perhaps the most well-known type of learning disability. This form of learning disorder is characterized by problems in oral reading and with distortions, substitutions, and omissions in both oral and silent reading (*DMS-IV,* 1994). Sixty to eighty percent of students identified as LD are males, the majority of whom experience problems in the area of reading. This high rate toward identifying males raises the issue of biases in the assessment/referral process. In fact, according to the U.S. Department of Education (1991), nearly half of all children receiving special education services are considered learning disabled.

Recent research studies (i.e. Flynn & Rehbar, 1994) have challenged the common belief that reading problems are higher among boys than girls. The findings from these studies showed no significant differences in the rates of reading disorders between boys and girls. This area is subject to much disagreement among and between professionals in the field of learning disabilities.

HISTORY

Scholars in the field of LD disagree about the number of constituent groups in the early history of LD (Mercer, 1987). For brevity, this chapter focuses on two different groups of theorists and the historical contributions of each as related to the clinical assessment of children and youth with learning disorders.

Historically, two major groups of theorists were instrumental in the development of the field of LD. These two groupings are arbitrary and include some overlap and even subgroups. This classification is used for the purpose of brevity. Perceptual motor theorists studied the relationship between visual or auditory perception and motor performance such as writing. Emphasis on brain-based perceptual and motor disabilities was the major concern for this group of professionals. Terms such as brain-injured, central nervous system dysfunctions, organic brain damage, and processing difficulties were often used by this group of theorists to describe individuals (Coles, 1978). Emphasis was usually placed on reading disorders based on letter/word reversals and difficulties in copying designs correctly. The second group, language theorists, were concerned with the language development of children (spoken and written). Language theorists believed that LDs were related to some maladaptation in the development of language or speech. Academic achievement was viewed in terms of the use of language. Such problems as incomplete speech development, difficulty with pronoun reference, and inability to apply various rules of grammar were believed to be the basis of LD.

Perceptual Motor (PM) Theorists

The development of PM theorists can be traced to Kirk Goldstein, who studied World War I veterans. His subjects had suffered either an open or closed head injury and were labeled as brain injured. The clinical/medical connection was emphasized in Goldstein's work. Goldstein, a student of Gestalt psychology, emphasized figure/ground relationships, part/whole identification, and figural reversal in copying designs that led to the use of the term brain injured to identify children with this type of problem. In 1988 (Kirk, 1988), this group of brain-injured children was incorporated into the category of LD. The works of Goldstein influenced Alfred Strauss and Hing Werner, who were working at the Wayne County Training School. Strauss and Werner studied children diagnosed as mentally retarded due to nongenetic (exogenous) factors. Strauss and Werner identified seven characteristics that could be used to identify LD children: perceptual disorders, perseveration, thinking disorders, behavior disorders, soft neurological signs, no history of Mental Retardation (MR), and history of neurological impairment (Bender, 1992). Various aspects of these seven characteristics were later found in the definition of LD. Strauss and Werner also made three additional major contributions to the field of LD. First they separated brain injury from retardation; second, they recommended differential teaching strategies based on the individual characteristics of the learner (Hallahan & Kauffman, 1976). Third and perhaps most important, Strauss and Werner served as mentors for such notable figures as Kephart and William Cruickshank. Kephart incorporated motor learning into perceptual-motor development and developed one of the earliest textbooks on teaching methods for brain-injured students. Many of his teaching suggestions are still used in classrooms today. In the 1960s and 1970s, Cruickshank applied Strauss and Werner's findings to nonretarded youth. Cruickshank's work focused on distractibility and hyperactivity (currently known as Attention-Deficit Hyperactivity Disorder; ADHD), and he developed comprehensive educational interventions for this type of children. Cruickshank's work can be directly linked to formulation of the definition for LD. His classic book published in 1961, *A Teaching Method for Brain Injured and Hyperactive Children* (Cruickshank, Bentzen, Rotzberg, & Tannhouser, 1961), was the most influential book during the 1960s and early 1970s concerning the education of children and youth with LD.

Early Language Theorists

Head, in 1926, published a series of articles on adult World War I veterans who had lost their ability to read as a result of a brain injury (Kirk, 1988). Head's work was independent of Goldstein's work but strengthens the hypothesis between brain injury and reading disorders. Samuel Orton's work at the Iowa State Psychopathic Hospital on left-brain hemisphere dominance suggested that dominance was lacking in children with language and learning problems. This lack of dominance was referred to as strephoseymbolio (twisted symbols). Orton, through his research, advocated the use of phonics and kinesthetics to teach this population. The use of touch and movement in teaching is still widely used by classroom teachers to help LD students.

The information processing model of input/output was postulated by Charles Osgood during the 1920s. Osgood's model was the foundation for the identification of the Fernald subtype of LDs. Grace Fernald, working at the University of California in the early 1920s, developed an instructional modality (multisensory) approach to teach LD students. Even though the approach is not supported by research, many teachers in special education incorporate remedial instruction based on tactile, auditory, visual, and kinesthetic procedures.

Samuel Kirk, who worked with Orton at the Wayne County Training School, conducted research on language usage in nonretarded children. He became a formative force in the development of federal policies during the late 1950s and 1960s. The development of the Illinois Test of Psycholinguistic Abilities (Kirk et al., 1968), which was supposed to identify deficits in visual/auditory-based abilities and led to instructional based teaching strategies, came from Kirk.

The modality training was further advanced by the work of Helmer Myklebust. Myklebust worked with deaf children and later expanded his work to include language and reading. He championed modality training using auditory and visual stimuli based on the strengths of the LD student. Even though used in today's classroom, studies on the use of the modality training approach have shown little evidence of improvement. According to Bender (1992), from the 1960s the LD movement could be characterized as a social-political field (Chalfant, 1985; Hammill & Larsen, 1974; Mercer, 1987; Ysseldyke, 1987). Among the factors affecting the development of LD as a profession were human factors, finding factors, and research. This period witnessed many new definitions of learning disability, as well as passage of DL 94-142 and the formation of professional and strong parent advocacy groups. Research focuses ranged from aptitude treatment models, to direct instructions, social misperceptions, and subtyping of various LD categories. The assessment of LD—especially the inclusions and exclusions causes—was subject to numerous debates and research efforts. Who is eligible for LD services was not only a social question, but also a legal issue often settled in courts. The objective of this section was to provide a brief historical overview of the field of LD; and due to space limitation, many leaders and expert professionals had to be omitted.

THE ASSESSMENT PROCESS

The current approach to identifying specific LDs is plagued with problems. The identification and assessment of children and youth with LDs is varied and confused due to the lack of consensus concerning appropriate eligibility criteria for assessment (Bender, 1992). Some assessment procedures address the various components of the definition of LD. Within the framework of the definition of LD assessment, specialists must address four major components: (1) ability/achievement-discrepancy clause, (2) an emphasis on psychological process, (3) addressing the hypothesis of an organic etiology, and (4) the exclusion clause (children with specific handicapping conditions such as mental retardation are omitted).

Working within this framework, clinicians must use a combination of assessment instruments that address the four major components of the LD definitions. The psychological process has drawn considerable attention and heated debates, especially in deficits-subtest grouping and using a process module to identify LD students. The most common diagnostic procedure, called the IQ-achievement discrepancy, involves establishing that a student's academic performance on standardized achievement tests is significantly below that expected from his/her IQ score. This approach is unreliable for diagnostic purposes for several reasons, such as norming of testing and standard score and grade equivalency scores, but a complete review of this topic is beyond the scope of this chapter. This step in the assessment process is characterized by trying to find a significant discrepancy between a given assessment instrument (intellectual test) and an achievement test, or a visual-motor assessment instrument or language test. A different approach to determining which children have LDs is the exclusion procedure. A student can be excluded from being identified as LD if he or she has a diagnosis of MR, if the LD is due to behavioral disorders or medical conditions, and if the learning problems are due to his or her cultural/environmental or economic factors. How do clinicians effectively quantify all of the above factors? This question must be answered satisfactorily by either clinicians or administrators before a student can be eligible for LD services in a school system.

Another major difficulty that plagues the process of identifying students as LD is the discrepancy criteria between ability achievement of one's score on a standardized intelligence test and the score he or she received on an individual achievement test. The difficulty here is who determines what is required for a significant or large discrepancy. This dilemma is further complicated because of the variation from state to state by school district; different tests normed on different populations; and many children who are identified as LD do not demonstrate any discrepancy (Rotter, 1988; Algozzine & Ysseldyke, 1987). How do clinicians distinguish between students who have a LD and students who are low-achieving for other reasons? This issue becomes especially problematic for the student in the higher grades.

Given the failure of assessment of perceptual-motor and language-based psychological processes, the long, cumbersome process of determining ability-achievement discrepancy, and many teachers' dissatisfaction with the types of information revealed by assessment specialists, a relatively new assessment model has evolved for instructional assessment purposes. Assessment for instructional purposes is typically related to instructions in the classroom. An assessment for instructional purposes is usually the responsibility of students' teachers, who often know the student best, excluding, of course, their parents. The various approaches used for assessment information for instructional planning are (a) normal-referenced achievement testing, (b) criterion-referenced assessment, (c) curriculum-based assessment, and (d) classroom-task analysis and error analysis.

Associated features of children who are diagnosed as LD are low self-esteem (or self-concept); a high dropout rate (nearly 40% of students quit school according to the *DSM-IV,* 1994); and behavior problems, especially with social adjustment. As part of the comprehensive assessment process of a student suspected of having an LD, careful attention should be given to the personality and social characteristics of the individual with LD. Research has clearly documented that among children who are LD, there is an array of social-emotional problems. Consequently, the skilled clinicians will attend to assessment methods whereby the social-emotional behavior problems of these students can be addressed. The *DSM-IV* (1994) indicates that as many as 25% of individual children with Conduct Disorders, Oppositional Defiant Disorder, Attention-Deficit Hyperactivity Disorder, and Dysthymic Disorders also have a Learning Disorder.

A clinician will need to have competencies not only in psychoeducational assessment but also in clinical assessment that merely goes beyond giving "a test." The term contextual variables, associated with the assessment of students with a possible LD, is of utmost importance. The variables that the assessment specialist must attend to are careful planning, critical developmental issues, the purpose of assessment (focus, goals/objectives), the referral problem, and defining the various behavior domains that will be assessed.

Assessment of Students with a Learning Disability

Sattler (1988) indicated that the clinician has three major objectives in the assessment of a learning disorder student: (a) to estimate general intelligence (used to gauge achievement and expected performance), (b) to determine the areas(s) of impairment, and (c) to discover areas of strengths that can be useful in the remediation process. Beitchman and Young (1997) recommended that as the first step in diagnosis, a child's current academic functioning be evaluated. This step is important because if the child is not functioning below the expected level for his/her age or grade then the child is not likely to require special assistance.

The Assessment Plan

The following variable should be carefully evaluated in any student who is referred as having a possible learning disability. The foundations for assessing any child suspected of having an LD, of course, are a valued and reliable measure of cognitive abilities and a comprehensive-achievement test. Assessment of cognitive abilities should include verbal-linguistic, visual-motor-planning, sequencing, executive functioning, and memory components, as well as components of a neuropsychological battery. Variables that should be considered in selecting an achievement or academic test are the psychometric properties of the instruments; the age of the child; and whether the instrument measures such domains as receptive and expressive vocabulary skills, written expressions, letter recognitions, patterns, and so on. For subskills within an academic domain—for instance, reading—the instrument should be able to assess word and cloze procedure, passage comprehension, reading rate, word or speech sounds (phonics), word attack skills, and oral and silent reading ability. Tests of arithmetic/math skills should include sections on oral and silent reading problems, number recognition, tracking ability, recall, recognition of the process called for in solving a problem (adding, subtraction, etc.), and single- and double-column problems, just to mention a few domains. Sattler (1988) and Beitchman and Young (1999) strongly suggest that the skilled clinician investigates child and situational variables that could be contributing factors for an LD. Situational variables include family and school demands on the child, self-concept, attention/concentration problems, and social skills and social emotional variables. Each of these mentioned variables or components should be given careful consideration as a component of a comprehensive evaluation because the results from each domain will be used to help determine a student's strengths and weaknesses and to develop an effective treatment program at school as well as at home.

Neurological investigations such as those by Hynd and Semrud-Clikerman (1989), Flowers (1993), and Logan (1996) have been able to identify structural and functional characteristics of the brains of LD children. In the search for neuroanatomical and neurofunctional differences between LD and non-LD children, especially regarding reading disorders, few if any of the studies can be considered as conclusive, according to Beitchman and Young (1999). Further, Beitchman and Young (1999) concluded that reading disabilities fall along a continuum and do not represent a discrete entity or findings from imaging technologies and at this time should be considered as tentative. A guide for assisting the clinicians in selecting various assessment instruments that can be used as part of a comprehensive battery for evaluating students for LD is provided in Figure 7.1.

Pitfalls

Many of the pitfalls in the diagnosis of LD can be overcome with proper planning and the proper diagnostic approach. Such planning of a diagnostic approach should involve the following components:

1. A comprehensive interview with all parenting figures and individual teachers complimented by a thorough developmental, school, social, medical, and mental health history

2. A developmentally appropriate interview with the child to assess his or her view of any difficulties as well as explanations of why and symptoms for possible comorbid conditions (anxiety, depression, ADHD, or unusual thinking)

3. When appropriate, a medical evaluation to determine health status and screen for sensory deficits or other physical and neurological difficulties

4. An appropriate cognitive assessment of ability and achievement

5. The use of both broad-spectrum and narrowly focused parent, child, and teacher rating scales

6. Adjunct assessment techniques for speech, language, and fine and gross motor and visual motor-perceptual functions.

A case example is provided that was used to assist a school district's planning and eligibility committee in determining if a student meets the criteria for LD.

Instrumental			Domains		
	Cognitive	Visual Motor	Academic/Achievement	Behavior	Attention/Memory
	Raven's Progressive Matrice	Berry Test of Visual Motor Integration	Personality Inventory for Children	Personality Inventory for Children	Wide-range Assessment of Memory & Learning
	WISC-III	Benton Facial Recognition Test	Woodcork Reading Mastery Tests-R	Behavior Ruling Profile	Test of Memory & Learning
	K-ABC			Child Behavior Checklist	
	S-B-IV	Benton Judgment of Line Orientation	Basic Achievement Skills Included	School Behavior Checklist	Brown Attention-Deficit Disorder Scale
	Woodcock-Johnson	Slosson Visual-Motor Performance Test	Test of Nonverbal Abilities		Conner Rating Scale
	S-FRIT			Self-Control Rating Scale	Continuous Performance Test
	K-AIT	Motor-Free Visual Perception Test		Child and Adolescent Symptom Inventory	Matching Familiar Figure Test
	DTLA-4	Minn-Perception-Diagnostic Test-R			
	Differential Ability Scales	Bender Visual Motor Gestalt Test		Devereux Behavior Rating Scale-School	Wechsler Memory Scale
	Naglieri Nonverbal Ability Test	Wide Range Assessment of Visual Motor Abilities			Children's Memory Scale

Figure 7.1 List of Assessment Instruments for Students Referred for a Possible Learning Disorder

CASE STUDY: COMPREHENSIVE INTERPRETIVE PSYCHOLOGICAL EVALUATION

Name: Michael
Date of Birth: November 27, 1990
Chronological Age: 7 years 8 months
School: Keystone
Date of Evaluation: August 12, 1998
Grade: First
Examiner: Dr. Vance

Referral Information

Michael was referred for evaluation by his mother and Dr. Andy, mainly because of learning problems in school, possible Attention-Deficit/Hyperactivity Disorder, and possible developmental delay, but also due to peer problems. The main goals of this evaluation were to answer the following questions: Is Michael in an appropriate classroom setting? Are special education services recommended for Michael? Are therapeutic interventions advised? Should Michael be monitored for future developments? Should a medical or other professional specialist also be seen?

Background Information

Michael is a Caucasian male, age 7 years 8 months. The background information presented here about Michael is based primarily on reports from his mother and his teacher. He lives with his biological parents and is one of two children in his residence. Michael is the youngest child in his family. His family economic status is upper class. As a child, his home environment was enriched. Cultural opportunities at home (e.g., availability of books, family trips to museums) are excellent. Both Michael's mother and his father graduated from college. When she was pregnant with Michael, his mother reported that she had no health problems, did not use any alcohol, and did not smoke cigarettes. Michael's birth was normal, with no unusual problems. Following birth, Michael experienced no unusual problems. During early childhood, Michael was described as hyperactive, difficult, and hypersensitive. He developed physical skills such as sitting, crawling, and walking later than most children. His early language development was slow in comparison to other children. His early motor development and skill acquisition were behind his agemates, and his social development was slow. His cognitive development (e.g., counting, learning the alphabet) was also behind that of those his age.

Michael attended preschool and went to kindergarten and is now in first grade at a parochial school. Since starting school he has been tutored. He is reported to enjoy school and to get along with his teachers. Michael's skill strength in school is reported to be his ability to please his teacher. In contrast, his weaknesses are reported to be concentration, handwriting, being careful and checking his work, and vocabulary, together with verbal expression. During the past 2 years Michael's grades have been mostly Cs.

Instruments

- Weschler Intelligence Scale for Children–Third Edition
- Wide Range Achievement Test R-3
- Children's Problem Checklist
- Child Behavior Checklist 91–Teacher's Report
- Minnesota-Percepto Diagnostic Test-R
- Draw-A-Person
- Behavior Disorder Identification Scale–Home Version
- Conners' Parent Rating Scale
- Conners' Teacher Rating Scale
- Slosson Full-Range Intelligence Test
- Clinical Interview with Mother
- Diagnostic Interview Schedule for Children

Test Results and Interpretation

Michael was given the WISC-III, a test that evaluates the present level of intellectual functioning of children and adolescents. He scored in the Low Average to Average range of intelligence (Verbal IQ = 88, Performance IQ = 94, Full Scale IQ = 90), ranking at about the 25th percentile relative to other 7-year-olds. The chances are very good (about 19 out of 20) that Michael's true Full Scale IQ is likely to fall between 85 and 95. The 6-point difference between his Verbal and Performance IQs is not statistically significant and indicates that his intelligence on these two scales is consistent. Therefore, Michael demonstrated about equal skill manipulating concrete and nonverbal materials.

The WISC-III yields four indexes. Two are large: Verbal Comprehension (VC), composed of four Verbal subtests; and Perceptual Organization (PO), composed of four Performance subtests. Two are smaller: Freedom from Distractibility (FD), composed of two Verbal subtests, and Processing Speed (PS), composed of two Performance subtests. Michael earned Indexes of 91 on VC (27th percentile), 93 on PO (32nd percentile), 78 on FD (7th percentile), and 93 on PS (32nd percentile).

Michael's Indexes on the two factors that include only Verbal subtests (VC and FD) differ significantly. He performed better on tasks that measure verbal comprehension and expression (27th percentile) than on tasks that require sequencing and number ability and are unusually susceptible to behaviors such as distractibility and anxiety (7th percentile).

He displayed below average capability on the FD factor, which may have been partly due to distractibility, because this behavior was specifically observed during both the oral arithmetic subtest and the test of immediate auditory memory. In fact, Michael evidenced distractibility during other tasks as well, and a concentration weakness was also noted for Michael at school. In addition, Michael's low FD score seems to indicate a problem in dealing with numbers. Michael's distractibility and limited attention span are possible explanations for his low FD score even though similar behaviors were observed during some other WISC-III subtests as well. Distractibility and limited attention span typically have a more adverse effect on tests of oral arithmetic and immediate memory than on tests of verbal concepts or nonverbal thinking.

Michael's Indexes on the two factors composed only of Performance subtests (PO and PS) do not differ significantly. He performed about as well on tasks that measure visual-motor coordination and nonverbal reasoning as he did on tasks that require highly speeded paper-and-pencil responding and that are unusually susceptible to behaviors such as low motivation, lack of concentration, and reflectiveness.

On Performance subtests, Michael had a significant strength on a test of design copying (75th percentile). Furthermore, he did well on a test that required him to rapidly copy simple symbols associated with shapes. On the whole, these two subtests assess reproduction of models. His score at the 66th percentile indicates a strength for this combined group. He performed better when reproducing models that were geometric designs or matching items rapidly (66th percentile) than when using planning ability to solve problems such as arranging picture sequences and scanning symbols (12th percentile).

Appearance and Behavior Characteristics

Michael appears younger than his stated age of 7 years. His height is average for his age, and his weight is average for his build. He has brown eyes, and his hair is dark brown. Michael was dressed appropriately, and his hygiene was good. He appeared pleasant and smiling. He spoke rapidly and talked in a monotone. He displayed awkward visual-motor coordination. Michael was very willing and compliant when he began the test session. Rapport was easy to establish, but difficult to maintain.

Michael appeared to demonstrate obsessiveness during the evaluation, when he continued trying to solve items after the time expired on the speeded tasks of arranging pictures to tell stories, arithmetic problem-solving, and assembling cut-up picture puzzles. He also seemed to demonstrate obsessiveness when he spent extra time making sure that he was precisely correct on a test of puzzle solving. Further, Michael indicated that a trivial detail was missing for some wrong answers on a test of finding missing parts in pictures. In addition, he gave additional unnecessary responses on several items that had already been adequately answered on a test of telling how two concepts are alike. In addition, he gave too much detail or irrelevant information when giving reasons and explaining answers on a test of social comprehension.

Michael demonstrated poor visuoperceptual skills during the evaluation when he rotated at least two designs more than 30 degrees on a test of copying abstract designs with blocks. Further, Michael showed poor visuoperceptual skills when he lost the square shape for some designs on a test of design copying. He also was unaware that some pairs of puzzle pieces were put together incorrectly on a test of puzzle solving. Further, he had orientation problems (assembled some shapes at an angle or upside down) on a test of puzzle solving. Further, Michael made errors in copying numbers or symbols on a test of rapidly copying simple symbols that are associated with shapes.

Michael showed immaturity during the evaluation when he had to be reminded to continue after coming to the end of a line on a test of rapidly copying simple symbols that are associated with shapes. Further, Michael evidenced immaturity when he did not understand the importance of working fast on a test of picture sequencing. In addition, he used materials in an inappropriate way on a test of picture sequencing. Further, Michael had to be reminded to continue after coming to the end of a page on a test of rapid scanning and decision-making about symbols.

Michael evidenced distractibility during the evaluation when he was distracted by stimuli in the environment on tests of incomplete pictures, oral arithmetic, and auditory short-term memory. Michael showed low risk-taking at times when he refused to guess if unsure of an answer on a test of social understanding, and when he rarely elaborated on an initial response, even when queried, on the verbal tests of word knowledge and social understanding. Michael showed poor coordination when he held the pencil awkwardly on a test of rapidly copying simple symbols that are associated with shapes, and when he was slowed down by apparent visuomotor coordination problems on the nonverbal tests of design copying and rapid symbol scanning. Michael displayed weak receptive language skills while being tested when he didn't seem to understand the wording of some questions on a test of general information, when he had difficulty understanding the meaning of "same" and "like" on a test of word similarities, and when he had trouble understanding the spoken directions for the task on a test of rapid symbol scanning.

Michael showed low motivation during the evaluation when he had to be urged to keep solving some items on the nonverbal tests of picture sequencing and puzzle solving. Michael showed a limited attention span during the evaluation when he had difficulty sustaining attention for the full 20 seconds per item on a test of incomplete pictures and had difficulty attending to some items during a test of immediate memory. Michael evidenced a problem working with numbers when he used finger writing to solve some items on a test of oral arithmetic. Michael displayed a weakness in visual memory when he responded to most items by going back and forth from the Target Group to the Search Group (sometimes several times per item) before marking Yes or No on a test of rapid symbol scanning. The physical environment of the testing session was optimal, and the results of the evaluation are considered valid.

Michael's academic achievement as measured by the Wide Range Achievement Test-R3 varied from a beginning first-grade level (Arithmetic) to a 2.2 grade level in Reading. Michael achieved the following standard scores: reading 104, spelling 86, and arithmetic 71. According to the discrepancy formula, Michael qualifies as a learning disabled student in the area of Arithmetic (19-point difference between achievement and ability, significant at the .01 level).

Visual motor integration skills, as measured by the Minnesota-Percepto-Diagnostic Test-R and as observed by the examiner, indicate that Michael's gross and fine motor-visual integration is delayed. He obtained a T-Score of 32. This places Michael at the 3rd percentile level relative to other 7-year-olds. He could not correctly execute a circle or a square. Visual motor integration skills appear to be on the development level of that of a 5-year-old.

Results from the Behavior Disorders Identification Scale (Home Version), with Mrs. Powell as the informant, showed that Michael obtained the following standard scores: Learning Self Control = 4, Interpersonal/Social = 6, Inappropriate Behavior = 13. This scale has a mean of 10 and standard deviation of 3. These results strongly suggest that Michael has skill deficiencies in the following domains: Learning Self Control, Interpersonal/Social, Displaying Inappropriate-Immature Behaviors, and Physical Symptoms (Fears).

On the Conner's Teaching Rating Scale, used to screen for ADHD problems, Michael obtained one elevated score, which was on the Perfectionism scale. All other subscale scores were below the cut-off screening score, including the Hyperactivity, ADHD Index, Inattentive Index, and the Conner's Global Index. The elevated score of the Perfectionism Scale indicates that Michael sets high goals for himself, is very fastidious about the way he does things and is obsessive about his works.

With his teacher as the informant for the Conners' Teaching Rating Scale, Michael obtained the following elevated T-Scores: Cognitive Problems = 78, Anxious-Shy = 74, Conners' ADHD Index = 68, Hyperactive-Impulsive = 72. These elevated scores support the behavior observations, interviews, and assessment data. Results from the Achenbach JCBCL Teacher's Report showed, according to his teacher, that Michael experienced difficulty with the following behavior domains: obsessions and compulsions, fears, inattention, and distractibility. Michael obtained significantly high scores on the following CBCL constructs: anxious/depressed, social problems, thought problems, and attention problems (T-Scores all above 60). The majority of these scales are of the internalizing grouping of an over anxious disorder. In fact, Michael obtained a cluster T-Score of 64 on the internalizing grouping.

On the DISC and the clinical interview, Michael and his mother reported the presence of a number of fears, obsessions, and compulsive symptoms such as persistent ideas and thoughts (thunder) that become intrusive and inappropriate and cause marked anxiety and distress. His repetitive behaviors are seen in his attachments to books, which he uses to help reduce his anxieties. The severity of these anxiety-problems is supported by his teacher's report on the CBCL and from behavioral observations.

Summary

Michael is a 7-year-old Caucasian male who was referred for evaluation by his mother and Dr. Andy because of concerns about learning problems in school, possible ADHD, and possible developmental delay. During the present evaluation, Michael evidenced distractibility, immaturity, and low risk-taking; seemed to display obsessiveness; evidenced poor coordination; demonstrated weak receptive language skills; and showed poor visual perceptual skills. On the WISC-III, Michael earned a verbal IQ of 88, a Performance IQ of 94, and a Full Scale IQ of 90. Michael performed about as well on tests of verbal comprehension and expression as he did on tests of nonverbal thinking and visual-motor coordination. Overall, Michael performed in the Low Average to Average range of intelligence. Michael had a relative strength in reproduction of models and had a relative weakness in number ability. When reproducing models of geometric designs or matching items rapidly, he did better than on planning problems.

Diagnostic Impression and Recommendations

Michael is a 7 year 8 month old boy who has a low average intelligence and processes a low average level of adaptive behavior skills. His social maturity level appeared to be lower than his chronological age. Diagnostically, Michael meets the *DSM-IV* criteria for Learning Disorders with comorbid conditions in the following areas: Learning Disorder–Arithmetic, Central-Processing Problems, Receptive-Expressive Language Disorder, and an extreme sensitivity to loud sounds. Comorbidity in the area of Anxiety Disorder and ADHD is noted.

Michael should be treated by Dr. Jones for his Anxiety Disorder. His mother and father should also be seen for therapy. Michael will need additional support structure and assistance in terms of tutorial help, extra study sessions at school, organizational assistance, and rehearsal with feedback. Instructions must begin at his level of readiness with appropriate educational assistance, or he might be overwhelmed in school. He learns best in a situation that is highly structured with few interfering stimuli where he can apply his language skills. He also thrives on warm personal attention. A discrete trial teaching approach would be very helpful for Michael. Cognitive rehearsing strategies including cognitive mapping, verbal rehearsing, and imagery would be helpful for Michael as a resource for solving problems. In addition, facilitating retrieval by crunching information, using memories, and categorizing presented materials (crunching = Michael, to-get-her). Having Michael verbally repeat directions to ensure comprehension and accuracy would be appropriate. Perhaps a multimodality approach that includes a combination of whole words (context) and sight by phonic would be helpful. A goal of teachers who are working with him (reading) should be to develop automatic memory, building in reinforcement and moving as fast as possible but as slow as necessary to master the basic elements. A note of caution: Michael experiences some delay in visual-motor integration development, as writing demands increase in both complexity and length overtime, this may become problematic for school success. A continuous charting of Michael's performance across all academic areas is suggested. A chart of suggested remedial teaching strategies specific to his problem areas follows. Michael is a delightful child, full of energy, and a joy to work with!

Booney Vance
SUBTEST SCORES SUMMARY

Verbal Subtests	Raw Score	Scaled Score	PR
Information (IN)	9	9	37
Similarities	8	8	25
Arithmetic (AR)	10	6	9
Vocabulary (VO)	19	10	50
Comprehension (CO)	9	6	9
(Digit Span DS)	7	6	9

Performance Subtests	Raw Score	Scaled Score	PR
Picture Completion (PC)	12	8	25
Coding (CD)	49	10	50
Picture Arrangement (PA)	11	7	16
Block Design (BD)	30	12	75
Object Assembly (OA)	13	8	25
Symbol Search (SS)	17	7	16

DIFFERENCES BETWEEN SUBTEST SCORES AND MEAN OF SUBTEST SCORES

Subtest	Scaled Score	Diff. from Mean	Signif. of Diff.	Freq.	S/W
VERBAL					
Information (IN)	9	1.50	ns	>25%	
Similarities (SM)	8	0.50	ns	>25%	
Arithmetic (AR)	6	−1.50	ns	>25%	
Vocabulary (VO)	10	2.50	.15	25%	
Comprehension (CO)	6	−1.50	ns	>25%	
Digit Span (DS)	6	−1.50	ns	>25%	
Mean of Six Verbal Subtest Scaled Scores = 7.50					
Scatter = 4 (p < .05, Freq = 82.9%)					
PERFORMANCE					
Picture Completion (PC)	8	−0.67	ns	>25%	
Coding (CD)	10	1.33	ns	>25%	
Picture Arrangement (PA)	7	−1.67	ns	>25%	
Block Design (BD)	12	3.33	.05*	25%	
Object Assembly (OA)	8	−0.67	ns	>25%	
Symbol Search (SS)	7	−1.67	ns	>25%	
Mean of Six Performance Subtests Scaled Scores = 8.67					
Scatter = 5 (p < .05, Freq = 77.6%)					

*significant at the .05 level

SHARED-ABILITY COMPOSITES ANALYSIS

	INDEX	PR	S/W
Bannatyne			
Verbal Conceptualization (SM+VO+CO)	89	23	
Spatial (PC+BD+OA)	96	39	
Acquired Knowledge (IN+AR+VO)	90	25	
Sequential (DS+AR+CD)	82	12	
Horn			
Fluid Intelligence (SM+DS+PC+PA+BD+OA)	87	19	
Crystallized Intelligence (IN+VO+CO+SM)	91	27	
Dean			
Abstract Thought (SM+BD)	100	50	S
Remote Memory (IN+PC)	91	27	
Auditory Memory (DS+AR)	78	7	
Social Comprehension (CO+PA)	80	9	
Kaufman			
WISC-R Freedom from Distract. (DS+AR+CD)	82	12	
Simultaneous Processing (PC+BD+OA)	96	39	
Verbal Reasoning (CO+SM)	84	14	

ADDITIONAL ISSUES

Lifelong Existence of LD

Learning disorders are usually a lifetime condition persisting beyond late adolescence and adulthood (Maughan, 1995). According to Beitchman and Young (1999), the general intelligence and the severity of the LD are the predictors of later difficulties at the adult stage; girls seemed to be at risk for having social and emotional problems (Bruck, 1985). The more one has continuing problems with literacy and math, the higher the incidence of reported depression. Later life difficulties for their diagnostic group are manifested in men's being more vulnerable to unemployment and women's being more likely to move into cohabitation and child-rearing earlier than their non-LD peers (Maughan and Hagell, cited in Maughan, 1995).

The results from the Australian Temperament Project, a longitudinal study of a representative group of children from grades K to 7 (Prior et al., 1999), which investigated the relationship of learning difficulties and behavior problems in preadolescence, showed that there was neither a significantly higher rate of LD in boys versus girls nor a higher rate of internalizing problems including depression, anxiety, and phobias. Children with an LD in only one academic domain were more likely to have an anxiety-based disorder, whereas students with more than one area of impairment were more likely to have disruptive-behavior disorders. A salient finding of Prior's et al. (1999) study was the stability and persistence of LDs, especially for boys. Evidence available concerning the extent to which LD persists into adulthood is consistent that both academic and social/emotional problems persist for 5 to 6 years after graduation from high school (Bender, 1992; Boetsch et al., 1996). It seems relatively clear that LDs are a lifelong phenomenon, and one would conclude that the public school efforts to cure LDs have not been successful.

Comorbidity

Comorbidity can be defined as the existence of two or more psychiatric problems/diagnoses in a given individual. Relationships between mental health problems and LDs have been well documented (Ferguson & Lynsky, 1997; Prior, 1996). There is an overlap/comorbidity between LD, especially reading disabilities and psychiatric disorders. Of course, poor academic achievement and poor school behavior often go hand in hand. The overlap between LD and mental health problems is estimated at approximately 40% to 50% depending on the kinds of problems considered (Hinshaw, 1992).

The question which always is debated about these sets of problems leads to which came first. Few large-scale longitudinal studies are available that trace the development path of LD and behavior problems (BP). Smart et al. (1996) showed that children identified at 7 to 8 years of age as having reading problems were more likely to have entered school with adjustment problems. Waring et al. (1996) found that both LD and BP students were at a higher risk for continuing problems in both areas as compared with students who have only a reading problem. According to the *DSM-IV* (APA, 1994), the school drop-out rate for children and adolescents with an LD is nearly 40%; unemployment for adults with an LD is significantly higher than non-LD adults; and 20% to

40% of children and adolescents with an LD have Conduct Disorders, Oppositional Defiant Disorders, ADHD, and Major Depressive Disorders.

Attention-Deficit/Hyperactivity Disorder

There is a high degree of overlap between LD, especially reading disorders and ADHD. Light et al. (1995), found that the shared genetic variation of ADHD and reading disabilities was at least 70%. Other researchers such as Holborrow and Berry (1986), Prior et al. (1999), and Shaywitz et al. (1986) reported rates varying from 10% to 60% of children with ADHD and concurrent reading problems. Good clinical practice dictates that clinicians should assess for the existence of ADHD with or without hyperactivity in LD children. Assessment for the presence of ADHD is important to help develop what interventions are required for the student.

Internalizing Disorder

The relationship between LD and internalizing disorders such as anxiety and depression has not received much documentation. In other words, there is a paucity of good data-based research studies of internalizing disorders involving direct comparisons of children and adolescents with and without LD, according to Beitchman and Young (1999). In a classic well documented review of the literature on emotional well-being and adolescents with LD from 1984 to 1993, Huntington and Bender (1993) focused on five variables: self-concept, attributions, anxiety, depression, and suicide. Huntington and Bender (1993), based on their review of a decade of research, concluded that adolescents with learning disabilities have less positive academic self-concepts than their nondisabled peers. Adolescents with LD attribute both success and failure more internally than do comparison groups. Adolescents with LD experience higher levels of trait anxiety and have a significant higher prevalence of minor somatic complaints than nondisabled peers and studies of children in classes for the learning-disabled. Studies of adolescents with LD report higher rates of depression on self-report measures, according to Huntington and Bender (1993).

Prior et al. (1999) reported on the relationship between specific types of LD and various types of disorders among clinical groups of children with LD. Prior et al. (1999) found that the comorbidity diagnosis rate was 52% among the LD clinical groups. The most frequent type of disorder among the spelling group of children was phobia/anxiety (50%, with 30% having coexisting ADHD). Among the arithmetic disorder students, 37% had phobias/anxiety followed by conduct disorder/oppositional defiant disorder (23%). Combining the LD groups showed that 52% had externalizing disorders; 32% had internalizing; and 16% had comorbid disorders.

Externalizing Disorders

Beitchman and Young (1999) suggested that there are development correlations between children with reading disorders and externalizing behavior. Frich et al. (1991), in an excellent data-based study among early school-aged children, documented an association between aggression and learning problems and their comorbidity with ADHD.

Williams and McGree (1996) and Moffett (1993) found that by adolescence there are clear links between antisocial behavior and variables related to LD. However, much of the investigated work by researchers between the variables of LD and externalizing disorder have been subject to controversy.

Three common hypotheses have been used to explain the relationship between LD and antisocial behavior. Grande (1988) formulated the school failure hypothesis, which simply implied that the acting out and up behavior for most LD students results from a lack of school success, which results in low self-esteem, frustration, and acting-out behavior. Zimmerman et al. (1979) used the detection hypothesis/differential treatment to explain the correlation of LD and externalizing behavior. They proposed that students who are LD engage in equal incidents of antisocial acts that are treated differently from non-LD peers by the justice system. Larson (1988) proposed a susceptibility explanation that suggested that LDs are accompanied by personality characteristics that predispose the student to delinquent behavior. McGee et al. (1986) did, however, suggest that children with reading disorders may have more preexisting externalizing problems. Beitchman et al. (1997) summarized the research on the association of reading disorders and behavior problems as "weak with some evidence that behavior difficulties predate reading disorders and no evidence that reading disabilities predate aggressive behavior" (p. 1026).

Social Skills

Social misperception is a term often associated with students who have an LD. This term is defined as one's ability to read and interpret discrete signs used to function socially accurately (Bryan, 1991). Parker and Asher (1987) suggested that a child's ability to function socially has important implications for his or her overall adjustment. Bryan (1991) reviewed the social problems associated with LD and indicated that LD students are not as socially competent as their normally achieving peers. Bryan (1991) suggested that these children have problems understanding others' affective states, especially in new and complex situations. Vaughn and Hogan (1990) concluded that many children with learning disorders have problems in several components of social competencies that begin early and worsen with age.

Many students with LD have difficulties making and maintaining positive interpersonal relationships with classmates and same-aged peers. This applies not only to their peers but also to the perceptions of teachers as well. Garrett and Crump (1980) found that teachers perceive students with LD as less desirable to have in the classroom than nonhandicapped children. Various researchers have found that compared with their non–learning disabled peers, students with LD were less accepted and more frequently rejected (Bryan, 1976), less popular (Bryan, 1978), less frequently selected to play (Hutton & Palo, 1976), and perceived as having lower social status (Stone La Greca, 1990). Vaughn et al. (1990) found that LD students were less accepted by peers even prior to being identified as LD. Merrill (1998) suggested that inadequate social skills and poor peer relationships during childhood for LD children may lead to a wide variety of problems late in life such as school drop-out, delinquency, unemployment, conduct-related discharges from the military services, and psychiatric hospitalization. Good clinical practice would mandate that the clinician keep abreast of the latest developments in the assessment of social skills and peer relations and include such instruments in his or her diagnostic battery, because an important outcome of using such data obtained from the assessment of social skills is to develop appropriate social-behavioral-intervention plans. Without interventions the consequences of poor social skills can be severe for many students with LD.

MEDICAL FACTORS IN LEARNING DISABILITIES

A thorough medical evaluation should be included as a part of the multidisciplinary approach team that evaluates children suspected of having learning disabilities. One reason this is an important part of the evaluation process is that learning disabled children have been found to have an increased frequency of health problems (Cowell, 1990). Another is that a variety of medical conditions is associated with impairments in cognitive and academic functioning. Graham (1991) has identified several pediatric disorders that are associated with cognitive and learning problems, including chromosomal abnormalities, congenital heart disease, asthma, diabetes, and childhood cancers. Greenblatt and Greenblatt (1997) add neurological disorders, head trauma, and cerebral palsy to the list. The relationship between medical problems and learning problems may reflect the direct effects of disease processes, a shared underlying pathology that affects both cognition and physical health, the adverse effects of medications or other treatment approaches, and/or the stress and disruption caused by medical problems. The determinants of individual outcomes of medically ill children are complex, difficult to predict, and dependent on multiple factors, such as coping skills, parental involvement, and other environmental factors (Wright & Masten, 1997). As a result, knowledge of the relationship between medical problems and learning problems is essential if intervention is to be well-informed, comprehensive, and effective.

One area in which medial and learning problems coincide is in the sequelae of prematurity and low birth weight. Strauss (2000) examined 26-year-long follow-up data on a cohort of 1,064 low–birth weight but full-term infants. Data indicated that low birth weight was associated with significant deficits in academic achievement, increased likelihood of referral for special education, and a decreased likelihood of obtaining professional or managerial level careers. Stewart et al. (1999) examined brain structure and neurocognitive and behavioral functioning in adolescents who had been born prematurely. Their findings indicated that 40 of the 72 prematurely born patients in their sample showed unequivocally abnormal MRIs, and another 15 had MRI findings of an equivocal nature, whereas only one abnormal and 5 equivocal MRI findings were identified in the control group who had been born full term. The adolescents who had been born prematurely had significantly more reading and adjustment problems than the control group. Middle, Johnson, Alderdice, Petty, and Macfarlane (1996) performed a follow-up survey on children aged 7 who had been born prematurely and at low birth weights. They found a significantly high rate of academic problems, increased need for additional educational support services, and increased utilization of health services in general. This finding was more pronounced for very low birth weight (below 1,500 grams) children. Very low birth weight children who had chronic lung disease (CLD) were found to have similar general health profiles to very low birth weight children who did not have CLD, but those with CLD were found to have significantly poorer academic impairment (Farel, Hooper, Teplin, Henry, & Kraybill, 1998). The extent to which prematurity and low birth weight contribute to learning problems as a result of neurological impairments, the effects of related medical conditions (such as CLD), and other factors have yet to be clearly determined, but the finding that these conditions are associated with higher rates of cognitive and academic problems seems well established.

Children who have been diagnosed with various forms of cancer have also been identified as being at greater risk for learning difficulties. Sloper, Larcombe, and Charlton (1994) reported that teacher ratings of children who were 5-year survivors of cancer indicated significantly more difficulties in concentration and in academic progress for these children. Data from Cool (1996) indicated that children who had received bone marrow transplant for treatment of cancer showed declining IQ scores, poorer academic achievement, and impaired fine motor skills. Arvidson, Kihlgren, Hall, and Lonnerholm (1999) also found that children who received bone marrow transplantation for treatment of childhood hematological malignances had higher rates of learning difficulties and specific problems on neuropsychological tests in the domains of attention, memory, and strategies. In both of these studies related to bone marrow transplantation, the earlier the age of diagnosis, the greater these adverse effects on cognition appeared to be. Fletcher and Copeland (1988) reviewed the literature on the effects of cranial radiation in acute lymphocytic leukemia (ALL) and concluded there was clear evidence that this therapy is associated with cognitive impairment, and also that earlier onset was associated with higher rates of cognitive adverse effects. Brown et al. (1998) found that cranial irradiation and chemotherapy treatment for ALL was associated with generally average performance on most cognitive abilities, but with specific impairments in nonverbal cognitive skills. These studies suggest that either the direct effects of cancer or the side effects of treatment of cancer, or a combination of these, result in significant learning difficulties. Although these lifesaving treatments are essential for the survival of childhood cancer patients, they present an additional challenge to childhood cancer survivors in the form of higher risks for cognitive and academic impairments.

Asthma has also been associated with educational problems in children. Graham (1991) summarized some of this literature and concluded that the educational progress of asthmatic children is somewhat retarded, but suggested that frequent absences from school or the effects of treatment with bronchodialators, rather than learning disabilities, was mostly responsible for these educational deficits. Celano and Geller (1993) also reviewed the literature on the association between asthma and learning problems. They acknowledged that this association has been suspected and that there is some evidence to support this idea, but concluded that there was insufficient evidence to confirm that children with asthma had a significantly higher risk for academic problems. However, Fowler, Davenport, and Garge (1992) reported that children with asthma had a 1.7-time greater risk of learning disability when compared to physically healthy children.

Other medical problems frequently associated with academic and learning problems are epilepsy (Bourgeois, 1998), headache (Wellage, 1998), HIV (Krener, 1991), and thyroid disorders (Graham, 1991). Despite the number of medical conditions that have been found to have an association with cognitive impairments, some medical conditions have been demonstrated not to have an association with learning disabilities. For example, Crawford, Kaplan, and Field (1995) reported that Type I diabetes is not associated with any cognitive, academic, or learning difficulties. In addition, Hobbs and Sexson (1993) reported that the literature on outcomes for children with end-stage liver and kidney disease who received organ transplants suggests neurocognitive benefits derived from organ transplantation for these children. In this instance, treatment appears to provide a beneficial effect on cognitive functioning.

A final way in which the relationship between learning disabilities and medical problems needs to be considered lies in the special health needs of learning disabled individuals. As previously mentioned, learning disabled children have been found to experience higher than average levels of health problems. There are also other ways that learning disabilities can be a factor in health care. For example, Rauch-Elenekave (1994) found that there was a high incidence of undetected learning disability among teenage mothers referred to a program for teens who experienced out-of-wedlock pregnancy. The experiences of school failure and the need for alternative sources of self-esteem and "success" (e.g., pregnancy in this case) were hypothesized as key reasons that these teens got pregnant. If their learning disabilities had been detected earlier and academic experiences could have provided a more constructive source of self-esteem, fewer of these teens may have experienced pregnancy. Robertson and Jackson (1996) noted that rates of smoking were equivalent for children with and without learning disabilities, but suggested that health promotion programs might be improved if special needs of a learning disabled population were factored into the program literature and design. Kelly and Gottesman (1997) also suggested that individuals with reading, writing, and other learning disabilities may be impaired in their ability to understand their medical conditions and participate fully in their medical care. They suggested that modification and accommodations in health care delivery might be needed to serve learning disabled individuals optimally. These ideas suggest that involvement of medical professionals includes much more than identifying or excluding medical causes of learning problems and also that learning disabilities affect an individual's access and treatment by the medical profession, meaning that a much broader appreciation of medical factors in learning disabilities is needed.

There is a need for additional research concerning medical factors in learning disabilities. It is essential to determine which additional medical conditions and treatment, other than ones currently recognized, may be associated with learning disabilities. It will also be important to determine whether the source of learning problems associated with medical problems is a result of the disease itself or of the treatments used to combat the disease and to look for ways to overcome these effects or develop strategies specifically for these conditions. Finally, the role of the stress of medical illness in interfering with academic progress needs to be clarified. Few studies have looked at the relative contributions of each of the factors. Increasing recognition of the special needs of learning disabled populations in receiving medical care is also an area that is only now being explored, and is an area where mental health professionals might provide guidance to providers of general medical services. Psychologists and other allied health professionals, physicians, educators, and parents all need to recognize the special vulnerability for learning impairment of medically ill children. Education about, early recognition of, and intervention for learning problems in medically ill children will only occur when this consistently happens.

APPROACHES TO TREATMENT AND INTERVENTIONS

Treatment and Remediation Approaches

Attempts to assist children with learning disabilities have ranged from providing extra tutorial help on a one-to-one basis to sophisticated programs directed at remediation of a visual-perceptual problem. In fact, an industry has arisen in the attempt to develop effectual approaches to the remediation of a learning disorder. Most remedial efforts today focus on direct instruction of subskills, according to Speat-Swerling and Sternberg (1996). However, despite the current focus on direct instruction, there seems to be a return to the focus on treating underlying processes as evidenced by the work of Tallal et al. (1996) and Merzenech et al. (1996).

Two major approaches of instruction for mainstream students with LD are remediation and compensation. The goal of remediation is the improvement of a weakness or deficit, whereas compensatory strategies are to bypass or make up for a weakness by using the strengths of the student. Remediation is used to teach students basic academic and social skills. Compensatory, when used, is often with older students, and teaching strategies are designed to bypass skill deficiencies in order to teach basic subject areas.

Process and multisensory training are prime examples of compensatory teaching. At one time this was a popular educational approach for students with LD. Process and multisensory methods of intervention involve the training psychological process, such as visual and auditory perception or training using multiple sensory modalities. Data-based studies have not been able to document the effectiveness of process and multi-sensory approaches as being effective (Hammill, 1990). Two major criticisms associated with these approaches are that they are for renewal from academics and take too much time that is not directly associated with teaching basic content materials.

REMEDIATION: SPECIFIC SKILL TRAINING

Within this category, there are a number of major approaches that professionals recognize as being effective in assisting students with LDs (see Figure 7.2).

Behavior-Based Approaches

Behavioral treatment interventions concentrate on measurable behaviors and represent several common remedial education approaches. The following categories reflect the major approaches within the treatment domain: direct instruction/curriculum-based instruction; behavioral intervention such as token economy; and behavioral-contracts, a time-out use of extinction and precision teaching and cognitive behavioral approaches that concentrate on changing one's cognition or thoughts. This approach has been found to be successful in remediating specific skills defects (Swanson, 1989; Borkowski, 1992; Scrugg & Mastropieri; Hallahan et al. 1979). Examples of cognitive behavior approaches used to treat LD students are self-instruction (Meichenbaum, 1975), scaffolded instruction (Englert et al., 1991), reciprocal teaching, self-monitoring, attribution training and teaching, milocognition, and rehearsal skills.

Behavior Modification	Cognitive	Environmental	Unproven
Token Economy	Self-Monitoring	Biofeedback	Patterning
Positive Reinforcement	Goal Setting	Assertive Technology	Procare Training
Timeout	Verbal Rehearsal		Auditory-Perceptual Training
Extinction	Attribution Training		
Reinforcing Incompatible Behavior	Problem Solving		Visual-Motor Training
	Relaxation Training		Megavitamins
Precision Tracking	Scaffolded Instruction		Trace Elements
Direction Instruction	Emotive Imagery		Special Diets
Ignoring	Cognitive Restructuring		Chiropractic Procedures
Shaping	Social Training		
Contingency Management			
Task Analysis			

Figure 7.2   Summary of Instructional Treatment Approaches for Children with a Learning Disorder

Bender (1992) suggested that behavioral treatment approaches are the most influential type of instructional treatment used in schools today. Many special education teachers, clinicians, regular instructors, and parents use behavior techniques with some frequency. For example, 90% of all learning disability teachers have reported using behavioral intervention strategies in their classes (Meheady et al., 1982). The cognitive behavioral model of learning is a very effective tool for conceptualizing the instructional process. The cognitive behavioral approach is based on an interactive learner perspective that gives the LD student more responsibility for planning and managing the solution for his or her educational problems. This approach promotes active involvement among the LD child, the educational task, and the teacher or therapist.

Unsupported Intervention Approaches

In any research-based field, we have a professional obligation and responsibility to keep abreast of the research regarding any treatment approach used with children and youth. In addition, we have a professional obligation to the consumers to discourage the use of various treatment/intervention approaches that are not supported by empirical data-based research until such evidence is forthcoming to support this treatment. For psychologists, the American Psychological Association's Ethical Principles warn against such activities, especially the use of testimonials for any treatment approach. Some parents who have a child who is handicapped become desperate in trying to "fix" the child and will seek almost any type of help. Sometimes these parents will accept a treatment even when such treatments have not shown promise, when the research literature has not documented their usefulness, and even when there is strong evidence against the use of such treatment programs. As professionals, we need to be sensitive to the needs of parents who may want to use an unproven treatment procedure to treat a disorder. The sharing of information on the efficacy of various treatment approaches to consumers in a caring manner, allowing them to make their own decisions, is our professional and moral obligation.

Bender, in his excellent 1992 book on learning disabilities, documents and provides a review of various unsupported treatment approaches.

On the basis of his excellent review, the following conclusions seem appropriate: (a) Research studies on visual/perceptual learning, auditory training, and multisensory learning have not demonstrated effectiveness; (b) there is no scientifically accepted evidence to support the use of patterning as a treatment approach for LD; and (c) various biochemical approaches (diets such as sugar-free megavitamins are trace elements) have not been supported by the majority of data based research studies.

Medication

Because many children with LD have co-occurrences of ADHD, a comprehensive medical evaluation is appropriate. Significant fears remain around the use of psychopharmacologic agents in the treatment of social and emotional difficulties of children (Del Mundo et al., 1999). However, the benefits of psychopharmacologic treatment of children have become increasingly established within the research literature and clinical practice (Pumariega et al., 2000). Of course, pharmacotherapy is never the sole modality in treating children and adolescents with co-occurring disorders. A well integrated multimodal treatment approach is recommended, requiring close communication among different clinicians, educators, and parents. When a concurrent disorder such as ADHD, Anxiety Disorder, or Major Depression contributes to the severity of the LD problem, clinical practice would suggest the use of medication when appropriate. However, Beitchman and Young (1999) consider the use of medication on a LD in the absence of comorbid problems as experimental.

SUMMARY

When Samuel Kirk in the early 1960s proposed the term *learning disabilities* as a compromise, I seriously doubt if he would have thought that there would be eleven different definitions for his term. The labeled LD student represents a complex constellation of behaviors and conditions. The four most common factors in defining a learning disability are IQ/achievement discrepancy, presumption of central nervous system dysfunction, psychological processing problems, and a learning problem not due to environmental disadvantage, mental retardation, or emotional problems. Clinicians use three general types of assessment instruments to evaluate students with LD: standardized achievement and intelligence tests, formative evaluation measures, and various types of inventories. Students with LD often have a high rate of concurrent disorders, such as ADHD, Major Depression Disorders, and Anxiety Disorders.

Treatment and intervention methods for academic problems as well as for socialemotional difficulties are process training behavior modification, cognitive behavior training, curriculum-based procedures, and medication. Once popular as an educational method for students with LD, process training is not used much in schools. Cognitive and behavior modification methods for treating the child's academic and social-emotional difficulties are the most popular intervention methods used by today's teachers.

Authorities have documented that LD often exists throughout the life span, and various programs are currently addressing the unique needs of this population. Future issues facing the field of learning disabilities are numerous. Professionals will continue to labor with changes in the definition of LD. Great research efforts will be made on identifying subgroups of children with LD. The hope for this type of documentation is that it will lead to a better match between learner's characteristics and instructional developing service models. A major question yet unanswered is, is there a need for providing education services to preschool children with learning problems? Will this issue become a legal and political problem? Professional improvements of teachers as well as the high rate of burn out are two issues that deserve to be addressed by universities and school-district staff personnel. Perhaps the professional improvement plan (PIP; currently used in West Virginia) could be used as one model to address professional improvement.

The role of parents, home schooling, and charter schools will have an impact on the field of LD. As for research, in what direction will this take place? The research focus, if any, will affect the field drastically. The field of learning disability, although relatively young, is a new, dynamic, and growing field where much work will be required. Tremendous advances have been made in the field of LD over the past 15 years. According to Maughan (1995), the most positive and successful outcomes have consistently emerged from studies in which LD children have received support and encouragement at home, specialized attention at school, and selected professional help consistent with their strengths and weaknesses. Best professional practice would mandate the importance of comprehensive multidisciplinary assessment, tailored to meet the individual intervention programs of LD students. Follow-up studies of students with LD in light of the recent findings regarding comorbidity and the existence of LD into adulthood are a must if the professionals in the field of learning disabilities are to understand the scope and depths of how LD affects a child or adult fully.

REFERENCES

Algozzine, B., & Ysseldyke, J. E. (1987). Questioning discrepancies: Retaking the first step 20 years later. *Learning Disability Quarterly, 10,* 301–302.

American Psychiatric Association. (1994). Diagnostic and statistical manual for mental disorders (4th ed.). Washington, DC: Author.

Aronbach, L. J. (1949). *Essentials of psychological testing.* New York: Harper & Brothers.

Arvidson, J., Kihlgren, M., Hall, C., & Lonnerholm, G. (1999). Neuropsychological functioning after treatment for hematological malignancies in childhood, including autologous bone marrow transplantation. *Pediatric Hematology and Oncology, 16,* 9–21.

Beitchman, M. D., & Young, A. R. (1997). Learning disorders with a special emphasis on reading disorders: A review of the past 10 years. *Journal of the American Academy of Child & Adolescent Psychiatry, 38, 8,* 1020–1031.

Bellack, A. S., & Hensen, M. (1988). Future directions. In A. S. Belleck & M. Hensen (Eds.), *Behavioral assessment: A practical handbook* (pp. 287–297). Elmsford, NY: Pergamon Press.

Bender, W. N. (1992). *Learning disabilities: Characteristics, identification, and teaching strategies.* Boston: Allyn & Bacon.

Bender, W. N., & Wall, M. E. (1994). Social-emotional development of students with learning disabilities. *Learning Disability Quarterly, 17,* 323–341.

Berg, M. (1988). Toward a diagnostic alliance between psychiatrist and psychologist. *American Psychologist, 41,* 52–59.

Berry, M. (1986). Toward a diagnostic alliance between psychiatrist and psychologist. *American Psychologist, 41,* 52–59.

Boetsch, E., Green, P. A., & Pennington, B. F. (1996). Psychological correlates of dyslexia across the life span. *Developmental Psychopathology, 8,* 539–562.

Bourgeois, B. F. (1998). Antiepeleptic drugs, learning, and behavior in childhood epilepsy. *Epilepsia, 39,* 913–921.

Brown, R. T., Madan-Swain, A., Walco, G. A., Cherrick, I., Levers, C. E., Conte, P. M., Vega, R., & Lauer, S. J. (1998). Cognitive and academic late effects among children previously treated for acute lymphocytic leukemia receiving chemotherapy as CNS prophylaxis. *Journal of Pediatric Psychology, 23,* 333–340.

Bruck, M. (1985). The adult functioning of children with specific learning: A follow-up study. In I. Sigel (Ed.), *Advances in Applied Developmental Psychology.* Boston: Allyne & Bacon.

Bryon, T. (1991). Social problems and learning disabilities. In B. Y. Wong (Ed.), *Learning about learning disabilities* (pp. 195–229). San Diego: Academic Press.

Carr, A. (1985). Psychological testing of personality. In H. Kaplan & B. Sadock (Eds.), *Comprehensive textbook of psychiatry* (pp. 514–535). Baltimore: William & Wilkins.

Celano, M. P., & Geller, R. J. (1993). Learning, school performance, and children with asthma: How much at risk? *Journal of Learning Disabilities, 26,* 23–32.

Chalfant, J. C. (1985). Identifying learning disabled students: A summary of the national task force. *Learning Disabilities Focus, 1,* 9–20.

Clohin, J., & Sweeney, J. A. (1986). Psychological assessment. In R. Michels et al. (Eds.), *Psychiatry 1* (pp. 241–269). Philadelphia: Sippincott.

Coles, G. S. (1978). The learning disability test battery: Empirical and social issues. *Harvard Educational Review, 48,* 313–340.

Conners, C. K. (1990). *Conners rating scale.* Toronto, Canada: Multi-Health Systems.

Cool, V. A. (1996). Long term neuropsychological risks in pediatric bone marrow transplant: What do we know? *Bone Marrow Transplant, 18* (Supplement), S45–S49.

Cowell, J. M. (1990). Dilemmas in assessing the health status of children with learning disabilities. *Journal of Pediatric Health Care, 4,* 24–31.

Crawford, S. G., Kaplan, B. J., & Field, L. L. (1995). Absence of an association between insulin-dependent diabetes mellitus and developmental learning difficulties. *Heraditas, 122,* 73–78.

Cruickshank, W. M., Bentzen, F. A., Rotzberg, R. H., & Tannhouser, M. T. (1961). *A teaching method for brain injured and hyperactive children.* Syracuse, NY: Syracuse Press.

Del Mundo, A., Pumariega, A. J., & Vance, H. B. (1999). Psychopharmacology in school-based mental health services. *Psychology in the Schools, 36*(5), 437–450.

Elber, H. W. (1964, September). Automated personality description with 16 PF data. In R. D. Dregor, *Computer reporting of personality test data.* Symposium American Psychological Association, Los Angeles, CA.

Exner, J. E. (1987). Computer assistance in Rorschach interpretation. In J. N. Butcher (Ed.), *Computerized psychological assessment* (pp. 218–235). New York: Basic Books.

Farel, A. M., Hooper, S. R., Teplin, S. W., Henry, M. M., & Kraybill, E. N. (1998). Very low-birthweight infants at seven years: As assessment of the health and neurodevelopmental risk conveyed by chronic lung disease. *Journal of Learning Disabilities, 31,* 118–126.

Finnly, J. C. (1966). Programmed interpretation of the MMPI and CPI. *Archives of General Psychiatry, 15,* 75–81.

Fletcher, J. M., & Copeland, D. R. (1988). Neurobehavioral effects of central nervous system prophytactic treatment of cancer in children. *Journal of Clinical and Experimental Neuropsychology, 10,* 495–537.

Flynn, J. M., & Rehbar, M. H. (1994). Prevalence of reading failure in boys compared with girls. *Psychology in the Schools, 31,* 66–71.

Fowler, M. G., Davenport, M. G., & Garg, R. (1990). School functioning of US children with asthma. *Pediatrics, 90,* 939–944.

Goldstein, G., & Hersen, M. (1992). *Handbook of Psychological Assessment.* New York: Pergamon Press.

Graham, P. J. (1991). Psychiatric aspects of pediatric disorders. In M. Lewis (Ed.), *Child and adolescent psychiatry: A comprehensive text* (pp. 977–994). Baltimore: Williams & Wilkins.

Greenblatt, E., & Greenblatt, R. M. (1997). Learning disabilities: Developmental disorders. In J. Noshpitz (Ed.), *Handbook of child and adolescent Psychiatry: Vol. 2* (pp. 235–252). New York: Wiley.

Hallahan, D. P., & Kauffman, J. M. (1976). *Introduction to learning disabilities: A psychobehavioral approach.* Englewood Cliffs, NJ: Prentice Hall.

Hammill, D. D. (1990). A brief history of LD. In D. Hamell & P. Myers (Eds.), *Learning disabilities: Basic concepts, assessment practices and instructional strategies* (pp. 1–14). Austin: Pro-Ed.

Hammill, D. D., & Larsen, S. (1974). The relationship of selected auditory perceptual skills and reading ability. *Journal of Learning Disability, 7,* 429–436.

Henshaw, S. P. (1992). Externalizing behavior problems and academic underachievement in childhood and adolescents casual relationships and underachievement mechanisms. *Psychological Bulletin, 111,* 127–155.

Hinlington, D. D., & Bender, W. N. (1993). Adolescents and learning disabilities at risk? Emotional well-being, depression, suicide. *Journal of Learning Disabilities, 26,* 159–166.

Hobbs, S. A., & Sexson, S. B. (1993). Cognitive development and learning in the pediatric organ transplant recipient. *Journal of Learning Disabilities, 26,* 104–113.

Holborow, P. L., & Berry, P. S. (1986). Hyperactivity and learning disabilities. *Learning Disabilities, 19,* 426–431.

Honaker, L. M., & Flower, R. D. (1990). Computer-assisted psychological assessment. In G. Goldstein & M. Hersen (Eds.), *Handbook of psychological assessment* (pp. 521–546). New York: Pergamon Press.

Honaker, L. M., & Harrell, T. H. (1988). *Microcomputer system for the Intake Evaluation Report.* Indiolantic, FL: Psychogistics.

Hynd, G. W., & Samuel-Aikerman, M. (1989). Dyslexia and brain morphology *Psychological Bulletin, 106,* 447–482.

Hynowitz, P., & Sweeney, J. A. (1985). Focal diagnostic psychological testing. *The Psychiatric Hospital, 16,* 91–95.

Johnson, J. H., & Williams, T. A. (1980). *Using a line computer technology in a mental health admitting system.* In J. B. Sidowski, J. H. Johnson, & T. A. William (Eds.), *Technology in mental health care delivery systems* (pp. 237–249). Norwood, NJ: ABLEX.

Kamphaus, R. (1993). *Clinical assessment of children's intelligence.* Boston: Allyn & Bacon.

Kanfer, F. H., & Saslow, G. (1969). Behavioral diagnosis. In C. F. Franks (Ed.), *Behavior therapy: Appraisal and status* (pp. 148–175). New York: McGraw-Hill.

Katz, M. M. (1989). The multivantaged approach. In S. Wetzler & M. M. Katz (2nd Eds.), *Contemporary approaches to psychological assessment* (pp. 16–42). New York: Brunner/Mazel.

Kauffman, A. S. (1979). *Intelligence testing with the WISC-R.* New York: Wiley.

Kelly, M. S., & Gottesman, R. L. (1997). Adults with severe reading and learning difficulties: A challenge for the family physician. *Journal of the American Board of Family Practice, 10,* 199–205.

Kirk, S. A. (1988). *Historical aspects of learning disabilities.* Unpublished Paper of Keynote Speech at Rutgers University.

Kirk, S. A., McCarthy, J. J., & Kirt, W. D. (1968). *The Illinois test of psycholinguistic abilities.* Urbana: University of Illinois Press.

Kovacs, M. (1992). *Children Depression Inventory.* Toronto, Canada: Multi-Health System.

Krener, P. G. (1991). HIV-Spectrum disease. In M. Lewis (Ed.), *Child and adolescent psychiatry: A comprehensive textbook* (pp. 994–1004). Baltimore: Williams & Wilkins.

Kurg, S. E. (1987). *Psychware Sourcebook 1987–1988.* Kansas City, MO: Test Corporation of America.

Larson, K. A. (1988). A research review and alternative hypothesis explaining the link between learning disability and delinquency. *Journal of Learning Disabilities, 21,* 363–369.

Lazarus, A. A. (1973). Multimodal behavior therapy: Treating the "basic id." *Journal of Nervous and Mental Disease, 156,* 404–411.

Light, J. G., Pennington, B. F., Gilgen, J. W., & Detries, J. C. (1995). Reading disabilities and hyperactivity disorders: Evidence of a common genetic etiology. *Developmental Neuropsychology, 11,* 323–335.

Logan, W. T. (1996). Neuroimaging and functional brain analysis. In J. H. Beitchman, N. J. Cohen, & R. Tannock (Eds.), *Language, learning and behavior disorder* (pp. 249–271). New York: Cambridge University Press.

McGee, R., Williams, S., Share, D. L., Anderson, J., & Silva, P. A. (1986). The relationship between specific reading retardation, general reading backwardness and behavior problems in a large sample of Dunedin boys. *Journal of Child Psychological Psychiatry, 27,* 597–610.

Maag, J. W. (1999). *Behavior management: From theoretical implications in practical applications,* San Diego: Singular.

Maddux, C. D., & Johnson, L. (1998). Computer-assisted assessment. In B. Vance (Ed.), *Psychological assessment of children* (pp. 87–105). New York: Wiley.

Meheady, L., Duncan, D., & Sainato, D. (1982). A survey of use of behavioral modification techniques by special indicators. *Teaching Education and Special Education, 5,* 9–15.

Meichenbaum, D. H. (1975, June). *Cognitive factors as determinates of LD: A cognitive functional approach.* Paper presented at NATO Conference on Learning Disorders: Theoretical Approaches, Korsor, Denmark.

Mercer, C. D. (1987). *Students with learning disabilities* (3rd ed.). Columbus, OH: Merrill.

Merrill, K. W. (1998). Assessing social skills and peer relations. In B. Vance (Ed.), *Psychological assessment of children* (pp. 246–276). New York: Wiley.

Merzenick, M. M., Jenkins, W. M., Johnson, P., Schreiner, C., Miller, S. L., & Talal, P. (1996). Temporal processing deficits of language-learning impaired children ameliorated by training. *Science, 271,* 77–80.

Middle, C., Johnson, A., Alderdice, F., Petty, T., & Macfarlane, A. (1996). Birthweight and health development at the age of seven years. *Child Care and Health Delivery, 22,* 55–71.

Moffitt, T. E. (1993). The neuropsychology of conduct disorders. *Psychopathology, 5,* 135–151.

Moreland, K. L. (1987). Computerized assessment: What's available. In J. N. Butcher (Ed.), *Computerized psychological assessment* (pp. 26–49). New York: Basic Books.

Motarazzo, J. D. (1986). Computerized clinical psychological test interpretation: Unvalidated plus all means no signs. *American Psychologist, 41,* 14–24.

Moughan, B. (1995). Annotation: Long-term outcomes of developmental reading problems. *Journal of Child Psychological Psychiatry, 36,* 357–371.

National Joint Committee on Learning Disabilities. (1988). *Defining learning disabilities* (p. 1). Washington, DC: NJCLD.

Parker, J. G., Asher, S. R. (1987). Peer relations and later personal adjustment: Are low accepted children at risk? *Psychological Bulletin, 102,* 357–389.

Pioddrowski, A. Z. (1964). A digital computer administration of inkblot test data. *Psychiatric Quarterly, 38,* 1–26.

Prior, M. (1996). *Understanding specific learning difficulties.* Sussex, England: Psychology Press.

Prior, M., Smart, D., Sanson, A., & Oberkloid, F. (1999). Relationships between learning difficulties and psychological problems in preadolescent children from a longitudinal sample. *Journal of the American Academy of Child and Adolescent Psychiatry, 38*(4) 429–436.

Pumariega, A. J., Del Mundo, A., & Vance, H. B. (2000). Pharmacotherapy in the context of children's mental health system of care. In B. J. Burns & K. Haagwood, *Community-based intervention for growth with serious emotional disorders.*

Pumariega, A. J., & Vance, B. (1999). School board mental health services: The foundations for system of care for children's mental health. *Psychology in the Schools, 5,* 371–378.

Rauch-Elnekave, H. (1994). Teenage motherhood: Its relationship to undetected learning problems. *Adolescence, 29,* 91–103.

Reynolds, C. R. (1984). Critical measurement issues in learning disabilities. *Special Education, 18,* 451–476.

Robertson, S. B., & Jackson, C. (1996). Initiation of smoking among children with and without learning disabilities. *Journal of Developmental and Behavioral Pediatrics, 17,* 248–252.

Rogers, H., & Saklofihe, D. H. (1985). Self-concept, laws of control and performance expectations of learning disabled children. *Journal of Learning Disabilities, 18,* 273–278.

Rogers, M. (1998). Psychoeducational assessment of culturally and linguistically diverse children and youth. In H. B. Vance (Ed.), *Psychological assessment of children: Best practices for school and clinical settings* (pp. 355–384). New York: Wiley.

Rotter, K. F. (1988). *The effects of cueing upon the ability to predict outcomes in learning disabled and non-learning disabled adolescents.* Unpublished doctoral dissertation, Rutgers University, New Brunswick, NJ.

Rourke, B. P., & Fuerst, D. R. (1996). Psychological dimensions of learning disabilities subtypes. *Assessment, 3,* 277–290.

Sattler, J. M. (1988). *Assessment of children* (3rd ed.). San Diego, CA: Author.

Sloper, T., Larcombe, I. J., & Charlton, A. (1994). Psychosocial adjustment of five-year survivors of childhood cancer. *Journal of Cancer Education, 9,* 163–169.

Spear, R., Swerling, L., & Sternvery, R. J. (1996). Educational practices for children with RD: In *Off track: When poor readers become "learning disabled"* (pp. 185–228). Bolder, CO: Westview Press.

Strauss, R. S. (2000). Adult functional outcome of those born small for gestational age: Twenty-six year follow-up of the 1970 British birth cohort. *Journal of the American Medical Association, 283,* 625–632.

Stewart, A. L., Rifkin, L., Amess, P. N., Kirkbride, V., Townsend, J. P., Miler, D. H., Lewis, S. W., Kingsley, D. P. E., Mosley, I. F., Foster, O., & Murray, R. M. (1999). Brain structure and neurocognitive and behavioral function in adolescents who were born very preterm. *The Lancet, 353,* 1653–1657.

Swason, H. L. (1989). Strategy instruction: Overview of principles and procedures for effective use. *Learning Disability Quarterly, 12,* 3–14.

Swerling, L., & Sternberg, R. J. C. (1996). Educational practices for children with RD. In *Off track: When poor readers become "learning disabled"* (pp. 185–228). Boulder, CO: Westview Press.

Tallal, P., Miller, S. L., & Bedi, G. (1996). Language comprehension in language: Learning impaired children improved with acoustically modified speech. *Science, 271,* 81–84.

Taylor, C. B. (1983). DSM-III and behavior assessment. *Behavior Assessment, 5,* 5–14.

Technology in mental health care delivery systems (pp. 237–249). Norwood, NJ: Ablax.

Tollefson, H., Tracy, B. D., Johnson, E. P., Buenning, M., Farmer, A., & Barke, C. R. (1982). Attribution patterns of learning disabled adolescents. *Learning Disabilities Quarterly, 5,* 14–20.

U.S. Department of Education. (1991). *Position paper on learning disabilities.* Washington, DC: Department of Education, Office of Special Education Program.

Vale, C. D., & Keller, L. S. (1987). Developing expert computer system to interpret psychological tests. In J. N. Butcher (Ed.), *Computerized psychological assessment* (pp. 325–343). New York: Basic Books.

Vance, B., & Awaad, A. (1998). Best practices in assessment of children: Issues and trends. In B. Vance (Ed.), *Psychological Assessment of Children* (p. 148). New York: Wiley.

Vaughn, S., & Hogan, A. (1990). Social competence and learning disabilities: A prospective study. In H. I. Swanson & B. Keogh (Eds.), *Learning disabilities: Research* (pp. 175–191). Hillsdale, NJ: Erlbaum.

Vaughn, S., & Hogan, A. (1990). Social competency and learning disabilities: A prospective study. In H. Swanson & B. K. Keogh (Eds.), *Learning disabilities: Theoretical and research issues* (pp. 175–191). Hillsdale, NJ: Erlbaum.

Wechsler, D. C. (1996). *Manual for the Wechsler Intelligence Scale for Children* (3rd ed.). San Antonio, TX: Psychological Corp.

Weiner, I. (1983). The future of psychodiagnosis revisited. *Journal of Personality Assessment, 47,* 451–459.

Wellage, L. C. (1998). Headache in children: Data from the 1988 Child Health Supplement to the National Health Interview Survey. *Dissertation Abstracts International, 58(7-B),* 3590.

Wetzler, S. (1989). Parameter of psychological assessment. In S. Wetzler & M. M. Katz (Eds.), *Contemporary approaches to psychological assessment* (pp. 3–15). New York: Brunner/Mazel.

William, S., & McGee, R. (1996). Reading in childhood and mental health in early adolescents. In N. J. Beitchman, W. L. Chonen, & R. T. Tannock (Eds.), *Language, learning, and behavior disorder: Clinical perspectives* (pp. 530–354). New York: Cambridge University Press.

Wright, M. O., & Masten, A. S. (1997). Vulnerability and resilience in young children. In J. D. Noshpitz (Series ed.) & S. Greenspan, S. Wieder, & J. Osofsky (Vol. eds.), *Handbook of child and adolescent psychiatry: Vol. 1. Infants and preschoolers: Development and syndromes* (pp. 202–224). New York: Wiley.

Ysseldyke, J. (1987). Classification of handicapped students. In M. C. Wang, M. C. Reynolds, & H. J. Walberg (Eds.), *Handbook of special education: Resource and practice* (pp. 81–103). New York: Peryanion Press.

Zimmerman, J., Rich, W. D., Keilutz, L., & Bender, P. K. (1979). *Some observation on the Link Between Learning Disabilities and Juvenile Delinquency* (LDJD-003). Williamsburg, VA: National Center for State Courts.

Chapter 8

COMMUNICATIVE DISORDERS

NANCY J. SCHERER

The major objectives of this chapter are to provide (a) an overview of profiles of language and speech impairment in children with specific language impairment, developmental delays, and autism; (b) a discussion of the developmental theoretical model of communication development; and (c) discussion of standardized and informal assessment procedures.

RATIONALE FOR COMMUNICATION ASSESSMENT

Why assess communicative performance? The answer to this question may seem obvious for the young child who is not talking, but what about the school-aged child who is struggling academically or the preschool child with severe behavior problems? For all these children, communication impairments may be an underlying deficit that contributes to these very different manifestations. Understanding and use of language is fundamental to human communication. As such, impairments in language development may have far-reaching effects. Language impairments may impact social development, academic learning, attention, memory, and even higher cognitive learning (Paul, 1995; Owens, 1995).

Early identification of language impairment is essential to lessen the potential effects of a language disorder. Assessment of language and speech is the first step in the identification of communication disorders. Accurate description of language performance serves several functions. First, it assists in determining whether a language impairment is present. Presence of a language impairment has bearing on other assessments performed as part of an interdisciplinary evaluation. Understanding and use of language is required for most assessment measures, and deficits in these domains would impact performance that relies on verbal skills. Second, language assessment can provide information pertaining to the type of communication impairment and whether the communication impairment exists alone or is associated with other developmental or learning impairments. Third, accurate diagnosis of communication impairments aids in determining eligibility for services and recommendations for the type and frequency of services.

DEVELOPMENTAL APPROACH

Communication development occurs as part of a complex maturational process such that milestones emerging early in life may bear little resemblance to milestones of later development. How then do we decide what to assess and how to assess these diverse milestones? Research in communication development has identified two processes: receptive and expressive language (Nelson, 1998; Paul, 1995; Owens, 1995). Although these processes remain important throughout development, the specific domains assessed within each process change with age. For example, the assessment of gestural communication is essential for assessment of expressive development in toddlers but is unnecessary for older, school-aged children. Likewise, written language assessment is important for the school-aged child but not for the preschooler.

Within each process of receptive and expressive language, several domains play a dominant role. These domains include vocabulary and grammar (including word order in sentences and inflectional morphology comprising word endings, e.g., dog/dogs, walk/walked). Additionally, expressive language has some unique components not part of receptive language, including rules governing language use or pragmatics and the production of speech sounds. Pragmatics include the rules for expressing basic communicative intent that emerges prior to a child's first words in the form of gesture and vocalization. For example, a child may point and vocalize to request a toy prior to being able to request the toy with a word. These early communicative gestures form the foundation for conversational use as language and speech are acquired. Speech sound development has its own acquisition timetable apart from language milestones. Considerable research has been completed on the age of acquisition of speech sound production, making this domain one of the most easily recognized and assessed (Smit, Hand, Freilinger, Bernthal, & Bird, 1980). Both standardized and informal measures assess these domains. Standardized tests often assess these domains broadly, whereas informal procedures probe individual domains in more depth.

In addition, the relationship between the receptive and expressive language processes and other cognitive and motor domains may assist professionals in differentiating between an isolated communication impairment and deficits involving other cognitive, learning, or psychosocial parameters. The presence of distinctive relationships between language, cognition, motor, and social development has been captured in the definitions of specific disorders such as specific language impairment, developmental delay, and autism.

PROFILES FOR IMPAIRMENT

Many disorders of communication development have been characterized by profiles of strengths and weaknesses that describe the relationship between receptive language, expressive language, speech, and other developmental domains such as cognitive development and motor development. These profiles provide a visual image of the relative synchrony among developmental domains and may assist in the diagnostic classification process. The term *profile* assumes that typical development is described by a flat profile and that atypical development shows some deviation from this flat profile. De-

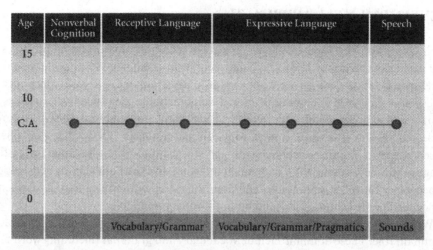

Figure 8.1   Prototypic Communication Profile for Typically Developing Children

veloping a profile for a child requires use of either age-equivalent or standard scores plotted in comparison to the child's mental or chronological age (Miller, 1981; Miller & Paul, 1995). Figure 8.1 shows a prototypic example of typically developing children who have language and speech performance commensurate with cognitive status and chronological age. This profile represents a prototypic picture of children without significant performance strengths or weaknesses, instead of the profile of an individual child who may show some deviation from this stylized profile.

A profile may be constructed following administration of standardized and informal tests and can assist the professional in two ways. First, the profile may be useful in determining the differential diagnosis of the impairment. Profiles are a way of comparing a child's performance to prototypic performance for a group or subgroup of children having a known diagnostic classification. For example, the profile of children with specific language impairment is different from the profile observed in children with developmental delay. Second, profiles may be used to describe the performance of individual children and highlight the domains requiring intervention.

DIAGNOSTIC PROFILES

Profiles for four diagnostic groups will be discussed: specific language impairment (SLI), specific language impairment—expressive (SLI-E), developmental delay, and autism. Specific language impairment (SLI and SLI-E) are considered disorders in which language and speech are isolated areas of deficit relative to other areas of strength. Additionally, language and speech impairments may coexist with other developmental and social deficits as in the disorders of autism and developmental delay.

Specific Language Impairment (SLI and SLI-E)

The profiles for specific language impairment are characterized by delays in receptive and expressive or expressive language development. These delays are outside the developmental range expected for the child's age and nonverbal cognitive performance. The

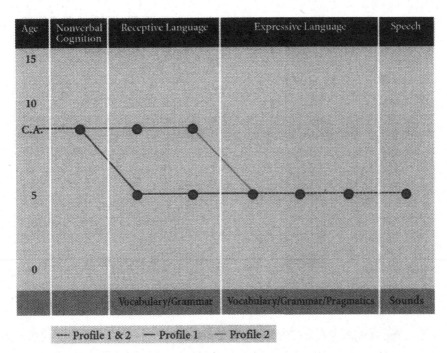

Age	Nonverbal Cognition	Receptive Language	Expressive Language	Speech
		Vocabulary/Grammar	Vocabulary/Grammar/Pragmatics	Sounds

--- Profile 1 & 2   — Profile 1   — Profile 2

Figure 8.2   Prototypic Communication Profile for Children with Specific Language Impairment (solid line) and Specific Language Impairment–Expressive (dotted line)

discrepancy between nonverbal and language domains is a hallmark of both forms of specific language impairment (Watkins, 1997). However, SLI and SLI-E differ in the child's receptive language performance. Children with SLI show receptive deficits, whereas children with SLI-E show receptive language commensurate with chronological age level (Paul, 1995). Figure 8.2 provides an example of a profile of SLI and SLI-E.

Developmental Delay

Most studies of children with developmental delay have been conducted on children with Down syndrome. Many children with Down syndrome show a delayed, flat profile across all developmental domains (Miller, Leddy, & Leavitt, 1999). However, 60 to 75% of children with Down syndrome show a greater expressive language delay than is predicted by other developmental performance. The two most commonly occurring profiles for children with Down syndrome are displayed in Figure 8.3. The features of the profile that differentiate the developmental delay profile from SLI and SLI-E profiles include the discrepancy between chronological age and nonverbal cognition. Children with developmental delay show a gap between chronological age and nonverbal cognitive performance, whereas no gap is present for children with SLI or SLI-E.

Autism

Speech and language impairments are a significant component of disorders on the autism spectrum. However, these impairments are most prominent in the area of language use or

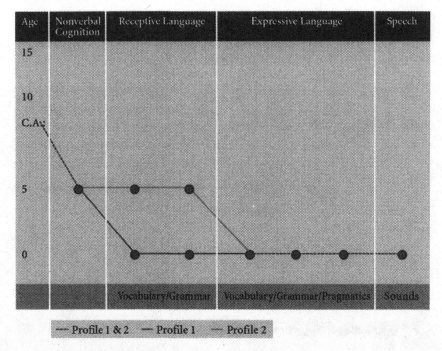

Figure 8.3   Communication Profiles

Note: Communication profiles for two of the most common subgroups of children with Down Syndrome. Children with receptive and expressive deficits below that expected based on nonverbal cognitive performance are represented by the solid line, and children with expressive deficits below that expected based on nonverbal cognitive performance are represented by the dotted line.

pragmatics (Scott, Clark, & Brady, 2000). This area of deficit is characteristic regardless of the severity of speech and language impairments. For example, children with autism who are high functioning show a similar profile to children who are lower functioning, the difference being the extent of the gap between chronological age and levels of language and developmental performance. Children with a diagnosis of Asberger's syndrome are often viewed as performing the closest to age norms, with the exception of pragmatic performance (Campbell, 1999). Figure 8.4 shows profiles for children with autism who show different levels of performance. The unique feature of the profiles for children on the autism spectrum is the significant deficit in pragmatics relative to performance in other language and nonverbal cognitive domains (Tager-Flusberg, 1989). This deficit is not observed in children with SLI, SLI-E, or developmental delay.

TYPES OF ASSESSMENT

Standardized Tests

Most standardized tests of communication development assess receptive and expressive language development, but they may assess additional areas including speech sound production, auditory memory, sequencing, phonemic awareness, and written language. The benefits of standardized instruments are the known validity and relia-

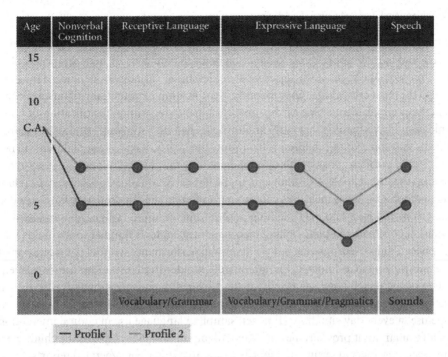

Age	Nonverbal Cognition	Receptive Language	Expressive Language	Speech
15				
10				
C.A.				
5				
0				
		Vocabulary/Grammar	Vocabulary/Grammar/Pragmatics	Sounds

— Profile 1   — Profile 2

Figure 8.4   Prototypic Communication Profiles for Children on the Autism Spectrum
Note: Profile designated by the dotted line represents children who are high functioning.

bility of the procedures, as well as scoring and normative comparisons that yield standard scores permitting comparison to performance or other standardized tests. Standardized tests are effective in determining whether there is an impairment present. However, they have been criticized for their inability to determine the specific areas of deficits contributing to the disorder, which is so essential for intervention planning (Huang, Hopkins, & Nippold, 1997; Merrell & Plante, 1997).

Informal Procedures

Standardized tests measure language performance through elicited items that often require a specific answer. Although these procedures provide a time-efficient means of assessing language performance, they do not sample language in typical communicative contexts (Nelson, 1998). Informal procedures can be used to supplement standardized tests by providing flexibility in presentation of test items not permitted during standardized presentations. Further, informal procedures may provide a sampling of the child's use of language that is not tested in standardized measures (Miller & Paul, 1995; Miller & Chapman, 1999). One frequently used informal procedure is a language sample. A language sample is a procedure in which conversational interaction between the child and clinician or parent is taped and analyzed for vocabulary, grammar, and appropriateness of language used (Miller, 1981). Informal procedures, such as language samples, are particularly important for children with behavioral concerns that may interfere with their test-taking behavior. Normative comparisons are available for language sampling as well as many other informal procedures, although standard scores are often not derived from these procedures.

Assessment of Infants and Toddlers

Most assessment measures for very young children are comprised of observational, elicited, and parent-report items. Reliance on items that must be elicited from young children is problematic because this age is most vulnerable to variable cooperation. However, it is also the most critical age range for early identification of potentially significant communication impairments. One of the greatest fallacies regarding identification of communication impairment is that early impairments will be outgrown. Although research supports that some young children will outgrow their early delays, many children will not (Paul, 1995). Further, considerable development has gone into early language assessment measures that are reliable and valid; and, in the hands of a qualified pediatric speech language pathologist, these measures can serve to differentiate children with language disorders from children who may catch up without intervention. Language assessment of toddlers necessitates sampling of language in natural contexts familiar to the child (Vinson, 1999). Clinical settings may not yield optimal performance without consideration of these natural language contexts. In other words, standardized tests alone are insufficient to adequately assess language development. Normed parent questionnaires have been developed that are reliable and provide the parents' perception of the child's optimal language use in every day situations. Further, sampling language use in natural interaction with a familiar adult provides the clinician with an observable sample of the child's performance in the clinical setting that may be compared to parent generated reports.

Table 8.1 shows a description of common language assessment areas and measures for children birth to 3 years of age. The table shows the testing areas that comprise a communicative assessment. The standardized tests include general measures of receptive and expressive language development sampling all domains within these two processes. In addition, standardized, normed parent-report questionnaires that sample language use in the home environment are available. Many informal procedures are available for children in this age group. Language sample analysis procedures are available with age norm comparisons. Informal procedures are also available for nonverbal cognitive development, play, communicative gesture, and language comprehension.

Assessment of Preschool-Aged Children

More standardized language measures are available for the preschool-aged child than for the toddler, however, poor compliance to test administration procedures is still a variable for this age group. Informal procedures, particularly language sampling, are required to augment standardized assessment measures to capture language use in naturalistic contexts. As with younger children, informal procedures may also be appropriate to measure nonverbal cognition, language comprehension, and play development. Table 8.1 displays frequently used language tests and informal procedures appropriate for preschool-aged children.

Assessment of School-Aged Children

Communication assessment for the school-aged child consists primarily of standardized, formal language tests. Most standard tests assess receptive and expressive language through a series of subtests that evaluate different domains within these two pro-

Table 8.1 Cognitive, Language, and Speech Assessment Protocols for Three Age Groups.

Birth to 3 years

Areas of Communication	Reason for Assessment	Test Measures
Cognition		
Developmental assessment	Differentiate language/non-language deficits.	Bayley Scales of Infant Development-2
Nonverbal skills	Play is a developmental task that parallels language development.	Play Assessment Piagetian concepts: Assessing Linguistic Behavior
Language		
Standardized tests: receptive/expressive	Comparison to normative sample. Sample language in structured tasks.	Sequenced Inventory of Communicative Development-2 (SICD), Rossetti Infant-Toddler Scale
Communication Intent	Explore diversity of gestural/vocal communicative attempts.	Communication & Symbolic Behavior Scale
Parent questionnaire	Sample use of language in home environment.	Communicative Development Inventory (CDI)
Language Sample	Use of language in natural communicative contexts.	Developmental Sentence Scoring (DSS), Systematic Analysis of Language Transcripts (SALT)
Speech		
Consonant Inventory	Sampling of repertoire of speech sounds.	Naming objects controlled for articulation features
Syllable Structure	Babbling and consonant-vowel combinations as a window to later articulation development.	
Stimulability	Ability to produce consonants in a hierarchy of complexity from isolation, syllables to words.	Use of hierarchy of cues to facilitate sound production.
Hearing	Hearing acquity and middle ear function.	Electrophysiologic assessment, otoacoustic emissions, behavioral audiometry, immittance testing.

(*continued*)

Table 8.1 Continued

Areas of Communication	Reason for Assessment	Test Measures
Preschool		
Cognition		
Developmental assessment	Differentiate language/non-language deficits.	Refer for WIPPSI or Leiter Informal Piagetian Assessment
Language		
Standardized tests receptive/expressive	Comparison to normative sample. Sample language in structured tasks.	SICD-R, Test of Language Development (TOLD:P3), Preschool Language Scale-3
Questionnaire	Sample use of language in home environment.	CDI for children with significant delay.
Language Sample	Use of natural communication context.	DSS, SALT
Speech		
Consonant Inventory	Sampling of repertoire of speech sounds.	
Syllable Structure	Sampling of consonant-vowel combinations.	
Single Word Articulation Test	Sampling of sounds in controlled words for accuracy compared to adult model.	Goldman-Fristoe test of Articulation (GFTA)
Connected Speech	Sample sound production in conversation and compare to single word production.	Language Sample, GFTA Stories
Stimulability	Ability to produce consonants in a hierarchy of complexity from isoltion, syllables to words.	
Hearing	Assess auditory acquity and middle ear function.	Electrophysiologic assessment, otoacoustic emissions, behavioral audiometry, immittance testing

School Age

Areas of Communication	Reason for Assessment	Test Measures
Cognition		
Developmental assessment	Differentiate language/non-language deficits.	Refer for WISC-III Nonverbal cognitive assessment
Language		
Standardized tests receptive/expressive	Comparison to normative sample. Sample language in structured tasks.	TOLD:P3, Clinical Evaluation of Language Fundamentals-3
Written Language Questionnaire	Written vocabulary, grammar, punctuation. Sample use of language in home and school environments.	Test of Written Language
Language Sample	Use of language in natural communicative contexts.	DSS, SALT
Speech		
Consonant Inventory	Sampling of repertoire of speech sounds.	
Syllable structure	Sampling of consonant-vowel combinations.	
Single word articulation test	Sampling of sounds in controlled words for accuracy compared to adult model.	Goldman-Fristoe test of Articulation (GFTA)
Connected Speech	Sample sound production in conversation and compare to single word production.	GFTA Stories
Stimulability	Ability to produce consonants in a hierarchy of complexity from isolation, syllables to words.	Language sample
Hearing	Assess auditory acquity and middle ear function.	Electrophysiologic assessment, otoacoustic emissions, behavioral audiometry, immittance testing

cesses. Each test selects specific subtests based on the model of language development proposed, and each assesses receptive and expressive language using subtests that require different levels of processing and response modalities. For example, the Test of Language Development (TOLD; Newcomer & Hammell, 1997) assesses expressive vocabulary by asking the child to define words, whereas the Clinical Evaluation of Language Fundamentals—Revised (CELF-3; Secord, Semel, & Wiig, 1995) assesses expressive vocabulary through a sentence completion task. The language complexity required to respond to these two different subtests may influence whether this domain is viewed as a strength or weakness for the child being assessed. In addition to standardized tests, language sampling of conversation and narration is still an important informal procedure that should augment formal test measures for the school-aged child.

Issues in the Difficult-to-Test Child

Children with behavioral, social, or motoric deficits may be unable to perform on standardized language tests that must be administered in a prescribed way. Among the most common are children who are nonoral. Whether because of gross motor or speech production limitations or lack of compliance, these children present challenges in the diagnostic process. These children, often preschoolers, have no recognizable speech or use few speech sounds. Formal standardized measures are ineffective in obtaining valid estimates of performance. Informal procedures are important to provide a realistic picture of language function because they permit flexibility in method of presentation and responses for children who are difficult to test.

CASE EXAMPLE

Referral Information

KR, aged 4 years 1 month, was referred for a speech and language evaluation as part of an interdisciplinary assessment of developmental and social/emotional status. KR had received an initial behavioral assessment 6 months earlier because of tantrums and the presence of inappropriate social interaction with peers and family. His parents conducted a behavioral intervention recommended at the time of the initial evaluation.

History

KR had an unremarkable birth and early developmental history. Speech and language delays were observed from the age of typical onset. At the time of the evaluation, KR was using fewer than 10 words and had a provisional diagnosis of autism at the preceding evaluation.

Assessment Plan

Language

General receptive/expressive: Standardized: Sequenced Inventory of Communicative Development (SICD-R)

| Language sample: | Conversational sample of communication during play |
| Parent questionnaire: | Communicative Development Inventory |

Speech

| Articulation: | Phonetic Inventory from language sample |

Developmental   Vineland Adaptive Behavior Scale

A copy of report of the assessment is included in the Appendix.

ASSESSMENT TO TREATMENT

Once the assessment process is completed, recommendations for monitoring or treating may be developed using the profile of communicative performance as a guide. The communication profile identifies areas of speech and language weaknesses that should be addressed in intervention planning. Treatment programs may be designed to remediate specific areas of deficit or to stimulate broad communicative processes. For some children, initial assessment may not provide an opportunity for augmentation of formal test measures with informal assessment information. Particularly for children who are difficult to test, a period of diagnostic intervention may be warranted. The purpose of diagnostic intervention is to administer informal assessment procedures that will complete the diagnostic profile and to evaluate the child's response to different treatment approaches. Following that period of diagnostic intervention, treatment planning may be completed.

LEADERS IN THE FIELD

The field of communicative disorders has its origins in psychology and linguistics. During the 1960s the field was dominated by assessment models that viewed communicative disorders within a pathology framework. That is, the purpose of early assessment models was to characterize a disorder by the deficits exhibited and to tie those deficits to a site of lesion. However, with the advances in research in child language development, new theoretical models were applied to assessment and intervention of children with language impairments. These new models utilized a developmental perspective that assessed both communicative strengths and weaknesses and viewed these according to age-related acquisition.

As the models accounting for language development and disorders changed from pathologies models to developmental models, assessment procedures followed. Current advances in the field of language assessment have focused on providing formal and informal procedures that assess critical milestones in language development. Developmental models proposed dual processes of receptive and expressive language. However, past assessment models had focused on expressive language while neglecting assessment of receptive language. Beginning with aspects of grammar, Miller and Yoder (1984) developed an assessment of the comprehension of the typical acquisition sequence of word order and grammatical forms using controlled pictures (e.g., verb tenses, prepositions, question forms). Chapman, Klee, and Paul (1986) and Miller and Paul (1995) published informal clinical procedures for aspects of language comprehension that were difficult to assess in a standard format. For example, Chapman developed procedures for testing the understanding of language forms through manipulation of objects, a task that favored performance of young children. The publication of these procedures permitted assessment of children at younger ages than was previously realized.

As more was learned about early language development, protocols were developed to assess these milestones in children with potential impairments (Bloom & Lahey, 1988). Standardized and informal procedures were developed for prelinguistic stages of development and the earliest stages of language development (Carpenter, Coggins, Olswang, & Stoel-Gammon, 1989; Wetherby & Prizant, 1993). Many new procedures that assessed language in naturalistic contexts were developed in response to the needs of young children (Paul, 1995; Pena, 1996; Miller & Chapman, 1999). These included procedures for the analysis of conversation, narration, and diagnostic therapy. These procedures, combined with standardized measures, have expanded the scope of language assessment to very young children and children who traditionally were difficult to assess.

SUMMARY

This chapter presented an overview of the communication assessment process. The developmental theoretical perspective and the implications for assessment were discussed. Profiling of communication abilities was introduced and used to present prototypic communication profiles for children with primary language impairment and those profiles showing language impairments associated with other developmental disabilities such as autism or developmental delay. Assessment measures (standardized and informal) were discussed for three age groups: birth to three, preschool and school-age and specific measures given as examples. Modification of assessment protocols for the difficult-to-test children were presented. Finally, a case example was presented to demonstrate the assessment planning process and show a sample clinical report.

Case Study

East Tennessee State University
School of Public and Allied Health
Department of Communicative Disorders
Speech-Language-Hearing Clinic
P.O. Box 70643
Johnson City, Tennessee 37614-0643

This 4 year 1 month old male was referred by the Department of Psychiatry and Behavioral Sciences for a speech and language evaluation as part of a complete evaluation. KR was accompanied to the evaluation by his mother and father, who served as informants. The family is currently living in Japan and KR's family speaks English. The major concern expressed today pertained to speech and language therapy recommendations.

When questioned regarding developmental milestones, his parents reported that his motor milestones were within normal limits (i.e., he sat unsupported between 7–9 months, crawled between 10–12 months, and walked alone between 10–12 months). According to his parents, KR engaged in babbling and sound imitation as a baby between 25–48 months. His first word occurred between 25–36 months, and two-word combinations occurred between 37–48 months. His parents remarked that KR depends on gestures to understand spoken messages and to relay messages to others. Discussing KR's play behavior, his parents reported that his interaction with adults and peers was limited and characterized by a need for routines.

KR is currently enrolled in preschool and has received speech therapy 3 times per week for two years. No additional information was available regarding his preschool placement.

TEST BEHAVIOR
During the evaluation, KR presented himself as a quiet child who was frequently distractible and required direction from the clinician. Verbal and tangible reinforcement was necessary for KR to attend to tasks. While attending to verbal tasks, he required contextual cues.

HEARING
According to his parents, KR had middle ear infections between 2–3 years of age. A hearing evaluation was conducted on June 26, 1998. His thresholds were obtained in sound field at 30 dB HL, which is in the borderline normal range. Testing was conducted in sound field instead of headphones due to behavioral performance. Individual ear information was not obtained; however, the overall impression was that Karl's hearing was adequate for speech and language learning.

LANGUAGE
The Sequenced Inventory of Communication Development-R (SIDC; Hedrick, Prather, & Tobin, 1984) was administered to assess receptive and expressive language. The SICD-R indicated that KR had an age score of 16 months in receptive language. One of KR's strengths on the receptive scale was that he responded appropriately by turning toward his mother's voice when she called his name. He also turned to localize the sound of a rattle. He responded to different sounds around the house. One of his weaknesses on this scale is that he did not respond by turning to localize high-pitched sounds. His score on the receptive scale was also affected by his limited understanding of words, including names of items of clothing, outdoor items, and acquaintances, as well as descriptive words. His score in expressive language placed him between the 12- and 18-month level. One of KR's strengths was that he vocalized when something he liked was taken away from him. KR continued to imitate sounds during interaction. He changed pitch while vocalizing, and he made specific word-like vocalizations, such as consonant-vowel combinations. One of his weaknesses on this scale was his limited verbal use. He did not use consistent sound combinations to label objects or people.

KR's parents completed the MacArthur Communication Development Inventory (CDI; Fenson et al., 1993) to assess receptive and expressive vocabulary size, as well as early grammatical production. This parent report indicated that KR had an understanding of 101 vocabulary words; however, he did not produce these words, which put him below the 5th percentile in each communication mode for children 16 months of age. The CDI also indicated that KR is below the 5th percentile for sentence complexity. KR's receptive vocabulary was characterized by understanding of short phrases such as "Do you want more?" and object, person, action (e.g., go, come), description (e.g., big), and location (e.g., in) words. KR understands *what* and *where* questions. KR used few early com-

(*continued*)

municative gestures. His mother reported: reaching for a toy, blowing kisses, and extending arms to be picked up. He did not use pointing to request objects or comment on them; nor does he use social gestures for *hi* and *bye*. He did engage in chase games, singing, and dancing, but not games requiring two participants. KR did demonstrate common actions associated with objects (e.g., put phone to ear); however he did not engage in pretend play (e.g., pretend to be parent, substitute one toy for another). Imitation of daily activities was emerging. Often, symbolic activities emerge first in play and then in language. KR did not show the symbolic function yet in play.

The Vineland Adaptive Behavior Scales (Sparrow, Balla, & Cicchetti, 1984) was administered to assess receptive and expressive communication, socialization, daily living, and motor skills. KR's standard scores (mean 100, standard deviation 15) in the adaptive behavior domains were Communication 50, Daily Living 75, and Socialization 63. His performance in the communication and socialization domain corresponded to a percentile rank of less than 1. His performance in the daily living domain corresponded to a percentile rank of 5. His performance in the motor skills domain corresponded to a percentile rank of 29. KR obtained an Adaptive Behavior Composite standard score of 65. His standard score corresponds to a national percentile rank of 1 and classifies his general adaptive functioning as Low. His communication impairment was his weakest area, whereas motor and daily living skills appeared to be a strength.

A language sample was collected and analyzed using the Systemic Analysis of Language Transcripts (SALT; Miller & Chapman, 1999). The transcript summary portion of SALT analysis showed the following:

- 46 intelligible words
- 69 total words
- 23 different words
- 66% intelligibility
- 36% responses to *wh* questions
- 2% responses to yes/no questions
- 1.0 Mean Length of Utterance (MLU)

KR's communication was most significantly affected by his reduced vocabulary, limited speech sounds, limited ability to initiate interaction with words or gestures, and lack of symbolic play. However, KR was beginning to use language at an imitation level. It is significant to note that 66% of KR's intelligible utterances were direct imitations. Also, the 23 different words that he used were direct imitations of an adult model. KR's responses to *wh* questions and yes/no questions were considered direct imitative answers modeled and prompted by the adult. For example, the clinician would ask, "What do you want?" and then the clinician would instruct KR after no response, "Tell me open." Only 33% of KR's words were not direct imitations, meaning that KR relied on models and prompting. KR was not yet combining words, as reflected by a Mean Length of Utterance (MLU) of 1.0, and was in Early Brown's Stage I, which has an expected age of 18 months. Brown's Stage I is characterized by one word utterances that are primarily nouns and verbs.

SPEECH

Articulation was also assessed from a language sample and a parent report. Results indicated that KR has a limited phoneme inventory. These sounds were primarily the early developing sounds, including nasal (m, n), stop (p, b), and glide (w) consonants. He used only neutral vowels: /a/ and /i/. KR showed oral-motor groping behaviors during his word attempts, often resequencing sounds. KR was very focused on oral productions by adults when he was attempting words. KR's syllable structure consisted primarily of VCV,

CV, and CVCV (consonant-vowel-consonant-vowel) combinations such as *mama* and *papa*. An examination of oral structures was not conducted. Normal symmetry of the face and lips was observed.

| | Phoneme Inventory | |
Manner of Production	Word Initial	Word Final
Stop		
Oral	p, b	p
Nasal	m	n
Glide	w	

A dynamic assessment procedure was performed to evaluate response to sign use versus oral language use. KR was so focused on oral production that he did not attend to the signs. Further, he became frustrated with attempts to assist him in sign formation.

SUMMARY

The results of this evaluation indicate that KR's receptive and expressive language forms are delayed compared to his chronological age and to other developmental parameters (e.g., motor development). His language performance was at approximately a 16- to 18-month level. With expressive levels he relied mostly on imitated productions. Play was characterized by no pretend elements but ritualized forms such as lining up blocks. KR demonstrated a limited phonemic inventory, primarily of stops (p, b), nasals (m, n) and glides (w). Hearing was within normal limits.

RECOMMENDATIONS

Based on results of the evaluation, it is recommended that the frequency of KR's therapy be increased to four to five times per week with sessions of at least 1 hour. The following therapy recommendations were made:

Vocabulary Skills

1. Increase vocabulary knowledge and production by selecting words that would be useful in his everyday environment (e.g., potty, ball, water, and make). Word selection may be chosen from the words comprehended in the MacArthur Communicative Development Inventory, which provides a vocabulary listing of early words. Vocabulary selected should emphasize words that begin with stops (p, b, t, d, k, g), nasals (m, n), and glides (w) which are earlier acquired sounds, but should also introduce some new sounds, particularly early developing fricatives (f, s, sh). Word selection should also incorporate function categories of a first lexicon. The goal should be to move from imitation to spontaneous production.

2. Expand the frequency and range of KR's communication intent expressed by his words. Present KR with a series of communicative temptations that are structured situations that can be set up nonverbally and are designed to entice child-initiated communication acts. For example, the box of Legos was used to tempt KR to tell the evaluators to "open" the box.

Social Skills

Emphasize social skills training by providing social situations to involve communication procedures (e.g., answering the telephone, greeting, and expressing empathy). The following abilities should be gradually incorporated to develop KR's communicative social skills:

(*continued*)

1. Turn-taking skills
2. Initiating Topic
   a. Commenting (I noticed that you enjoyed playing with the Legos.)
   b. Asking questions (Would you like to play with Legos today?)
3. Sustaining Topic
   a. Answering questions (I would like to play with the Legos.)
   b. Imitations (You like to play with Legos.)
   c. Expanding sentence to include new words (We could build a house or a car with Legos.)
4. Clarification of Miscommunication
   a. Expansion through modifiers (These blocks are small and blue.)
   b. Extension through association (These blocks are the same as your blocks at home.)
5. Communication Repair When Breakdowns Occur
   a. Request for clarification (Would you repeat that, please?)
   b. Repeat sentence heard to clarify (You said that you didn't get to play with Legos at home often?)

REFERENCES

Bayley, N. (1993). *Bayley Scales of Infant Development—II.* San Antonio, TX: Psychological Corp.

Bloom, M., & Lahey, P. (1988). *Language disorders in children.* New York: Wiley.

Campbell, D. (1999). Asberger's syndrome: Strategies for diagnosis and treatment. Advance for Speech-Language Pathologists and Audiologists, vol. 9, no. 39. King of Prussia, PA: Merion Publications.

Carpenter, R. L., Coggins, T. E., Olswang, L. B., & Stoel-Gammon, C. (1989). *Assessing linguistic behavior.* Seattle: University of Washington Press.

Chapman, R., Klee, T., & Paul, R. (1986). *Assessing language comprehension in children.* Needham Heights, MA: Simon & Schuster.

Fenson, L., Dale, P., Reznick, S., Thal, D., Bates, E., Hartsung, J., Pethick, S., & Reilly, J. (1993). *MacArthur Communicative Development Inventories.* San Diego: Singular.

Goldman, R., & Fristoe, M. (1986). *Goldman-Fristoe Test of Articulation.* Circle Pines, MN: American Guidance Service.

Hedrick, D., Prather, E., & Tobin, A. (1984). *Sequenced Inventory of Communicative Development* (Rev. ed.). Seattle: University of Washington Press.

Huang, R. J., Hopkins, J., & Nippold, M. (1997). Satisfaction with standardized language testing: A survey of speech-language pathologists. *Speech, Language and Hearing Services in the Schools, 28,* 12–29.

Hughes, D., Fey, M., & Long, S. (1992). Developmental sentence scoring: Still useful after all these years. *Topics in Language Disorders, 12,* 1–12.

Linder, T. (1993). *Transdisciplinary play-based assessment.* Baltimore, MD: Brookes.

Miller, J. (1981). *Assessing language production in children.* Boston: Allyn & Bacon.

Miller, J., & Chapman, R. (1999). *Systematic analysis of language transcripts.* University of Wisconsin-Madison, Language Analysis Laboratory.

Miller, J., & Paul, R. (1995). *The clinical assessment of language comprehension.* Baltimore: Brookes.

Miller, J., Leddy, M., & Leavitt, L. (1999). *Improving the communication of people with Down syndrome.* Baltimore: Brookes.

Miller, J., & Yoder, D. (1984). *Language comprehension test.* Baltimore: University Park Press.

Merrell, A. W., & Plante, E. (1997). Norm-referenced interpretation in the diagnostic process. *Speech, Language and Hearing Services in the Schools, 28,* 50–58.

Nelson, N. W. (1998). *Childhood language disorders in context.* Boston: Allyn & Bacon.

Newcomer, P., & Hammill, D. (1997). *Test of Language Development: Primary* (3rd ed.). Austin, TX: Pro-Ed.

Owens, R. E. (1995). *Language disorders: A functional approach to assessment and intervention.* Boston: Allyn & Bacon.

Paul, R. (1995). *Language disorders from infancy to adolescence.* St. Louis, MO: Mosby.

Pena, E. (1996). Dynamic assessment: The model and its language applications. In K. Cole, P. Dale, & D. Thal (Eds.), *Assessment of communication and language* (pp. 281–308). Baltimore: Brookes.

Rossetti, L. (1990). *Rossetti Infant-Toddler Language Scale.* East Moline, IL: LinguiSystems.

Secord, W. A., Semel, E., & Wiig, E. H. (1995). *Clinical Evaluation of Language Fundamentals* (Rev. ed.). San Antonio, TX: Psychological Corp.

Scott, J., Clark, C., & Brady, M. (2000). *Students with autism.* San Diego: Singular.

Smit, A. B., Hand, L., Freilinger, J. J., Bernthal, J. E., & Bird A. (1980). Iowa articulation norms project and its Nebraska replication. *Journal of Speech and Hearing Disorders, 55,* 779–798.

Sparrow, S., Balla., D., & Cicchetti, D. (1984). Vineland Adaptive Behavior Scales. Circle Pines, MN: American Guidance Service.

Tager-Flusberg, H. (1989). A psycholinguistic perspective on language development in the autistic child. In G. Dawson (Ed.), *Perspectives on the nature of autism* (pp. 92–109). New York: Guilford Press.

Vinson, B. P. (1999). *Language disorders across the lifespan.* San Diego: Singular.

Watkins, R. (1997). The linguistic profile of SLI. In L. Adamson & M. A. Romski (Eds.), *Communication and language acquisition: Discoveries from atypical development* (pp. 161–179). Baltimore: Brookes.

Wechsler, D. (1967). *Manual for the Wechsler Preschool and Primary Scale of Intelligence.* San Antonio, TX: Psychological Corp.

Wechsler, D. (1991). *Manual for the Wechsler Intelligence Scale for Children* (Rev. 3rd ed.). San Antonio, TX: Psychological Corp.

Wetherby, A., & Prizant, B. (1993). *Communication and symbolic behavior scales.* Riverside, CA: Riverside.

Chapter 9

PERVASIVE DEVELOPMENTAL DISORDERS

DAVID A. SABATINO, H. BOONEY VANCE, AND GERALD FULLER

INTRODUCTION

Pervasive Developmental Disorders (PDD) include a group of one broadband and four specific childhood mental disorders, each of which has unique recognizable and therefore diagnosable features. The two general characteristics, which stretch across all of the specific diagnostic entities in this group of disorders, are impairments in (a) social interaction and (b) communications. These disabilities include (a) sensory disabilities (moderate/severe hearing problems or deafness); (b) physical disabilities frequently resulting from neurological impairments or enervation or from structural problems related to the understanding of aurally received speech, to vocal motor speech production, and to the formation or association of central language concepts; (c) social learning and cultural/familial related disabilities; and (d) frequent unexplained emotional problems such as severe childhood depression with withdraw, or a number of hysteric or even psychotic conditions. All four of these specific conditions have the capability of producing similar behaviors; thus multidisciplinary differential diagnosis is required. The most common diagnostic problem, however, is that of differentiating PDDs from mental retardation, as both share similar symptoms. Both PDD and mental retardation are capable of interfering with communications and inhibiting social responsiveness. Although they may be comorbid, the vast difference between them is that a mentally retarded child's intellectual and adaptive (social) behaviors should be very similar in developmental age or functional level. In sharp contrast, there is a significant difference between the intellectual development of the children with PDDs in either their communications or their social responsiveness.

The characteristics associated with PDDs are frequently subtle. Differential diagnosis requires persons from several disciplines interacting to enhance a diagnosis, promoting communication among the team membership. The multidisciplinary team members should reflect a combination of clinical and human development training and experience. This team of multidisciplinary professionals may include a speech and language pathologist, a child clinical psychologist, a social worker, a child psychiatrist, an audiologist, and a pediatrician. If the child has achieved school age, school psychologists, special educators, and other school personnel (remedial and developmentally prepared) professionals are needed.

The *Diagnostic and Statistical Manual of Mental Disorders—Fourth Edition* (American Psychiatric Association, 1994) defines a PDD as a "severe and pervasive impairment in several areas of development" (p. 65). Along with the common symptoms just mentioned, most children with PDD also display repetitive stereotypic behaviors that are "distinctly deviant." In autism these stereotypic behaviors are below the person's mental level of development. Under the broad rubric of Pervasive Developmental Disorders, DSM lists four contributing conditions and a fifth Not Otherwise Specified entry. The four categories are Autistic Disorder, Rett's Disorder, Childhood Disintegrative Disorder, and Asperger's Disorder. The fifth diagnostic category is simply Pervasive Developmental Disorder Not Otherwise Specified (NOS). A number of the pervasive developmental disorders are secondary to other medical conditions, such as chromosomal disorders.

AUTISM

The prevailing belief in the 1940s and 1950s was that autism was in itself a form of childhood psychosis. Early on, autism required differential diagnosis to distinguish between it and childhood schizophrenia. However, the history of autism is characterized by an absence of unifying theories, as evidenced by the misuse of the term—as if it were synonymous with many other conditions affecting human development, social interactions, and the need for communications. Autism has been described by a number of different observers whose observations were based on small samples of children in particular environments. Therefore, different observers have drawn divergent generalizations about this condition, producing a range of possible behaviors that may be included in a description of this childhood developmental disorder. Consequently, the diagnostic entity *autism* is simply not currently being used with precision. It is frequently overused and misused as an umbrella term interchangeable with other diagnostically undifferentiated conditions and developmental disorders.

By the late 1950s a Kannerian description of autism offered it as a subtype of childhood psychosis. By the 1970s the field had overwhelmingly embraced the term, labeling nearly all children with severe behavioral disorders as "autistic." It is ironic that those who work with children displaying disconnected social and communication developments will enter the new millennium searching for a meaningful classification structure that will probably include a number of clinical subtypes. These subtypes will probably be more related to developmental levels of functional behavioral performance than to the behavior itself. It could be that there are subtypes of PDDs, many more than the four listed in the *DSM-IV*. However, each subtype will recognize that within age boundaries, certain performance levels will exist; hence, it may be as simple as seeing childhood conditions as mild, moderate, and severe across a number of given behaviors. Thus, a child would be diagnosed descriptively given the uniqueness of presenting behaviors and the level to which the child is able to use those behaviors to interact socially and communicate with others. Whatever the future holds, it must not return to the simplistic, etiologically based concepts offered by Kanner and Rimland. Given this growing interest and improved methodology, there is hope that the future of individuals with autism will be brighter (Eaves & Awadh, 1997).

Prevalence

Autism, with its paradoxical signs and symptoms, occurs at a low prevalence rate. With the broader diagnostic standards currently in vogue, prevalence estimates have generally been on the increase. Older estimates of Autistic Disorder usually fell in the range of 7 to 14 cases per 10,000 (Locke, Banken, & Mahone, 1994). There is currently, however, a striking range of prevalence estimates: 2 to 21 for every 10,000 children (Kaplan, Sadock, & Gregg, 1994; Ritvo & Freeman, 1978). Such large fluctuations do not bode well for planning services, determining etiology, or, more fundamentally, validating autism as an identifiable syndrome (Eaves & Awadh, 1997).

Quay and Werry (1986) write that childhood psychosis/autism is a rare mental disorder that "receives an emphasis that is out of all proportion to the number of children affected" (p. 185). The fascination that professionals, parents, and laity have with this rare condition is disproportional to its incidence in the population. The reason may be that many incorrectly substitute the term autism for mental retardation. Autism holds promise for normal or full restoration following treatment, whereas mental retardation does not. The majority of the general population associate autism with movie characterizations, such as Dustin Hoffman's character in *Rainman*. Such films show the promise of a person with unique but intriguing differences from the norm reflected in the condition of autism. They see the reflection of a brilliant mind that is just underneath a unique display of inhibiting social and communicative behaviors. Reaching the brilliance of the person provides hope for a treatment breakthrough. Would that every parent could have that hope, and that every professional could offer it.

Historic Significance

The study of autism has only a 50-year-old history. Like most conditions that affect children, and especially those for which there is no adult counterpart, diagnostic descriptions were uncommon until Kanner (1943) consolidated the symptoms and produced a description of Infantile Autism separate from childhood schizophrenia and other forms of psychoses affecting children. The first issue of the *Journal of Autism and Childhood Schizophrenia* (e.g., Kanner, 1971) discussed various attempts to identify and treat children who were thought to be psychotic. The works of Maudley, a British psychiatrist, were cited by Kanner as among the first to acknowledge insanity in children (Kanner, 1971). Maudley was criticized extensively for suggesting that something as "unnatural" as insanity could exist in children. According to Kanner (1971), Maudley provided the basis for a system classifying mental disorders in children. Hence, he established the very existence of *insanity* in children. Maudley presented a six-point classification scheme that laid the groundwork for other professionals to investigate insanity (mental disorders) in children. A number of early books addressing the issue of childhood psychosis appeared by the beginning of the twentieth century. In the early 1900s Sante de Sanctis described a subpopulation of children as having *dementia pral-*

cocissina, which was a developmental detoriation often found in children confronting psychosis. Sanctis' findings opened the door and served as a benchmark for other investigators to make comparative observations regarding the developmental status of children presenting emotional problems. Suddenly it was just as possible for a child to display developmental regression from a mental disorder as it was from a physical disorder (as cited in Rosenberg, Wilson, Maheay, & Sindelar, 1992).

In the early 1900s, Bleuler coined the term *schizophrenia* to replace dementia praecox. Bleuler's new term described a cluster of behaviors exhibited by adults with psychosis, but failed to address childhood schizophrenia substantially (Shaw & Lucas, 1970). Bleuler's contribution was threefold. First, he provided a prognosis of hope; second, he suggested that the very roots of schizophrenia in adults might have its source in childhood; and third, he identified a cluster of relevant behaviors that might be useful for making a diagnosis of childhood schizophrenia. The first attempt to document Bleuler's diagnostic criteria of schizophrenia to a preadult population was conducted by Potter (1933). Potter's landmark work stipulated six conditions requiring documentation in the establishment of a diagnosis of childhood schizophrenia (Wherry, 1972). Potter's six criteria for a diagnosis of childhood schizophrenia were the following:

1. Generalized retraction of interest in the environment
2. Dereistic (i.e., deviating from normal logic) thinking, feeling, acting
3. Disturbance of thought, manifested through blocking, preservation, incoherence, and mutism
4. Defects in emotional rapport
5. Rigidity and distortion of affect
6. Alterations of behavior (e.g., bizarre behaviors, stereotypical acts)

Potter's leadership in developing diagnostic reference criteria behavior in the early 1940s led other investigators to report on a variety of new information expanding knowledge related to childhood psychoses. Bradley and Bowen (1941) proposed an operational definition of childhood schizophrenia through a description of overt symptoms. These researchers compared the behavior of psychotic and nonpsychotic children on eight observable symptoms that characterized schizophrenic children. The importance of Bradley and Bowen's identification process was that the diagnosis was to be based upon observable behaviors. Bradley and Bowen (1941) indicated that four of the eight behaviors—seclusiveness, bizarre behavior, regressive interests, and sensitivity—were primary in making an appropriate diagnosis. Secondary behaviors, such as irritability, daydreaming, decrease of interests, and physical inactivity, were necessary for the diagnosis of childhood schizophrenia, rounding out the eight total symptoms.

Bender (1942) reported that childhood schizophrenia could be related to the perception of body distortions. She attempted to ascertain these distortions through children's drawings and response as an important emotional aspect of childhood development. Her research produced data on the relationship between the age of onset and the identification of perceptual distortions and impairments in the self in childhood schizophrenia. She established three distinct age periods and related behavioral responses: birth to three years, early and middle childhood, and preadolescence. Bender gave the diagnostician much needed knowledge concerning the developmental status at the age of presentation of the child's illness. No longer could differential diagnostic practices exclude the importance of the child's developmental status regardless of their chronological age. In PDDs, certain developmentally sensitive behaviors are typical, whereas others are typical only at a certain stage in the developmental process. This fact has often been obscured by the devastation of the illness.

Kanner (1943) is credited with first using and describing the term *autistic* as applied to children. Originally the term had been used to describe forms of withdrawal fantasy shown by schizophrenics. That usage caused a confusion that still exists. Kanner described nine features associated with autism in his classic paper titled "Autistic Disturbance of Affective Contact":

1. Inability to develop relationships

2. Delay in the acquisition of language

3. Noncommunicative use of spoken language after it develops

4. Delayed echolalia

5. Pronominal reversal

6. Repetitive and stereotypical play

7. Maintenance of sameness

8. Good rote memory

9. Normal physical appearance

These nine symptoms were later reduced into two categories (maintenance of sameness in children's repetitive behavior; and extreme aloneness, with onset within the first two years of life; Arrons & Gittens, 1992).

ASPERGER'S DISORDER

In the early 1940's, Austrian psychiatrist Hans Asperger described a pattern of abnormal behavior in a group of adolescents. Asperger labeled these adolescents as austistic psychopaths and provided detailed descriptions of these youths. According to some experts (e.g., Arrons & Gittens, 1992), Asperger and Kanner described the same condition. Asperger (1944) described four children ages 6 to 11 who had difficulties in social skills but were within the normal range of cognitive and verbal skills. Asperger referred to these children's disorder as *Autistischen Psychopathen in Kindesalter,* or Autistic Personality Disorder in Childhood (Klin & Volkmar, 1997). Asperger described the following features:

1. Impairment in nonverbal communication

2. Idiosyncrasies in verbal communication

3. Egocentric preoccupation with special interests

4. Intellectualization of affect

5. Poor body awareness/clumsiness
6. Behavior difficulties/conduct problems
7. Onset (not before the third year of life)
8. Gender patterns

Although Asperger's and Kanner's descriptions of their respective children shared many commonalties, these two professionals were unaware of each other's work. In fact, Asperger's works remained unknown in the English-language literature until Wing reported on a series of case reports (Klin & Volkmar, 1997). According to Klin and Volkmar, Kanner's description "became associated with the characteristically lower intellectually functioning autistic child, and Asperger's (1944) description was of highly intellectually functional, more verbal, older children with autism" (p. 95).

Tantam (1988) proposed a subcategory for autistic people who were sociable, lightly clumsy, and verbally skilled, and who had highly developed special interests. He referred to this syndrome as Asperger's Syndrome. Other terms and subtypes of psychosis peculiar to childhood have emerged since the late 1940s. Rank (1949) referred to them as atypical children. Ornitz and Ritvo (1976) and Wing and Gould (1979) suggested the term *symbolic psychosis*. As late as 1977, Corbett, Harris, Taylor, and Trimble coined the term *disintegrative psychosis*. Disintegrative psychosis is used to describe autistic children with symptoms occurring between ages 3 and 5 with severe regression in all areas of functioning occurring after normal early development (Quay & Werry, 1986).

CHANGES IN CONCEPTUAL CONSIDERATIONS

The 1940s and 1950s introduced the concept of children who presented with two overriding unique behaviors. First, their communication appeared impaired in language mediation and association and was not used to address others but to clarify self. Second, much of their behavior was stereotypical, with perseveration, randomness, and, much like their speech, more self-directed than directed to include others. The disorganization in thought and the absence of purposeful behaviors caused early observers to believe that PDDs, especially autism, were in fact a form of childhood schizophrenia or other forms of children's psychosis. Professionals in the late 1960s altered this conceptual view. Kanner (1971) and Rimland (1971) took two etiologically divergent positions but both agreed that autism was a unique disorder and that it thus must be differentiated diagnostically from childhood schizophrenia, symbiotic psychosis, childhood psychosis, and atypical development. Nevertheless, practitioners and researchers seized upon the term, and by the mid-1970s the vast majority of children with severe behavioral disorders and limitations in communications were being diagnosed with Infantile Autism. No listing (classification) was provided for autism in the first or second editions of the *DSM*. It was not until 1987, when the revised third edition of the *DSM* was published (*DSM-III-R,* 1987), that Autistic Disorder, rather than autism, was offered to the professional community. Childhood onset PDD, Heller's syndrome, atypical PDD, and disintegrative psychosis were all relegated to the one ambiguous category known as

Pervasive Developmental Disorder Not Otherwise Specified. Symptom clarity that could enable differential diagnosis was in the late 1980s still very crude. The childhood schizophrenia classification could be used only if the child met the criteria for adult forms of schizophrenia. Rimland (1994) captured the reason that so many practitioners gravitate toward the use of the term autism despite the absence of clarity and precision. He noted, "'Childhood Schizophrenia' was not an attractive term to parents or professionals; 'autism' sounded much better" (p. 19). There were also political purposes behind the shifts in definitions and the diagnostic practices that were based upon them. For instance, Schopler and Mesibov (1986) wrote that the definition promoted by the National Society for Autistic Children was primary intended to obtain propitious social policy for children with Autistic Disorder and their families. When differing criteria are used to identify subjects with Autistic Disorder, it is difficult, if not impossible, to reconcile the conflicting results that are frequently reported in the literature (Eaves & Awadh, 1997).

Unfortunately, until the confusion over definitions and diagnoses is overcome, there will be little progress in the discovery of effective treatment approaches for children with autism. To date, the most effective interventions have not been unique to children with autistic disorder. Rather, the same treatments are found to be similarly effective with a wide array of moderate and severe developmental disabilities in children and young people. In lieu of research on instructional programs designed for autistic children, most practitioners assume "that the principles that apply assessment and treatment of . . . one population are also relevant to [autism]" (Koegel & Koegel, 1999, p. 16).

Given the current heterogeneity of behavior symptoms across individuals, a prominent recent trend in the literature has been the search for meaningful subgroups of individuals with autism (e.g., Borden & Ollendick, 1994; Eaves, Ho, & Eaves, 1994; Sevin et al., 1991, Wing & Attwood, 1987). There are important reasons for attempting to subclassify individuals in a heterogeneous group. First, different subgroups may have different etiologies. Second, like various forms of cancer and fevers, different subgroups may demand different treatments. Finally, course and prognosis may vary, depending upon the etiology and treatment of the subgroup.

Basically, three subtypes of autism have been found, according to Wing (1997). The three types are aloof, passive, and active-but-odd. The validity of these three groups has received support from Eaves and Awadh (1997). Each subtype tends to be associated with particular uniqueness in clinical behaviors.

Aloof group. According to Wing (1997), this group corresponds closely to the typical clinical picture of autism. This group is the most distant from social contact and usually rejects unsolicited physical or social contact. For this group the use and understanding of verbal and nonverbal communication are severely impaired. Wing suggests that individuals in this group remain mute most of their lives. Rapidly cycling mood changes are common in this group. Individuals demonstrate stereotypical behavior and show little symbolic pretend play, either on their own or with their parents.

Passive group. Wing (1997) indicates that this group does not make spontaneous social approaches, except to fulfill needs. However, individuals do accept other's approaches without protest. This group joins in games and activities but takes a passive role. Echolalia is often present, and speech patterns are better developed than those for the aloof group. Stereotypical movement and odd response to sensory stimuli may be minimal or absent. According to Wing, the passive group is likely to be the best behaved and most easily managed of the three groups. Usually this group may be diagnosed in early years because the main signs of impairment are delayed.

Active-but-odd group. This group makes spontaneous approaches to other people, but only in a group setting.

CURRENT DEFINITIONS OF AUTISM

It may clarify the issue of definition of the Pervasive Developmental Disorders if five of the major contributing definitions of autism, worldwide, are examined. Autism was selected because it represents the most frequently referenced and most commonly used PDD. Five definitions have been the most popular over the last 20 years.

Creak and the British Working Party

Creak's (1961, 1964) definition represented the combined thought of the British Working Party, a group of 13 clinicians and researchers who found themselves in disagreement with Kanner. Their position of disagreement was that autism does not represent a distinct diagnostic category as Kanner maintained. Their intent was to provide practitioners the capability of identifying early forms of childhood psychosis as (a) gross and sustained impairment of emotional relationships with people; (b) apparent unawareness of personal identity to a degree inappropriate for age; (c) pathological preoccupation with particular objects or certain characteristics of objects, without regard to functioning; (d) a tendency to maintain or restore sameness; (e) abnormal perceptual experience; (f) frequent acute, excessive, and seemingly illogical anxiety; (g) speech either lost, never acquired, or failing to develop; (h) distortion in motility pattern; and (i) background of intellectual retardation in which periods of normal or exceptional intellectual function or skill may appear. Although the definition is now dated, the authors of two currently popular assessment instruments (Schopler, Reichler, & Renner, 1988; Krug, Arick, & Almond, 1980) used those symptoms developed in response to Creak's definition in the development of their scales. Consequently, the continued use of this instrument contributes to the current impact of Creak's and the British Working Party's definition.

Autism Society of America

The current definition adopted by the Autism Society of America (ASA) is an outgrowth of the definition written by Ritvo and Freeman (1978). The latest version is published in each newsletter issue of the ASA *Advocate.* According to a recent issue (1996, May-June), autism "typically appears during the first three years of life." Further, the ASA considers autism to be a neurological disorder with the following behavioral symptoms: (a) disturbances in the rate of appearance of physical, social, and language skills; (b) abnormal sensations (i.e., sight, hearing, touch, balance, smell, taste, reaction to pain, and the way the body is held); (c) delayed or missing speech and language, though specific thinking capacities may be present; and (d) abnormal relating to people, objects, and events. Severely disabled individuals may exhibit extreme self-injury, repetitive behavior, and aggression.

Rutter

The position taken by Rutter is that without a systematic structure through which diagnostic practices can be routinely reviewed, the definition will be on a case basis; hence, each case will be based on different criteria. He requested that a common operational definition of autism be adopted and used diagnostically by all practitioners stabilizing a population of autistic children that the professional community can agree on. Rutter's (1978) definition of autism contained four essential diagnostic criteria: (a) onset before 30 months of age; (b) impaired social development with a number of special characteristics that are not consistent with the child's intellectual level; (c) delayed and deviant language development, also with a number of special characteristics that are not consistent with the child's intellectual level; and (d) insistence on sameness (e.g., stereotyped play patterns, aberrant preoccupations, or resistance to change). Rutter "strongly recommended that, in order to ensure comparability, all investigators define their samples in this way" (p. 156).

Diagnostic and Statistical Manual of Mental Disorders (DSM)

There are many reasons why the *DSM* has undergone three distinct revisions over the past sixteen years. The *DSM* was developed by mental health clinicians as a guide to obtain diagnostic consistency. Since the bulk of mental health practitioners are adult focused, the *DSM* has emphasized conditions in adults and de-emphasized conditions in children. It is now commonly used by widely diverging disciplines and professionals (e.g., legal) to resolve differences in definitions, to resolve legal disputes, to develop appropriate treatment plans, to ensure the stability of diagnostic practices by insurance providers, and to enable researchers to describe atypical populations with mental disorders in a consistent manner. In the most recent *DSM* (*DSM-IV*, 1994), the sections on mental disorders in children are more complete. The following discussion highlights the differences and definitions of autism since 1980 in the *DSM-III*, *DSM-III-R*, and the *DSM-IV* (1994).

The authors of the *DSM-III* (1980) chose not to use such terms as atypical children, symbiotic psychosis, and childhood psychotic disorders because these conditions in children bore little relationship to the psychotic disorders observed in adults. Instead, the term Pervasive Developmental Disorder was adopted by American Psychiatry Association because it described "most accurately the core clinical disturbance in children with mental disorders and the variation in their development. Many basic areas of psychological development are affected at the same time and to a severe degree" (*DSM-III*, 1980, p. 86). Included among the Pervasive Developmental Disorders were Infantile Autism, Childhood Onset Pervasive Developmental Disorder, and Atypical Pervasive Developmental Disorder.

Childhood Onset Pervasive Developmental Disorder (COPDD) occurs after 3 months of age but before 12 years of age. Unlike those for Infantile Autism, the criteria for COPDD focused heavily on affective disturbances: excessive anxiety, unexplained rage, and self-mutilation. The label Atypical Pervasive Developmental Disorder was to be used when criteria were not met for Infantile Autism or COPDD (Eaves & Awadh, 1997).

A comparison of Rutter's (1978) and the *DSM-III*'s (1980) definitions reveals that the definitions have much in common, although there are differences in the criteria that are highlighted as primary, in the features offered as examples of primary criteria, and in associated features. For instance, Rutter's primary criterion of "insistence on sameness" becomes one example of the autistic child's "bizarre responses to various aspects of the environment" in the *DSM-III* (p. 183). Further, Rutter agreed that delusions and hallucinations were unlikely to develop in children with autism, but he did not include this exclusionary statement in his definition, as did the authors of the *DSM-III*. Below is a summary of the diagnostic criteria for Autistic Disorder as presented in the *DSM-III-R* (APA, 1987).

At least 8 of the following 16 items must be present. At least two items from (1), one item from (2), and one item from (3) must be included:

1. Qualitative impairment in reciprocal social interaction as manifested by:
   a. Marked lack of awareness of the existence of feelings of others
   b. No or abnormal seeking of comfort at times of distress
   c. No or impaired imitation
   d. No or abnormal social play
   e. Gross impairment in ability to make peer friendship

2. Qualitative impairment in verbal and nonverbal communication, and in imaginative activity as manifested by:
   a. No mode of communication
   b. Markedly abnormal nonverbal communication
   c. Absence of imaginative activity
   d. Marked abnormalities in the production of speech, including volume, pitch, stress, rate, rhythm, and intonation
   e. Marked abnormalities in the form or content of speech, including stereotyped and repetitive use of speech
   f. Marked impairment in the ability to initiate or sustain a conversation with others, despite adequate speech

3. Markedly restricted repertoire of activities and interests manifested by:
   a. Stereotyped body movements
   b. Persistent preoccupation with parts of objects
   c. Marked distress over changes in trivial aspects of environment
   d. Unreasonable insistence on following routines in precise detail
   e. Markedly restricted range of interests and a preoccupation with one narrow interest

4. Onset during infancy or childhood (*DSM-III-R,* 1987).

The 1987 revision of the *DSM-III* made three important changes. First, the labels within Pervasive Developmental Disorders changed. Infantile Autism was changed to

Autistic Disorder; COPDD was dropped; and Atypical Pervasive Developmental Disorder became Pervasive Developmental Disorder Not Otherwise Specified. The diagnostic disposition of affective disturbances previously emphasized in COPDD (e.g., excessive fearfulness, giggling for no apparent reason, and wrist biting) appeared as associated features in Autistic Disorder (Eaves & Awadh, 1997). Second, the number of primary criteria was reduced from six to four. That is, the criteria excluding features associated with schizophrenia (e.g., delusions, hallucinations) were dropped, and the two criteria involving language development and speech were combined into one criterion. Third, the diagnostic criteria of the *DSM-III-R* increased significantly in specificity and explicitness. The 16 items describing the criteria were accompanied by behaviorally worded examples, making the determination of their presence or absence easier. Beyond that, the definition specified for the first time a number of items that must be present in order to make the diagnosis. Finally, the age of onset was expanded from age 30 months to include the entire childhood period.

The changes in the definition of autism substantially increased the prevalence of autism (Hertzig, Snow, New, & Shapiro, 1990; Spitzer & Siegel, 1990). For instance, Hertzig et al. (1990) showed that among 75 children with Pervasive Developmental Disorders, 41% met the *DSM-III* criteria for Infantile Autism, whereas 71% of the same children met the *DSM-III-R* criteria for Autistic Disorder.

More changes took place with the publication of the *DSM-IV* (1994). First, three subtypes of Pervasive Developmental Disorders were added: Rett's Disorder, Childhood Disintegrated Disorder, and Asperger's Disorder. With regard to Autistic Disorder, the three primary criteria were retained. However, the number of behavioral descriptors were reduced from 16 to 12, several of the descriptors crossing criteria. A summary of the *DSM-IV* definition of Autistic Disorder follows.

At least 6 of the following 12 descriptors must be present. At least two items from (1), one item from (2), and one item from (3) must be included to complete the diagnosis:

1. Qualitative impairment in reciprocal social interaction as manifested by
   a. Marked impairment in the use of multiple nonverbal behaviors
   b. Failure to develop peer relationships appropriate to developmental level
   c. Lack of spontaneous seeking to share enjoyment, interest, or achievements with others
   d. Lack of social or emotional reciprocity

2. Qualitative impairment in communication
   a. Delay in, or total lack of, the development of spoken language
   b. Marked impairment in the ability to initiate or sustain a conversation in individuals with adequate speech
   c. Stereotypical or repetitive use of language or idiosyncratic language
   d. Lack of various, spontaneous, make-believe play or social imitative play appropriate to developmental level

3. Restricted repetitive and stereotyped patterns of behavior, interests, and activities
   a. Encompassing preoccupation with one or more stereotyped and restricted patterns of interest that is abnormal in intensity or focus

    b. Apparently inflexible adherence to specific, nonfunctional routines or rituals

    c. Stereotyped or repetitive motor mannerisms

    d. Persistent preoccupation with parts or objects

4. Delays or abnormal functioning in social interaction, language as used in social communication, or symbolic and imaginative play prior to 3 years of age

5. The disturbance is not better accounted for by Rett's disorder or childhood disintegrative disorder (*DSM-IV*, 1994)

Although it is too soon to complete a summary evaluation of the *DSM-IV* changes to the classification of PDDs, there are preliminary points of likely concern. First, the addition of three new subtypes of PDDs will probably draw criticism, if only because their construct validity has yet to be demonstrated. Second, the reduction in the number of items used to describe the three primary criteria for autistic disorders is likely to cause consternation among clinicians and researchers alike. The reduction in items, taken together with the fewer behavioral examples offered in the new definition, could cause another round of changes in the prevalence estimates (Eaves & Awadh, 1997). Further, the change in definition does little to assuage, and probably exacerbates, preexisting problems in comparing research results across studies that employ different definitions of autism (Eaves & Awadh). Finally, the age of onset has changed; and the requirements for delayed or abnormal functioning in social interaction, language, or symbolic play must be present before the third year has been added. Eaves and Awadh suggested that other issues are likely to arise, and they contend that it seems doubtful that a gold standard for the diagnosis of autistic disorders will ever exist.

Special Education Services

When the Individuals with Disabilities Education Act (IDEA) was reauthorized in 1990, autism was made a separate category of disability and was defined as

> a developmental disability significantly affecting verbal and nonverbal communication and social interaction, generally evident before age 3, that adversely affects educational performance. Other characteristics often associated with autism are engagement in repetitive activities and stereotyped movements, resistance to environmental changes or changes in daily routines, and unusual responses to sensory experiences. The term does not apply if a child's educational performance is adversely affected primarily because the child has a serious emotional disturbance. (34 C.F.R., Part 300, Sec. 300.7 [b] [1])

Although autism is often considered a mental disorder, mental health providers must consider the educational definition to assist parents in obtaining special education services for their children.

AUTISM-RELATED DISORDERS

There are three autism-related disorders that appear in the *DSM-IV.* These are (a) Rett's Disorder, (b) Childhood Disintegrated Disorder, and (c) Asperger's Disorder.

Fragile X Syndrome is often considered a similar disorder, or one that should be ruled out whenever autistic symptoms are present (American College of Medical Genetics, 1994).

Rett's Disorder

For a diagnosis of Rett's Disorder to be made, the *DSM-IV* requires the following symptoms to be observed:

1. Degeneration of motor skills after about age 5 months
2. Deceleration of head growth between 5 and 48 months
3. Loss of voluntary motor ability in the hands between about 5 and 30 months, followed by stereotyped hand movements such as writing
4. Limited social interaction
5. Poorly coordinated gait
6. Severely impaired receptive and expressive language abilities
7. Severe psychomotor retardation

Rett's Disorder occurs only in females and may result in severe to profound mental retardation.

Childhood Disintegrated Disorder

Children with this disorder appear normal for at least the first 2 years of life. A *DSM-IV* diagnosis requires significant loss of skills in at least two of the following areas (acquired before the age of 10 years):

1. Expressive or receptive language
2. Social skills and adaptive behavior
3. Bowel or bladder control
4. Play skills
5. Motor skills

The major difference between autism and Childhood Disintegrative Disorder is the loss of motor skills (Medicine Net, 1997).

Asperger's Disorder

Children with this disorder have many of the symptoms of autism but lack cognitive or language impairments. They often display concrete and literal thinking, have excellent memories, and are thought of as eccentric. In addition, *DSM-IV* requires display of at least two of the following problems:

1. Lack of normal peer relationships
2. Inability to share with others
3. Lack of emotional or social reciprocity
4. Stereotyped behaviors
5. Ritualistic behaviors
6. Repetitive motor movements
7. Preoccupation with parts of objects

In the past, many children with Asperger's Disorder were diagnosed as having "high-functioning autism." Many adults with Asperger's Disorder are capable of working and living independently.

Fragile X Syndrome

Although not identified by *DSM-IV* as an autism-like disorder, Fragile X Syndrome often produces symptoms similar to those of autism. These symptoms include poor eye contact; rapid, repetitive speech; and difficulty adjusting to change (Gene Care, 1996). Fragile X Syndrome usually results in mental retardation and distinctive physical characteristics such as prominent ears. The condition results from a chromosomal error in which the X chromosome (which carries the genes for female sexuality) breaks or has a weak arm. About 1 in every 1,200 males and 1 in every 2,500 females will develop Fragile X Syndrome. Males usually have more severe symptoms than females (American College of Medical Genetics, 1994). Diagnosis of Fragile X Syndrome is made by examining a sample of the patient's chromosomes under a microscope and by analyzing DNA. Chromosome analysis can identify carriers of the condition as well.

ASSESSMENT

Current assessment of Pervasive Developmental Disorders is complex, requiring differential diagnosis and a multidisciplinary point of view. The difficulty for diagnosticians has been the absence of agreement on symptoms necessary to generate a diagnosis. Although classification systems have become slightly more descriptive, they are still vague and defy diagnosticians' need for specific behavioral descriptors. Currently, the assessment of children with autism typically involves the use of several avenues of information. One is the traditional interview and direct observation of the child's behavior in various environments, including those both familiar and unfamiliar to the child. Likewise, interactions with caregivers and noncaregivers may be an essential aspect of the diagnostic process. Standard diagnostic practices include standardized developmental scales and both verbal and nonverbal intelligence tests; specific measures of functional language, visual and auditory processing, language development, memory and learning, and other cognitive development scales; adaptive behavior scales; and the use of general and specific developmental rating scales (i.e., autistic scales). Multiple rating scales should be used with a number of different informants defining the specific environment within which the observations are made.

Informal Observation

Observations should be made of the child's free play, interpersonal interaction, language (verbal and nonverbal) responses to language cues, manual motor speech production, response to environmental interactions, and adaptive behaviors, including the identification of unique perseverative, stereotypic, and ritualistic behaviors. Children with autism may show delayed language development, may not manifest a need for interpersonal communications, and may not understand spoken language or even respond to environmental (nonspeech) sounds. A common language-related characteristic is echolalia or meaningless parroting (repetitive reproduction) of someone else's words and phrases. Other language distortions may include rambling, irrelevant or bizarre speech, and misuse or omission of pronouns and connecting words (Sattler, 1988). Interpersonal interactions and affect are often assessed in structured and unstructured play settings, and information on adaptive behavior may be obtained from interviewing parents, child care workers, and teachers. The speech produced frequently has syntactic errors and uniqueness in suprasegmental structures of language, including intonation.

Structured processes for gathering observational data from primary and secondary caregivers (informants) were developed by behavioral scientists in the 1950s and 1960s. These approaches involve identifying the target behaviors in need of change and collecting data on those behaviors. When used to monitor treatment efficacy, the preintervention behaviors reported by informants are referred to as *baseline behaviors;* those behaviors that will become the focus of the intervention are known as *target behaviors.* One technique that is helpful in identifying antecedent events is the *structured diary.* It is used to record the antecedent events (events that precede the targeted behavior), the behavior, and the consequences (events that follow the behavior). A variety of formats can be used but should include the date and time the behavioral incident began, the antecedents of the behavior in question, a description of the behavior, the consequences of the behavior, and the individual's response to the consequences.

A time block chart is useful for recording the numbers of behaviors that occur within a specified time period, such as 10-minute intervals. Such a chart lists time periods down the left-hand side and days or dates across the top. Observers enter a plus (+) if the behavior occurred during the time period and a minus (–) if it did not. A *tally frequency count* keeps track of the total number of occurrences of the targeted behaviors, and during *measurements* record the length of time over which a particular behavior occurred. Finally, a *functional analysis* records information about antecedents and consequences of a behavior to identify behaviors that are reinforcing for the individual.

Powers (1997) suggested the following guidelines, based on frequency of the behavior, for determining which data collection procedure to use:

1. *For behavior that occurs less than 5 times a day,* use a structured diary to record information on the frequencies and functions of the behavior.

2. *For behavior that occurs between 5 and 10 times a day,* use a tally system supplemented with structured diaries in which the behavior is recorded based on a time sample basis or a priority basis. For example, a time sample might require recording and observation of the target behavior every 5 minutes. Priority recordings are notations of the most significant or severe behavior that occurs in a given period of time.

3. *For behavior that occurs more than 10 times a day,* a tally system may be too cumbersome, and a time block chart may be more practical.

Development-Based Assessment

According to Klin et al. (1997), "children with pervasive developmental disorders present unique issues for assessment" (p. 411). Many children with autism and related conditions typically exhibit problems in multiple areas of development, language, cognitive development, adaptive social and interpersonal behavior, social skills, affect, and moods.

Sparrow, Carter, Raeusim, and Morris (1995) developed a comprehensive developmental assessment approach that emphasized the need to identify available resources as well as the implications of the child's deficits and needs for his or her real-life adaptations. This assessment approach is valuable because it provides behavioral data across a number of developmental domains and examines for consistency across environmental settings. It is often observed that children with Pervasive Developmental Disorders are inconsistent in behavioral responses across various domains, even in similar environments with the same caregivers.

Klin et al. (1997) suggest that the following principles define the development assessment approach:

- Assessment of multiple areas of functioning (intellectual communication, functional skills, etc.)
- Adaptation of a developmental perspective
- Variability of skills (strengths/deficits, or profile of assets and deficits rather than a summary of scores)
- Variability across setting (home, school, day care, etc.)
- Functional adjustment (adjustment to real-life demands, everyday life wants)
- Delays and deviance (departure from normal expectations)

For additional detailed discussion on development-based assessment, the reader is referred to Klin et al. (1997).

Behavioral Assessment

Powers (1997) indicated that "behavioral assessment is an ongoing process designed to guide treatment planning by providing predictive, formative, and summative behavioral information" (p. 448). Thus, behavior assessment emphasizes description of stimuli (antecedents) and the child's ability to direct (control) his or her behavior. Although the relationship between a behavior being displayed and the child's social rule learning is unclear, it must be emphasized that the therapeutic practice currently producing the greatest efficacy has been structured behavioral modification. Four steps are recommended in using behavior assessment techniques (Powers, 1997):

1. Identifying and describing target behavior
2. Determining antecedent and consequent events which controls the behavior
3. Designing and implementing a treatment program
4. Evaluating outcome of treatment program

Another purpose of behavioral assessment is defining the target behavior as controlled by environment; this is sometimes referred to as the molar and molecular level of analysis (Powers, 1997). Multidimensional assessment (Evans, 1986) is the identification of the child's strengths and needs using multiple sources of data to guide treatment planning and effective instructional/behavioral management strategies. A major concern of behavioral assessment and intervention is that target behavior is functional in nontreatment settings and must be generalized and maintained over time. Stokes and Osnes (1988) identified a practical/predictive strategy involving assessment of three broad behavioral areas. These three areas are natural functional conveniences (reinforcers), training opportunities, and identification of the stimuli that serve as functional mediators of newly learned behavior. This approach expands behavior assessment from analysis of target behavior to include social context. Powers (1997) believes that employing such an assessment strategy can lead to a better understanding of treatment effectiveness and treatment failures.

SPECIFIC SCALES FOR AUTISM

Scales used for specific diagnostic purposes with autism are the Autism Diagnostic Interview (LeCouteur et al., 1989), Rimland's Diagnostic Checklist for Behavior-Disturbed Children (Rimland, 1964), and the Behavior Rating Scale for Autistic and Atypical Children (Ruttenberg, Dratman, Fraknoi, & Wenar, 1966). Frequently used descriptive scales include the Childhood Autism Rating Scale (Schopler et al., 1988), the Behavior Observation Scale (Freeman, Ritvo, Guthrie, Schroth, & Ball, 1978), and the Ritvo-Freeman Real Life Ratings (Freeman, Ritvo, Yokota, & Ritvo, 1986).

Childhood Autism Rating Scale (CARS)

The CARS is a 15-item scale used to identify children (over age 2) with autism and to distinguish mild-to-moderate from severe autism. The scale was developed over a 15-year period using more than 1,500 cases. The examiner rates the child on each item using a 7-point scale. The rating indicates the degree to which the child's behavior deviates from that of a normal child of the same age. Children who score above a given point are identified as having autism. The item content of the CARS is based on a broad view of autism from multiple diagnostic systems, including the *DSM*. The research literature (Sevin et al., 1991; Morgan, 1988; Teal & Wiebe, 1986) indicates that the CARS has variable reliability and is valid for several purposes. Internal consistency has been reported at .94, and median inter-rater reliability is in the .60 range. The CARS demonstrated a correlation of .67 with the Autism Behavior Checklist (ABC). However, the CARS correctly identified 98% of the children with autism, whereas the ABC identified 88% of the sample. Teal and Wiebe suggest using as a criterion for severe autism a total score greater than 36 and five or more scales rated 3 or higher. A discriminant analysis of the CARS comparing autistic children with trainable mentally retarded children produced 100% predictive accuracy (Teal & Wiebe, 1986).

Autism Screening Instrument for Educational Planning—Second Edition (ASIEP-2)

This scale helps to evaluate children with autism and to develop appropriate instructional plans. It can be used with children 18 months of age and over. The scale looks at five aspects of behavior, including the Autism Behavior Checklist, Sample and Vocal Behavior, Interaction Assessment, Education Assessment, and Prognosis of Learning Rate. Each subtest employs a different format, and each is individually normed. The scale yields percentiles and summary scores for each subtest.

Behavior Rating Instrument for Autistic and Other Atypical Children—Second Edition (BRIAAC-2)

This instrument has seven scales, beginning with most severe autistic behavior and progressing to behavior comparable to that of a normal 3.5- to 4.5-year-old. It can be administered to children of all ages. The scale measures Relationship to an Adult; Communication, Drive for Mastery; Vocalization and Expressive Speech; Sound and Speech Reception; Social Responsiveness; and Psychobiological Development. Two additional scales assess nonvocal communication for those children who use manual communication (Ruttenberg, Kalish, Wenar, & Wolf, 1977). The BRIAAC-2 is based primarily on Kanner's definition of autism. It appears to have good internal consistency, inter-rate reliability, and validity (Morgan, 1988). Spearman rank correlation coefficients ranged from .85 to .88 for the four scales, and inter-rate correlation ranged from .85 to .93 (Parks, 1983). Internal consistency of the eight scales range from .54 to .86.

Autism Diagnostic Observation Schedule (ADOS)

The ADOS consists of eight tasks presented to the child by the observer over a 20- to 30-minute time frame. The content of these tasks can vary according to the age and developmental level of the subject. The tasks include construction and unstructured presentation of toys, as well as a poster task, a book task, drawing, demonstration, and conversation. Eleven target behaviors are coded from these tasks according to a 3-point qualitative severity scale in four different areas: mood and nonspecific abnormal behaviors, communication/language, reciprocal social interaction, and stereotyped behaviors. The inter-rate reliability was found to be adequate, although some coefficients from a test-retest study by the authors of the test were as low as .57.

Behavior Observation Scale (BOS)

This scale contains a checklist of 35 behaviors intended to differentiate autistic from mentally retarded and normal children. The observation procedure involves observing the child for 27 minutes (nine intervals of 3 minutes each). Each of the items is scored from 0 to 3 based on the frequency of the observed behaviors (Freeman & Schroth, 1984). Reliability data on the BOS were collected on 89 children: 36 were autistic, 30 were mentally retarded and matched to the autistic group by mental age, and 23 were normal. Interobserver agreement was computed for the ratings. Correlation coefficients were greater than .85 on 55 of the 67 behaviors (Parks, 1983).

Autism Diagnostic Interview (ADI)

This scale was designed to assess the major characteristics of autism and to differentiate autism and Pervasive Developmental Disorders from other disorders such as mental retardation. It was developed to conduct interviews with the principal caregivers of children who are at least 5 years old with a mental age of at least 2 years. The interviewing task is to obtain detailed descriptions of the child's behavior in three general areas: restricted and stereotyped behaviors, reciprocal social interaction, and communication and language. The child's behaviors are scored on a scale ranging from 0 to 3, where a score of 0 indicates that the particular behavior is not present and a 3 suggests the behavior is present to a severe degree. The ADI authors report that validity and reliability demonstrate strong psychometric properties. The scores also differentiate between autistic and mentally retarded subjects (Lord, Storoschuk, Rutter, & Pickels, 1993). The authors report adequate evidence of inter-rate reliability. The correlation ranged from .91 for language/communication to .96 for reciprocal social interaction.

Autism Behavior Checklist (ABC)

The ABC is a 57-item behavioral rating scale. The initial development and norms were based on the ratings of 1,049 professionals. Each item is rated for presence/absence, with 1 to 4 points assigned to symptom presence based on an empirically derived weighting plan. The items make up five scales: sensory, relating, body and object use, language, and social self-help. Test scores can be compared to normative groups by age and diagnosis. The mean total scores for autistic groups are 78; other diagnostic groups have a mean of 45. The ABC is part of the ASIEP-2 described earlier. It was developed using items and information from existing autism scales. It has been reported to have good reliability and content validity. The scale's accuracy is very good. In a study by Wadden, Bryson, and Rodger (1991), the ABC accurately discriminated 91% of the children, with 87% autistic and 96% nonautistic. Split-half reliability was found to range from .74 to .87 (Volkmar et al., 1988; Krug et al., 1980). Krug et al. also reported inter-rate reliability of 95%, whereas Volkmar et al. found 70%. The authors of the test recommend a cut-off score of 67.

Diagnostic Checklist for Behavior-Disturbed Children, Form E-2 (E-2)

This form consists of 80 parent-completed questions measuring behaviors in the following areas: speech/language, social interaction, motor skills, reaction to stimuli, medical history, intelligence, family environment, and physiological dates. The first 17 questions concern the child's age, sex, birth order, age of onset of problems, anomalies in perception, and reactions to sensory stimuli. Another 41 questions concern behavioral patterns associated with autism: spontaneous motor and imitative ability, ritual acts, visual and auditory problems, withdrawal, social interaction, and physical appearance. Another 17 questions concern speech: its absence or presence, age of speech appearance, ability to communicate, echolalia and use of personal pronouns. Four questions concern the child's parents, and the last question invites the parents to read over their answers and select 10 questions best describing their child. The scale measures behavior through age 5. Each symptom of autism that is endorsed by the parent is assigned a positive point, and each question answered in the nonautistic direction is given a negative point. A score of +20 or higher is considered indicative of autism. The author has a large database to support the validity of the E-2. Teal and Wiebe (1986) found that E-2 scores correctly classified 85% of autistic children and 95% of retarded children. Reliability has not been extensively studied.

Parent Interview for Autism (PIA)

This scale is grouped into the following subscales: Social Relation, Affective Responses, Motor Limitation, Peer Interactions, Object Play, Imaginative Play, Language Understanding, Nonverbal Communication, Motor Behaviors, Sensory Responses, and Need for Sameness. Parents are asked to rate the frequency of the behavior for each item on a 5-point scale. Internal consistency for the scales ranges from a low of .55 for Object Play to a high of .83 for Relating. Test-retest correlation ranges from .48 to .90.

Ritvo-Freeman Real-Life Rating Scale (RLRS)

This scale was developed to identify the behaviors that characterize autism more accurately. It can be used after observation of a 30-minute play period. Unusual sensory behaviors are emphasized. Adequate subscale and total inter-rate reliability was found (Sevin, Matson, Coe, Fee, & Sevin, 1991). Correlation with the CARS total score was .77. Three of the five subscales—Social Relationships, Sensory, and Language—had adequate-to-high internal consistency.

Pervasive Developmental Disorder Rating Scale (PDDRS)

This is a screening device designed to measure three factors: arousal, affect, and cognition. The three factors were based on 325 children. The PDDRS provides both a stan-

Table 9.1   Representative Rating Scales for Assessment of Autism

Autism Behavior Checklist Scales (ABC; Krug, Arick, & Almond, 1980).

Autism Diagnostic Interview (ADI; LeCouteur, Rutter, Lord, Rios, Robertson, Holdgrafer, & MacLellan, 1989).

Autism Diagnostic Observation Schedule (ADOS; Lord, Rutter, Goode, Heemsbergen, Jordan, Mawhood, & Schopler, 1989).

Autism Screening Instrument for Educational Planning (ASIEP; Krug, Arick, & Almond 1980).

Behavior Observation Scale (BOS; Freeman, Ritvo, Guthrie, Schroth, & Ball, 1978).

Behavior Rating Scale for Autistic and Atypical Children (BRIAAC; Ruttenberg, Dratman, Fraknoi, & Wenar, 1966).

Childhood Autism Rating Scale (CAR; Schopler, Reichler, & Renner, 1988).

Diagnostic Checklist for Behavior-Disturbed Children (E2; Rimland, 1968, 1971).

Parent Interview for Autism (PIA; Stone, & Hogan, 1993).

Pervasive Developmental Disorder Rating Scale (PDDRS; Eaves, 1993).

Ritvo-Freeman Real-Life Rating Scale (RLRS; Freeman, Ritvo, Yokota, & Ritvo, 1986).

dard score (Mean = 100, SD = 15) for each of the three areas and a composite score. Percentile ranks are also provided for each of the three domains and the composite score.

About the Specific Scales for Autism

There are a number of specialized testing scales available to diagnose autism. Some are more widely used, such as the CARS, than others. This instrument has been repeatedly documented as a reliable screening instrument. CARS scales are still considered to be experimental in nature, whereas others are still seen to be in the research-and-development stages. See Table 9.1 for a representation of rating scales. It is important to recognize that a diagnosis should not be made with a single instrument. A battery of tests that is well thought-out and covers as many areas of functioning would be the best choice.

DIFFERENTIAL DIAGNOSIS

In the diagnosis of Pervasive Developmental Disorders, it is critical to differentiate them from other disorders, such as deafness, language impairment, mental retardation, and other childhood mental disorders.

Autism versus Asperger's Disorder

Autistic disorders are highly similar to Asperger's disorder. Both disorders manifest evidence of impairments in social interaction. This is noted by deficiencies in nonverbal behavior (eye-to-eye gaze and facial expression) and in a lack of social or emotional reciprocity. The child with an autistic disorder also demonstrates marked impairment in communication, which is not present in Asperger's disorder. In addition autistic chil-

Table 9.2   Differential Diagnosis of Autism and Asperger's

Criteria	Autism	Asperger's
Language	Delayed and deviant language development	Absence of delayed and deviant language development
Motor	Absence of clumsiness	Presence of clumsiness
Cognitive	Presence of cognitive delay	Absence of cognitive delay
Interests	Very restrictive	Less restrictive
Bizarre Behaviors	Many bizarre behaviors	Fewer bizarre behaviors
Social	Lack social intentionally and reciprocity	Demonstrate more social intentionality and reciprocity
Relationship	Show none or less affection, do not seek comfort	Show more need for affection, often seek comfort

dren manifest delays in cognitive development, whereas children with Asperger's do not. Thus, autistic children exhibit overt impairments in the ability to initiate or sustain social conversations. They also lack the ability to engage in spontaneous and social initiative play. It may be useful to characterize the child with an autistic disorder as one with a basic incapacity to attach and relate interpersonally.

In contrast, children with Asperger's disorder appear by nature to be oversensitive youngsters who possess communicative skills but have drawn into themselves as a defensive position due either to their hypersensitivity or to severely problematic interpersonal experiences (Szatmari, Bartolucci, & Bremmer, 1989; Szatmari, Archer, Sandra, Streiner, & Wilson, 1995). See Table 9.2 for a complete guide to differentiation between these two disorders.

Autism versus Schizophrenia

The separation of schizophrenia and autism did not occur until the appearance of the *DSM-III*. Before 1980, the two disorders were grouped together under the term *Childhood schizophrenia*. However, this older classification scheme has continued, so that the term childhood schizophrenia is often wrongly referred to as autism. One difference is that the child with schizophrenia manifests hallucinations or delusions, which are prominent during a period of 1 month or more (*DSM-IV,* 1994). One other important difference is the age of onset. Children who begin to show symptoms before age 3 are diagnosed as having an Autistic Disorder, and those of ages 5 to 15 more closely resemble schizophrenia (Green, Campbell, & Hardesty, 1984; Watkins, Asarnow, & Tanguay, 1998). In addition, autism is characterized by normal or above-average motor development, good physical health, and no history of mental illness in the family. In contrast, poor physical health and a family history of psychosis characterize childhood schizophrenia. See Table 9.3 for a detailed list of differences between the two groups.

Table 9.3   Differential Diagnosis of Autism and Schizophrenia

Criteria	Autism	Schizophrenia
Onset	Before age 3	After 3 years of age
Development	Absence of a normal period of development	Presence of normal period extending beyond 2 years
IQ	Majority of cases subnormal, 70% less than 70 IQ	Mostly dull normal, 15% less than 70 IQ
Prenatal Complications and Cerebral Dysfunction	More common occurrence	Less common occurrence
Premorbed Abnormality	More pervasive and developmentally catastrophic	Less pervasive and developmentally catastrophic
Hallucinations and Delusions	Not present or transitory	Present and more permanent
Play	Show no symbolic play (pretend)	Show symbolic play (pretend)
Socioeconomic	Overrepresentation of upper SES groups (Artifact)	More common in lower SES groups
Health	Good physical health	Poor physical health
Family	No history of mental illness	Often a family history of psychosis

Autism versus Mental Retardation

A majority of mentally retarded children are quite sociable and communicative, whereas children with autism show no or little social interest in relating with others (Jacobsen & Ackerman, 1990). Autistic children tend to have fewer facial abnormalities than mentally retarded children. Also, autistic children tend to have better motor coordination than mentally retarded children. The test performance of the autistic child is quite erratic and variable in performance, while the performance of the mentally retarded child is relatively even with little variability. See Table 9.4 for a complete listing of behaviors that differentiate these two groups.

INTERVENTIONS

Major goals of intervention/treatment programs for individuals with autism should relate to the assessment of the person's level of functioning within each area of impairment. Thus, as clinicians we must strive to ameliorate difficulties and help the individual with autism cope to the highest degree possible. Specific goals of treatment should include the following:

- Fostering development of social and communication skills
- Enhancing learning and problem solving

Table 9.4   Differential Diagnosis of Autism and Mental Retardation

Criteria	Autism	Mental Retardation
Relationships	Relate poorly to others regardless of Mental Age level	Usually related to others in accordance with their Mental Age
Language	Do not use language to communicate with others	Use language they do have to communicate with others
Test Performance	Very erratic and variable performance for both inter and intra test performance	Relatively even performance or profile with little variable performance
Skill Development	More developed when matched by age and IQ	Less developed when matched by age and IQ
Daily Living	Modes of information acquisition are *not* readily accessible and deployable	Modes of information acquisition are more readily accessible and deployable
Sensory Stimulation	Lack of learning via social interaction and integration of sensory stimulation	Demonstrate some learning via social interaction and integration of sensory stimulation
Motor Coordination	Good motor coordination	Often poor motor coordination
Appearance	Often attractive with few or no physical anomalies	Less attractive with more physical anomalies

- Decreasing behaviors that interfere with learning and access to opportunities for normal experiences
- Helping families cope with the diagnoses of autism

Unfortunately, curriculum interventions (method and content of instruction) have taken a backseat to other methods (psychological, medical, behavioral, etc.) of treatment. Schopler (1994) identified 28 approaches to treatment of individuals with autism. As Olley and Reese (1997) pointed out, these 28 approaches enjoyed a brief time in headlines of newspapers. They were featured on television programs, but few of the approaches had objective evidence for their effectiveness. Furthermore, few of these 28 approaches specified exactly what behavior it was that they expected to improve (outcome produced). In other words, "the majority of the 28 do not have an explicit curriculum" (p. 484). Yet, curriculum is an essential component of any effective education, intervention, or treatment program. Olley and Reese provided an excellent overview of some major published approaches on curriculum and classroom structure for children and youth with autism. They included such programs as the developmental approach, Treatment and Education of Autistic and Related Communication Handicapped Children (TEACCH), cognitive criteria (a daily life theory that originated in Japan), behavioral, ecological, and IMPACT. Please note that there is no pure example of any of the models mentioned, and each curriculum combines components from the others' approaches. Most of the dual-curricula approaches contain similar instructions in areas of content such as communication training, play and social skills, self-management, adaptive behavior, skills for working groups, and transition skills to adulthood. Most curriculum intervention strategies are characterized by combining two intervention aspects: (a) a clear structure approach and (b) direct teaching procedures.

To teach children with autism effectively, teachers and other professionals must consider the children's cognitive characteristics. According to Quik (1995), these children (a) are likely to think in pictures instead of words, (b) have difficulty retrieving information from memory, (c) cannot follow long sequences of verbal information, (d) cannot mentally manipulate more than one idea at a time, (e) cannot attend to or use information through a single sensory modality, (f) cannot generalize, and (g) experience perceptual confusion. To account for these difficulties, educational interventions for students with autism should be highly structured and should emphasize teaching the students to communicate effectively and interact with others socially, to adequately make changes, and to master simple tasks that can be used in work and social environments outside the classroom. As early as possible, students with autism should also be taught vocational and community living skills (Engel, 1994).

Engel (1994) describes the following strategies for teaching high-functioning students with autism:

1. For children with poor organizational skills, break tasks down into small steps.

2. For students who have difficulty with abstract concepts, use concrete instruction. If abstract thinking is necessary, provide visual cues such as gestures or written words.

3. For children with unusual or problem behavior, reduce stress by providing a way for the child to remove himself physically from stressful situations.

4. Be aware that misbehaving children are not intentionally trying to be disruptive, and don't take their misbehavior personally.

5. For children who use and interpret language literally, avoid ambiguous words and phrases such as idioms and metaphors.

6. For children who cannot interpret nonverbal and other social cues, be as concrete as possible.

7. For children who don't seem to fully understand oral language, speak clearly and concisely.

8. For children who are upset by variations in routine, prepare advance notice of impending changes.

9. For children who are distractible, minimize environmental stimulation by reducing lighting or making changes in seating arrangements.

10. For children who engage in verbal repetitions, require written verbal responses to calm the child and stop the repetitive behavior. For children who do not read or write, role-play the repetitive verbal behavior by taking the child's part and having her respond.

11. For the child with communication difficulties, avoid asking the child to relay important messages to teachers or parents about school events and rules. Direct communication and phone calls are more effective.

12. For children who are socially isolated, recruit a classmate who will be an occasional partner for games and other activities.

We believe that the combination of structured classroom training in communication and social skills with behavioral modifications is the most effective way of teaching children with autism. Gains in language and cognition have been found using the two approaches in combination, and with observable decreases in maladaptive behaviors. Also, parent training in concepts and skills of behavioral modification and at-home follow-up therapy through training in other areas have multiple effective results. Teachers must have a highly structured classroom with the expectation that children with autism will learn specific skills before going to the next level of learning.

Behavioral Intervention

Failures in intervention/treatment studies are rarely reported. Also, studies reporting behavior intervention used either single-case designs, or the sample sizes were very small. Thus, generalization from the findings is especially reduced. Consistent successful results were reported for behavior intervention programs that, according to Bregman and Gerdtz (1997), support the efficacy of behavior intervention treatment programs for individuals with autism.

Bregman and Gerdtz (1997) indicated that "during the past 10 years behavior interventions have become the predominant treatment approach for promoting the social, adaptive, and behavioral functioning of children and adults with autism" (p. 620). Behavior intervention treatment strategies have proven successful in reinforcing adaptive responses and suppressing maladaptive ones, such as aggression, self-injury, destructive behavior, noncompliance, and stereotyped movements, which are the core features of autism. According to Bregman and Gerdtz, behavioral treatment programs can enhance personal independence, develop responsible choice through skill development and habilitative training, and increase prosocial behavior, relaxation, self-control, and leisure.

Bregman and Gerdtz (1997) divide behavior intervention strategies into broad categories. These categories are (a) antecedent intervention (what happens prior to a behavior) used in an effort to avert a problem, (b) consequence (programs) procedures used following the target behavior, and (c) skill development, which is used to teach an alternative or more appropriate behavior, thereby reducing the maladaptive behavior. What is yet unresearched is the interaction of behavior intervention strategies with specific problem behaviors. Bregman and Gerdtz believe that the use of computers will enhance obtainment of data for behavior treatment programs with individuals having Pervasive Developmental Disorder. See Table 9.5.

There is substantial evidence that children with a wide variety of development delays and disorders (e.g., autism and mental retardation), have a greater chance for successful outcomes from resulting interventions when they are younger (Guralnick, 1998). Early intervention programs have indeed been judged effective for children with autism (Kazdin, 1993) over the past several years, and are difficult to evaluate outcomes.

Table 9.5 Behavior Intervention Strategies

Methods Used to Increase Behavior	Methods Used to Decrease Behavior
Shaping	Satiation
Modeling	Punishment
Behavior Rehearsing	Time out
Reinforcement Schedules	Desensitization
Ratio, Interval	Alternative Response
Positive Reinforcement	Response-Contingent
Token Economy	Confinement
Contingency Contracting	Loss of Privilege
Program Restructuring	Reprimands
	Overcorrection
Direct Teaching	Differential Reinforcement
	Response Cost
	Penalizing
	Ignoring
	Extinction

Common Elements of Effective Intervention Programs

Over the last 20 years a number of programs have been intensively researched regarding interventions/strategies for young children with autism and for their families (Kazdin, 1993; Bregman & Gerdtz, 1997). These programs vary in their individual philosophical approaches and strategies but each one was to publish and share information about the characteristics of their subject sample, methodologies, use, and outcomes. Dawson and Sterling (1997) reviewed eight models of early intervention program for children with autism. They have described six common elements that appear to be effective in early intervention programs. A few of the programs reviewed by Dawson and Sterling were the May Institute TEACCH, the University of California at Los Angeles Young Autism Program, and the Walden Preschool and Douglas Developmental Disabilities Center. The six common elements identified are summarized below:

1. *Curriculum content.* The curricula of the programs emphasize five basic skill domains, including the following abilities: (a) to attend to environmental elements that are essential for learning, especially to social stimuli; (b) to imitate others; (c) to comprehend and use language; (d) to play appropriately with toys; and (e) to interact socially with others.

2. *Highly supportive teaching environments and generalization strategies.* The programs first try to establish core skills in highly structured environments and then work to generalize these skills to more complex, natural environments.

3. *Predictability and routine.* Since the behavior of children with autism is easily disrupted by changes in environment and routine, the programs adopt strategies to assist the child with transitions from one activity to another.

4. *Functional approach to problem behavior.* Since young children with autism often show problem behaviors, the programs first try to prevent the development of these behaviors by structuring the environment. If problem behaviors persist, the programs use a functional approach that involves the following steps: (a) recording the behavior, (b) developing a hypothesis about the function that behavior serves for the child, and (c) changing the environment to support appropriate behavior which allows the child to cope.

5. *Plans for transition for preschool classroom.* The programs teach survival skills that children will need in order to function independently in preschool or school classrooms later on.

6. *Family involvement.* The programs include parents as a critical component in the intervention for young children with autism. Family involvement is an important factor for success of a program because parents can provide unique insights into creating an intervention plan and can provide additional hours of intervention. Including parents in the intervention can also help children achieve greater maintenance and generalization of skills and can help reduce parents' stress levels.

The Family in Treatment

Bettelheim (1967) noted that historically the treatment of children with autism resulted in separating children from their parents, and often by placing them into a treatment facility. Within the past two decades we have seen a major shift from isolation of the child to comprehensive family treatment—in some cases, involving the parents as cotherapists (Campbell, Schopler, Cueva, & Hallin, 1996). The pioneering works of Schopler and Reichler (1971) and Campbell and Schopler (1999) ushered in professional collaboration of parents in the treatment of children with autism. This collaboration approach was designed as much to assist parents as it was to understand and help children. Schopler and Reichler (1971) document that parents of autistic children were as much the victim of the disorder as were their children.

Lovaas (1987) demonstrated that parents could become effective therapists. In addition, family involvement in the treatment program can foster mutual parental and professional support and continuity in the treatment program, and has strongly motivated the parents to help their children (Moes, 1995) because they are in a team framework and are not working alone. This type of family therapeutic program often prevents hostility and over-regulation of the child with autism by family members. Family therapy is an essential component of the total intervention program for the treatment of children with PDDs.

Educational Intervention

Any treatment program, regardless of the individual disorder, needs to be comprehensive and designed to meet the needs and levels of functioning for each person. This is especially true for children with PDDs because this condition is usually lifelong, and treatment modalities must change with age and development. Leaders in the field of PDD such as Campbell et al. (1996) have suggested that perhaps the most important treatment component for children with PDD is special education programs in the schools. Special education should begin at a very early age (Early Intervention Programs), focusing initially on language and speech development, and should target the most challenging behavior deficits. Perhaps the main focus on language and speech therapy is to maximize communication of the child, verbal or otherwise, in order to foster a need for socialization. Various treatment procedures have been used to help children with PDDs develop language. A comprehensive discussion of all the treatment modalities is beyond the scope of this chapter (see Vance, Fuller, & Awadh, 1995).

Social skill training has also received considerable attention in the treatment of children with autism. The modality treatment approach focuses on developing social competence and social skills in children with social cognitive deficits. A continuum of intervention strategies and programs is important as the child progresses in school and earns independence. Such programs are designed to meet the needs of each child, usually shifting from a one-on-one intervention to interventions in larger groups, whether the intervention is speech, language development, physical therapy, occupational therapy, or vocational preparation leading to independent communication and social functioning. As the program changes to meet changing developmental needs, it is also important to help the child move from highly structured environments to more inclusive environments in more general educational settings. These programs help the child with autism function as independently as possible.

An important ingredient to individualizing interventions for children with PDDs is that the interventions be based on information gathered from comprehensive assessment processes. The assessment procedure should pinpoint and clearly identify specific strengths and weaknesses of the child as well as the needs of the family and child. As part of the intervention program, guidelines should be available for monitoring the progress of the child and parents. Accurate documentation of the child's progress, based on specific intervention strategies through a trial period, is often necessary to determine efficacy. If intervention strategies do not work, the intervention or its application should be changed as the intervention/treatment plan is developed. Continued reassessment of children with autism and their family dynamics is necessary in plotting the child's progress and developmental status. Reassessment is recommended at least once a year. Results should be compared to functional levels, not to age-expected norms. As with any intervention program, the treatment technique selected should ensure that there is scientific evidence for the continued support of its use. A team approach should be used to ensure that multiple interventions and strategies providing various descriptors are coordinated into an integrated treatment plan, and that there is collaboration across all disciplines and between the team and the family. Figure 9.1 provides information from data-based research studies about the effectiveness of various intervention strategies used with children and youth with autism.

Language Intervention

It is beyond the scope of this paper to provide a comprehensive discussion of the variety of strategies used to enhance language and communication development of children with PDDs. Communication skills may be the main factor in predicting the extent to which individuals with autism can adjust and participate in society. The pervasive na-

Supported	Nonsupported
Intensive Behavioral Interaction Program for Young Children	Developmental Individual Difference (DIR)
Applied Behavioral Analyst Strategy	Sensory Integration Theory (SIT)
Functional Analyst of Children Behavior	Auditory Integration Training (AIT)
Sign Language	Facilitated Communication Music Therapy Touch Therapy
Visual Communication Approach	Hormone Therapy
Intensive Parent Training	Intravenous Immuneglobin Antiyeast Therapies Vitamin or Trace Therapies Diet Therapy Psychotherapy

Figure 9.1   Summary of Proven Treatment/Intervention Strategies That Have Been Supportive by Research Data for Children

ture of these disorders affects not only receptive and expressive language development but also nonverbal behavior (social interaction, behavior regulation, and collaborative learning). Language intervention programs include prelinguistic enhancing, language development and augmentative and alternative communication. Cohen and Swettenham (1997) provide the interested reader with four excellent chapters on language intervention approaches for individuals with autism.

In most instances the type of intervention and strategies used for intervention with individuals with autism are primarily guided by what is useful in promoting, developing, and adapting to the environment. As professionals work with individuals with autism and their families, they need to be realistic about what can be accomplished using current information. There are no magical cures, and many so-called breakthrough programs such as facilitated communication lie outside the realism of accepted practice, and are not supported by rigorous scientific studies (Myles & Simpson, 1994).

Pharmacotherapy

A number of medications have been suggested as possible treatments for children with autism. Over the past decade, a large number of well-designed research studies have evaluated the efficacy of using medications for treating autism in children and adults (McDougle, 1997; Campbell et al., 1990; Pumariega, Del Mundo, & Vance, 2000). Most of these studies were randomized controlled treatments that used double-blind and placebo-controlled designs (McDougle, 1998). As research on autism has expanded in recent years, most researchers agree that there are biological bases for this disorder. This consensus has led to the development of a number of new medications to treat PDDs, especially autism and Asperger's.

Level	I. Low Yield: Low Risk	II. Moderate Yield: Moderate Risk	II.	III. Moderate Yield: High Risk		III. High Risk: Low Yield
Drugs		SSRIs	ADD drugs	Atypical Neurolepics	Mood Stabilizers	
	Buspar Trazodone Naltrexone	Prozac Praxil Zoloft Luvox Anafranil (?)	Ritalin Dexedrine Adderall Tenex Clonidine	Risperdal Zyprexa Seroquel Clozaril (?)	Lithium Tegretol Valproic Acid New Seizure Meds	Mellaril Thorazineserentin Loxitane Navane Haldol Prolixin
Results	Decreased:	Decreased:	Decreased:	Decreased:	Decreased:	Decreased:
	SIB Aggression Violence Stereotypy	SIB: Sexual Aggression Violence Stereotypy OCD Depression Social Withdraw	Aggression Hyperactivity Stereotypy Depression	Violence Aggression SIB Psychosis Activity	Mania-Bipolar Aggression SIB Activity	Aggression Violence SIB Psychosis
	Increased:	Increased:	Increased:	Increased:	Increased:	Increased:
	Mood Psychological Development	Energy Mood	Attention Activity Mood	Mood	Mood	

Figure 9.2   Effectiveness of Various Agents When Used with Children Who Are Autistic

In 1994, the Autistic Research Institute (ARI-Form 34EE) published data gathered from 8,700 parents of children with autism on the effectiveness of various psychotropic medications. The parents responded to a 6-point scale (made worse, 5–6; made better, 3–4; had no effect, 1–2). An interesting finding was that methylphenidate (in Ritalin, the drug most commonly prescribed) and risperidone have demonstrated promise in the treatment of uncontrollable behaviors. The use of selective serotonin reuptake inhibitors (SSRIs) for treating challenging behaviors associated with autism has increased within the last three years. McDougle (1998) has demonstrated the efficacy of SSRIs in diminishing obsessive-compulsive, stereotypic behavior and improving social reciprocity and learning in both controlled and uncontrolled studies. Vance and Pumariega (2000) reported a single case study using fluoxetine (Prozac) on a child with severe PDD. This study demonstrated the efficacy of fluoxetine in decreasing stereotypic behaviors. A dramatic increase in social reciprocity was also achieved, as observed by both teachers and parents. A relative new agent Secretin, a polypeptide hormone secreted by the pancreas, has received increased attention as an agent for treating autism; Secretin has not been approved as a treatment agent for any medical conditions; no controlled studies supporting its efficacy have been reported. For children and youth with autism and Asperger's disorder, pharmacotherapy is a valuable addition to a comprehensive treatment and habilitation program that can improve a variety of associated symptoms and enhance developmental progression (Pumariega et al., 2000; Del Mundo, Pumariega, & Vance, 1999). Figure 9.2 summarizes the use of agents with autistic children.

The etiology of autism is multifactorial, and there is no known cure. McDougle (1997) stated that "the appropriate use of medication, in the context of a comprehensive individualized treatment program, can enhance the autistic person's ability to benefit from educational and behavior modification interventions" (p. 719). The quality of life for people with autism and their family members can be improved with appropriate psychopharmacology and individualized compulsive psychosocial treatment plans. Research over the past 20 years has yielded little information regarding the pathophysiology of autism (McDougle, 1997). A major concern in the psychopharmacological treatment of autism is that about one third of children with autism develop seizure disorders at some point in their lifetime (Volkmar & Nelson, 1990). McDougle (1997) provides a comprehensive treatment on the subject of effective pharmacotherapy for individuals with autism.

CONTROVERSIAL AND UNORTHODOX INTERVENTIONS

The history of treatment of autism is punctuated by claims of cures and miracle solutions. As a result, a long list of controversial and unorthodox interventions has come into and gone out of fashion over the years. Some of these treatments may be beneficial, as claimed in anecdotal reports by parents and professionals. To date, however, the efficacy of these treatments is still in question.

Facilitated Communication

Of all the unorthodox treatment, none has been as controversial or received as much media attention as facilitated communication (FC). The Autism Society of America (1996) defines facilitated communication as follows:

> A technique by which a "facilitator" supports the hand, arm, or shoulder of a communicatively impaired individual, this method assists the person with impairment to extend an index finger and either point to or press the keys of a typing or other communication device. If successful, the individual who was previously unable to communicate can do so by typing or spelling out words.

Initially, FC was heralded as a miracle cure and was purported to show that many individuals previously thought to be functioning in the below-normal range actually had average or even above-average intelligence. However, the majority of studies on FC have demonstrated conscious or unconscious influence by the facilitator. Although this approach is still experimental and lies outside the realm of accepted practice (Myles & Simpson, 1994), it may hold promise, especially as an avenue to explore greater care of technology. A number of professional organizations have adopted and published statements in which they identify FC as a technique that has not been scientifically validated. Some of these include the American Association of Pediatrics, the American Association on Mental Retardation, and the American Psychiatric Association.

Dimethylglycine

Dimethylglycine (DMG) is a food supplement resembling vitamin B_{15}. It does not require a prescription and can be purchased in health food stores. Some parents have claimed that use of DMG results in improvements in speech, eye contact, social behaviors, and attention span.

Gluten- and Casein-Free Diets

Such diets avoid bread or other foods containing protein from wheat (gluten) as well as protein from milk and diary produce (casein). These proteins are thought to cause allergic responses and hyperactivity. The theory is that the body of the individual with autism lacks the ability to break down these proteins, allowing enzymes to enter the brain via the bloodstream, which produces negative developmental effects.

Foods and Food Coloring

Some parents believe that eliminating certain foods and food coloring can reduce autistic behaviors. For example, some parents believe that eating apples, oranges, and other citrus fruits, as well as chocolate and certain other foods, will result in severe behavior problems for children with autism. Some parents also believe that synthetic pigments used in food coloring can result in hyperactivity.

Case Study: Comprehensive Integrative Psychological Evaluation

Name: Bob
Age: 2 years 5 months
Gender: male
School: none
Date of Evaluation: 10/30/98 and 11/01/98
Date of Report: 11/05/98
Date of Birth: 05/10/96
Grade: not applicable

REASON FOR REFERRAL
Bob's mother wanted a second opinion regarding her son's diagnosis of autism by the development pediatric unit at the local hospital. In addition, she was seeking information about treatment and intervention opinions.

INSTRUMENTS ADMINISTERED
  • Clinical intervention with parents
  • Observation on three different days
  • Adaptive behavior
  • Review records
  • Preschool Evaluation Scale
  • Gilliam Autistic Rating Scale
  • Child Behavior Checklist for Ages 2 to 3

- Preschool Language Scale—Third Edition
- Autism Screening Instrument for Educational Planning
- Achenbach's Child Behavior Checklist

DEVELOPMENT HISTORY AND BEHAVIOR OBSERVATION

Bob was the third live birth of three pregnancies. His mother exhibited hypertension during the last trimester. At 37 weeks, the decision was made to hospitalize her; labor was induced with Pitocin after 24 hours. Delivery occurred within several hours after the amniotic sac broke. Gas was used during the second stage of labor. Bob was born with placenta strangulation, but resuscitation was not necessary. His Apgar score was above 7 (normal).

According to Bob's parents, all developmental milestones, including speech, developed normally up until 18 months of age. Bob began to regress in language skills and did not explore his environment interactively. At 24 months Bob's tantrums worsened, his eye contact disappeared, and his speech reverted to grunts and growls. His gross and fine motor skill development at age 2 was normal; his hearing was also normal. Self-help skills were delayed. Bob was seen by his pediatrician in October 1998 and was diagnosed with autism. His head circumference was only 48 cm, placing him at the 10th percentile.

His development status at age 2 years 5 months was characterized by an absence of communication, few single sounds, no new words learned since 18 months. He would imitate and point to objects he wanted but would fail to respond to his name and had limited eye contact and total disregard for emotional attachment. Bob interacted aggressively with his siblings. When disciplined he became violent and uncontrollable (aggressive, destroyed household items). His level of social and peer interaction behavior was delayed. His behavior was often described as overacting to stimulation of people, and he was developmentally delayed, characterized by lack of sharing. He showed no separation anxiety and was easily agitated, acting out physically without impulse control. When acting aggressively, he was a physically strong child. He disliked wearing clothes. Throughout the observation periods, many stereotypic behaviors were noticed (finger tapping, rolling backward and forward, self-biting, picking at skin or scabs). These behaviors served as self-stimulating. Bob had temper tantrums that lasted 40 minutes. During this time, he broke items, turned over furniture, his others, and was self-injurious. He did not respond positively to consistent firm limits but could be reinforced through verbal redirection, which reduced the intensity of his behavior outbreaks.

ASSESSMENT RESULTS

Bob's mother completed the Preschool Evaluation Scale (PES), which is a measure of adaptive/developmental skills. This scale has six subtests measuring various developmental domains. The PES has a mean of 10 and a standard deviation of 3. Bob's scores were the following.

Subscales	Standard Scores	Percentile Scores
Language muscle skills	16	89
Small muscle skills	15	95
Cognitive thinking	7	15
Expressive language	5	5
Social/emotional	7	15
Self-help skills	10	50

Development delays were especially noticeable in the areas of cognitive thinking and expressive language and in the social/emotional domain.

(*continued*)

The Preschool Language Scale—Third Edition is used to ascertain receptive and expressive language skills in infants and young children. The two subscales—auditory comprehension and expressive communication—are combined to provide a total language score. The output pressures are reported both as standard scores with a mean of 100 and standard deviation of 15 and as age equivalent scores. Bob obtained a comprehension standard score of 82 with a percentile rank of 12. On expressive communication, Bob obtained a standard score of 57 with a percentile rank of > 1. His total language score was 60, with percentile rank of > 1. Bob's total language age equivalent was at the 9-month level. He displayed severe language communication delays in the areas of expressive language.

The Achenbach's Child Behavior Checklist for ages 2 to 3 was administered with Bob's mother as the informant. Results from this instrument were highly indicative of clinical abnormality in two behavioral areas displaying externalizing broad band behaviors. Bob scored high on the emotional obsessive-compulsive and on the inattentive subtests. He produced high scores on items such as has a low tolerance for frustration, cannot sit still and is restless, avoids eye contact, fights, is aggressive and hurts others, shows little fear of danger, and displays violent temper reactions. His scores on three measures were at the 99th percentile level for children his age. In other words, he scored higher than 99% of all children in the standardization sample of these three subtests.

The Adaptive Behavior Scale (ABS) of the AAMD is a behavior rating scale that is often used with children suspected of having challenging behaviors. The ABS has a mean of 10 with a standard deviation of 3. Bob's results from his mother's ratings are:

Scales	Mean = 10	Mean = 100
Self-help skills	8	90
Communication skills	3	65
Social skills	4	70
Academic skills	1	55
Occupational skills	—	—
Atypical skills	1	55

Please note the similarities between the scores of the ABS and the PES. The Atypical Behavioral Scale is a subscale of the ABS that asks questions related to violence, destructiveness, stereotyped behavior, odd mannerisms, self-abuse, unusual vocal habits, and hyperactive tendencies. Bob obtained a highly significant clinical score on this domain.

Results from the Gilliam Autism Scale are a measure of skills and behaviors indicative of the possibility of autism. The scale consists of four subtests and a total score, which provides an autism quotient. Bob's mother was present as he completed this instrument. Scores are reported as T-scores with a mean of 10 and a standard deviation of 3. A T-score is a form of standard score. Results obtained from the GAS are as follow:

Subtests	Standard Scores	Percentage	Degree of Severity
Stereotyped behaviors	15	96	high
Communication	16	97	high
Social interaction	15	96	high
Development	9	48	average
Autism quotient	126	85	high

Two subscales from the Autism Screening Instrument for Educational Planning—Second Edition (ASIEP-2) were administered to Bob. ASIEP-2 is designed to help professionals identify individuals who might be autistic. Its format is a checklist of nonadaptive behaviors. The two subscales administered were the autistic Behavior checklist and the sample of vocal behavior. The Autism Behavior Checklist tests the following domains of behavior: sensory relations, body and object use, and social self-help skills. Bob obtained a score of 79, which suggested positive behavioral symptoms of autism. The sample of vocal behavior subscale measures speech characteristics associated with the diagnosis of autism (e.g., repetitive, noncommunicative, unintelligible, and babbling). His language age equivalence score is on the 11-month age level with an obtained score of 70 (indicating high probability of autistic behavior).

DIAGNOSTIC IMPRESSIONS AND SUMMARY

Bob is a male age 2 years 5 months who displayed hyperkinetic behaviors throughout the evaluation process. Results from all available sources—observation, interviews, and rating scales—suggest that Bob meets the diagnosed criteria for Autistic Disorder. He presents many challenging behaviors that are a source of stress to his family. Bob is in constant motion, full of energy, and his verbal behavior is random babble. His development, according to his mother, has regressed after 18 months (decompensation) in the past month or so. On the Achenbach CBCL he obtained clinically significant scores on the Social Problems, Attention Problem, Thought Problem, and the Aggressive Behavior Scales. Self-injurious behaviors were noted during assessment, observation, and training periods. Improvement in eye contact should be given a priority at the beginning of treatment.

Treatment of individuals with autism should be aggressive and intensive. Initial attention must be directed to his self-injurious behavior using redirection: ignoring incompatible behaviors and reinforcing positive ones. The goals of treatment and instruction for Bob should be mastering a multiplicity of specific behaviors, such that Bob can gradually master enabling skills, broad skills, and ultimately communication and social domains skills.

DIAGNOSIS

AXIS   I: 1. Pervasive Developmental Disorder NOS

2. R/O Anxiety Disorder

3. R/O Attention Deficit Hyperactivity Disorder

4. R/O Attention etiology like Seizure Disorder

Rule out Retts Disorder (females only usually). Rule out Childhood Disintegrative Disorder (regression after two years of normal development). Rule out an organic brain disorder negative (CT, scan and MRI). Rule out Fragile X Syndrome.

AXIS   II: Deferred

AXIS   III: Deferred

AXIS   IV: Psychostressors, chaotic family situation, mother has PhD, mother working full time, both parents have histories of depression.

AXIS   V: GAF

Past year GAF unknown

Current GAF of 40

TREATMENT PLAN AND RECOMMENDATIONS

1. Obtain medical, physiological development baseline examination, CBC, SMAA, thyroid function test, TSH, urine analysis, EKG and EEG to R/O seizure disorder. Obtain Conners Rating Scale and CBCL.

2. Obtain chromosome analysis to R/O chromosome abnormality like Fragile X.

(continued)

3. Structure environment at home and school including special education, speech and language instruction, teaching adaptive skills.

4. Behavior therapy reduces unwanted symptoms, promotes speech, social interaction and assertiveness. It increases self-reliance and self-care skills and facilitates exploration.

5. Parent education to provide guidance and education and to deal with emotional reaction such as guilt or denial. Parents can contribute to child's learning of language and self-care and adaptive skills and arrange for special education and for adjunctive services and make long-term plans for the child.

6. Training and behavior management skills are essential for tolerable home environment and for maximizing the child's potential.

7. Obtain informed consent for the trial of Luvox. Start with 12.5 mg before bedtime for one week, then increase to 25 mg before bedtime. Monitor for medication side effects. Patient's mother consented for the trial of Luvox.

8. Discussed with mother importance of outpatient clinic follow-up to monitor for medication side effect and progress in social and language acquisition.

9. Mother to communicate patient's progress.

10. Reevaluate after a year.

SUMMARY

It is most difficult to summarize a changing body of information about a subject that has only been described as a human condition for less than a century, especially when that human condition is devastating, not only to the individuals it affects, but to their entire family as well. Pervasive Developmental Disorders connect the human condition in the two areas of greatest sensitivity to humankind: communications and social interaction. Therefore, not only do the children who should be exploring and interacting with their world feel alone, cutoff, and abandoned, but so also do those around them. That in itself would be at least as devastating as congenital deafness, but the entire socialization process is also threatened. In addition, there appear to be other information processing problems that present additional challenges to all other learning activities (social, functional, academic, and vocational).

The facts are these: (a) the scientific community has simply not produced much usable data on PDD, and more is unknown at this point than is known; (b) education and the healing arts are also without a definitive theory, hence specifics in practice have been more trial and error than proven interventions; and (c) diagnostically, countless children must go unrecognized each year simply because few clinicians have had much experience at all with PDDs. It is most difficult to find training or professional preparation in cases of populations that truly need a multidisciplinary diagnosis and treatment team. The only conclusion that can be drawn is that much is yet to be learned, and much is yet to be known.

Until information gaps are closed, what can be expected? We can expect that further differentiation and delineation of these conditions will occur. And, in the sense of having a shattered crystal ball, we can expect that a number of new conditions will be described that share the primary two features: (a) communications disorders and (b) social interactive disorders. The diagnostic process is still one of describing the unique behaviors that seem to define the conditions. The crudeness of that practice is apparent. Many childhood disorders produce impairments or limitations in communications and social interactiveness. What then of the interventions? What we have learned is that preschool efforts appear to be most helpful. We have also learned that the more family-based the treatment is, the better. The practice of treating the communication problems first and then the limitations in social interaction next—focusing on these two behavioral aspects before intervening with others—may make considerable sense. However, we are without any real evidence of treatment efficacy.

Where should we be going in the near future? We badly need a national database and information clearinghouse. We need collective research across existing centers. We need advanced special-topics institutes nationwide and central postgraduate multidisciplinary training programs offered at leading universities with PDD centers. We need to develop a full range of programs that offer hope from cradle to the grave. We need to use a combination of the old sensory stimulation approaches in conjunction with advances in technology to cue language and behavior, offering highly structured teaching techniques within therapeutic environments. We need to see the promise of many interventions and to avoid dependency upon a magical or mystical cure. What we have learned about complex behavioral problems is that a cure is rarely found, and the game is best advanced on the ground a yard at a time through teamwork. In the end we would propose that there will be no substitute for teamwork, and the family is still the centerpiece.

REFERENCES

American College of Medical Genetics. (1994). Fragile X Syndrome. Diagnostic and career listing. http://www.org/genetics/acmg/pol.16.htm.

American Psychiatric Association. (1994). *Diagnostic and statistical manual of mental disorders* (4th ed.). Washington, DC: Author.

American Psychiatric Association. (1987). *Diagnostic and statistical manual of mental disorders* (3rd ed., revised). Washington, DC: Author.

American Psychiatric Association. (1980). *Diagnostic and statistical manual of mental disorders* (3rd ed.). Washington, DC: Author.

Arrons, M., & Gittens, T. (1992). *The handbook of autism: A guide for parents and professionals.* London: Tavistock & Routledge.

Asperger, H. C. (1944). Die Autistenchen Psychopathen in Kindesatter. *Archis fur Psychiatri und Nervenkranheiten, 117,* 76–136.

Bender, L. (1942). Schizophrenia and childhood. *The Nervous Child, 1,* 138–140.

Bettelhiem, B. (1967). The empty fortress: Infantile Autism and the birth of self. New York: Free Press.

Blalock, G. (1991). Paraprofessionals: Critical team members in our special education programs. *Intervention in School and Clinic, 26,* 200–214.

Borden, M. C., & Ollendick, T. H. (1994). An examination of the validity of social subtypes in autism. *Journal of Autism and Development Disorders, 24,* 23–37.

Bradley, C., & Bowen, M. (1941). Behavior characteristics of schizophrenic children. *Psychiatric Quarterly, 15,* 298–315.

Bregman, J. D., & Gerdtz, J. (1997). Behavior interventions. In D. Cohen & F. R. Volkmar (2nd Eds.), *Handbook of Autism and pervasive developmental disorders* (pp. 607–630). New York: Wiley.

Campbell, M. C., Andenor, L. T., Small, A. M., Locasreco, J. J., Linch, N. S., & Ehoroco, M. C. (1990). Naltrexone in autistic children: A double blind and placebo controlled study. *Psychopharmacology Bulletin, 26*, 10–19.

Campbell, M., Rapport, J., & Simpson, G. (1999). Antipsychotics in children. *Journal of the American Academy of Child and Adolescent Psychiatry, 38*, 537–545.

Campbell, M., Schopler, E., Cueva, J. E., & Hallin, A. (1996). Treatment of autistic disorder. *Journal of the American Academy of Child and Adolescent Psychiatry, 2*, 134–143.

Cohen, S. B., & Swettenham, J. (1997). Theory of the mind: Its relationship to executive function and central coherence. In D. Cohen & F. R. Volkmar (2nd Ed.), *Handbook of autism and pervasive developmental disorders* (pp. 880–893). New York: Wiley.

Corbett, J., Harris, R., Taylor, E., & Tremble, M. (1977). Progressive disintegrative psychoses of childhood. *Journal of Child Psychology and Psychiatry, 18*, 211–219.

Creak, M. (1961). Schizophrenia syndrome in childhood: Progress report of a working party. *Cerebral Palsy Bulletin, 3*, 501–504.

Creak, M. (1964). Schizophrenia in children: Further progress report of a working party. *Developmental Medicine and Child Neurology, 6*, 530–535.

Dawson, S., & Sterling, J. (1997). Early intervention in autism. In M. J. Gurolnick (Ed.), *The effectiveness of early intervention* (pp. 307–326). Baltimore, MD: Brooks.

Del Mundo, A. S., Pumariega, A. J., & Vance, H. B. (1999). Psychopharmacology in school based mental health services. *Psychology in the Schools, 36*, 437–450.

Eaves, I. M. (1986). Response structure and the triple response-mode concept. In R. D. Nelson & S. C. Hayes (Eds.), *Conceptual foundations of behavior assessment* (pp. 131–155). New York: Guilford Press.

Eaves, R. C. (1993). *Pervasive Developmental Disorder Rating Scale.* Opelika, AL: Small World.

Eaves, R., & Awadh, A. M. (1997). The diagnosis and assessment of autistic disorders. In H. B. Vance (2nd ed.), *Psychological assessment of children: Best practices for clinical and school settings* (pp. 390–430). New York: Wiley.

Eaves, R., Ho, H. H., & Eaves, D. M. (1994). Subtypes of autism in cluster analysis. *Journal of Autism and Developmental Disorders, 24*, 3–22.

Engel, A. J. (1994). The Montgomery Country Public School System: Preschool for children with Autism. In J. L. Harris & J. S. Handleman (Eds.), *Preschool education program for children with autism* (pp. 38–70). Austin, TX: Pro-Ed.

Evans, I. M. (1986). Response structure and the triple-response-made concept. In R. D. Nelson & S. C. Hayes (Eds.), *Conceptual foundation of behavioral assessment* (pp. 131–155). New York: Guilford Press.

Freeman, B. J. (1966). Diagnosis of the syndrome of autism: Questions parent ask. http://www.autism society.org/pachanges/getstart diagnosis.httml

Freeman, B., & Schroth, P. (1984). The development of the Behavioral Observation System (BOS) for Autism. *Behavioral Assessment, 6*, 177–187.

Freeman, B., Ritvo, E., Guthrie, D., Schroth, P., & Ball, J. (1978). The Behavior Observation Scale for Autism. *Journal of the American Academy of Child Psychiatry, 24*, 290–311.

Freeman, B., Ritvo, E., Yokota, A., & Ritvo, A. (1986). A scale for rating symptoms of patients with the syndrome of autism in real life settings. *Journal of the American Academy of Child Psychiatry, 25*, 130–136.

Gene Care. (1996). Fragile X DNA testing. http://www.genecare.com/fx.shtml.

Green, W., Campbell, M., & Hardesty, A. (1984). A comparison of schizophrenia and autistic children. *Journal of the American Academy of Child Psychiatry, 23*, 399–407.

Guralnick, M. J. (1998). Effectiveness of early intervention for vulnerable children: A developmental perspective. *American Journal of Mental Retardation, 102,* 314–345.

Hertzig, M. E., Snow, M. E., New, E., & Shapiro, T. (1990). DSMITT and DSM-IIT-R: Diagnosis of autism and pervasive developmental disorder in nursery school children. *Journal of the American Academy of Child and Adolescent Psychiatry, 29,* 123–126.

Jacobsen, J., & Ackerman, L. (1990). Differences in adaptive functioning among people with autism and mental retardation. *Journal of Autism and Developmental Disorders, 20,* 205–219.

Kanner, L. (1943). Autistic disturbance of affective contact. *The Nervous Child, 2,* 217–250.

Kanner, L. (1971). Childhood psychosis: A historical overview. *Journal of Autism and Childhood Schizophrenia, 1,* 14–19.

Kaplan, H., Sadock, R., & Gregg, J. (1994). *Synopsis of psychiatry: Behavioral science clinic psychiatry* (7th ed.). Baltimore: William & Wilkins.

Kazdin, A. E. (1993). Replication and extension of behavioral treatment of autistic disorders. *American Journal of Mental Retardation, 92,* 377–380.

Klin, A., Carter, A., Volkmar, F. R., Cohen, D. J., Marans, W. D., & Sparrow, S. S. (1997). Assessment issues in children with autism. In D. Cohen & F. R. Volkman (2nd ed.), *Handbook of Autism and Pervasive Developmental Disorders* (pp. 411–447). New York: Wiley.

Klin, A. & Volkmar, F. C. (1997). Asperger's Syndrome. In D. Cohen & R. R. Volkmar, (2nd ed.), *Handbook of Autism and Pervasive Developmental Disorders* (pp. 94–122). New York: Wiley.

Koegel, R. I., Fres, W. D., & Surratt, A. U. (1994). Self management of problematic social behavior. In E. Schopler & C. B. Mesibou (Eds.), *Behavioral issues in Autism* (pp. 81–94). New York: Plenum Press.

Koegel, R. L., & Koegel, L. K. (1999). Teaching children with autism. Baltimore: Brookes.

Krug, D., Arick, J., & Almond, P. (1980). Behavior checklist for identifying severely handicapped individuals with high levels of autistic behavior. *Journal of Child Psychology and Psychiatry, 21,* 221–229.

LeCouteur, A., Rutter, M., Lord, C., Rios, P., Robertson, S., Holdgrafer, M., & MacLellan, J. (1989). Autism diagnostic interview. A standardized investigator-based instrument. *Journal of Autism and Developmental Disorders, 19,* 363–388.

Locke, B. J., Banken, J. A., & Mahone, C. H. (1994). The grouping of autism: Etiology and prevalence at fifty. In J. L. Matson (Ed.), *Autism in children and adults: Etiology, assessment, and interventions* (pp. 35–57). Pacific Grove, CA: Brook/Cole.

Lord, C., Rutter, M., Goode, S., Heemsbergen, J., Jordan, H., Mawhood, L., & Schopler, E. (1989). Autism Diagnostic Observation Schedule: A standardized observation of communicative and social behavior. *Journal of Autism and Developmental Disorders, 19,* 185–212.

Lord, C., Storoschuck, S., Rutter, M., & Pickels, A. (1993). Using the ADI-R to diagnose autism in preschool children. *Infant Mental Health Journal, 14,* 234–252.

Lovaas, O. I. (1987). Behavioral treatment and normal educational and intellectual function in young autistic children. *Journal of Consulting Psychology, 55,* 5–9.

McDougle, C. (1998). Psychopharmacology. In D. Cohen & F. Volkman (Eds.), *Handbook of Autism and Pervasive Developmental Disorders* (pp. 707–729). New York: Sulinweley & Sons.

McDougle, C. J. (1997). Psychopharmacology. In D. Cohen & F. R. Volkmar (2nd ed.), *Handbook of Autism and Pervasive Developmental Disorders* (pp. 707–729). New York: Wiley.

Medicine Net. (1997). Autism. http://www.Medicinenet.com/mainmence/encyelop/artuile/art.a/autism.htm.

Moes, D. (1995). Parent education and parenting stress. In R. L. Koegel & L. K. Koegel (Eds.), *Teaching children with autism* (pp. 79–93). Baltimore: Brookes.

Morgan, S. (1988). Diagnostic assessment of autism: A review of objective scales. *Journal of Psychoeducational Assessment, 6,* 139–151.

Myles, B. S., & Simpson, R. L. (1994). Facilitated communication with children diagnosed autistic in public school settings. *Psychology in the Schools, 3,* 208–220.

Olley, J. G., & Reeve, C. (1997). Issues in curriculum and classroom structure. In D. Cohen, & F. R. Volkmar (2nd ed.), *Handbook of Autism and Pervasive Developmental Disorder* (pp. 448–459). New York: Wiley.

Ornitz, E. M., & Ritvo, F. (1976). The syndrome of autism: A critical review. *American Journal of Psychiatry, 13,* 609–621.

Ozonoff, S. (1997). Causal mechanism of autism: Unifying perspective from an information processing framework. In D. Cohen & F. R. Volkmar (2nd ed.), *Handbook of Autism and Pervasive Developmental Disorders* (pp. 868–879). New York: Wiley.

Parks, S. (1983). The assessment of autistic children: A selective review of available instruments. *Journal of Autism and Developmental Disorders, 13,* 255–267.

Potter, H. (1933). Schizophrenia in children. *American Journal of Psychiatry, 12,* 1253–1268.

Powers, M. D. (1997). Behavioral assessment of individuals with autism. In D. Cohen & F. R. Volkmar (2nd ed.), *Handbook of Autism and Pervasive Developmental Disorders* (pp. 448–459). New York: Wiley.

Pumariega, A. J., Del Mundo, A. S., & Vance, H. B. (2000). Psychopharmacology in the context of children mental health system of care. In B. Burns, K. Huagord, & M. English (Eds.), *Community-based intervention for youth with severe emotional disorders* (pp. 187–200). New York: Oxford.

Quay, H. C., & Werry, J. S. (1986). *Psychopathological disorders of childhood.* New York: Wiley.

Quik, K. (1995). *Teaching children with Autism: Methods to enhance learning communication and socialization.* Albany, NY: Delman.

Rank, B. (1949). Adoption of psychoanalytic techniques for the treatment of young children with atypical development. *American Journal of Orthopsychiatry, 19,* 130–139.

Rimland, B. (1964). *Infantile autism.* Englewood Cliff, NJ: Prentice-Hall.

Rimland, B. (1968). On the objective diagnosis of infantile autism. *Acta Paedopsychiatrica, 35,* 146–161.

Rimland, B. (1971). The differentiation of childhood psychoses: An analysis of checklists for 2,218 psychotic children. *Journal of Autism and Childhood Schizophrenia, 1,* 161–174.

Rimland, B. (1994). The modern history of Autism: A personal perspective. In J. L. Matson (Ed.), *Autism in children and adults: Etiology, assessment and intervention* (pp. 1–11). Pacific Grove, CA: Brovka/Cole.

Ritvo, R., & Freeman, B. J. (1978). National society for autistic children definition of the syndrome of autism. *Journal of Autism and Developmental Disorders, 8,* 162–170.

Rosenberg, M. B., Wilson, R., Maheay, L., & Sindelar, P. J. (1992). *Educating students with behavior disorders.* Boston: Allyn & Bacon.

Ruble, L. (1996). Conference notes: 1993 international conference on autism. http://www.autism society.org/pachanges/getstart.diagnosis.html.

Ruttenberg, B., Dratman, M., Fraknoi, J., & Wenar, C. (1966). An instrument for evaluating autistic children. *Journal of the American Academy of Child Psychiatry, 5,* 453–478.

Ruttenberg, B., Kalish, B., Wenar, C., & Wolf, E. (1977). *Behavior Rating Instrument for autistic and other atypical children* (Rev. ed.). Philadelphia: Developmental Center for Autistic Children.

Rutter, M. (1978). Diagnosis and definition of childhood autism. *Journal of Autism and Developmental Disorders, 8,* 139–161.

Sattler, J. C. (1988). *The assessment of children intelligence.* San Diego: Author.

Schopler, E. (1994). Behavioral priorities for autism and related disorders and related developmental disorders. In S. Schopler & G. B. Mesibou (Eds.), *Behavior issues in Autism* (pp. 55–77). New York: Plenum Press.

Schopler, E., & Mesibou, G. B. (1986). Introduction to social behavior in autism. In E. Schopler & G. B. Mesibou (Eds.), *Social behavior in autism* (pp. 1–11). New York: Plenum Press.

Schopler, E., & Reicher, R. J. (1971). Parents as cotherapist in the treatment of psychotic children. *Journal of Autism and Childhood Schizophrenia, 1*, 87–102.

Schopler, E., Reichler, R., & Renner, B. (1988). *The Childhood Autism Rating Scale.* Los Angeles: Western Psychological Services.

Schopler, E. (1994). Behavior priorities for autism and related developmental disorders. In E. Schopler, & G. B. Mesibou (Eds.), *Behavioral issues in Autism* (pp. 55–77). New York: Plenum Press.

Seigel, B., Anders, F. F., Cialanello, R. D., Bienenstock, B., & Kralmer, H. C. (1986). Empirically derived subclassification of the autistic syndrome. *Journal of Autism and Developmental Disorders, 16*, 275–293.

Sevin, J., Matson, J. Coe, D., Fee, V., & Sevin, B. (1991). A comparison and evaluation of three commonly used autism scales. *Journal of Autism and Developmental Disorders, 21*, 417–431.

Sevin, J. A., Matson, J. L., Cole, D., Love, R. S., Motese, M. J., & Benevidez, D. A. (1991). Empically dervised subtypes of pervasive developmental disorders: A cluster analysis. Unpublished manuscript.

Shattock, P. (1996). Back to the future: An assessment of some of the unorthodox forms of biomedical interventions currently being applied to autism. http://oseres.sunderland.ac.uk/durham 95.html.

Shaw, C. R., & Lucas, A. R. (1970). *The psychiatric disorders of childhood.* New York: Appleton-Century-Crofts.

Sparrow, S., Carter, A. S., Raeusim, G., & Morris, R. (1995). Comprehensive psychological assessment throughout the life span: A developmental approach. In D. Cicchett & D. J. Cohen (Eds.), *Developmental psychopathology* (Vol. 1, pp. 81–108). New York: Wiley.

Spitzer, R. L. & Siegel, C. (1990). The DSM-IIT field trial of pervasive developmental disorders. *American Journal of Child and Adolescent Psychiatry, 29*, 855–862.

Stokes, T. T., & Osnes, P. G. (1988). The developing applied technology of generalization and maintenance. In R. U. Homer, G. Dunlap, & R. I. Kolgel (Eds.), *Generalization and Maintenance* (pp. 5–19). Baltimore, MD: Brookes.

Stone, W., & Hogan, K. (1993). A structural parent interview for identifying young children with autism. *Journal of Autism and Developmental Disorders, 23*, 639–652.

Szatmari, P., Bartolucci, G., & Bremmer, R. (1989). Asperger's Syndrome and Autism Comparisons on early history and outcome. *Developmental Medicine and Child Neurology, 31*, 709–720.

Szatmari, P., Archer, L., Sandra, F., Streiner, D., & Wilson, F. (1995). Asperger's Syndrome and Autism differences in behavior, cognition and adaptive functioning. *Journal of the American Academy of Child and Adolescent Psychiatry, 34*, 1662–1671.

Teal, M., & Wiebe, M. (1986). A validity analysis of selected instruments used to assess autism. *Journal of Autism and Developmental Disorders, 16*, 485–496.

Tantaum, D. (1988). *A mind of one's own.* London: National Autistic Society.

Vance, H. B., & Pumariéga, A. J. (in press). Fluoxetine treatment of a child with severe PDD: A single case study. *Journal of Psychiatry.*

Vance, H. B., Fuller, G. B., & Awadh, A. (1995). Autism: Assessment and intervention. In D. Sabatino & B. Brooks (Eds.), *Contemporary interdisciplinary intervention for children with emotional and behavioral disorders* (pp. 699–730). Durham, NC: Carolina Academic Press.

Volkmar, F. (1987). Diagnostic issues in the pervasive developmental disorders. *Journal of Child Psychology and Psychiatry, 28*, 365–369.

Volkmar, F., Cicchette, D., Dykens, E., Sparrow, S., Leckman, J., & Cohen, D. (1988). An evaluation of the Autism Behavior Checklist. *Journal of Autism and Developmental Disorders, 18,* 81–97.

Volkmar, F. R., & Nelson, D. S. (1990). Seizures disorders in autism. *Journal of the American Academy of Child and Adolescent Psychiatry, 1,* 127–129.

Wadden, N., Bryson, S., & Rodger, R. (1991). A closer look at the Autism Behavior Checklist: Discriminant validity and factor structure. *Journal of Autism and Developmental Disorders, 21,* 529–538.

Watkins, J., Asarnow, R., & Tanguay, P. (1998). Symptom development in childhood onset schizophrenia. *Journal Child Psychology and Psychiatry, 291,* 865–878.

Wherry, J. 5. (1972). The childhood psychoses. In H. C. Quay & J. S. Wherry (Eds.), *Psychopathological-Disorders of Children* (pp. 173–223). New York: Wiley.

Wing, L. (1997). Syndromes of autism and atypical development. In D. Cohen & F. R. Volkmar, (2nd ed.), *Handbook of Autism and Pervasive Developmental Disorders* (pp. 148–172). New York: Wiley.

Wing, L., & Attwood, A. (1987). Syndromes of autism and atypical development. In D. J. Cohen & A. Donnelan (Eds.), *Handbook of Autism and Pervasive Developmental Disorders* (pp. 3–19). New York: Wiley.

Wing, L., & Gould, J. (1979). Severe impairment of social interaction and associated abnormalities in children: Epidemiology and classification. *Journal of Autism and Childhood Schizophrenia,* 11–29.

World Health Organization. (1990). *The ICD-b classification of mental and behavioral disorders. Diagnostic criteria for research.* Geneva: Author.

World Health Organization. (1993). *The ICD-II diagnostic criteria for research.* Geneva: Author.

Chapter 10 ———————————————————————————————

DISRUPTIVE BEHAVIOR DISORDERS: ASSESSMENT AND INTERVENTION

JOHN E. LOCHMAN, HEATHER E. DANE, THOMAS N. MAGEE, MESHA ELLIS, DUSTIN A. PARDINI, AND NANCY R. CLANTON

In this chapter, we give an overview of the nature of Disruptive Behavior Disorders in children and adolescents, and we explore factors that serve to cause and maintain this form of psychopathology. The chapter examines relevant assessment measures for children with these behavioral problems, and a case example illustrates the use of several of these assessment methods. Empirically supported interventions for children with aggressive behavioral problems will be reviewed, with special focus on behavioral and cognitive-behavioral interventions. Finally, important clinical issues related to assessment and intervention are discussed.

DISRUPTIVE BEHAVIOR DISORDERS

The Disruptive Behavior Disorders include Conduct Disorder and Oppositional Defiant Disorder (American Psychiatric Association, 1994). Conduct Disorder, Oppositional Defiant Disorder, aggression, and delinquency are all terms that refer to antisocial behaviors that indicate an individual's inability or failure to conform to his or her societal norms and authority figures, or to respect the rights of others (Frick, 1998a; Lochman, in press-a; Lochman, Magee, & Pardini, in press). These behaviors can range from chronic annoying of others and argumentativeness with adults to stealing, vandalism, and physical harm to others. Although these behaviors cover a broad spectrum of problems, they are often highly correlated, with relatively few youths showing only one type of conduct problem (Frick et al., 1993). This relatedness of behaviors suggests there is often a single dimension of antisocial behaviors and conduct problems (Lochman et al., in press).

Antisocial behaviors of children and adolescents have long been a major concern of society. This attention seems justified given the increased attention society has given to juvenile correction facilities; early intervention programs such as Fast Track, devel-

The preparation of this chapter has been supported by grants from the National Institute of Drug Abuse and the Center for Substance Abuse Prevention within the Substance Abuse and Mental Health Services Administration.

oped by the Conduct Problems Prevention Research Group (1992, 1999a, 1999b); and the enormous financial costs of youth crime. In addition, conduct problems in children represent the childhood behavioral problems most referred to mental health professionals, especially for boys (Frick, 1998b). Aggressive and disruptive behavior is one of the most enduring dysfunctions in children; and if left untreated, it frequently results in high personal and emotional cost to the child, the family, and to society in general. As a direct result, much research has investigated the causes, treatment, and prevention of conduct problems.

As a clinical syndrome with a broad list of symptoms, it is logical to expect much heterogeneity within the group that falls under the umbrella term of conduct problems. In addition to heterogeneity in the type of conduct problems manifested, children with conduct problems can differ also in the causal factors involved, the developmental course of the problems, the response to treatment, and the interaction between any of these.

Although there is a strong agreement that children with conduct problems are a very heterogeneous group, there is significantly less consensus about the most appropriate method of classifying conduct problems into meaningful subtypes. One of the most widely used and accepted classifications of disruptive behavior disorders is the criteria in the *Diagnostic and Statistical Manual of Mental Disorders—Fourth Edition* (APA, 1994). The criteria employs a two-dimensional approach with an explicit symptom list for making a diagnosis. This system divides conduct problems into two syndromes. Conduct Disorder (CD) and Oppositional Defiant Disorder (ODD). CD is defined as:

> A repetitive and persistent pattern of behavior which violates the rights of others or major age appropriate societal norms or rules. These behaviors fall into four main groupings: aggressive conduct that threatens physical harm to other people or animals, nonaggressive conduct that causes property loss or damage, deceitfulness and theft, and serious violations of rules. Three or more characteristic behaviors must have been present during the past 12 months. (p. 85)

ODD is defined as:

> A recurrent pattern of negativistic, defiant, disobedient, and hostile behavior toward authority figures that persists for at least 6 months and is characterized by the frequent occurrence of at least four of the following behaviors: losing temper, arguing with adults, actively defying or refusing to comply with requests or rules of adults, deliberately doing things that will annoy other people, blaming others for his or her own mistakes or misbehavior, being touchy or easily annoyed by others, being angry and resentful, or being spiteful or vindictive. (p. 91)

The *DSM-IV* also distinguishes between children who begin showing conduct problems in early childhood from those who begin showing conduct problems closer to adolescence. If any symptoms are present prior to age 10, with the child meeting criteria for CD, he or she is classified Childhood-Onset Type. However, if criteria are met for CD and no symptoms are present prior to age 10, the child is classified Adolescent-Onset Type.

In addition to differentiating between CD and ODD, there have also been several attempts to further delineate dimensions of Conduct Disorders. The *DSM-III* and *DSM-III-R* (APA, 1980, 1987) made distinctions among children with CD on the two dimensions of socialization and aggressiveness. First, socialization refers to children's capability of forming social relationships. The "group-type" CD youth commits antisocial acts primarily with delinquent peers, whereas "solitary-type" children do not form lasting relationships and commit antisocial acts primarily alone. Second, distinctions were made between children who exhibited aggressive behaviors as part of their pattern of antisocial behavior and those who did not. CD has also been classified into the two dimensions of overt versus covert types, and of destructive versus nondestructive types.

CD and ODD are conceptually related to each other. Research indicates that CD is a developmentally advanced form of ODD, and that there are similar correlates for both ODD and CD. Both children with ODD and children with CD come from lower socioeconomic strata (Frick et al., 1992; Keenan, Loeber, Zhang, & Stouthamer-Loeber, 1995), are more likely to have a parent with a history of antisocial personality disorder (Faraone, Biederman, Keenan, & Tsuang, 1991; Frick et al., 1992), and have parents who use ineffective disciplinary practices (Frick et al., 1993).

Although some appearances of aggressive behavior are relatively common in mild forms during early childhood years, aggressive and antisocial behaviors become more clinically significant if the instances are highly intense, if they occur with high frequency, or if they are characterized by notably violent elements in childhood and later adolescent years (Lochman, in press-a). Undoubtedly, the frequency with which children or adolescents manifest clinically significant and impairing levels of conduct problems is greatly determined by the definition used for such conduct when surveying populations. The *DSM-IV* notes a prevalence ranging between 2% and 16% for ODD (APA, 1994). For CD, rates of 6% to 16% for males and 2% to 9% for females have been cited (APA, 1994). Conduct problems occur more often in boys than in girls, at a rate of approximately 3 to 1 (Kazdin, 1998; Lochman & Szczepanski, 1999). Both CD and ODD, therefore, occur more commonly in males than in females, but ratios vary widely as a function of both the age of the child and the definition of the disorder (APA, 1994; Hinshaw & Anderson, 1996). The higher rate for boys is primarily evident for childhood-onset CD; the male to female ratio evens out among adolescent conduct problem youths. Characteristic symptom patterns tend to differ developmentally as well. Childhood-onset conduct problems tend to reflect aggressive behavior, whereas adolescent-onset conduct problems tend to reflect more delinquent behavior (vandalism, theft; Zoccolillo, 1993).

These prevalence rates are only approximations of CD, however. The criteria for delineating individual symptoms appear somewhat arbitrary. Children and adolescents with subclinical conduct problems, failing to meet diagnostic criteria, are often significantly impaired. Loeber (1990) hypothesized that aggressive behavior in elementary school–aged children is part of a developmental trajectory that can lead to adolescent delinquency and CD. Childhood-onset CD is expected to be preceded by physical aggression and poor peer relationships in the elementary school years. Longitudinal research has documented this evolution of disorder by finding that children's aggressive behavior and their rejection by their peers can be additive risk markers for subsequent maladjusted behavior in the middle school years (Coie, Lochman, Terry, & Hyman,

1992), and that aggressive behavior is a risk marker for early substance use, overt delinquency, and police arrests in the later adolescent years (Coie, Terry, Zakriski, & Lochman, 1995; Lochman & Wayland, 1994). Children are more at risk for continued aggressive and antisocial behavior if they display aggressive behavior in multiple settings within their home, school, and neighborhood, and if they develop "versatile forms of antisocial behavior by early to mid-adolescence" (Lochman, in press-a; Lochman & Szczepanski, 1999).

One of the most distressing qualities of conduct disorders is their enduring stability over the course of childhood and adolescence and even potentially into adulthood. Conduct disorders may be one of the most enduring forms of psychopathology in children (Frick, 1998a). Longitudinal research has indicated that CD is often a precursor of Antisocial Personality Disorder (APD) in adulthood (Frick, 1998a). It is estimated that approximately half of children with CD develop significant APD symptomatology. Two factors that predict the development of APD are the number of CD symptoms the child exhibits and early age of onset of symptoms (APA, 1994).

FACTORS ASSOCIATED WITH ODD AND CD: ETIOLOGY AND CORRELATES

For adolescents with childhood-onset Conduct Disorder, the developmental trajectory leading to the disorder may start very early among infants with irritable, difficult-to-soothe temperaments (Loeber, 1990), and who are less adaptable to change (Lochman, in press-a). These temperamentally difficult children are at risk of failing to develop positive attachments with caretakers, for displaying high rates of hyperactive behavior and poor attentional control in the preschool years, and for becoming involved in increasingly coercive interchanges first with parents and later with teachers. Moffitt (1993) has suggested that life-course persistent delinquents, or "early starters," are at risk early in life because of both biological and family factors. In some children, family dysfunction may be sufficient to initiate this sequence of escalating aggressive behavior. Poor, crime-ridden neighborhoods also add to the environmental risk factors leading to seriously aggressive behavior (Frick, 1998a; Greenberg, Lengua, Coie, Pinderhughes, & the Conduct Problems Prevention Research Group, 1999). Loeber (1990) hypothesized that children then begin to generalize their use of coercive behaviors to other social interactions, leading to increasingly aggressive behavior with peers and adults by early elementary school and to dysfunctional social-cognitive processes. Because of their aggressive behavior, these children can often be socially rejected by their peer group, and can then become more withdrawn and isolated. Their academic progress can also deteriorate during these years, partially because of worsening relationships with teachers and peers. By early to middle adolescence, these youth are then prone to meeting their affiliation needs by gravitating toward deviant peer groups, and these deviant groups can be become an additional proximal cause for delinquent behavior (Coie et al., 1995; Patterson, Reid, & Dishion, 1992).

Despite our ability to diagnose Oppositional Defiant Disorder and Conduct Disorder in children and adolescents reliably, there still remains considerable heterogeneity among individuals diagnosed with these disorders (Kazdin, 1995), leaving no single means for classifying variant groups of deviant youth. (Lahey, Loeber, Quay, Frick, & Grimm, 1992). This dilemma has created a burgeoning area of research examining various factors that may modify the developmental trajectory of antisocial behavior in children and adolescents (Hinshaw, Lahey, & Hart, 1993). Because longitudinal studies suggest that a majority of children who engage in delinquent acts do not continue to exhibit antisocial behaviors as adults (Moffitt, 1993; Robins, 1978a), some theorists have begun looking at factors that facilitate the development of deviant behavior and help predict life-course persistent antisocial behavior. This burgeoning area of research has given clinical psychologists a greater understanding of the factors to assess when evaluating a child or adolescent who is exhibiting conduct problems. In particular, issues associated with comorbidity, child traits, peer relationships, and familial factors have provided a greater understanding of how and why antisocial behavior continues to develop across the lifespan.

Comorbidities

ADHD symptoms. Because youth with oppositional and conduct problems commonly display behaviors that can be described as impulsive and overactive, it is not surprising that many of these children also meet criteria for Attention-Deficit/Hyperactivity Disorder (ADHD). In a recent study looking at community samples of children with CD, investigators reported that 75% to 90% of children had co-occurring ADHD (Abikoff & Klein, 1992). Similarly, several longitudinal studies have provided substantial evidence suggesting that children who exhibit symptoms of hyperactivity and impulsivity are at greater risk for developing later substance abuse disorders, conduct disorders, and antisocial personality disorders, when compared to control children (Gittelman, Mannuzza, Shenker, & Bonvagura, 1985; Mannuzza, Klein, Konig, & Giampino, 1989). Children with ADHD symptoms also seem to be at increased risk for committing serious violent crimes and becoming institutionalized, when compared to matched controls (Satterfield, Hoppe, & Schell, 1982). Even more concerning is longitudinal evidence suggesting that children with both comorbid conduct problems and ADHD symptoms are at greater risk for serious antisocial behavior in adolescence and adulthood than are youth with conduct problems alone (Moffitt, 1990; Loeber, Brinthaupt, & Green, 1990; Lynam, 1998). This accumulation of research has led many mental health professionals to advocate the early identification and treatment of children who exhibit both conduct problems and hyperactivity/impulsivity, because they are viewed as a subgroup of youths that contains future chronic offenders (Lynam, 1996).

Internalizing disorders. Children with conduct problems also tend to display symptoms associated with anxiety and depressive disorders, which could potentially alter the course of their antisocial behavior (Miller-Johnson, Lochman, Coie, Terry, & Hyman, 1998; Young et al., 1995). For example, there is some indication that children with both conduct and depressive problems are more likely to abuse substances in adolescence compared to youth with conduct problems alone (Miller-Johnson et al., 1998); other researchers have noted that internalizing symptoms may partially mediate the relationship between early conduct problems and later substance use (Young et al., 1995). Moreover, it seems that the relation between conduct problems and depressive symptoms may be partially accounted for by peer rejection (Panak & Garber, 1992). Specifically, children who exhibit antisocial behavior often aggravate their peers and are likely to be rejected by them as a result, thereby producing their depressive symptoms. Although it is clear that there is a significant co-occurrence between disruptive behavior disorders and internalizing symptoms, more longitudinal studies in this area are needed to expand our understanding of how, and if, internalizing disorders modify the developmental trajectory of conduct problems in children and adolescents.

Learning problems. Children with ODD and CD also tend to have academic problems, but the reason for these difficulties, as well as the potential ramifications in terms of the developmental course of conduct problems, remains unclear. For example, Frick et al. (1991) noted that while 20% to 25% of children who meet criteria for CD are underachieving in school relative to their IQ or chronological age, these problems seem to be related to symptoms associated with ADHD. On the other hand, adolescents who begin exhibiting conduct problems seem to have learning difficulties that are not accounted for by presence of ADHD (Hinshaw, 1992). Similar studies have found that children with disruptive behaviors are at greater risk for dropping out of school, but this relation is partially mediated by grade retention and special classroom placement (Vitaro, Brendgen, & Tremblay, 1999). Regardless of the developmental mechanisms involved, it is clear that children with conduct problems are at risk for developing severe academic problems; thus school functioning is an important aspect of any comprehensive ODD or CD evaluation.

Child Factors

Timing of onset. Because longitudinal studies suggest that a majority of children who engage in delinquent acts do not continue to exhibit antisocial behaviors as adults (Moffitt, 1993; Robins, 1978a), recent classification systems have begun looking at factors that may predict life-course persistent antisocial behavior. The most encouraging evidence for a chronic and severe pattern of delinquency comes from the distinction between childhood- and adolescent-onset conduct disorder, which was included in the *DSM-IV* (APA, 1994). In particular, several studies have reported that youth who engage in the most persistent, severe, and violent antisocial behavior are most likely to initiate their delinquent behavior in childhood rather than adolescence (Blumstein, Farrington, & Moitra, 1985; Lahey et al., 1998; Loeber, 1988; Moffitt, 1993). Robins, Tipp, and Pryzbeck (1991) also noted that youths who first display antisocial behavior in childhood are two times more likely to meet adult diagnostic criteria for antisocial personality disorder than are youths who first exhibit delinquent behavior in adolescence. Although these studies provide significant evidence for subtyping delinquent juveniles based on age of onset, some investigators have suggested that there still may be considerable heterogeneity among juveniles who exhibit antisocial behavior in childhood (Frick, 1998a; Lynam, 1998).

Callous-unemotional traits. Recently, investigators have begun examining the role that psychopathic traits play in the development and expression of antisocial behavior in children (Lilienfeld, 1998; Lynam, 1998). Many of these studies have focused on the callous (e.g., lack of empathy, manipulativeness) and unemotional (e.g., lack of guilt, emotional constrictedness) traits that represent the cornerstone of the psychopathic personality (Cleckly, 1976; Hare, 1993). Evidence suggests that the presence of callous-unemotional (CU) traits may delineate a subgroup of antisocial juveniles who exhibit a more severe and chronic pattern of delinquent behavior. For example, adjudicated adolescents with high levels of CU traits are more likely to exhibit childhood-onset antisocial behavior (Silverthorn, Frick, & Reynolds, 1999) than are youth without these traits. A similar study by Caputo, Frick, and Brodsky (1999) reported that juveniles incarcerated for violent sex offenses had higher levels of CU traits than did youth convicted of other violent offenses and nonviolent offenses. Moreover, Christian, Frick, Hill, Tyler, and Frazer (1997) noted that clinic-referred children with conduct problems and CU traits tended to have a greater number and variety of conduct problems, more police contacts, and a stronger family history of Antisocial Personality Disorder than did children with conduct problems alone. These findings are important given that the number and variety of conduct problems (Loeber, 1990), early police contacts (Quay, 1987), family history of APD (Lahey et al., 1995), early onset of conduct problems (Moffitt, 1993) and violent sex offending (Brannon & Troyer, 1995) have all been consistent predictors of poor outcomes in delinquent youth.

Gender differences.   The prevalence of conduct problems and severe antisocial behavior in boys is significantly higher than in girls, with most studies reporting a gender ratio of approximately 4 to 1 (Silverthorn & Frick, 1999). Although this statistic suggests that ODD and CD are sex-linked disorders, recent investigations have noted relatively few gender differences in disruptive behaviors during the preschool years (Keenan & Shaw, 1997) and a dramatic decrease in the discrepancy between boy's and girl's antisocial behavior in adolescence (McGee, Feehan, Williams, & Anderson, 1992). In addition, the gender differences during adolescence seem to be associated primarily with aggressive behavior, whereas prevalence rates of nonaggressive symptoms are nearly equivalent across genders during this developmental period (Offord, Adler, & Boyle, 1986; Offord, Boyle, & Raccine, 1991). Some investigators have hypothesized that the differences in aggressive behavior between adolescent boys and girls may be due to differential manifestations of aggression, with boys showing the more traditional verbal (e.g., threatening) and physical (e.g., hitting, punching) forms of aggression, and girls displaying a more relational type of aggression (e.g., excluding others, starting rumors) that is not typically assessed in children with conduct problems (Crick & Grotpeter, 1995). Although the reason for these gender differences is unclear, it is evident that girls do not typically begin exhibiting severe patterns of antisocial behavior until adolescence, unlike the two-trajectory model of boys' conduct problems outlined in the *DSM-IV.* Despite this difference in initial manifestation of conduct problems, adolescent-onset antisocial girls show many of the same risk factors and persistent antisocial behavior as childhood-onset boys, leading some investigators to propose a third developmental pathway for girl's antisocial behavior that has been referred to as delayed-onset CD (Silverthorn & Frick, 1999).

Social cognitive processes.   A recent accumulation of research has suggested that children who exhibit antisocial behavior can be differentiated from their peers on a number of social-cognitive variables. Initially, Dodge, Pettit, McClaskey, & Brown (1986) proposed that aggressive children have difficulties in five different stages of social information processing, including (a) encoding social cues; (b) making interpretations and attributions about social information; (c) generating possible solutions to interpersonal problems; (d) deciding which plan to enact based on the perceived consequences; and (e) enacting the chosen plan. Since Dodge's initial proposal there has been a substantial amount of evidence indicating that children with conduct problems do exhibit cognitive deficits in processing social information at each of these stages. For example, studies have found that children exhibiting antisocial behavior are more likely than normal children to attend to hostile (Gouze, 1987) and irrelevant (Lochman & Dodge, 1994) cues, to attribute hostile intentions to others (Lochman & Dodge, 1994), to generate problem solutions that are more action oriented and involve less verbal assertion and negotiation (Lochman & Lampron, 1986; Dunn, Lochman & Colder, 1997; Lochman, Meyer, Rabiner, & White, 1991), to expect positive consequences for aggressing (Perry, Williard, & Perry, 1990), and to lack perspective taking skills and emotional empathy during social interactions (Cohen & Strayer, 1996). In live interactions with peers, aggressive children have distorted perceptions and perceive peers' behavior to be more aggressive than it was and to underperceive their own aggressiveness (Lochman, 1987; Lochman & Dodge, 1998). Aggressive children have social goals that place high value on dominance and revenge and relatively little value on affiliation, and these distinctive social goals have been found to have a direct effect on children's selection of solutions to social problems (Lochman, Wayland, & White, 1993). In addition, youth with conduct problems are less adept at enacting positive interpersonal behaviors than children without conduct problems (Dodge, Pettit, McClaskey, & Brown, 1986).

Peer Variables

Social rejection.   An accumulation of evidence has suggested that children with disruptive behaviors are at risk of being rejected by their peers. Several investigators have found that although these factors are related, both childhood aggressive behavior and peer rejection independently seem to predict delinquency and conduct problems in adolescence (Lochman & Wayland, 1994; Coie et al., 1992). In a similar vein, aggressive children who are socially rejected tend to exhibit more severe behavior problems than do children who are either aggressive only or rejected only (Bierman & Wargo, 1995). Despite the compelling nature of these findings, race and gender may moderate the relationship between peer rejection and negative adolescent outcomes. For example, Lochman and Wayland (1994) found that peer rejection ratings of African American children within a mixed-race classroom did not predict subsequent externalizing problems in adolescence, whereas peer rejection ratings of Caucasian children were associated with future disruptive behaviors. Another study found that although peer rejection predicted serious delinquency in boys, it failed to do so with girls in the sample (Miller-Johnson, Coie, Maumary-Gremaud, Lochman, & Terry, 1999). Consequently, clinicians should be aware that social rejection seems to perpetuate the development of antisocial behavior in children with conduct problems; but this relation may be modified by factors such as gender, and the use of sociometric ratings systems in the classroom may be biased against African American boys placed in predominantly Caucasian classrooms.

Deviant peer groups.   As children with conduct problems enter adolescence, they tend to associate with deviant peers. It is believed that many of these teens have been continually rejected from more prosocial peer groups because they lack appropriate social skills and, as a result, turn to antisocial cliques as their only means for social support (Miller-Johnson et al., 1999). Unfortunately, these affiliations tend to exacerbate and reinforce their antisocial behavior, thereby modifying the developmental course of their conduct problems. For example, studies have shown that the relationship between childhood conduct problems and adolescent delinquency is at least partially mediated by deviant peer group affiliation (Vitaro, Brendgen, Pagani, Tremblay, & McDuff, 1999), whereas other findings indicate that there is a two- to four-fold increase in the likelihood of committing antisocial acts in a deviant peer context (Keenan et al., 1995). Overall, this evidence suggests that an evaluation of the antisocial behavior of an adolescent's peer group could provide important information about the development of a child's antisocial behavior over time.

Familial Factors

Parenting practices.   Various parenting behaviors are also associated with the development of antisocial behavior in children and adolescents. In particular, parenting practices that are characterized by vague commands, poor monitoring, low levels of warmth and parental involvement, and rigid control and harsh punishment tend to be associated with increases in conduct problems in children (Forehand & Long, 1988; Patterson, 1986; Pettit, Harrist, Bates, & Dodge, 1991; Lochman & Lenhart, 1993). Also, parent/child interactions that are characterized by increased levels of verbal and physical aggression have been linked to higher levels of children's conduct problems and delinquency (Vissing, Strauss, Gelles, & Harrop, 1991), whereas increased levels of marital conflict seem to be associated with the development of reactive aggression in children (Lochman & Craven, 1993, March). Interestingly, some recent studies have found that children's temperamental characteristics, such as activity level and fear, may moderate the relationship between harsh parenting practices and antisocial behavior (Colder, Lochman, & Wells, 1997). Subsequently, clinicians must take into account the complex interactions between parenting styles and child characteristics when attempting to understand the developmental course of conduct problems in youth.

ASSESSMENT: DIAGNOSIS AND FORMULATION

Research findings on the nature and correlates of disruptive behavior disorders can be extended to the development of a comprehensive, empirically based assessment. Before discussing areas of functioning and types of assessment tools that may be useful, it is important to reiterate a few main points of any clinical evaluation. First, disruptive behavior disorders are a heterogeneous grouping, therefore the exact assessment battery will need to be tailored to the specific presenting problem and the child being evaluated.

Various measures and domains may be more or less informative, depending on the case. Second, patterns of behaviors associated with disruptive behavior disorders often will vary based on context (e.g., school vs. home). Recognition of this highlights the importance of using multiple informants and multiple modalities during the evaluation. Also, behaviors associated with disruptive behavior disorders may not be seen during the formal clinical evaluation (e.g., because of low frequency or social desirability). For this reason, gathering information at multiple points in time may also be useful. Finally, the development of disruptive behaviors is often the result of a complex interaction of multiple causal factors (Kamphaus & Frick, 1996). As such, when developing a conceptual framework of the problem, it is important to consider a multitude of domains related to child functioning. Let us now consider which specific domains must be examined during an assessment of disruptive behavior disorders.

The first major area to explore is the presence of core symptoms. For ODDs, core symptoms include a pattern of defiant, negativistic, and hostile behaviors (such as blaming others, defying authority, deliberately annoying others, and vindictiveness; APA, 1994). Core symptoms related to CD include aggression to people or animals, destruction of property, deceitfulness or theft, and serious violations of rules (APA, 1994). Factors related to the presence of core symptoms include severity or degree of impairment, situational variability, and age of onset. Determination of age of onset is especially important for a few reasons. First, it is important when considering the duration and chronicity of the problem behaviors. Second, the current edition of the *DSM-IV* distinguishes between Childhood-onset and adolescent-onset subtypes of CD. As mentioned earlier, these subtypes often have different etiologies and consequent approaches to treatment, therefore, it is important to differentiate between the two in the clinical evaluation.

Various aspects of family functioning have been found to be related to the development of disruptive behavior disorders (Frick, 1994). A good assessment of parental functioning should be included in a comprehensive clinical assessment for disruptive behavior disorders. Aspects of parental socialization practices found to be especially important include parental involvement in the child's activities, parental supervision of the child, and the use of harsh or inconsistent discipline (Loeber & Stouthamer-Loeber, 1986). Additional meaningful aspects of family context include parental psychiatric adjustment and marital instability/divorce (Frick, 1994). Similar aspects of family dysfunction correlate with ODD and CD; however, children presenting with CD will often experience a greater number or severity of these circumstances, or both (Kamphaus & Frick, 1996).

Peer relationships represent another key area in the assessment of disruptive behavior disorders. As mentioned earlier, children with disruptive behavior disorders often experience peer rejection and often associate with a deviant peer group. As such, how the child perceives his or her relationships with peers, as well as how peers perceive the child, is an important factor to examine in a comprehensive evaluation.

Due to the high degree of overlap between conduct problems and learning disorders, any evaluation for disruptive behavior disorders should include a psychoeducational component. Overall, children with ODD or CD are more likely to experience academic difficulties than are children without conduct problems. Aspects of academic functioning especially likely to be affected are verbal IQ and achievement scores (Kronenberger & Meyer, 1996). Studies have also found that differences in academic functioning exist among children with conduct problems. Children with status or passive offenses are likely to have higher intellectual abilities than those committing aggressive acts (Kronenberger & Meyer). In light of these findings, a psychoeducational evaluation is an important part of an evaluation of disruptive behavior disorders.

Research has shown that the social cognitive style of children with conduct problems often differs from that of children without these problems (Lochman, Lampron, Burch, & Curry 1985; Lochman, Whidby, & FitzGerald, in press). As such, an evaluation of attributional style, cue-encoding abilities, and problem-solving abilities is as important for clinical assessment as for basic research on social cognitive processes, and can be readily assessed in clinical assessment protocols (Lochman et al.). Other areas to be addressed include beliefs and expectations about outcomes, social goals, social perspective–taking abilities, and empathy skills. On a related note, the child's self-report of feelings and subjective experiences may also provide valuable insight (Kamphaus & Frick, 1996).

As with any clinical evaluation, obtaining good medical, developmental, and family histories is critical to an accurate diagnosis. Since the ODD and CD diagnoses are based on behavioral rather than biological/medical criteria, a full medical exam is not necessary. A perfunctory exam, however, serves as a screening device and will alert the examiner to possible alternative explanations for the problem behaviors. A thorough developmental history will also alert the examiner to any circumstances occurring early in the child's life that may be relevant to the development of conduct problems. Research has found that disruptive behavior disorders are more prevalent in families with a history of mood disorders, ODD, CD, ADHD, Antisocial Personality Disorder (APD), and substance abuse (Kamphaus & Frick, 1996). Obtaining background information about the mental health of relatives of the child being evaluated may provide supporting evidence for a disruptive behavior disorder diagnosis or may provide the examiner with additional hypotheses about the nature of the problem.

Information regarding the social climate surrounding the child may also provide valuable information critical to the conceptualization of disruptive behavior disorders. Factors relating to the child's school environment, family economic situation, and surrounding neighborhood have all been found to be related to conduct problems and therefore should be examined (Kamphaus & Frick, 1996, Lochman, Whidby, & Fitzgerald, in press). These factors may be directly related to conduct problems or may be indirectly related through factors such as substance use or abuse. In either case, investigating the social climate of the child is important.

A variety of assessment tools may be useful in assessing disruptive behavior disorders. Each has unique strengths and weaknesses, and each has different domains for which it may be more or less appropriate. Behavior rating scales are one of the most popular methods of assessing child behavior in clinical evaluations. This type of measure allows the examiner to gather information from multiple informants in a relatively short time period, is easy to administer, and can allow detection of low-frequency behaviors. Omnibus scales in particular provide a quick and easy method of screening for the presence of comorbid disorders. In addition to being efficient, behavior rating scales in many cases also have good normative data, allowing the assessor to determine if certain behaviors are developmentally appropriate. For instance, a certain degree of oppositional behavior is common in preschool and adolescence. Age-based normative data allow the assessor to determine if the severity of the oppositional behaviors goes beyond what might be expected for these age groups. Controversy exists regarding the appropriateness of using gender-based normative data; in general, comparison to age-based norms is preferred over comparison to gender-based norms (Kamphaus & Frick, 1996). Other points to consider when deciding if a behavior rating scale is appropriate to use include the following: (a) whether the measure provides enough coverage of the core symptoms to be able to differentiate among subtypes, and (b) whether the scale measures what it purports to. It is important to examine the item content of a scale to verify that the scale measures what it claims to and that it is not based on outdated conceptualizations. Examples of behavior rating scales commonly used in the assessment of disruptive behavior disorders include the Behavior Assessment System for Children (BASC; Reynolds & Kamphaus, 1992) and the Child Behavior Checklist (CBCL; Achenbach & Edelbrock, 1983; Achenbach, 1991).

Structured interviews also provide valuable information about the presence of conduct problems. Whereas behavior rating scales are quick and provide good coverage of the basic symptoms of disruptive behavior disorders, structured interviews allow for the collection of more detailed information and are more likely to provide enough coverage of core symptoms to differentiate among subtypes of these disorders. Structured interviews go beyond superficial behaviors and allow the clinician to gather information regarding the severity, age of onset, and situational variables related to conduct problems. Less structured interviews may also be useful in determining attributions and reasoning behind behaviors. Like behavior rating scales, many structured interviews also include valuable normative information and are tied to diagnostic criteria. Disadvantages to structured interviews exist, however. They are often time consuming and, in some cases, require specialized training of the interviewer. Examples of structured interviews used include the Diagnostic Interview Schedule for Children (DISC; Costello, Edelbrock, Dulcan, Kalas, & Klaric, 1987) and the Child Assessment Schedule (CAS, Hodges, 1987).

Although behavior rating scales and structured interviews provide a great deal of important information, this information is filtered through the perceptions of others (e.g., teachers, parents). Another method of collecting data, direct observation, allows the clinician to see the child's problem behaviors without being influenced by the opinions of others. Because the child may not exhibit the concerning behaviors at the clinic, direct observation in various settings (e.g., at home, at school) and over multiple time periods will provide a more accurate view of typical daily functioning. Additionally, observation of the child within multiple interpersonal relationships (e.g., with peers, with parents) is important. As with structured interviews, a trade-off exists between more in-depth information and more time required to make a detailed direct observation.

Sociometric data provide important information regarding the nature of children's peer relationships. Typically, sociometric information is gathered in the classroom by the teacher and involves children rating their classmates based on variables such as, "fights the most," "liked the most," and "disliked the most" (Hughes, 1990; Gresham & Little, 1993). This technique can provide information regarding peer acceptance, rejection, and social status and may be especially important for subtyping socialized versus undersocialized children with conduct problems, which in turn may be important when designing interventions. Though clinically useful, sociometric data do have drawbacks: a great deal of normative data does not exist for many of these measures, and informed consent typically needs to be obtained from the peer group that is providing the sociometric nominations and ratings.

A fourth technique useful in the clinical evaluation of conduct problems is the use of vignettes and hypothetical situations designed to assess social cognitive processes. Although these techniques were originally developed for research purposes, they have been effectively used for clinical assessment as well (Lochman, Whidby, & FitzGerald, in press). The child is presented with an ambiguous situation or story and is asked to tell about what would happen next (social problem solving) or what the intentions of the characters in the stories were (attributions). This technique is especially useful in assessing social problem-solving style, and it can give the clinician insight on the child's current repertoire of problem-solving strategies. An example of this technique is the Problem Solving Measures for Conflict (PSM-C) (Lochman & Lampron, 1986; Dunn, Lochman, & Colder, 1997).

An array of areas to address in the evaluation of disruptive behavior disorders and techniques useful in assessing these domains has been presented. Before moving to a case example, let us first reiterate a few issues related to any comprehensive evaluation that are worth mentioning in relation to assessing conduct problems specifically. Although at times difficult to do, alternative explanations for conduct problems should be explored and ruled out. Often, primary and secondary causes are intertwined and as such cannot be separated easily; however, examining the severity of symptoms and temporal sequencing of problem behaviors can help with this determination (Kamphaus & Frick, 1996). Delineating which symptoms are primary and which are secondary is extremely important in the formulation of an effective treatment plan.

Additionally, although a comprehensive evaluation would ideally include information regarding a wide selection of domains related to the development of conduct problems collected from multiple informants using multiple modalities over multiple time periods, the scope of the evaluation will be affected by practical factors. With this in mind, the clinician should select those measures and methods most relevant to the evaluation on a case-by-case basis. Each child is unique; therefore, each evaluation will be unique. Perhaps the most important thing to keep in mind when conducting an evaluation of problem behaviors is that the best assessment is one that leads to the development of specific treatment objectives. Specific strengths and weaknesses of the child should be outlined in such a way that leads to identifiable recommendations for treatment.

CASE STUDY

For this case study, we will overview the types of diagnostic, behavioral, and cognitive measures that we typically use to assess children with disruptive behavior disorders. In addition to these basic assessment measures, we assess children's social-cognitive processes, which serve as a focus for our cognitive-behavioral intervention work. Case examples of the use of a social problem-solving measure and of a cue-encoding measure (relevant for attributional biases) with these types of child clients can be found in Lochman, Whidby and FitzGerald (in press).

Background Information

Billy Sherman was 11 years 5 months when his mother referred him to an outpatient mental health clinic for a comprehensive psychological assessment upon the urging of his teacher and his probation officer. According to his mother, Billy displayed significant problems related to property destruction, tantrums, physical and verbal aggression, and defiance. Before the referral, Billy had been released to his mother's custody after being temporarily placed in the local juvenile detention center. Billy had been charged with disorderly conduct and criminal mischief after breaking into a store and stealing video games.

Prior to his legal trouble, Billy was placed in an alternative school due to the level and intensity of his disruptive behavior. According to his mother, Billy had been suspended several times, and school officials frequently threatened expulsion. Billy reportedly disobeyed authority figures, picked fights with peers, and threw temper tantrums whenever he did not get his way. Ms. Sherman also complained about Billy's excessively high activity level in the school environment as well as at home.

Billy was also having significant academic difficulties. Ms. Sherman reported that he had been struggling with reading and comprehension since entering school. Ms. Sherman indicated that Billy's work speed and comprehension level were significantly below those of his classmates. Billy frequently required a tremendous amount of individualized attention. Ms. Sherman reported that he often did not complete his work unless someone was working closely with him. Billy began receiving Chapter 1 special services for reading when he was 5 years old. He had to repeat first grade due to reading problems and difficulty copying from the chalkboard. A fifth-grade student at the time of the evaluation, Billy continued to have difficulty copying from the chalkboard, reading, and remembering words.

According to his mother, Billy was diagnosed with ADHD when he was 6 years old and had consistently taken medication for his hyperactivity since being diagnosed. Despite Billy's history of disruptive behavior, he was reported to possess a number of positive interpersonal qualities. In one-on-one interactions, Billy was described as having a friendly smile and being quite likable and very mannerly.

Billy reportedly came from a very unstable home environment. Billy and his mother lived in at least five different cities during the course of his life. Whereas his mother was a consistent caregiver for Billy, Mr. Sherman did not maintain contact with him. Apparently, Mr. and Ms. Sherman's marriage involved a number of physical assaults. The couple divorced before Billy's birth.

Ms. Sherman indicated a strong family history of mental illness. For example, Billy's uncontrollable and violent behavior was noted to be the same type of behavior that his maternal uncles displayed when they were his age. Billy's uncles were reported to be mentally unstable, engaging in activities such as unaggravated assault and screaming at passing cars. Ms. Sherman denied ever sexually abusing Billy or knowledge of abuse by others, but there was suspicion that an older neighbor abused Billy when he was in preschool.

Ms. Sherman, a homemaker, attained a twelfth-grade level education. Ms. Sherman reported that she received regular prenatal care during her pregnancy with Billy and that she did not suffer from any major complications. However, Ms. Sherman reported experiencing severe stress during her pregnancy because of family difficulties. Billy was born 1 month prematurely. As reported by Ms. Sherman, Billy met all of his developmental milestones within normal age limits. During his first year, Billy had occasional high fevers that sometimes caused seizures.

Assessment of Core Symptoms

Billy's emotional and behavioral functioning was assessed through diagnostic structured clinical interviews with Ms. Sherman, Billy's teacher at the time, and Billy (DISC-2 3; Shaffer, Fisher, Piacentini, Schwab-Stone, & Wicks, 1991) and rating scales completed by Ms. Sherman, Billy's teacher at the time, his probation officer, and himself (BASC, Reynolds & Kamphaus, 1992; CBCL; Achenbach, 1991). On the DISC-2 3, Billy's teacher, probation officer, and Ms. Sherman reported a high number of symptoms related to inattention, overactivity, and impulsivity. Regarding symptoms of overactivity and impulsivity, it was reported that Billy often seemed "on the go," talked too loud, acted without thinking, bothered other children when they were working, and often fidgeted and talked excessively. Ms. Sherman added that Billy had a short attention span, and his teacher added that he did not listen or follow instructions, was disorganized, easily distracted, and made careless mistakes. On the BASC, Ms. Sherman, Billy's teacher, and his probation officer indicated that Billy displayed significant problems with hyperactivity and maintaining attention compared to his same-aged peers. These symptoms were consistent with a diagnosis of ADHD Combined Type.

A diagnosis of ADHD was supported by previous psychological evaluations that noted that many of these behaviors had caused consistent problems for Billy since he was approximately 6 years old and resulted in a diagnosis of ADHD. These behaviors were also shown to cause significant problems for Billy at home and school and across a variety of situations. In particular, Billy's problems with overactivity and inattention interfered with his ability to follow directions, complete schoolwork, and get along with peers.

Other areas of concern expressed by Ms. Sherman, Billy's teacher, and his probation officer were behaviors that violated the rights of others as well as major societal norms. On both the diagnostic interview and rating scales, all informants indicated that compared with his same-aged peers, Billy had significant problems with aggression and conduct. Specifically, all respondents reported that Billy was often cruel to other people, lied to stay out of trouble, and intimidated others. Ms. Sherman added that Billy bullied other children at school, had problems with certain authority figures, and threw extensive tantrums. In addition, according to a response to a question on the CBCL, Billy's teacher indicated that he often threatened to hurt others. These behaviors were consistent with a diagnosis of CD. Because these behaviors had been present since before the age of 10 years, he met the criteria for the childhood-onset type of CD. In addition, the behaviors were adversely affecting Billy's relationship functioning at home, at school, and with peers.

Billy's social functioning was assessed through ratings (Social Skills Rating System, Gresham & Elliott, 1990) by Ms. Sherman and his teacher and through a sociometric exercise. Both respondents rated Billy's social skills as below average when compared to same-aged peers. Ms. Sherman also indicated that Billy had a clinically significant tendency to evade others and avoid social contact. On the BASC, all respondents indicated that Billy had problems with atypical behaviors. (Elevated scores in this area have been related to immature behavior that is often seen in children with disruptive behavioral disorders.) In clinical interviews, both Ms. Sherman and his teacher reported that Billy was immature and insecure, and that he was unaccepting of responsibility and lacked insight into the effects of his behaviors. He was, in addition, a reportedly shy, very passive, poor communicator, and he often appeared to be distant, as if he was daydreaming. In group interactions with peers, Billy was often rejected and routinely ostracized. Both his mother and teacher reported that Billy very seldom talked to other children and preferred to be alone. Billy also displayed great deficits on measures used to assess his social problem-solving skills as well as his attributional biases. Furthermore, a sociometric exercise indicated that Billy was both withdrawn and aggressive with peers. One third of his classmates nominated him as "fights most" and "most shy" while one fourth of his classmates nominated him as "meanest."

On the BASC, Billy indicated that he was having difficulty related to feeling rejected and misunderstood by others. On a sentence completion task, Billy stated he would like to know "how life [is] . . . going to be me since I don't have no friends." He also completed sentences stating "At home . . . nothin' goes right for me" and "My greatest worry is . . . about my father." Billy was given the Childhood Depression Inventory (CDI; Beck, Steer, & Garbin, 1988) to assess depressive symptoms. His scores in the Negative Mood and Ineffectiveness Indexes were classified in the Very Much Above Average range when compared to children his age. Although his overall scores on the CDI were not indicative of a diagnosable depressive condition, Billy's scores were elevated and suggested he was having difficulty negotiating his daily interactions in his environment.

Assessment of Intellectual and Academic Abilities

Billy's performance on psychoeducational measures suggested that his perceptual organization and nonverbal skills were significantly better developed than his verbal comprehension. Billy's extremely low verbal scores indicated that he was in need of individualized special education services. Thus, it was not surprising that he had great difficulty in school. On the WISC-III (Wechsler, 1991), Billy achieved a Verbal Scale IQ score of 73 and a Performance Scale IQ Score of 91. His verbal performance was classified in the Borderline range while his perceptual organizational skills fell in the Average range. Billy's reading, math, and writing scores indicated achievement consistent with what would be expected based on his assessed intellectual abilities. Consequently, intervention aimed at facilitating Billy's development of strategies to overcome his behavioral challenges, his problem-solving difficulties, and increasing his basic skills and knowledge was clearly indicated.

INTERVENTIONS

This careful assessment of the child with Oppositional Defiant Disorder or Conduct Disorder will lead to an individualized treatment plan for the child. Historically, psychosocial treatment of conduct-disordered youth was perceived to be difficult and not very productive (Lochman, in press-a). However, randomized clinical trials have begun to identify empirically supported treatments for children with CD and ODD. Brestan and Eyberg (1998) systematically reviewed the treatment research literature for children with conduct problems, and they identified two parent training intervention programs as having well-established positive effects (Patterson, Reid & Dishion, 1992; Webster-Stratton, 1994) and ten other programs as being probably efficacious.

Cognitive-Behavioral Interventions

Researchers have identified four types of cognitive-behavioral interventions. The first is child behavior modification, which focuses the intervention directly on the child in order to change or modify existing aggressive behavior. Similarly, parent behavior modification is focused on changing parent interaction with the child in order to regulate or decrease aggressive behavior. Interventions can also be school-based, as with school behavior modification. In this type of intervention, teachers are taught how to decrease aggressive child behavior through their interactions with the child in a manner similar to the parent intervention. Finally, the mixed behavior modification encompasses focusing on the child, parent, and school all in one intervention.

Late Elementary to Middle School Intervention Programs

Anger Coping Program.   The Anger Coping Program is a cognitive-behavioral intervention program focusing on child behavior modification. It is a group intervention using 18 structured sessions to help children recognize and decrease aggressive behavior. The groups are usually comprised of four to six aggressive children of varying social and cognitive strengths and weaknesses.

In this section we will briefly summarize the goals and objectives in each session of the Anger Coping Program. See Lochman, Lampron, Gemmer, and Harris (1987) and Lochman, FitzGerald, and Whidby (1999) for a detailed guide to this intervention. The goals comprising each session include: Session 1, explaining the purpose of the group and the rules and structure of the program, Session 2 and 3, self-talk training, Sessions 4 and 5, establishing the perspective-taking concept, Session 6, recognizing physiological signs of anger, Session 7, incorporating goal setting, Sessions 8 through 18, solving social problems.

In Session 1 the goal is predominantly to acquaint members and establish the structure of the group sessions. To explain the purpose of the group, we usually describe it as a way to learn self-control or anger control. Next it is important to go over the rules expected to be followed by the group. These rules generally include items involving confidentiality, physical contact, paying attention and participating, shouting, and so forth. At this point, we also ask the children in the group if they have any suggestions for session rules. Next, the behavioral contingency system is explained. Using this contingency, children can receive points during group sessions for good behavior (i.e., complimenting or helping someone) that accumulate and can be traded in for a more tangible reward later on. In addition, the children can lose points for bad behavior, such as shouting. A group leader can call a "strike" if a child is misbehaving; if the child accumulates three strikes, he loses a point. After these rules are explained, group members play a game to get acquainted (Lochman & Wells, 1996).

The self-talk sessions teach children how to remind themselves verbally not to use aggression (e.g., "Stop! Think! What can I do?"). Group members participate in a variety of activities, such as a verbal taunting game that helps them handle others' teasing behavior by using these self-talk statements. Whereas the self-talk sessions help children deal with automatic anger feelings, the perspective-taking sessions teach the children to not automatically become angry in perceived problem situations. The perspective taking sessions use pictures of ambiguous situations to stimulate group discussions of a variety of nonhostile intentions the person in the picture may have. Then the group may practice perspective taking with other group members using role-playing. Group leaders emphasize attending to nonhostile cues in ambiguous situations. In this way, their understanding of others' perspectives and of how easily intentions can be misjudged can be practiced and demonstrated.

To help group members understand when they need to utilize the self-talk and perspective-taking techniques, they must learn how to recognize physiological signs of anger. To do this, the group watches a video of other children acting angry. Then they are asked if they can describe what signs in the video pointed to the fact that those children were angry. Group members are encouraged to discuss the physical signs of anger in the children, such as clenched fists, scowling faces, and objects being thrown. Then group leaders can introduce internal signs of anger, such as rapid heartbeat and tight muscles. After group members can recognize their own physiological signs of anger, they are taught to use these signs as a cue to start problem solving instead of getting angry. Children are taught steps to problem solving, such as problem identification, choices, and consequences. Then children model and practice role-playing using these steps. In addition, over several sessions group members can videotape themselves role-playing a scenario they have created in which they are modeling the use of these steps (Lochman & Wells, 1996).

The outcome effects for the Anger Coping Program show that children who participated display reduced disruptive-aggressive behavior, increased on-task behavior, less parent- and teacher-rated aggression, and higher self-esteem (for a full review of outcome research see Lochman, Dunn, & Klimes-Dougan, 1993). These results are based on studies utilizing pre- and postassessments as well as comparisons between participants in the program and controls (Lochman, Dunn, & Wagner, 1997). The long-term effects of the program indicate that participants maintained many of the gains pertaining to on-task behavior and self-esteem, but some of the behavioral gains were not maintained (Lochman, 1992). However, in comparison to control groups and nonaggressive boys, participants in the Anger Coping Program had higher self-esteem, gave more relevant problem-solving solutions on a problem-solving task, and in a 3 year follow-up study showed lower rates of drug abuse, including the use of alcohol and marijuana (Lochman, 1992).

Coping Power Program.   The Coping Power Program is an extended version of the Anger Coping Program that is designed to boost the limited preventative outcome effects of the Anger Coping Program. To accomplish this, 15 more sessions were added to the basic Anger Coping Program for a total of 33 sessions for the Coping Power Program Child Component. The additional group sessions include emotional awareness, relaxation training, social skills training, social and personal goal setting, and handling peer pressure. In addition, the Coping Power Program includes individual sessions every four to six weeks to ensure the individualization of the treatment pertaining to the participant's social life. A Parent Component is also included in the program and is designed to cover the same time period as the Child Component. The parents meet for 16 sessions addressing parental use of reinforcement and positive attention, establishment of clear rules and expectations, correct and effective use of punishment, family communication, positive school experiences for the child, and stress management. Parents are instructed on what their child is learning in each session so that they can help facilitate and reward the practice of these new skills at home (Lochman & Wells, 1996; Lochman, in press-b).

The outcome research for the Coping Power Program indicates greater reductions in off-task classroom behavior. In one study, 183 teacher-rated aggressive boys were randomly placed in (a) a Child Component, (b) a combination of both the Child and Parent Components, or (c) an untreated control group. Though this is still an ongoing study, preliminary results indicate improvements in social competence, social information processing, locus of control, temperament, and lowered aggression. Parental increases have been found regarding parenting practices, anger, and marital relationship. Most of these child effects were still evident at a 1-year follow-up study, but certain parental effects and reduced child aggression were only evident in the combined Parent and Child Components, indicating the increased efficacy of using a combined treatment (Lochman, in press-b).

Intervention Programs for Young Children

Fast Track Program.   The Fast Track Program is a multisite intervention designed to integrate a targeted intervention for children with behavior problems with a universal prevention program in order to address child, family, school, and community levels in one intervention (Conduct Problems Prevention Research Group, 1992, 1999a, 1999b). The program will continue to provide intervention as children move through elementary, middle and early high school. This program is based on the premise that it is often difficult for children with behavior problems to generalize their treatment in the classroom where teachers and peers might not reinforce small steps in reducing aggression. Therefore, a Promoting Alternative Thinking Strategies (PATHS) component is used for all children so that aggressive and nonaggressive children will understand a common treatment. In addition, the treatment is designed to promote social competence in all children, leading to an improved classroom atmosphere and improved peer relationships. Understanding and communicating emotions is a main focus of the intervention in the early elementary school years. For example, children are taught to understand the difference between feelings and behaviors as well as how feelings can change throughout the day. Children then focus on positive social behavior, which encompasses another focus of the intervention. Positive behaviors, such as using good manners, making friends through good communication, and sharing, are taught and reinforced throughout these lessons. The other sessions in the early years emphasize self-control and steps to problem solving. Children are taught learning techniques, such as picturing a stop light for their emotions. For example, when they feel frustrated, they are encouraged to "go to the red light," to stop and think before they act—a modified idea from the Yale–New Haven Middle School Social Problem Solving Program (Weissberg, Caplan, & Bennetto, 1988).

The outcome effects of this intervention program indicate significant effects on peer ratings of aggression, disruptive behavior, and classroom atmosphere. In addition, at the end of first grade, moderate positive social effects were reported on children's social, emotional, and academic skills. Moderate positive effects were also reported for interactions with peers, social status, conduct problems, and special education placement for high-risk aggressive children.

The Montreal Delinquency Prevention Program.   This is a two-year intervention using both a child and parent component. The parent component is based on a treatment by the Oregon Social Learning Center (Patterson, 1982), and the child component teaches social skills and self-control. The intervention is given to children with behavior problems in the second and third grade (Tremblay, Masse, Pagani, & Vitaro, 1996). The outcome effects for those who received the intervention by age 12 showed reduced adjustment problems in school and reduced instances of trespassing and stealing compared to untreated controls (Tremblay et al., 1996). In addition, participants were also less likely to be involved with antisocial friends (Vitaro & Tremblay, 1994). Many of these effects have been documented at age 15 as well, showing that the intervention has preventative effects lasting until adolescence.

Dinosaur School.   This program was designed to reduce aggression for 4- to 7-year-olds with early-onset conduct problems. This intervention also uses a child and parent component; however, the Dinosaur School is the child component of a larger treatment program. The treatment program addresses weaknesses that children with conduct problems typically display, such as those with social skills, perspective taking, problem solving, and emotions, such as stress, loneliness, and anger. The parent component utilizes videotapes to help model effective parenting. Results indicate that participants in the Dinosaur School that received the child component had significantly fewer conduct problems reported at home and increases in problem solving skills compared to a control group receiving no intervention. In addition, at a 1-year follow-up study, most parents rated the behavior of their children as normal and not significantly in the behavioral problem range (Webster-Stratton & Hammond, 1997).

Intervention Programs for Adolescents

Anger Control Training.   This program teaches aggressive adolescents emotional arousal training in order to recognize anger feelings and manage them appropriately. The program consists of several components, including stress management, peer relation training, cognitive restructuring, and behavioral self-management. Preliminary research on the efficacy of this program in use with delinquent high school students found that the behavioral self-management component decreased the number of teacher reports of disruptive classroom behavior and increased students' problem-solving skills and self-control (Feindler, Marriott, & Iwata, 1984). Further research conducted with aggressive adolescents at a residential treatment facility suggested an improvement in the participants' abilities to recognize and manage anger feelings appropriately, as rated by staff members within the treatment facility. However, these results should be interpreted with caution because subjects were not randomly assigned to treatment conditions (Feindler, Ecton, Kingsley, & Dubey, 1986).

Adolescent Transitions Program.   This program was initially designed to help reduce the escalation of problem behaviors in later adolescence of adolescents displaying such problems at earlier ages. Dishion and Andrews (1995) tested the individual components of the program to gain results on the overall effectiveness the program in preventing further problem behaviors. This study targeted 158 at-risk families and then divided them into either a control group, parent focus condition, teen focus condition, parent and teen focus condition, or self-directed change condition (in which the participant received only materials and not direct individual treatment). The parent focus, teen focus, and parent/teen focus conditions all had positive effects indicated by reports and observations of reduced home conflict. In addition, the parent focus alone produced reductions in longitudinal measures of tobacco use as well as immediate improvements in classroom behavior. However, iatrogenic effects were found for those conditions in which teens were placed in groups with other problem-behavior teens. Those groups showed increases in tobacco use and disruptive classroom behavior. These iatrogenic effects were found at immediate and 1-year longitudinal follow-ups. The authors indicate the need to continually refine and test the current intervention methods, especially with respect to those that aggregate high-risk adolescents into groups, so that problem behaviors can be prevented and not augmented (Dishion & Andrews, 1995).

ISSUES AND IMPLICATIONS

The assessment and intervention research reviewed in this chapter indicates that there are promising and useful measures and treatments for children with disruptive behavior disorders. To further refine and develop clinical work in this area, attention should be directed at certain assessment-related and treatment-related issues that can guide our research and program development over the coming decade.

Assessment Issues

Perhaps the most critical need of assessment approaches is to address individual differences with children who present with ODD and CD. For example, it is important to understand how these behavioral patterns might develop differently for boys versus girls, for children with reactive versus proactive aggressive behavior, and for children with callous-unemotional traits. Recognizing the potential importance of differing causal and maintaining factors for various subgroups of conduct problem children such as these, the interventions will need to be tailored to meet the unique needs of different subtypes of children with conduct problems.

Assessment approaches need to map the targeted goals of intervention programs directly. For empirically supported treatments, intervention goals and activities are explicit and are relatively structured. Thus, we need to assess behaviors and processes toward which we will direct intervention. With this information, even fairly structured interventions can be adjusted to emphasize areas of greatest assessed weaknesses. For example, some aggressive children have clear, generalized, and highly deficient attributional and problem-solving skills, but other aggressive children have prominent deficits only in select aspects of problem solving. Cognitive-behavioral treatment should be delivered differently to these two types of children, because they have different patterns of social-cognitive difficulties.

Disruptive behavior disorders are determined by a number of different causal factors. Thus, assessment should be broad enough to assess this range of causal and maintaining factors. Optimal assessment thus addresses child behavioral, social and cognitive functioning, as well as parent functioning and broader contextual factors. The child's immediate context, involving factors such as parenting style and teacher's reactions, has obvious effects on the child's behavior. However, broader contextual factors such as neighborhood quality and cultural beliefs can have direct impacts on a parent's approaches to parenting, and thus can indirectly affect children's behavior. We need to attend to the cultural and ethnic relevance of our assessment measures carefully as well.

The assessment measures used in our clinical settings should be empirically linked to the types of developmental psychopathology with which we are intervening. These assessment measures should not only become a routine component of the initial evaluation process, but should also be used at the end of treatment to measure outcomes. In that sense, each case is a case study, or part of a collection of case studies. When children and their families are carefully assessed before and after treatment, the clinician can better understand the nature of the causal processes within the specific type of case being seen, can become more adept at readily adapting the treatment program to meet client's individual needs effectively, and can measure the effectiveness of their work across cases.

Clinical Issues

Multicomponent interventions.   The intervention research with aggressive children indicates that cognitive-behavioral interventions with components that address both children's social-cognitive processes and parents' parenting practices produce broader positive effects and better maintenance of behavioral improvements over time than do interventions that focus on children or parents alone (Kazdin, Siegel & Bass, 1992; Lochman, in press-b, Webster-Stratton and Hammond, 1997). Thus, optimal intervention planning would include structured, empirically supported interventions for children and parents. Interventions that have both child and parent components can address a wider set of risk and protective factors than can interventions with single components. Other intervention components—including teacher consultation, teacher training to implement programs directly in the classroom, and academic tutoring—can also augment and reinforce the effects of comprehensive interventions for children with early-onset conduct problems (Conduct Problems Prevention Research Group, 1999a).

Individualizing intervention.   Cognitive-behavioral interventions should be individualized in at least two ways. First, even though there is a guiding social cognitive model indicating the targeted goals for structured interventions, the interventions need to be adapted to meet the specific deficits and strengths of specific aggressive children. As we learn more about meaningful subtypes of children with aggressive, disruptive disorders (e.g., Frick, 1998a; Dodge, Lochman, Harnish, Bates, & Pettit, 1997), and we determine how different subtypes of children have different patterns of social-cognitive difficulties, then we can generate individualized treatment plans that emphasize certain aspects of cognitive-behavioral treatments more than others for particular children. Second, another way in which programs can be flexibly provided is by adjusting the delivery of a cognitive-behavioral protocol to meet emerging clinical issues. For example, when children begin discussing a current social problem, clinicians should respond by shifting their agenda for the session, and modeling and reinforcing problem-solving skills rather than sticking rigidly to the planned activities for the day. It is critical that clinicians keep in mind the overall objectives of the program, and the objectives of each session, so that the clinicians' flexible responses to children's problems and to group process problems can still have direct impact on the targeted social-cognitive difficulties of aggressive children.

Ethnic and community context.   Interventions must be delivered in ways that make them relevant and appropriate to the varying types of populations that can be found in urban, suburban, and rural settings. Lochman, Whidby, and FitzGerald (in press) noted that the effects of a cognitive-behavioral intervention like the Anger Coping Program could be limited by certain cultural constraints. Within African American, low-income populations, children's abilities to accept and use nonaggressive strategies to solve problems may be limited by their parents' modeling of physical aggression through their greater use of corporal punishment, and by their parents' direct advice to retaliate when confronted by certain types of threatening situations. These parental responses can often be the result of the parents' desire to protect their children within a threatening, violent environment within a low-income community. Intervention may need to advocate the use of "code switching" explicitly among these African American youth (Lochman, Whidby, & FitzGerald, in press), so that children can acquire a different code of behavior depending on the environment they are in (e.g., a violent, crime-ridden neighborhood vs. a relatively orderly school).

Developmental appropriateness.   Children's cognitive, social, and emotional developmental level should be carefully considered before using or adapting cognitive-behavioral interventions. Many of these interventions were originally developed for children or adolescents within certain age ranges, and the supportive intervention research may have been limited to those age ranges. Thus, the use of a structured intervention program with children outside that age range may be ineffective, because the targeted skills and program activities are not developmentally appropriate. To make the

Anger Coping Program relevant for children in the early years of elementary school, activities have to be more concrete, highly engaging, and briefly presented and must make frequent use of stimulating books, puppets, and arts-and-crafts activities. The intervention has to be highly structured because children at this age are active and are less able to engage in constructive group behavior such as turn-taking, sitting in one's seat, and making relevant comments. The intervention must also recognize that normative levels of perspective taking and sequential problem solving are much lower at this age range (Lochman, FitzGerald, & Whidby, in press; Lochman, Whidby, & FitzGerald, in press). In a similar vein, the Anger Coping Program can be adapted for use by older adolescents, but this requires more emphasis on discussion time and more attention to the risks posed by peer pressure and deviant peer groups. Lochman, FitzGerald, and Whidby discussed the types of content and structural changes that should be made with both young children and older adolescents.

Applications to school-based, outpatient, and residential settings.   The Anger Coping Program was originally developed and evaluated in school-based settings, and this method of intervention delivery has certain clear advantages. These advantages include (a) an opportunity for early screening, early intervention, and prevention with children with emerging disruptive behavior disorders; (b) an opportunity to work on children's interpersonal behavior problems within one of the settings where many of these problems occur; (c) a ready and easy opportunity to consult with children's teachers on a regular basis, thus extending the reach of the intervention by directing contingencies for children's behavior in the classrooms and by reinforcing teachers' skills in facilitating the development of children's social-cognitive skills; (d) inclusion of school personnel, such as school counselors and school psychologists as co-leaders, thus increasing the likelihood that the intervention will be accepted by other staff within the school setting and that the intervention will be maintained over time; and (e) attendance rates for children in their groups than are often higher than those of seen in an outpatient setting. However, we have found that the structure for the Anger Coping Program can be easily used in outpatient settings as well, and this has certain other advantages, including (a) the inclusion of parents in parent groups that meet at the same time as the child groups; (b) an extension of group meeting time, often to 90 minutes, permitting more intensive work within the group sessions; and (c) opportunities to provide the Anger Coping Program as part of an integrated treatment plan, which can include medication and other psychosocial treatments for comorbid conditions such as ADHD and anxiety disorders. Similar advantages occur when children are in residential or inpatient settings, and the Anger Coping Program appears to be an appropriate component treatment in these settings (Lochman, Curry, Dane, & Ellis, in press; Lochman, White, Curry, & Rumer, 1992). In all of these settings, we have found that many of the Anger Coping Program activities can be adapted for use in individual therapy, and we believe that periodic adjunctive individual therapy sessions are useful with ongoing group treatment as well. Research on other social problem-solving interventions have demonstrated the efficacy of these cognitive-behavioral interventions with inpatient and outpatient children (Kazdin, Esveldt-Dawson, French, & Unis, 1987; Kazdin et al., 1992).

Group process issues.   When these cognitive-behavioral interventions are delivered within the context of group therapy, the therapists have to be attentive to the development of negative group processes of possible iatrogenic effects that can occur when group members reinforce each other's deviant beliefs (e.g., Dishion & Andrews, 1995). At the stage of composing a group, we have found that the likelihood of creating a productive group increases when the children selected have the kinds of problems-solving deficits that are the focus of the Anger Coping Program; when some group members can serve as solid peer models for how to enact more competent verbal assertions and negotiation strategies; and when group members have at least a minimal level of motivation to work on their anger management difficulties. During the course of group sessions, we attempt to enhance a positive group process by including positive feedback time from all group members at the end of group sessions; we include group-wide contingencies for earning group reinforcements that thus promote cooperative behavior among group members, and we encourage the group to plan prosocial group activities that can positively impact others outside the group (e.g., creating drug prevention posters that focus on handling peer pressure which can be mounted in their school). When disagreements and conflicts develop between group members during sessions, these can be opportunities to model and reinforce the social-cognitive skills that are the focus of these cognitive-behavioral interventions, including finding ways to cool down, listening to the other person's point-of-view, getting a better understanding of the perspective of their peers, and using verbal assertion and negotiation skills under controlled conditions, while the group leaders provide coaching.

SUMMARY

This chapter outlined the characteristics of children with Conduct Disorder and Oppositional Defiant Disorder. These disorders involve stable, chronic behavioral patterns, and can lead to progressively more antisocial behaviors during the adolescent years. The research literature indicates that aggressive children have identifiable personal and familial characteristics, including hyperactive behavior, poor academic functioning, poor peer relationships, distorted and deficient social-cognitive processes, parents who use harsh and inconsistent punishment, and neighborhood problems. Thus, assessment should not only assess the Conduct Disorder and Oppositional Defiant Disorder symptoms, but also causal and associated factors of each. The chapter overviewed a range of the assessment methods directed at these factors and illustrated how some of these have been assessed in a case study. Cognitive-behavioral interventions have been found to reduce aggressive behavior in children and adolescents effectively, and several examples of these programs are illustrated for different age levels. Finally, implications for assessment—especially the need for attention to individual differences—and implications for intervention were raised. To further enhance the effectiveness of intervention, future intervention research and intervention development should address the use of multicomponent interventions, the need to individualize interventions and attend to the children's ethnic and community contexts, and group process issues, and should effectively adapt interventions to children treated in different settings, and at different developmental periods.

REFERENCES

Abikoff, H., & Klein, G. (1992). Attention-deficit hyperactivity and conduct disorder: Co-morbidity and implications for treatment. *Journal of Consulting and Clinical Psychology, 60,* 881–892.

Achenbach, T. M. (1991). *Integrative guide for the 1991 CBCL/4–18, YSR, and TRF profiles.* Burlington: University of Vermont Department of Psychiatry.

Achenbach, T. M., & Edelbrock, C. (1983). *Manual for the Child Behavior Checklist and Revised Child Behavior Profile.* Burlington: University of Vermont.

American Psychiatric Association. (1994). *Diagnostic and statistical manual of mental disorders* (4th ed.). Washington, DC: Author.

Beck, A. T., Steer, R. A., & Garbin, M. G. (1988). Psychometric properties of the Beck Depression Inventory: Twenty-five years of evaluation. *Clinical Psychology Review, 8,* 77–100.

Bierman, K. L., & Wargo, J. B. (1995). Predicting the longitudinal course associated with aggressive-rejected, aggressive (non-rejected), and rejected (non-aggressive) status. *Development and Psychopathology, 7,* 669–683.

Blumstein, A., Farrington, D. P., & Moitra, S. (1985). Delinquency careers: Innocents, desisters, and persisters. In M. Tonry & N. Morris (Eds.), *Crime and justice* (pp. 187–219). Chicago: University of Chicago Press.

Brannon, J. M., & Troyer, R. (1995). Adolescent sex offenders: Investigating adult commitment-rates four years later. *International Journal of Offender Therapy and Comparative Criminology, 39,* 317–326.

Brestan, E. V., & Eyberg, S. M. (1998). Effective psychosocial treatment of conduct-disordered children and adolescents: 29 years, 82 studies, and 5,272 kids. *Journal of Clinical Child Psychology, 27,* 180–189.

Caputo, A. A., Frick, P. J., & Brodsky, S. L. (1999). Family violence and juvenile sex offending: Potential mediating role of psychopathic traits and negative attitudes toward women. *Criminal Justice and Behavior, 26,* 338–356.

Christian, R. E., Frick, P. J., Hill, N. L., Tyler, L., & Frazer, D. R. (1997). Psychopathy and conduct problems in children: II. Implications for subtyping children with conduct problems. *Journal of the American Academy of Child and Adolescent Psychiatry, 36,* 233–241.

Cleckly, H. (1976). *The mask of sanity* (5th ed.). St. Louis, MO: Mosby.

Cohen, D., & Strayer, J. (1996). Empathy in conduct-disordered and comparison youth. *Developmental Psychology, 62,* 366–374.

Coie, J. D., Lochman, J. E., Terry, R., & Hyman, C. (1992). Predicting early adolescent disorder from childhood aggression and peer rejection. *Journal of Consulting and Clinical Psychology, 60,* 783–792.

Coie, J. D., Terry, R., Zakriski, A., & Lochman, J. E. (1995). Early adolescent social influences on delinquent behavior. In J. McCord (Ed.), *Coercion and punishment in long-term perspectives* (pp. 299–244). Cambridge, England: Cambridge University Press.

Colder, C. R., Lochman, J. E., & Wells, K. C. (1997). The moderating effects of children's fear and activity level on relations between parenting practices and childhood symptomatology. *Journal of Abnormal Child Psychology, 25,* 251–263.

Conduct Problems Prevention Research Group. (1992). A developmental and clinical model for the prevention of conduct disorder: The Fast Track Program. *Development and Psychopathology, 4,* 509–527.

Conduct Problems Prevention Research Group. (1999a). Initial impact of the Fast Track prevention trial for conduct problems: I. The high-risk sample. *Journal of Consulting and Clinical Psychology, 67,* 631–647.

Conduct Problems Prevention Research Group. (1999b). Initial impact of the Fast Track prevention trial for conduct problems: II. Classroom effects. *Journal of Consulting and Clinical Psychology, 67,* 648–657.

Costello, E. J., Edelbrock, C. S., Dulcan, M. K., Kalas, R., & Klaric, S. (1987). *Diagnostic interview schedule for children (DISC).* Pittsburgh: University of Pittsburgh Press.

Crick, N. R. (1995). Relational aggression: The role of intent attributions, feelings of distress, and provocation type. *Development and Psychopathology.*

Crick, N. R., & Grotpeter, J. K. (1995). Relational aggression, gender, and social-psychological adjustment. *Child Development, 66,* 710–722.

Dishion, T. J., & Andrews, D. W. (1995). Preventing escalation in problem behaviors with high-risk young adolescents. Immediate and 1-year outcomes. *Journal of Consulting and Clinical Psychology, 63,* 538–548.

Dodge, K. A., Lochman, J. E., Harnish, J. D., Bates, J. E., & Pettit, G. S. (1997). Reactive and proactive aggression in school children and psychiatrically impaired chronically assaultive youth. *Journal of Abnormal Psychology, 106,* 37–51.

Dodge, K. A., Pettit, G. S., McClaskey, C. L., & Brown, M. M. (1986). Social competence in children. *Monographs of the Society for Research in Child Development, 51*(2, Serial No. 213).

Dunn, S. E., Lochman, J. E., & Colder, C. R. (1997). Social problem-solving skills in boys with conduct and oppositional disorders. *Aggressive Behavior, 23,* 457–469.

Faraone, S. V., Biederman, J., Keenan, K., & Tsuang, M. T. (1991). Separation of *DSM-III* attention deficit disorder and conduct disorder. Evidence from a family genetic study of American child psychiatry patients. *Psychological Medicine, 21,* 109–121.

Feindler, E. A., Ecton, R. B., Kingsley, D., & Dubey, D. R. (1986). Group anger-control training for institutionalized psychiatric male adults. *Behavior Therapy, 17,* 109–123.

Feindler, E. A., Marriott, S. A., & Iwata, M. (1984). Group anger control training for junior high school delinquents. *Cognitive Therapy and Research, 8,* 299–311.

Forehand, R., & Long, N. (1988). Outpatient treatment of the acting child. Procedures, long term follow-up data, and clinical problems. *Advances in Behavior Research and Therapy, 10,* 129–177.

Frick, P. J. (1994). Family dysfunction and the disruptive behavior disorders: A review of recent empirical findings. In T. H. Ollendick & R. J. Prinz (Eds.), *Advances in clinical child psychology* (Vol. 16, pp. 203–226). New York: Plenum.

Frick, P. J. (1998a). *Conduct disorders and severe antisocial behavior.* New York: Plenum.

Frick, P. J. (1998b). Callus-unemotional traits and conduct problems: Applying the two-factor model of psychopathy to children. In D. J. Cooke et al. (Eds.), *Psychopathy: Theory, research, and implications for society* (pp. 161–187). Netherlands: Kluwer Academic.

Frick, P. J., Kamphaus, R. W., Lahey, B. B., Loeber, R., Christ, M. A. G., & Hart, E. L. E. (1991). Academic underachievement and the disruptive behavior disorders. *Journal of Consulting and Clinical Psychology, 59,* 289–294.

Frick, P. J., Lahey, B. B., Loeber, R., Stouthamer-Loeber, M., Christ, M. A., & Hanson, K. (1992). Familial risk factors to oppositional defiant disorder and conduct disorder: Parental psychopathology and maternal parenting. *Journal of Consulting and Clinical Psychology, 60,* 49–55.

Frick, P. J., Lahey, B. B., Loeber, R., Tannenbaum, L. E., Van Horn, Y., Christ, M. A., Hart, E. A., & Hanson, K. (1993). Oppositional defiant disorder and conduct disorder: A meta-analytic review of factor analyses and cross-validation in a clinic sample. *Clinical Psychology Review, 13,* 319–340.

Frick, P. J., O'Brien, B. S., Wooton, J. M., & McBurnett, K. (1994). Psychopathy and conduct problems in children. *Journal of Abnormal Psychology, 103,* 700–707.

Gittelman, R., Mannuzza, S., Shenker, R., & Bonuagura, N. (1985). Hyperactive boys almost grown up. *Archives of General Psychiatry, 42,* 937–947.

Gouze, K. R. (1987). Attention and social problem solving as correlates of aggression in preschool males. *Journal of Abnormal Child Psychology, 17,* 277–289.

Greenberg, M. T., Lengua, L. J., Coie, J. D., Pinderhughes, E. E., & the Conduct Problems Prevention Research Group. (1999). Predicting developmental outcomes at school entry using a multiple-risk model: Four American communities. *Developmental Psychology, 35,* 403–417.

Gresham, R. M., & Elliott, S. N. (1990). *Social skills rating system.* Circle Pines, MN: American Guidance Service.

Gresham, F. M., & Little, S. N. (1993). Peer-referenced assessment strategies. In T. H. Ollendick & M. Hersen (Eds.), *Handbook of child and adolescent assessment* (p. 165–179). Needham Heights, MA: Allyn & Bacon.

Hare, R. D. (1993). *Without conscience. The disturbing world of the psychopaths among us.* New York: Pocket.

Hinshaw, S. P. (1992). Externalizing behavior problems and academic underachievement in childhood and adolescence: Causal relationships and underlying mechanisms. *Psychological Bulletin, III,* 127–155.

Hinshaw, S. P., & Anderson, C. A. (1996). Conduct and oppositional defiant disorders. In E. J. Mash & R. A. Barkley (Eds.), *Child psychopathology* (pp. 113–152). New York: Guilford Press.

Hinshaw, S. P., Lahey, B. B., & Hart, E. L. (1993). Issues of taxonomy and co-morbidity in the development of conduct disorder. *Development and Psychopathology, 5,* 31–50.

Hodges, V. K. (1987). Assessing children with a clinical research interview: The Child Assessment Schedule. In R. J. Prinz (Ed.), *Advances in behavioral assessment of children and families.* Greenwich, CT: JAI Press.

Hughes, J. (1990). Assessment of social skills. Sociometric and behavioral approaches. In C. R. Reynolds & R. W. Kamphaus (Eds.), *Handbook of psychological and educational assessment of children: Personality, behavior, and context* (pp. 423–444). New York: Guilford Press.

Kagan, J., & Snidman, N. (1991). Temperamental factors in human development. *American Psychologist, 46,* 856–862.

Kamphaus, R. W., & Frick, P. J. (1996). *Clinical assessment of child and adolescent personality and behavior.* Boston: Allyn & Bacon.

Kazdin, A. E. (1995). *Conduct disorders in childhood and adolescence* (2nd ed.). Thousand Oaks, CA: Sage.

Kazdin, A. E. (1998). Conduct disorder. In R. J. Morris & T. R. Kratochwill (Eds.), *The practice of child therapy, 3rd ed.* (pp. 199–230). Boston: Allyn & Bacon.

Kazdin, A. E., Esveldt-Dawson, K., French, N. H., & Unis, A. S. (1987). Problem-solving skills training and relationship therapy in the treatment of antisocial child behavior. *Journal of Consulting and Clinical Psychology, 55,* 76–85.

Kazdin, A. E., Siegal, T. C., & Bass, D. (1992). Cognitive problem-solving skills training and parent management training in the treatment of antisocial behavior in children. *Journal of Consulting and Clinical Psychology, 60,* 733–747.

Keenan, K., Loeber, R., Zhang, Q., & Stouthamer-Loeber, M. (1995). The influence of deviant peers on the development of boys' disruptive and delinquent behavior: A temporal analysis. *Development and Psychopathology, 7,* 715–726.

Keenan, K., & Shaw, D. (1997). Development and social influences on young girls' early problem behavior. *Psychological Bulletin, 121,* 95–113.

Kronenberger, W. G., & Meyer, R. G. (1996). *The child clinician's handbook.* Boston: Allyn & Bacon.

Lahey, B. B., Loeber, R., Hart, E. L., Frick, P. J., Applegate, B., Zhang, Q., Green, S. M., & Russo, M. F. (1995). Four-year longitudinal study of conduct disorders: Patterns and predictors of persistence. *Journal of Abnormal Psychology, 104,* 83–93.

Lahey, B. B., Loeber, R., Quay, H. C., Applegate, B., Shaffer, D., Waldman, I., Hart, E. L., McBurnett, K., Frick, P. J., Jensen, P. S., Dulcan, M. K., Canino, G., & Bird, H. R. (1998). Validity of *DSM-IV* subtypes of conduct disorder based on age of onset. *Journal of the American Academy of Child and Adolescent Psychiatry, 37,* 435–442.

Lahey, B. B., Loeber, R., Quay, H. C., Frick, P. J., & Grimm, J. (1992). Oppositional defiant and conduct disorders: Issues to be resolved for *DSM-IV. Journal of the American Academy of Child and Adolescent Psychiatry, 31,* 539–546.

Lilienfeld, S. O. (1998). Methodological advances and developments in the assessment of psychopathy. *Behaviour Research and Therapy, 36,* 99–125.

Lochman, J. E. (1987). Self and peer perceptions and attributional biases of aggressive and nonaggressive boys in dyadic interactions. *Journal of Consulting and Clinical Psychology, 55,* 404–410.

Lochman, J. E. (1992). Cognitive-behavioral interventions with aggressive boys: Three-year follow-up and preventive effects. *Journal of Consulting and Clinical Psychology, 60,* 426–432.

Lochman, J. E. (2001). Conduct Disorder. In W. E. Craighead & C. B. Nemeroff (Eds.), *Encyclopedia of psychology and behavioral science.* New York: Wiley.

Lochman, J. E. (In press-a). Preventive intervention with precursors to substance abuse. In W. J. Bukoski & Z. Sloboda (Eds.), *Handbook of drug abuse theory, science, and practice.* New York: Plenum Press.

Lochman, J. E. (In press-b). Parent and family skills training in targeted prevention programs for at-risk youth. *Journal of Primary Prevention.*

Lochman, J. E., & Craven, S. V. (1993, March). *Family conflict associated with reactive and proactive aggression at two age levels.* Paper presented at the biennial meeting of the Society for Research in Child and Adolescent Psychopathology, Santa Fe, NM.

Lochman, J. E., Curry, J. F., Dane, H., & Ellis, M. (In press). The Anger Coping Program: An empirically supported treatment for aggressive children. *Residential Treatment for Children and Youth.*

Lochman, J. E., & Dodge, K. A. (1998). Distorted perceptions in dyadic interactions of aggressive and nonaggressive boys: Effects of prior expectations, context, and boys' age. *Development and Psychopathology, 10,* 495–512.

Lochman, J. E., & Dodge, K. A. (1994). Social-cognitive processes of severely violent, moderately aggressive, and nonaggressive boys. *Journal of Consulting and Clinical Psychology, 62,* 366–374.

Lochman, J. E., Dunn, S. E., & Klimes-Dougan, B. (1993). An intervention and consultation model from a social-cognitive perspective: A description of the Anger Coping Program. *School Psychology Review, 22,* 456–469.

Lochman, J. E., Dunn, S. E., & Wagner, E. E. (1997). Anger. In G. Bear, K. Minke, & A. Thomas (Eds.), *Children's needs II.* Washington, DC: National Association of School Psychology.

Lochman, J. E., FitzGerald, D. P., & Whidby, J. M. (1999). Anger management with aggressive children. In C. Schaefer (Ed.), *Short-term psychotherapy groups for children* (pp. 301–349). Northvale, ND: Jason Aronson.

Lochman, J. E., & Lampron, L. B. (1986). Situational social problem-solving skills and self-esteem of aggressive and nonaggressive boys. *Journal of Abnormal Child Psychology 14,* 605–617.

Lochman, J. E., Lampron, L. B., Burch, P. R., & Curry, J. E. (1985). Client characteristics associated with behavior change for treated and untreated boys. *Journal of Abnormal Child Psychology 13,* 527–538.

Lochman, J. E., Lampron, L. B., Gemmer, T. C., & Harris, S. R. (1987). Anger-coping interventions for aggressive children: Guide to implementation in school settings. In P. A. Keller & S. Heyman (Eds.), *Innovations in clinical practice: A source book,* vol. 6 (pp. 339–356). Sarasota, FL: Professional Resource Exchange.

Lochman, J. E., Magee, T. N., & Pardini, D. (In press). Cognitive behavioral interventions for children with conduct problems. In M. Reinecke & D. Clark (Eds.), *Cognitive therapy over the lifespan: Theory, research and practice.* Cambridge, England: Cambridge University Press.

Lochman, J. E., Meyer, B. L., Rabiner, D. L., & White, K. J. (1991). Parameters influencing social problem-solving of aggressive children. In R. Prinz (Ed.), *Advances in behavioral assessment of child and families,* vol. 5 (pp. 31–63). Greenwich, CT: JAI Press.

Lochman, J. E., & Lenhart, L. A. (1993). Anger coping intervention for aggressive children: Conceptual models and outcome effects. *Clinical Psychology Review, 13,* 785–805.

Lochman, J. E., & Szczepanski, R. G. (1999). Externalizing conditions. In V. L. Schwean & D. H. Saklofske (Eds.), *Psychosocial correlates of exceptionality* (pp. 219–246). New York: Plenum Press.

Lochman, J. E., & Wayland, K. K. (1994). Aggression, social acceptance, and race as predictors of negative adolescent outcomes. *Journal of the Academy of Child and Adolescent Psychiatry, 33,* 1026–1035.

Lochman, J. E., Wayland, K. K., & White, K. K. (1993). Social goals: Relationship to adolescent adjustment and to social problem solving. *Journal of Abnormal Child Psychology, 21,* 135–151.

Lochman, J. E., & Wells, K. C. (1996). A social-cognitive intervention with aggressive children: Prevention effects and contextual implementation issues. In R. D. Peters & R. J. McMahon (Eds.), *Prevention and early intervention: Childhood disorders, substance use and delinquency* (pp. 111–143). Thousand Oaks, CA: Sage.

Lochman, J. E., Whidby, J. M., & FitzGerald, D. P. (In press). In P. C. Kendall (Ed.), *Child and adolescent therapy* (2nd ed.). New York: Guilford Press.

Lochman, J. E., White, K. J., Curry, J. F., & Rumer, R. (1992). Antisocial behavior. In V. B. Van Hasselt & D. J. Kolko (Eds.), *Inpatient behavior therapy for children and adolescents* (pp. 277–312). New York: Plenum Press.

Loeber, R. (1988). Natural histories of conduct problems, delinquency and associated substance abuse: Evidence for developmental progressions. In B. B. Lahey & A. E. Kazdin (Eds.), *Advances in clinical psychology,* vol. 11 (pp. 73–124). New York: Plenum Press.

Loeber, R. (1990). Development and risk factors of juvenile antisocial behavior and delinquency. *Clinical Psychology Review, 10,* 1–42.

Loeber, R., Brinthaupt, V. P., & Green, S. (1990). Attention deficits, impulsivity, and hyperactivity with or without conduct problems: Relationships to delinquency and unique contextual factors. In R. J. McMahon & R. D. Peters (Eds.), *Behavior disorders of adolescence: Research, intervention, and policy in clinical and school settings* (pp. 39–61). New York: Plenum Press.

Loeber, R., & Stouthamer-Loeber, M. (1986). Family factors as correlates and predictors of juvenile conduct problems and delinquency. In M. Tonry & N. Morris (Eds.), *Crime and justice* (Vol. 7, p. 29–149). Chicago: University of Chicago Press.

Loney, B., & Frick, P. J. (2000). Dual process theory: Integrating the emotional and response modulation deficit perspective of psychopathic behavior. Manuscript submitted for publication.

Loney, B. R., Frick, P. J., Ellis, M., & McCoy, M. G. (In press). Intelligence, psychopathy, and antisocial behavior. *Journal of Psychopathology and Behavioral Assessment.*

Lynam, D. R. (1996). Early identification of chronic offenders: Who is the fledgling psychopath? *Psychological Bulletin, 120,* 209–234.

Lynam, D. R. (1998). Early identification of the fledgling psychopath: Locating the psychopathic child in the current nomenclature. *Journal of Abnormal Psychology, 107,* 556–575.

Mannuzza, S., Klein, R. G., Konig, P. H., & Giampino, T. L. (1989). Hyperactive boys almost grown up. IV: Criminality and its relationship to psychiatric status. *Archives of General Psychiatry, 46,* 1073–1079.

Mccord, J., Tremblay, R. E., Vitaro, F. & Demarias-Gervais, L. (1994). Boys' disruptive behavior, school adjustment, and delinquency: The Montreal prevention experiment. *International Journal of Behavioral Development, 17,* 739–752.

McGee, R., Feehan, M., Williams, S., & Anderson, J. (1992). DSM-III disorders from age 11 to age 15 years. *Journal of the American Academy of Child and Adolescent Psychiatry, 31,* 50–59.

Miller-Johnson, S., Coie, J. D., Maumary-Gremaud, A., Lochman, J. E., & Terry, R. (1999). Relationship between childhood peer rejection and aggression and adolescent delinquency severity and type among African American youth. *Journal of Emotional and Behavioral Disorders, 7,* 137–146.

Miller-Johnson, S., Lochman, J. E., Coie, J. D., Terry, R., & Hyman, C. (1998). Comorbidity of conduct and depressive problems at sixth grade: Substance use outcomes across adolescence. *Journal of Abnormal Child Psychology, 26,* 221–232.

Moffitt, T. E. (1990). Juvenile delinquency and attention deficit disorder: Boys' developmental trajectories from age 3 to 15. *Child Development, 61,* 893–910.

Moffitt, T. E. (1993). Adolescence-limited and life-course persistent antisocial behavior: A developmental typology. *Psychological Review, 100,* 674–701.

O'Brien, B. S., & Frick, P. J. (1996). Reward dominance: Associations with anxiety, conduct problems, and psychopathy in children. *Journal of Abnormal Child Psychology, 24,* 223–240.

Offord, D. R., Adler, R. J. M., & Boyle, M. H. (1986). Prevelance and sociodemographic correlates of Conduct Disorder. *The American Journal of Social Psychiatry, 6,* 272–278.

Offord, D. R., Boyle, M. H., & Racine, Y. A. (1991). The epidemiology of antisocial behavior in childhood and adolescence. In D. J. Pepler & K. H. Rubin (Eds.), *The development and treatment of childhood aggression* (pp. 31–54). Hillsdale, NJ: Erlbaum.

Panak, W. F., & Garber, J. (1992). Role of aggression, rejection, and attributions in the prediction of depression in children. *Development and Psychopathology, 4,* 145–165.

Patterson, G. R. (1982). *Coercive family process.* Eugene, OR: Castalia.

Patterson, G. R. (1986). Performance models for antisocial boys. *American Psychologist, 41,* 432–444.

Patterson, G. R., Reid, J. B., & Dishion, T. J. (1992). *Antisocial boys.* Eugene, OR: Castalia.

Perry, D. G., Williard, J. C., & Perry, L. C. (1990). Peers' perceptions of the consequences that victimized children provide aggressors. *Child Development, 61,* 1310–1325.

Pettit, G. S., Harrist, A. W., Bates, J. E., & Dodge, K. A. (1991). Family interaction, social cognition, and children's subsequent relations with peers at kindergarten. *Journal of Social and Personal Relationships, 8,* 383–402.

Quay, H. C. (1987). Patterns of delinquent behavior. In H. C. Quay (Ed.), *Handbook of juvenile delinquency* (pp. 118–138). New York: Wiley.

Reynolds, C. R., & Kamphaus, R. W. (1992). *Behavior assessment system for children (BASC).* Circle Pines, MN: American Guidance Services.

Robins, L. N. (1978a). Study predictors of adult antisocial behavior: Replications from longitudinal studies. *Psychological Medicine, 8,* 611–622.

Robins, L. N., Tipp, J., Pryzbeck, T. (1991). Antisocial personality. In L. N. Robins & D. A. Regier (Eds.), *Psychiatric disorders in America* (pp. 224–271). New York: Free Press.

Satterfield, J. H., Hoppe, C., & Schell, A. (1982). A prospective study of delinquency in 110 adolescent boys with attention deficit disorders and 88 normal adolescent boys. *American Journal of Psychiatry, 139,* 795–798.

Shaffer, D., Fisher, P., Piacentini, J., Schwab-Stone, M., & Wicks, J. (1991). *NIMH diagnostic interview schedule for children—version 2.3.* New York: New York State Psychiatric Institute.

Silverthorn, P., & Frick, P. J. (1999). Developmental pathways to antisocial behavior: The delayed-onset pathways in girls. *Development and Psychopathology, 11,* 101–126.

Silverthorn, P., Frick, P. J., & Reynolds, R. (1999). *Timing of onset and correlates of severe conduct problems in adjudicated girls and boys.* Manuscript submitted for publication.

Tremblay, R. E., Masse, L. C., Pagani, L., & Vitaro, F. (1996). From childhood physical aggression to adolescent maladjustment. In R. D. Peters & R. J. McMahon (Eds.), *Preventing childhood disorders, substance abuse, and delinquency* (pp. 268–289). Thousand Oaks, CA: Sage.

Vissing, Y. M., Strauss, M. A., Gelles, R. J., & Harrop, J. W. (1991). Verbal aggression by parents and psychosocial problems of children. *Child Abuse and Neglect, 15,* 223–238.

Vitaro, F., Brendgen, M., Pagani, L., Tremblay, R. E., & McDuff, P. (1999). Disruptive behavior, peer association, and conduct disorder: Testing the developmental links through early intervention. *Development and Psychopathology, 11,* 287–304.

Vitaro, F., Brendgen, M., & Tremblay, R. E. (1999). Prevention of school dropout through the reduction of disruptive behaviors and school failure in elementary school. *Journal of School Psychology, 37,* 205–226.

Vitaro, F., & Tremblay, R. E. (1994). Impact of a prevention program on aggressive-disruptive children's friendships and social adjustment. *Journal of Abnormal Child Psychology, 22,* 457–475.

Webster-Stratton, C. (1994). Advancing videotape parent training: A comparison study. *Journal of Consulting and Clinical Psychology, 62,* 583–593.

Webster-Stratton, C., & Hammond, M. (1997). Treating children with early-onset conduct problems: A comparison of child and parent training interventions. *Journal of Consulting and Clinical Psychology, 65,* 93–109.

Wechsler, R. D. (1991). *Wechsler Intelligence Scale for Children—Third Edition.* New York: Psychological Corp.

Weissberg, R. P., Caplan, M. Z., & Bennetto, L. (1988). The Yale-New Haven Middle School Social Problem Solving (SPS) Program. New Haven, CT: Yale University Department of Psychology.

Wootton, J. M., Frick, P. J., Shelton, K. K., & Silverthorn, P. (1997). Ineffective parenting and childhood conduct problems: The moderating role of callous-unemotional traits. *Journal of Consulting and Clinical Psychology, 65,* 301–308.

Young, S. E., Mikulich, S. K., Goodwin, M. B., Hardy, J., Cheryl, M. L., Zoccolillo, M. S., & Crowley, T. J. (1995). Treated delinquent boys' substance use: Onset, pattern, relationship to conduct and mood disorders. *Drug and Alcohol Dependence, 37,* 149–162.

Zoccolillo, M. (1993). Gender and the development of conduct disorder. *Development and Psychopathology, 5,* 65–78.

Chapter 11

ATTENTION-DEFICIT/ HYPERACTIVITY DISORDER

CHARLES D. CASAT, DEBORAH A. PEARSON, AND
JEANETTE PIERRET CASAT

INTRODUCTION

Attention-Deficit/Hyperactivity Disorder (ADHD) is a common neuropsychiatric disorder, typically identified in childhood, with uncertain (possibly multiple) etiologies, and an overlapping symptom presentation, resulting in significant impairments in family, social, academic, and cognitive spheres. Core difficulties are found in deficiencies in age- and situation-inappropriate focusing and persistence of attention to tasks, deficiencies in impulsivity or inhibition of behavioral responding, and excessive or situationally inappropriate levels of activity (Barkley, 1998; Tannock, 1998). ADHD is the most commonly diagnosed behavioral disturbance of childhood, affecting 3% to 5% of the general, nonreferred, school-aged population, and representing more than 50% of referrals to clinics for mental health evaluations (Cantwell, 1996). This figure translates to approximately 2,000,000 children with handicapping impairment, making ADHD a significant public health problem. Males appear to have a 2.5 to 3.5 odds ratio of being diagnosed with ADHD in comparison with females in nonreferred samples, and this increases to 10 to 1 in clinical samples (Biederman, 1998). The diagnosis is more frequent in those groups with social-economic disadvantages and other family-environment risk factors (Biederman, Faraone, Mick, & Lelon, 1995). The syndrome occurs across all cultures studied. The question of overdiagnosis of ADHD in the United States has been raised frequently. For instance, in Europe the diagnosis is made at a rate approximately one fourth as frequently as in the United States. Of particular concern is the possible overapplication of the diagnosis of ADHD among ethnic minorities in the United States, and especially among African American males (Reid, 1995). ADHD often co-occurs with other significant symptoms and impairments in functioning, including learning disabilities, oppositional, conduct, and anxiety and mood symptoms, which further complicates approaches to remediative interventions.

Despite the skepticism expressed by some who question the validity of the diagnosis of ADHD, there is substantial evidence indicating a familial/genetic predisposition for the larger group of children with the disorder. An additional body of recent corroborating data from neuroimaging studies supports the hypothesis that ADHD symptoms are subsumed, in part, by demonstrable functional deficits in areas of the frontal lobes. This hypothesis is further supported by neuropsychological data indicating deficits in the frontal lobe functioning.

A variety of treatments has been tried over the past few decades, ranging from environmental manipulation to behavioral strategies, such as behavioral modification techniques; cognitive-behavioral and social skills training interventions; recreational therapy; parent training; family therapy; adjunctive medication use with a welter of different agents (some successful, many not); and implementation of specialized interventions for learning disabilities. Many treatments of questionable validity and benefit have been tried, including diet therapy, megavitamin therapy, biofeedback, visual training, sensory integration training, chiropractic training, and herbal remedies. Multimodal interventions are often recommended and are frequently necessary to meet the identified needs of individual children adequately.

Skilled, comprehensive assessment is the key to serving the needs of children with ADHD, as well as those of their families. Assessment informs further interventions; and, in turn, the interventions minimize the effects of deficits and promote healthy growth and development. Early identification is ideal; before maladaptive styles become chronic, pervasive, and resistant to change, and before secondary negative self-estimates develop that reduce motivation and result in a diminished sense of self-efficacy and personal competence. There is some sense of urgency about these efforts, as research suggests a range of negative social, educational, occupational, and mental health outcomes in adulthood for individuals with ADHD.

The balance of this chapter will focus on the particulars of identification, assessment, and interventions for children with ADHD. Etiology and causation; ethnic/cultural factors; comorbidity; biologic correlates; genetics; relevant federal laws; rating scales and assessment tools; collaboration of the child's team that includes the parent, teacher, school psychologist, physician; and treatment planning and implementation are presented. Case examples will be given to illustrate the integration of assessment with interventions.

EVOLUTION OF THE DIAGNOSIS OF ADHD

Definition of ADHD as a disorder has undergone a great deal of revision in conceptualization through the twentieth century, and especially in the last 30 years, reflecting shifting views of the disorder, its essential nature, and the postulated pathophysiology. Such shifts are mirrored in successive iterations of the *American Psychiatric Association's Diagnostic and Statistical Manuals of Mental Disorders* (*DSM,* American Psychiatric Association 1968, 1980, 1987, 1994). An early reference to children with notable characteristics of aggression, defiance, and lack of "inhibitory volition" occurring before 8 years of age, is found in a paper by Still (1902). Focus for many years revolved around those children with evidences of brain injury, and with sequelae of overactivity, poor attention and concentration, and an impulsivity uncharacteristic for most children of like age. By the 1950s, there was a shift toward emphasis on milder, undetected events, such as birth trauma—early infectious, toxic, or traumatic brain insults that were thought to manifest during later development as difficulties in behavioral control and learning deficiencies (Pasamanack, Rogers, & Lilienfeld, 1956). This view gave rise to the term *minimal brain damage*. Although evidence for such brain insult remained elusive in most cases, this term remained prominent throughout the 1950s and 1960s, with an eventual shift of the concept toward the idea of a *minimal brain dysfunction*. Such a conceptualization was fueled by the work of Laufer, Denhoff, & Solomons (1957), who coined the term *hyperkinetic impulse disorder* and hypothesized an underlying neurological deficit centered in the thalamus. Eventually, this view of undetected brain damage was widely challenged (Birch, 1964, Rutter, 1977), although the emphasis on the excessive impulsivity activity levels was codified in the *DSM-II* (APA, 1968) as the Hyperkinetic Reaction of Childhood Disorder and remained until 1980.

During the 1970s there was a remarkable expansion of empirical research on ADHD, with the publication of almost 2,000 studies by the end of the decade (Barkley, 1998). This new interest was accompanied by the shift away from the preoccupation in the field on some sort of underlying brain damage and a consequent emphasis on motor hyperactivity toward a focus on inattentiveness and distractibility as the core deficits that characterized children with this disorder. The accompanying rise in the use of symptom rating scales (Conners, 1969; Goyette, Conners, & Ulrich, 1978; Werry & Sprague, 1970) was important in achieving a beginning comparability between findings of various studies. Equally, the emergence of criterion-based diagnosis (APA, 1980; Loney, 1983) was an important advance in the study of the nature of ADHD and its treatment. As a result of the operationalization of criteria, a subtyping of Attention Deficit Disorder emerged during the 1980s with separation into Attention Deficit Disorder with Hyperactivity (+H) or without Hyperactivity (–H). A parallel line of research by Dykman and colleagues during this period (Dykman, Ackerman, & Holcomb, 1985) led to distinguishing children with ADHD from those with learning disability (LD) or a combination of the two deficits.

With publication of the *DSM-III-R* (APA, 1987) the previous subtyping of ADD into with Hyperactivity and without Hyperactivity was eliminated in favor of a system that offered 14 criterion symptoms and a single threshold (8 or more symptoms present) required to establish diagnosis. Despite *DSM-III-R* reversion to a unitary set of criteria, the late 1980s and early 1990s saw a continued interest in investigation of possible subtyping of ADHD. A series of studies during that period suggested the validity of with Hyperactivity and without Hyperactivity differentiation (Lahey et al., 1994). Largely as a result of those investigations, the *DSM-IV* (APA, 1994) again classified attention deficit disorder with reference to predominantly inattentive type, predominantly hyperactive type, or combined type. Extensive empirical study was undertaken in preparation for the new ADHD criteria prior to release of the *DSM-IV*, with the generation of descriptors selected by factor analyses and field testing of the proposed criteria at multiple sites in North America. Subsequent study comparisons of *DSM-III-R* and *DSM-IV* diagnoses of ADHD have corroborated the validity of the inattentive, hyperactive/impulsive, and combined subtypes (Morgan, Hynd, Riccio, & Hall, 1996). Further, a high level of correlation (93%, $p < 0001$) is reported between those individuals who received a *DSM-III-R* diagnosis of ADHD who also received a *DSM-IV* diagnosis of ADHD, thus confirming good diagnostic continuity between the two classification systems (Biederman et al., 1997).

Current Concepts of ADHD

Table 11.1 lists the *DSM-IV* criteria for the diagnosis of ADHD. Diagnosis is established by the presence of a minimum of 6 of 9 criterion symptoms from either the Inattentive Type or Overactive/Impulsive Type, or by the presence of a minimum of 6 symptoms from each group for the Combined Type. To achieve *caseness* for ADHD, there must additionally be demonstration that the difficulties have persisted for a minimum

Table 11.1   *DSM-IV* Diagnostic Criteria for ADHD

A. Either (1) or (2)

Six or more symptoms that have persisted for at least 6 months to a degree that is maladaptive and inconsistent with developmental level:

1. Inattentive Type:
   1. Often fails to give close attention to details or makes careless mistakes in schoolwork
   2. Often has difficulty in sustaining attention in tasks or play activities
   3. Often does not seem to listen when spoken to directly
   4. Often does not follow through on instructions and fails to finish work
   5. Often has difficulty in organizing tasks or activities
   6. Often avoids or dislikes tasks that require sustained mental effort
   7. Often loses things necessary for tasks or play activities
   8. Often is easily distracted by extraneous stimuli
   9. Often is forgetful in daily activities

2. Hyperactive-Impulsive Type:
   1. Often fidgets with hands or feet or squirms in seat
   2. Often leaves seat in classroom or other situations where remaining seated is expected
   3. Often runs about or climbs excessively in situations where it is inappropriate
   4. Often has difficulty in play or engaging in leisure activities quietly
   5. Often is "on the go" or often acts as if "driven by a motor"
   6. Often talks excessively
   7. Often blurts out answers before the questions have been completed
   8. Often has difficulty awaiting turn
   9. Often interrupts or intrudes on others

B. Some inattentive or hyperactive/impulsive symptoms were present before age 7 years

C. Some impairment from the symptoms is present in two or more settings

D. There must be evidence of clinically significant impairment in social, academic or occupational functioning

E. The symptoms do not occur exclusively during the course of a Pervasive Developmental Disorder, Schizophrenia, or Other Psychotic disorder and are not better accounted for by another mental disorder (e.g., Mood Disorder, Anxiety Disorder, Dissociative Disorder, or a Personality Disorder)

Code Based on Type:

314.00 Attention Deficit/Hyperactivity Disorder, Predominately Inattentive Type

314.01 Attention Deficit/Hyperactivity Disorder, Predominately Hyperactive-Impulsive Type

314.01 Attention Deficit/Hyperactivity Disorder Combined Type (If both A1 and A2 are met).

of 6 months, that they are cross-situational (that is, that they occur in two or more domains of the child's life, such as at home and at school), and that there is interference with functioning in one or more important areas of the child's life. Although the importance of age of onset has been disputed recently (Barkley & Biederman, 1997), presence of some symptoms of ADHD must be apparent before 7 years of age. As pointed out earlier, the *DSM-IV* expands on the idea that the core symptoms revolve around inattention and distractibility and their consequences, although the presence of a subtype of ADHD with predominating symptoms of hyperactivity and/or social impulsivity is acknowledged.

There is a limited literature on gender-related differences in ADHD. The literature is clear on the preponderance of males in clinically referred samples (10.1), perhaps in part because of the higher levels of aggression in males that drive the referral process (Biederman, 1998). Recently published work by Sharp et al. (1999) has indicated that among a selected sample of girls with ADHD Combined Type, the symptoms were indistinguishable from those of previously studied boys with ADHD, and that response to stimulant medication is comparable. There is also a suggestion that there is a higher familial prevalence of ADHD in the relatives of girls with ADHD, but this requires additional replication and extension. The potential for underidentification of ADHD in girls and the later arrival in treatment requires further examination, as it has substantial outcome implications (Arnold, 1996; Biederman, 1998).

Differences in functioning can be demonstrated between school children with and without ADHD, and between the ADHD diagnostic subtypes. Those children with the combined subtype of ADHD have more difficulties in severity and pervasiveness of symptoms (Gaub & Carlson, 1997a). More severe symptoms also correlate with conditions of greater psychosocial adversity, such as living in low-income families, having fathers with alcohol abuse problems, higher levels of family dysfunction, and more psychiatric comorbidity, especially with disruptive behavioral disorders (Biederman et al., 1997; Scahill et al., 1999). These findings suggest that adverse conditions may play a part in the perpetuation of symptoms and in the development of other, especially externalizing, disorders in ADHD children (August, Braswell, & Thuras, 1998).

The diagnostic criteria for ADHD are said to be polythetic, that is, that any six of nine symptoms within either group are sufficient to render a diagnosis, creating a situation wherein the symptoms of children with the same ADHD diagnosis may appear significantly different. Using positive and negative predictive values, symptom utility estimates have been derived for the criterion symptoms of ADHD, as seen in Table 11.1. All are quite robust and indicate that a high degree of differentiation is achievable with the *DSM-IV* criteria.

A conceptual model for understanding ADHD that has received considerable attention in recent years is that of Barkley (1997). Barkley focuses on ADHD primarily as a disorder of inhibition of behavioral responses. This may manifest in difficulties in resisting highly determined (prepotent) responses, in the orderly cessation of ongoing responses, and/or of poor management of interfering (distracting) stimuli. In contrast to recent, atheoretical, empirically based conceptualizations, Barkley's model draws upon the work of Bronowski, among others (Barkley, 1997), and sets forth a unifying theory of dysfunction in cortical (primarily prefrontal lobe) executive functioning. Barkley identified four key executive functions (a) nonverbal working memory, (b) verbal working memory (as internalization of speech), (c) the self-regulation of affect/ motivation/arousal, and (d) reconstitution, which have in common that they are covert, internalized forms of behavior (pp. 154–155). Intact capacity for response inhibition is necessary to permit change through internalization of trial action sequences. In Barkley's model, it is response inhibition that is deficient, leading to faulty behavioral inhibition control that negatively impacts the 4 key executive functions, which in turn produce observable performance deficit outcomes such as the following (p. 237):

1. Disinhibited task-irrelevant responses
2. Impaired execution of goal-directed responses
3. Limited novelty/complexity of motor responses
4. Insensitivity to response feedback
5. Diminished goal-directed persistence
6. Behavioral inflexibility
7. Reduced task re-engagement following disruption
8. Poor control of behavior by internally represented information

Further deficits are noted in ADHD children (pp. 238ff)

1. Delays in development of internalization of speech
2. Deficits in forethought and anticipatory set
3. Impaired sense of time—the future and temporal durations
4. Diminished self-reflection
5. Deficits in hindsight
6. Deficient cross-temporal organization of behavior
7. Defective capacity for sequencing of events and responses to them
8. Limitation of imitation and vicarious learning
9. Deficient compliance with rules and instructions
10. Delays in the development of conscience and moral reasoning
11. Impairment in self-regulation of emotions and arousal
12. Impairments in social perspective taking
13. Deficiency in sustaining task motivation without immediate reinforcers
14. Deficient suppression of irrelevant motor actions during goal-directed tasks

Recent evidence from neuroimaging studies has supported the notion of frontal lobe dysfunction in ADHD. Imaging methods include structural imaging and functional imaging techniques. Structural neuroimaging techniques include computerized tomography (CT) and structural magnetic resonance imaging (sMRI) techniques, and functional neuroimaging techniques include positron emission tomography (PET), single positron emission tomography (SPECT; Zametkin & Liotta, 1997), functional magnetic resonance imaging (fMRI; Casey et al., 1997), and magnetic source imaging (MSI, Breier et al., 1999). While some studies failed to detect differences between ADHD and control subjects (Zametkin & Liotta, 1997), other reports (Casey et al., 1997; Castellanos et al., 1996) have demonstrated significant loss of right/left caudate asymmetry, a smaller right globus pallidus, and a small right frontal volume in the ADHD group, compared with normal, age-matched controls. This volumetric reversal in caudate nucleus assymetry has recently been reconfirmed in a study by Semrud-Clikeman et al. (2000). Casey et al. (1997) found performance on a laboratory task of inhibition correlated with measures of prefrontal cortex, caudate, and globus pallidus. Functional MRI in 7 adolescent males with ADHD and 9 control subjects engaged in a task requiring inhibition of a planned motor response (stop task) revealed subnormal activation of the right inferior prefrontal cortex and left caudate in the ADHD subjects (Rubia et al., 1999). Functional imaging studies with SPECT are not currently available for children. However, PET results have been reported. For instance, Zametkin et al. (1993) reported decreases in brain metabolism in selected areas among adolescents with ADHD. Improvement in this technology may encourage future studies and further elucidate pathophysiology using this methodology. Although the use of PET and SPECT procedures with young children is limited by their use of radioactive isotopes, other techniques such as fMRI are completely noninvasive, and as such have considerable promise for use with young children.

Genetic studies have provided further evidence for the neurobiological basis of ADHD. The familial linkage was first demonstrated by Cantwell (1972) and Morrison and Stewart (1973) in separate studies that reported higher rates of ADHD in the biological parents than among the adoptive parents of adopted children with ADHD. Several twin studies have given evidence of genetic contributions to ADHD; both Neuman et al. (1999) and Goodman and Stevenson (1989) reported greater concordance of ADHD in monozygotic than in dizygotic twins. To date, no agreement has been reached on the mode of inheritance, although there is general consensus that ADHD inheritance is genetically complex, with heterogeneity and influences from environmental factors (Neuman et al., 1999).

Recent molecular genetics studies have suggested an association between ADHD and several dopamine receptor genes (DRD2, DRD4, and possibly DRD5), with a repeat variant allele in subjects with ADHD compared to controls (Cook et al., 1995; Smalley et al., 1998; Daly et al., 1999; Faraone et al., 1999). The significance of the repeat allele is not completely understood, but it represents a type of genetic mutation that has been identified in as many as 20 diseases in the last decade (Margolis et al., 1999). Expanded repeat alleles are either in gene segments that are transcribed and remain represented in mature RNA, or are transcribed but then excised from the primary RNA. Such repeat expansions, when they occur, tend to be unstable, becoming longer with successive generations, and have been termed *expansion mutations*. The work of Faraone et al. (1999) suggests an association between the DRD4 gene with 7-repeat allele and ADHD, although it is too early to consider the DRD4 as a positive marker for ADHD. Other genes potentially implicated in the transmission of vulnerability to ADHD include dopamine beta hydroxylase (DBH; Day et al., 1999), and the dopamine transporter gene (DAT1; Winsberg & Comings, 1999). Winsberg and Comings have suggested an association between DAT1 and methylphenidate response. This evidence remains tentative, but anticipates future investigations.

Comorbidity of ADHD and other Conditions

Both epidemiologic studies and clinical practice have shown evidences of high rates of comorbidity between ADHD and other psychiatric disorders (Angold & Costello, 1993, Biederman et al., 1991, Spencer et al., 1999). In clinical practice, the rate of comorbidity is especially high, in part because of the selective nature of the referrals. Explanations for the high rates of comorbidity include suggestions of genetic/familial predisposition and low birth weight vulnerability. The comorbidity may also be inflated by halo effects that occur when information is gathered by rating scales, and by overlapping of symptoms especially with regard to externalizing disorders, such as Oppositional Defiant Disorder and Conduct Disorder (Abikoff, Courtney, Pelham, & Koplowicz, 1993). Analysis of the overlap of symptoms of ADHD and internalizing disorders, such as Generalized Anxiety Disorder (GAD), Bipolar Disorder (BPD) and Major Depressive Disorder (MDD), showed that the influence of shared symptoms is small: 75% of GAD, 79% of MDD, and 56% of BPD diagnoses were maintained after the overlapping ADHD symptoms were removed (Biederman, Faraone, Mick, Moore, & Lelon, 1996; Biederman, Faraone, Mick, & Lelon, 1995; Milberger, Biederman, Faraone, Murphy, & Tsuang, 1995). Comorbidity is seen with internalizing disorders, such as anxiety and mood disorders, externalizing disorders (including Oppositional Defiant Disorder and Conduct Disorder), and additionally with Tourette's syndrome (Comings & Comings, 1993) and Specific Learning Disorders (Biederman, Faraone, Milberger, et al., 1996; Faraone, Biederman, Lehman, et al., 1993; Chen, Faraone, Biederman, & Tsuang, 1994). In mental health settings, there is high level of overlap of ADHD with Oppositional Defiant Disorder (30–67%, August, Realmuto, MacDonald, Nugent, & Crosby, 1996; Carlson, Tamm, & Gaub, 1997; Kuhne, Schachar, & Tannock, 1997; Spencer, Biederman, & Wilens, 1999). This combination of symptoms is thought to predispose to the development of Conduct Disorder and later to Antisocial Personality Disorder. Further, vulnerability to the development of substance abuse is thought to be mediated through conduct disorder and later antisocial personality disorder (Tartar, 1988; Biederman, Wilens, et al., 1997; Kandel et al., 1997; Aytaclar et al., 1999; Chilcoat & Breslau, 1999).

ADHD is also one of most common behavioral disorders seen in children with mild to moderate mental retardation (MR), with prevalence rates estimated at 9% to 33% of children in special education classrooms (Ando & Yoshimura, 1978; Das & Melnyk, 1989; Epstein, Cullinan, & Gadow, 1986; Hunt & Cohen, 1988; Pearson, Norton, & Farwell, 1997). Interestingly, a recent study (Pearson et al., in press) demonstrated that children with MR and ADHD have a similar pattern of psychiatric comorbidity that is found in children with ADHD in the general school-aged population. These children also have high rates of symptoms of anxiety, depression, learning difficulties (even relative to other children with mental retardation), social problems, and family problems. Although ADHD is so common in this population, it is only within the last decade that more has become known about ADHD in children with MR (Pearson et al., 1997; Pearson et al., 1996), due in large part to the fact that subaverage intelligence (IQ level

< 80) was traditionally used as an exclusion criterion in studies of ADHD (Barkley, 1990a; Gadow & Poling, 1988) prior to that point.

In recent years there has been an intense interest in the relationship between ADHD and comorbid Bipolar Disorder (Bowring & Kovacs, 1992; Wozniak et al., 1995; Biederman, Faraone, et al., 1997), with estimates of comorbid occurrence being as high as 21% in a tertiary clinical setting. Although it is likely that there is such a comorbidity, the numbers may be inflated by methods of case determination, by the clinical setting from which the sample is drawn, and by a lack of commonly agreed-upon symptoms for defining Bipolar Disorder, especially among prepubertal children. Prospective studies of the offspring of lithium-responding parents currently underway at several sites in the United States may eventually elucidate this relationship. In the interim, clinicians should be conservative in applying the label of Bipolar Disorder to children with ADHD.

The potential for occurrence of comorbid conditions in children with ADHD underscores the requirement for comprehensive assessment methods, with careful inquiry in areas of symptoms and functioning apart from those relating to ADHD. As comorbidity can influence treatment response and eventual outcome, clinicians must have an acute awareness of this possibility in assessment, treatment planning, interventions, and counseling advice to parents.

ADHD Comorbidity with Specific Learning Disabilities

The clinician should exercise particular diligence in practicing awareness of the high co-occurrence of learning disabilities and ADHD. A learning disability is defined by Fletcher, Shaywitz, and Shaywitz (1999) as a disorder of cognition that manifests itself as a problem in understanding and using spoken or written language. Learning disabilities encompass disorders of listening, thinking, talking, reading, writing, spelling, and doing arithmetic. Specific Reading Disorder (SRD, still referred to as dyslexia) is the most common learning disorder in childhood, with an estimated prevalence of 5% to 17.5% (Shaywitz, 1998). Reading difficulty is familial, with a heritability rate of 23% to 65% among children of a parent with SRD. There is MRI evidence of functional disruption of neural systems underlying SRD, with underactivation in Wernicke's area, the angular gyrus, and the striate cortex, and overactivation of the inferior frontal gyrus (Shaywitz et al., 1998). While SRD is the most common and best studied of the specific learning disorders, the category also includes other specific learning disorders such as Specific Arithmetic Disorder, and Specific Writing Disorder (APA, 1994). There is an estimated comorbidity of 20% to 80% between ADHD and learning disorders (Cantwell & Baker, 1991; DuPaul & Stoner, 1994, Fletcher et al., 1999). Recent work by Klorman et al. (1999) using neuropsychological testing methods has shown that executive functioning deficits in ADHD are separate from those of SRD. This work is substantiated by another study of Purvis and Tannock (1997) using a method requiring subject recall of a lengthy narrative. Results indicated that the subjects with ADHD had higher-order executive functioning deficits, whereas the SRD group had deficits in basic semantics of language processing, and the comorbid ADHD/SRD group exhibited both deficits. It has been suggested that there is a causal connection between SRD and ADHD. Studies using structural equation modeling analysis have concluded that it is likely the ADHD symptom of inattentiveness plays a part in the occurrence of SRD, whereas conversely, the contribution of SRD to ADHD may also be detected (Rowe & Rowe, 1992). To date, no study has answered the question definitively, although there is inference that the relationship may indeed be reciprocal (DuPaul & Stoner, 1994; Fletcher et al., 1999).

Clinical Assessment of ADHD

Thorough evaluation is central to the development of a thoughtful and individualized treatment plan for intervention for the child or adolescent with ADHD. In this case, assessment must be multi-informant, multitrait, and multimodal to be valid. Major elements of the assessment include review of past medical and educational records, gathering of observations and standardized information from the child's teachers and parents, an interview with the parent or guardian, and a developmentally appropriate interview with the child. If there is need or indication, further medical or educational evaluation may be required to complete the assessment.

Parent Interview

The parent is the person who generally will have the most information about the child. As pointed out by Dulcan and the American Academy of Child and Adolescent Work Group on Quality Issues (1997), inquiry should be made regarding the following:

1. Reasons for seeking evaluation at this time
2. *DSM-IV* symptoms of ADHD, duration of symptoms, and resulting impairment, including school, family, and peers
3. *DSM-IV* symptoms of comorbid (or alternate) psychiatric diagnoses, including possible substance abuse
4. History of pediatric, psychologic, psychiatric, or neurological treatment for ADHD, including medication trials
5. Developmental history, including evidences of deficits or lags
6. Parenting style and disciplinary attitudes
7. Past parental attempts at behavioral management for identified difficulties
8. Medical history, including seizures, thyroid disease, head trauma, genetic or metabolic disorder, lead exposure, fetal alcohol exposure, use of medications that might cause the symptoms (such as theophylline, antihistaminics, steroids, etc.)
9. Family history of psychiatric disorders (including ADHD), tic disorders, neurologic disorders, substance abuse, and developmental and specific learning disorders
10. Current family situation, including changes in family constellation, family stressors, and crises
11. Summary explanation of the benefits parent wishes to come out of the evaluation for the child and family

Interview with the Child

The interview with the child should include the development of a working trust and rapport, and a developmentally appropriate inquiry and observational assessment of the following:

1. Orientation and style of adaptation to the office environment
2. Observable symptoms of ADHD
3. The child's perception of his/her performance at home, with parents, siblings, and other family members
4. The child's perceptions of academic achievement and competence, cooperation with the teacher and other authority figures, peer relations, and acceptance
5. The child's ability to identify and manage emotions and affects
6. The child's capacity for self-monitoring and self-regulation
7. Symptoms of other disorders, such as
   a. Defiance, obstructiveness, and withholding
   b. Irritability and aggression
   c. Anxiety
   d. Obsessive tendencies
   e. Sadness, withdrawal
   f. Oddities of speech, language, thought content
   g. Tics, stereotypies, or oddities of behaviors
8. Fine and gross motor coordination
9. Clinical impression of intelligence

Documentation of Physical Health

Physical health history and health within the past 12 months must be documented as a part of the evaluation. This should include information on chronic medical conditions, head trauma, physical evidences of possible abuse, immunizations, medications, and visual and hearing acuity. When a high level of suspicion warrants, further medical and/or neurological examination may be indicated and should be arranged through the family's physician, or through a health department.

School Information

School records and teacher observations constitute invaluable sources of information vital to establishing the cross-setting symptoms and difficulties. This information might include the following:

1. Verbal reports of behavior, personal classroom organization, peer relations, social skills, and academic progress
2. Results of individual and standardized academic achievement testing
3. Results and recommendations from other speech and language, occupational therapy, Individuals with Disabilities Education Act (IDEA), or Section 504 evaluations

Use of Rating Scales

Rating scales represent attempts to gather standardized observations of various aspects of the child's functioning and behavior. The best scales are reliable, valid, and treatment-sensitive. Their use increases the scope of information gathered and allows beginning comparison of a child's age-scaled behaviors with those of like-aged children. As noted by Conners (1998), the advantages of rating scales include the following:

1. They extend the evaluator's base of information in a cost-efficient manner.
2. They capture data on infrequent behaviors that might not occur in a single interview.
3. They are standardized in terms of methodical inquiry.
4. The most useful instruments have extensive norming by sex and age.

Rating scales also have disadvantages:

1. *Leniency errors* or *severity errors,* which represent forms of rater bias
2. *Halo errors,* in which the rater responds to other items biased by the rater's judgement on a particular behavioral item
3. *Recency error,* in which the rater is influenced by the most current observations
4. *Test/re-test errors,* in which the rater shows inconsistency in assigning rating values across a span of time
5. *Inter-rater errors,* wherein two raters may concurrently rate the same behavior differently

The obvious caveat regarding rating scales is that they must not be solely relied upon to establish a diagnosis of ADHD. There is always the possibility of false-positive and false-negative identification that results from over-reliance on the use of rating scales, and eventuates in false labeling or overlooking of treatment needs. Nonetheless, rating scales should play a legitimate and constant role in evaluation and treatment monitoring when used in concert with other sources of information about the child.

Rating scales may be classified generally into broad-band scales and narrow-band scales, according to the scope of focus of each. While the list is not exhaustive, examples of broad-band instruments include the Child Behavior Checklist, and the Teacher Report Form (Achenbach, 1991), the parent and teacher versions of the Behavioral Assessment System for Children (Reynolds & Kamphaus, 1992), and the Personality Inventory for Children (PIC; Lachar, 2000). Each of theses instruments uses multiple behavioral descriptors that are respondent-scored on a Likert-type scale, and all have extensive psychometrics. The results are generally stated in terms of T-scores (a mean of 50 and a standard deviation of 10) and percentile ranks, for estimation of internalizing and externalizing problems. Additionally, these measures have subscales that identify narrower-range attributes such as aggression, inattentiveness, anxiety, withdrawal/depression, and so forth. The value of these broad-band rating scales lies in their ability to survey a wide range of behaviors, thus fulfilling the multitrait demand characteristic of a good evaluation approach. The interested professional should become well acquainted with one or more of these broad-band screening instruments for work with children and adolescents.

Narrow-band rating scales are generally constructed to address only one area of behavior. Scales may be found for measurement of attention, overactivity, impulsivity, anxiety, depression, obsessive-compulsive traits, and more. As with the broad-band scales, these have an important use in systematic gathering of information both to aid in decision-making for diagnosis and treatment planning, and for monitoring the progress of interventions. Examples of such scales used for ADHD are the Conners Abbreviated Parent Rating Scale, Conners Abbreviated Teacher Rating Scale, IOWA Conners Rating Scale, ACTeRS, SNAP, DuPaul Rating Scale, and TOVA (Barkley, 1990b, Hinshaw, 1994). Norms are available for each scale, and psychometrics have been evaluated for reliability and validity.

Concern has been raised about potential overestimation of ADHD risk when narrow-band scales are applied to minority populations. Recent studies have noted a variant factor structure for the Conners Teacher Rating Scale (Reid et al., 1998), suggesting the scale does not fit white and minority populations equally well. Casat, Reid, Norton, Anastopoulos, and Temple (2000) found there was an odds ratio of 2.5 times higher likelihood of an African American male exceeding the threshold of 2.0 SD on the IOWA Conners than for Caucasian males in a survey sample of 3,997 urban elementary school children. This issue is of particular importance when using screeners as a means of risk identification in school-based mental health programs, because nearly half of the student population in the largest metropolitan areas comprises culturally different groups (American Council on Education, 1988).

Neuropsychological Tests

Numerous pneuropsychological tests have been employed to study components of attention in research studies investigating ADHD. These include Matching Familiar Figures Test, Stroop Test, Porteus Mazes, Paired Associate Learning Test, Tower of Hanoi, and Wisconsin Card Sort Test. Although use of these instruments has helped to clarify the functional deficits associated with ADHD, and although the instruments are correlated with other indicators of ADHD, they are not diagnostic per se, and have limited use in clinical settings (DuPaul, Anastopoulos, Shelton, Guevremont, & Metevin, 1992; Cantwell, 1996). Similarly, there was a significant use of the Freedom from Distractibility (FFD) Factor, derived from WISC-R subtests, comprised of Arithmetic, Digit Span, and Coding. The FFD received equivocal endorsement for identification of ADHD (Barkley, 1990b; Rispens et al., 1997).

With the development of the WISC-III, a four-factor structure has been endorsed, with realignment of subtests and the designation of a new subtest, the Symbol Search, that is included in the new Processing Speed factor, together with Coding. The FFD factor remains on the WISC-III and is derived from the Arithmetic and Digit Span subtests. Although the WISC-III *Manual* (Wechsler, 1991, p. 214) and some investigations (Mayes, Calhoun, & Crowell, 1998; Mealer, Morgan, & Luscomb, 1996) suggest that children with ADHD have deficits relative to their peers on the FFD factor, there is considerable controversy regarding the ability of the FFD factor to detect attention problems and to serve as a screening factor for ADHD. For instance, Reinecke, Beebe, and Stein (1999) and Riccio et al. (1997) note that the FFD factor does not correlate with other measures of attention, and that low scores on the FFD factor are also associated with other problems, such as learning disabilities and academic failure. Given this situation, although a review of WISC-III subtests is often helpful in identifying specific functional deficits, it is not recommended that the FFD factor be used for diagnostic purposes. In fact, even the WISC-III *Manual* does not recommend using WISC-III profiles for this purpose (Wechsler, 1991).

Other Clinical Tests

Currently the diagnosis of ADHD is established through clinical means; no laboratory tests are available to corroborate the diagnosis. Versions of the computerized Continuous Performance Task (CPT) have been employed by some (e.g., Gordon, 1986) as a part of the ADHD diagnostic process to measure response times, inclusion errors, and exclusion errors that correlate with characteristics of children with ADHD, and especially those with the Overactive/Impulsive and Combined types. Despite the CPT's popularity as a research tool, its relationship to the sustained attention deficits observed in ADHD, and hence its application to clinical practice, remains unclear (Corkum & Siegel, 1993). Similarly, miniaturized actometry, available in the form of nondominant wrist-attachable devices, may be used to measure movements. Correlations with ADHD children's activity levels are found in the quantification of recorded movements across time periods during the day and during sleep. However, as with the CPT, actometry is largely a research measure not to be used in diagnosis, although it may be used rarely in the adjustment of a child's medication regimen. A list of commonly used psychological tests and rating scales is found in Table 11.2.

TREATMENT PLANNING

The *DSM-IV* endorses multiaxial assessment in five domains, each of which contains complementary information that is pertinent to understanding the individual patient within a comprehensive, biopsychosocial conceptual model (APA, 1994). Assessment encompasses rendering of primary diagnoses according to the 5 axes

- Axis I   Principal clinical disorder; other disorders that may be the focus of clinical attention
- Axis II   Personality disorders: mental retardation
- Axis III   General medical disorders that may affect the current picture
- Axis IV   Psychosocial and environmental problems
- Axis V   Global assessment of functioning (GAF) currently and in the past 1 year

Use of the multixial system promotes systematic consideration of the symptoms, related medical conditions, environmental and psychosocial influences, and level of functional

Table 11.2 Examples of Test Instruments, Diagnostic Interviews, and Rating Scales Used in Comprehensive Evaluation of Children and Adolescents Presenting with Symptoms of ADHD

A. *Intellectual Assessment*

Wechsler Intelligence Scale for Children–3rd Edition (WISC-III), ages 6–16 or

Stanford-Binet Intelligence Scale–4th Edition

B. *Language Screening*

Peabody Picture Vocabulary Test–3rd Edition (PPVT-III), receptive language

Expressive One-Word Picture Vocabulary Test (EOWPVT), expressive language

C. *Visual Motor Integration*

Beery Developmental Test of Visual Motor Integration (Beery VMI)

D. *Academic Achievement (to rule out LD)*

Screening: Wide Range Achievement Test–3rd Edition (WRAT-III)

In-depth: Woodcock-Johnson–Revised (WJ-R) or

Peabody Individual Achievement Test (PIAT) or

Wechsler Individual Achievement Test (WIAT)

E. *Neuropsychological Functioning*

Trail Making Test (A & B)

Continuous Performance Test

Purdue Pegboard

F. *Adaptive Functioning*

Vineland Adaptive Behavior Scales

G. *Parent Behavioral Questionnaires*

Conners Parent Rating Scale (CPRS; primarily ADHD-related symptomatology)

Child Behavior Checklist (CBCL; multidimensional screening)

Personality Inventory for Children–3rd edition (PIC-R; multidimensional screening, also includes informant response style scales and info regarding cognitive style of child and family relations)

Behavioral Assessment System for Children (BASC)

H. *Teacher Behavioral Questionnaires*

Conners Teacher Rating Scale (CTRS, primarily ADHD-related symptomatology)

Teacher Report Form (TRF, multidimensional screening)

Behavioral Assessment System for Children (BASC)

I. *Projective Measures*

Roberts Apperception Test

Thematic Apperception Test

J. *Structured and Semistructured Diagnostic Interviews*

Kiddie Schedule for Affective Disorders and Schizophrenia (K-SADS)

Diagnostic Interview for Children and Adolescents–IV (DICA-IV)

Diagnostic Interview Schedule for Children–IV (DISC-IV)

Child and Adolescent Psychiatric Assessment (CAPA)

K. *Ratings of Psychopathological Severity*

Child and Adolescent Functional Rating Scale (CAFAS)

Children's Global Assessment Scale (C-GAS)

impairment and facilitates treatment planning. It should be noted that learning and communication disorders are entered on Axis I, whereas mental retardation is recorded on Axis II. The DSM axes are completed by the professional individual or team leader. Professionals should be thoroughly familiar with the structure and use of the *DSM-IV.*

Treatment planning is also a part of assessment, utilizing all information gathered earlier from the multimodal, multi-informant, multimethod inquiry, coming to a comprehensive identification of the patient and his/her family's problems, needs, and relevant child and family strengths. Ideally, treatment planning should include the presence of professionals from multiple disciplines. However, in practice this ideal is often substituted by the availability of reports from several individuals. This process should produce a written master treatment plan (MTP) that identifies diagnoses on all axes; a list of treatment needs and goals, together with a list of interventions for addressing the identified needs; and a list of those designated to carry out each part of the treatment plan. The MTP should also have a timeline for reviewing progress toward achieving those goals. The parent/guardian must be a part of the MTP process. This will ensure that the needs and goals selected by the professionals suit the needs and goals of the family, which will enhance treatment participation and compliance with recommendations and therapies by empowering the family as a full partner in the changes that must occur.

Special Treatment Planning Considerations in School Settings

The federal government has several relevant acts that require schools to comply with assessment, due process for involvement of families, treatment planning and documentation that must be adhered to for children with disabilities identified in primary and secondary educational settings. These include provisions of the Individuals with Disabilities Education Act (IDEA, 1975, re-enacted in 1997), and Section 504 of the Rehabilitation Act of 1973. IDEA establishes the rights of children with a variety of handicaps to an appropriate education and to necessary related services. The law mandates the evaluation of educational needs and the development of an individualized educational plan (IEP) for each qualified student. A multidisciplinary team must conduct educational, psychological, medical, and social-work evaluations. It specifies 11 categories of handicapping, including Seriously Emotionally Disturbed (SED), Specific Learning Disability, and Other Health Impaired (OHI). IDEA provides for a wide range of services, including speech and language therapy, occupational and physical therapy, diagnostic and school health services, counseling and transportation.

Whereas IDEA provides needed services outside the regular classroom setting, Section 504 of the Rehabilitation Act of 1973 requires evaluation and analysis of student needs with respect to those things required in regular education, with reasonable accommodations in the classroom to provide equal access to educational opportunities. Section 504 does not require an IEP, but a Student Accommodation Plan should be developed. Components of a Student Accommodation Plan might include (a) instructional modifications to improve attention, work production, and social adjustment, (b) behavioral management for problematic situations, (c) instruction in study strategies or social skills, (d) consultation with parents, (e) instructional aids (computer-assisted instruction), (f) alternative discipline method, (g) modified assessment procedures, and (h) monitoring medication and providing physician feedback. This act provides protection against discrimination on the basis of one's disability. Subpart D governs participation in preschool, elementary, and secondary school programs, and has a significant impact on the school district's responsibilities to provide a free and appropriate public education for all students with disabilities.

Integrating Treatment with Assessment

Interventions must begin with a review of the information available and the identified needs arising from the assessment process. The clinician must meet with the parents to review this information, and together a hierarchy of treatment goals must be established. Two immediate goals stand out (a) to educate the family about the nature of the difficulties and to answer the inevitable questions of concerned parents, and (b) to establish a rapport with child and family that will facilitate the cooperative implementation. Most parents are interested in cooperating with the proffered recommendations but may harbor anxieties about the adequacy of their parenting and their own contributions to the genesis of the problems. A few parents will either overtly or covertly reject the findings and treatment plan recommendations and will register skepticism, disbelief, or outright hostility, creating a barrier to resolution of the difficulties. It is important to inquire about the parents' concerns and to answer patiently and fully, because the treatment alliance, as well as the treatment plan, may lie in the balance at this juncture. Families may be especially apprehensive about the use of medications because of personal belief systems misinformation, or antimedication bias in the their community or culture.

Treatment should address needs in the following domains

- Psychological
- Cognitive
- Personal management
- Family relations
- Parenting skills
- School setting
- Peer relations
- Community

Specific target symptoms, strengths, and weaknesses of the patient, family, school, and community, as well as the presence of comorbid conditions, must be considered when selecting treatment strategies (Dulcan & the American Academy of Child and Adolescent Psychiatry, 1997). It is likely that no one intervention, in isolation, will adequately resolve all the needs identified in the MTP.

Validated and Empirically Supported Treatments for ADHD

Psychosocial Treatments

Several evidence-based treatments (Chambless & Hollon, 1998) with demonstrated efficacy have been developed for use with children who have symptoms of ADHD, and who additionally often have associated difficulties with lagging social skills, defiance of social rules, and frequent verbal or physical aggression. Among these are Problem-Solving Skills Training (PSST) and Parent Management Training (PMT; Kazdin & Weisz, 1998). PSST develops a child's reasoning and social skills in a step-by-step fashion for successful social decision-making and resolution of interpersonal situations. Emphasis is placed on how children fashion possible social responses, implement solutions, and assess results in interpersonal situations. Prosocial behaviors are developed through instruction, modeling, practice, role-playing, reinforcement, and invoking consequences. This sequence is repeated during treatment with increasingly complex situations and response patterns. Manualized programs are available to encourage thoroughness and reproducibility (Kazdin & Weisz, 1998). Extended gains have been shown, with continuation over a 1-year follow-up. Studies have suggested that PSST is more effective with older children than with children ages 5 to 7. The outcome has been poorer for children with extensive comorbid pathology, greater family stress and dysfunction, parental psychopathology, and poor reading and academic achievement.

PMT is one of the most thoroughly-researched therapy interventions (Weisz & Kazdin, 1998). The key premises of PMT are to train parents to alter and shape their behavior and that of their children, with emphasis on identification and employment of antecedants, behaviors, and consequences (Kazdin, 1997). Focus is drawn to identification of the unwanted behaviors and the shaping of prosocial behaviors that reduce the likelihood of occurrence of undesired behaviors, such as verbal aggression and physical hitting. Techniques used in teaching PMT derive from principles of reinforcement, punishment, and behavioral extinction, and include the use of prompts, scheduling of consequences, and incentives. PMT is conducted with the parents, who then implement the program in the home (Kazdin, 1997). Generally, the PMT may last from 12 to 25 sessions. Changes may be maintained for periods of 1 to 3 years, although results are diminished by the presence of family chaos and discord, parental stress, single-parent families, externalizing parental psychopathology and harsh parental disciplinary practices (Kazdin, 1997). In practice, PMT should be integrated into other interventions for the best outcome. As with other therapies, there is high risk for premature termination. Adolescents may respond less well to the effects of PMT than younger children (Dishion & Patterson, 1992). Outcome is further adversely affected by low socioeconomic status, presence of high levels of family stress, single-parent status, younger ages of parenting, and parent history of externalizing psychopathology and antisocial behaviors (Kazdin, 1997).

Another example of a more popularized parent training program dealing with behavioral issues in children with ADHD is the Systematic Training for Effective Parenting program (STEP; Dinkmeyer, McKay, & Dinkmeyer, 1997). A basic tenet of the STEP program is that children must accept responsibility for their actions or incur the consequences. Using very practical examples, the parents are taught how to set up effective strategies. An example of such a strategy might be as follows. The parent tells the child that it is his or her job to take out the trash. If the child doesn't do it, the parent will assume that the child would like the parent to do it. Of course, the parent will need to be paid for such a service, and the pay will come from the child's allowance. After all, it is the child's responsibility to see that the task gets done, so he or she must provide the resources to have someone else do it. Parents are also told how to communicate respect and encouragement to their children, as well as to foster cooperation and problem-solving approaches.

An attractive aspect of the STEP program is its easy accessibility. Many community-based agencies (e.g., churches, daycare centers) run classes, typically lasting for seven weekly sessions, and the manuals are readily available in the popular press, as well as in videotape format and Spanish versions. In recent years, the original version, which was focused primarily on the school-age child, has been expanded to versions aimed at children under 6 years of age (Dinkmeyer, McKay, Dinkmeyer, Dinkmeyer, & McKay, 1997) and teenagers (Dinkmeyer, McKay, McKay, & Dinkmeyer, 1998).

PHARMACOTHERAPY

There is a long list of medications that have been tried or are currently used as adjunct interventions for treatment of the symptoms of ADHD (see Table 11.3). The introduc-

Table 11.3   Medications Used or Tried for Treatment of ADHD Symptoms

Stimulant drugs licensed for ADHD indication:

Methylphenidate	Adderall
Pemoline	
Dextroamphetamine	

Other drugs with demonstrated effectiveness but not licensed for the ADHD indication:

Phenelzine	Tranylcypromine
Imipramine	Bupropion
Desipramine	Clonidine

Drugs with possible effectiveness in ADHD, but no controlled clinical trials:

Fluoxetine	Sertraline
Guanfacine	Nicotine
Nortriptyline	Methamphetamine
Protryptiline	Venlafaxine

Precursor drugs without proven effectiveness:

Levodopa	Phenylalanine
Carbidopa	Tyrosine

Other marketed drugs with no effectiveness or contraindicated:

Fenfluramine

Drugs in current development:

Tomoxetine (Eli Lilly and Co) unlicensed TCA analog

SLI381 (Shire) R-stereoisomer of Adderall

(Alza)

R-Methylphenidate (Celgene) R-stereoisomer of methylphenidate

Oral release osmotic system (OROS) (Alza) long-acting methylphenidate (Wilens & Spencer, 2000)

tion of medications into the treatment plan must be done with the express permission of the parents. Guidelines for addition of medication for ADHD symptoms include considerations of the following:

1. Completion of detailed assessment to determine that symptoms are those of ADHD (i.e., rule out symptoms of inattention that might be due to an affective or adjustment disorder)

2. Discussion of the place of medication in a comprehensive treatment approach, and alternative treatments

3. Description of rationale for medication choice, initial dosages, and schedule for medicating

4. Description of possible initial effects: adverse response (initial worsening of symptoms and severity); no apparent response (no change in symptoms or severity); and therapeutic response (an improvement, with lessening of target symptoms and severity)

5. Description of possible side effects

Medications are among the most powerful treatments for ADHD. However, not all children or adults will respond favorably to medication use. With stimulants, for instance, the estimated initial response rate is about 65% to 75% (Greenhill et al., 1998), although this rate may be increased by trials of a second or third stimulant, reaching an eventual 90% of children for whom there is a positive response (Elia, Borcherding, Rapoport, & Keysor, 1991), assuming compliance has been adhered to in taking the medication. Utility may also be decreased by unacceptable levels of side effects (e.g., with stimulant use, the occurrence of headaches, stomach cramping, or significantly delayed sleep onset at night). Frequently, the medication dosing levels and administration schedule must be adjusted, based on systematic observation and feedback, to achieve the best result for the individual child.

Stimulant medications, such as methylphenidate (Ritalin), dextroamphetamine (Dexedrine, Dextrostat), and pemoline (Cylert, Adderall) are among the most studied agents in modern pharmacotherapeutics. The first use was reported by Bradley (1937), with the use of benzedrine (racemic amphetamine) among a group of children hospitalized with aggression, disruptive behavioral style, and poor concentration. Since then, more than 140 double-blind, placebo-controlled investigations have been completed in school-aged children, mostly using methylphenidate and dextroamphetamine, with a nearly universal demonstration of efficacy for symptoms of ADHD (Greenhill et al., 1998). Effect sizes of 0.8 to 1.0 SD for activity levels and inattention have been reported for methylphenidate and dextroamphetamine (Elia et al., 1991), while effects of 0.6 to 0.8 SD have been noted on cognitive measures (Spencer et al., 1996). However, an interesting disparity was noted by Sprague and Sleator (1977) that optimal behavior (e.g., reduced hyperactivity) was achieved at higher doses of methylphenidate (0.6 mg/kg), whereas lower doses of medication (0.3 mg/kg) were associated with more optimal cognitive performance. These findings highlight the necessity of monitoring school performance carefully when titrating stimulant medication, in order to avoid overmedicating with respect to optimal cognitive performance.

Typically, the stimulant medications have a short length of action, in the range of 2.5 to 4 hours, necessitating multiple dosing of the drugs throughout the child's day for continued effectiveness. The stimulants are not protein-bound, do not deposit in the tissues or build up constant bloodstream levels, and are washed out each day. No demonstrated tolerance occurs with continued use, other than adjustments required because of weight increase over time. Although rebound irritability has frequently been reported in clinical practice, this has not been demonstrated in controlled group trials. The stimulants appear to have specific effects on decreasing distractibility and activity levels, diminishing impulsivity, and decreasing cognitive variance (Tannock, Schachar, & Logan, 1995), and indirect effects on improvement in pro-social behaviors has been demonstrated. Effects on improvement in classroom learning measures of reading and math have been reported (Pelham, Bender, Caddell, Booth, & Morrer, 1985). Additionally, the stimulants have an effect on decreasing levels of aggressive behaviors that may accompany children with comorbid. Oppositional Defiant Disorder and Conduct Disorder (Hinshaw, 1991). Effectiveness does not diminish significantly in situations of children with ADHD and comorbid anxiety symptoms (Pliszka,1992; Tannock et al., 1995). A less complete response to stimulants is found in children with ADHD and comorbid depression. To date, this has not been explored (Pliszka, 1998).

Whereas short-term effects of stimulants have been amply demonstrated, the long-term impact has been studied less. However, at least one study with dextroamphetamine (Gillberg et al., 1997) and the recent large NIMH Multimodal Treatment of ADHD (MTA) study with methylphenidate (MTA Cooperative Group, 1999a) have reported continued effectiveness of these medications beyond 1 year's exposure.

Because of the short behavioral life of a single dose of the stimulants, sustained release preparations have been developed for both methylphenidate and dextroamphetamine. This is advantageous especially in situations where compliance is a problem because of older children's negative attitudes toward taking medication as a result of peer ridicule in the school setting. These medications may have a behavioral effect for 6 to 8 hours (the length of the school day), although the onset of effect may be delayed as much as 1 hour after administration, in contrast to the 30 minutes it takes for the onset of action with regular-preparation stimulants. New stimulants in development, such as SLI381 (R-Adderall), may also have an extended behavioral effect.

Side effects most commonly encountered with stimulant use include appetite suppression, stomach cramping, headaches, and delayed sleep onset or other sleep interference (see Table 11.4 for a more complete list of medication side effects). The issue of growth suppression has been raised repeatedly with stimulant use. One prospective, long-term follow-up of probands with ADHD revealed no significant decrement in attained height (Mannuzza et al., 1991). A second prospective, 4-year follow-up study of growth-related outcomes among 132 ADHD children who had taken stimulant medications for management, and 113 normal controls, showed no evidence of pubertal delay, weight deficits, or relationship between measures of poor nutrition and short stature, and modest height deficits for the ADHD group in comparison with controls (Spencer et al., 1996).

Rebound effects for children coming off a dose of a stimulant medication (typically in the mid-to-late afternoon) have been a source of concern for parents and clinicians. Such rebound is marked by irritability and an exaggeration of overactivity. It is possible

Table 11.4 Potential Side Effects Associated with Stimulant Treatment

Nervousness

Loss of appetite

Anorexia

Insomnia

Nausea

Dizziness

Headache

Feels "heart is racing"

Facial or body tics (involuntary muscle jerks)

Staring

Unusual blinking

Skin rash

Hair loss

Depression

that what is being observed and reported is, in part, a resurgence of the basic underlying ADHD symptoms. Although this is not a significant issue for most children taking stimulants (Johnson et al., 1988), its occurrence in individual children may require adjustment of the dosing schedule, with, for instance, the addition of a smaller dose at 3 to 4 P.M. or use of an extended-release preparation of the stimulant for management, as the irritability is uncomfortable for the child and may negatively impact the child's relationships.

Stimulants, ADHD, and Comorbid Tic Disorders

Several early reports suggested that although stimulants produced improvements in inattentive and hyperactive symptoms, they either induced or exacerbated tics in children with ADHD and tic disorders (Borcherding et al., 1990; Golden, 1988; Gualtieri & Patterson, 1986). However, more recent reports, typically using larger samples, suggest that even long-term use of stimulants used in typical clinical doses do not produce or exacerbate tics to any greater extent than do placebos (Gadow, Sverd, Sprafkin, & Nolan, 1999; Law & Schachar, 1999).

There has been a significant increase in the prescription of stimulant medications in the 1990s (Zametkin, 1999; Jensen et al., 1999), even among preschool children (Zito et al., 2000). Jensen et al. estimated that 4.5 to 6.8 million children were receiving stimulant medications in 1995. Greenhill (1998) enumerated possible explanations for this rise, including increased duration of treatment, more diagnosis of ADHD in females and in adolescents, changing attitudes toward stimulant use, school pressures to prescribe, prescription for associated conditions such as ODD and CD, and recent treatment of ADHD in adults.

There is potential for abuse inherent in the prescription and use of stimulant medications, and especially for dextroamphetamine, which is highly sought after and has a street market value among substance abusers. However, little corroborating evidence is found to support the belief that stimulant use in a prescribed, closely managed manner will lead to later substance abuse, given the intervening variable of the development of conduct disorder. However, there should be frank discussions between the prescribing physician and the parents regarding abuse or diversion potential, and the need for close monitoring of the medications.

Stimulants and Comorbid Tourette's Syndrome

Tourette's syndrome (TS) is a neuropsychiatric disorder characterized by chronic motor and vocal tics that become apparent in childhood. There is a comorbidity of 50% for ADHD in individuals with TS (Peterson & Cohen, 1998). An early report (Lowe et al., 1982) cautioned against the use of stimulants for ADHD symptoms in those individuals with TS. This is problematic, however, considering that symptoms of ADHD can be severe enough to obviate participation in the regular classroom. In recent years, several groups have revisited the use of stimulants in TS, with the recommendation that methylphenidate and dextroamphetamine can be used to good advantage to reduce ADHD symptoms, although careful titration from lower dosages is prudent (Castellanos et al., 1997; Peterson & Cohen, 1998; Gadow et al., 1999; Law & Schachar, 1999). Exacerbation of tics appears dose-related (Castellanos et al., 1997), and not all children will respond to stimulant use (Gadow et al., 1999). Effects of stimulants on ADHD symptoms appear to be maintained with long-term use (Gadow et al., 1999). One exception may be that of children with mental retardation: using a fairly large ($N = 27$) sample, Handen et al. (1991) found that children with mental retardation and ADHD were at a higher risk for developing tics with methylphenidate treatment than were other children.

Tricyclic Antidepressants

The tricyclic antidepressants (TCA), first introduced in the 1960s, and including imipramine (IMI), desipramine (DMI), and nortriptyline (NTI), has been studied less than the stimulants during the 1980s and 1990s, but it appears to have significant benefit in addressing ADHD symptoms. Werry and Sprague (1979) reported that the efficacy of IMI was equal to that of MPH, and superior to placebo. Studies with DMI (Donnelly et al., 1986; Biederman, Baldessarini, Wright, Knee, & Harmatz, 1989) indicated significantly superior response over placebo for children with ADHD. Positive response has been reported in other retrospective or open bottle studies of ADHD with NTI (Wilens, Biederman, Geist, Steingard, & Spencer, 1993) and protriptyline (Wilens, Biederman, Abrantes, & Spencer, 1996) treatment. Several studies have also reported additional effects on decreases in irritability and aggression with tricyclic acid (TCA) use (Donnelly et al., 1986, Biederman et al., 1989). Concern with the occurrence of possible TCA-related adverse cardiovascular events, including unexplained cardiac fatalities in children taking TCAs, has in recent years led to the decline in use of these medications in ADHD and other childhood mental disorders (Wilens et al., 1996; Geller, Reising, Leonard, Riddle, & Walsh, 1999). When TCAs are used, parents should be made aware of the risks; a detailed individual and family cardiovascular history should be undertaken; and guidelines regarding monitoring of vital signs and ECG parameters should be adhered to strictly (Wilens et al., 1996).

Non-Tricyclic Antidepressants

This group includes monoamine oxidase inhibitors (MAOIs) such as phenelzine, tranylcypromine, and bupropion, and selective serotonin reuptake inhibitors (SSRIs) such as fluoxetine, sertraline, venlafaxine, nefazodone, and fenfluramine (Emslie et al., 1999). Among these, only the MAOIs phenelzine, tranylcypromine, and the aminoketone derivative bupropion have undergone controlled, double-blind trials. Zametkin, Rapoport, Murphy, Linnoila, and Ismond (1985) reported efficacy for tranylcypromine and phenelzine in ADHD symptoms similar to that found with methylphenidate. The practical drawback of MAOI use in children however is that children require close monitoring and employment of a tyramine-free diet to avoid a potentially severe hypertensive interaction with tyramine; consequently, MAOIs are not safe or feasible in routine clinical use for children with impulse control problems.

Bupropion has been tested in children with ADHD in at least two double-blind controlled studies that have demonstrated clinical efficacy (Barrickman et al., 1995; Conners et al., 1996). There are no cardiac side effects from bupropion, but there is a seizure-inducing potential that is dose-related, although this is of slight clinical concern when daily bupropion dosage is kept below 450 mg/day. This drug, as with other antidepressants, may be considered in situations where ADHD management is complicated by comorbid depressive disorder.

There are reports of use of other antidepressants for the treatment of ADHD, including case reports or reports of small open trials with fluoxetine (Barrickman, Noyes, Kuperman, Schumacher, & Verda, 1991) and venlafaxine (Hedges et al., 1995). However, on the basis of the current literature, these cannot be recommended as being specifically effective.

Other Medications in ADHD

Clonidine is an alpha-2 agonist that has shown benefit in treatment of ADHD symptoms in open and controlled trials (Hunt et al., 1986; Steingard, Biederman, Spencer, Wilens, & Gonzalez, 1993; Findling & Dogin, 1998). However, a recent meta-analysis (Conner, Fletcher, & Swanson, 1999) would indicate that its use be relegated to that of a second- or third-line intervention because of its small effect size (.44 SD) in trials reviewed. Clonidine has been suggested as having particular use in children with ADHD and comorbid tic disorder (Steingard et al., 1993). Additionally, clonidine has been used for management of aggression (Leckman et al., 1991) and is widely prescribed for management of primary or stimulant-related sleep disturbance in children with ADHD (Findling & Dogin, 1998). Questions have been raised about the potential for clonidine-related hypotension and cardiac arrhythmias, including sinus tachycardia and conduction defects detectable on ECG (Chandran, 1994). This concern has been debated recently in light of the extensive co-prescription of clonidine and methylphenidate (Wilens & Spencer, 2000; Wilens et al., 1999). Although practitioner alertness is advised when using a methylphenidate-clonidine combination medication regimen, extensive clinical practice has shown the effectiveness of this combination, and the reported difficulties have been of a low order of magnitude.

Guanfacine is an alpha-2 agonist analog of clonidine, also adopted from general medical use as an anti-hypertensive medication for control of symptoms of ADHD

(Hunt, Arnsten, & Asbell, 1995). To date, no controlled trials with guanfacine have been performed. It may be employed where symptoms of impulsivity and aggression are prominent. In contrast to clonidine, guanfacine administration induces little drowsiness with continued usage in most children. However, similar to clonidine, it is thought of as a second- or third-line drug for children with an uncomplicated clinical presentation.

Venlafaxine has been tested in open trials in adults with ADHD and may hold some promise for children who have failed other drugs, as is the case with nicotine. Fenfluamine use is contraindicated in ADHD. Antipsychotic medications such as chlorpromazine, thioridazine, and haloperidol have been used in the past but have little place in current treatment and run the risk of a range of side effects with protracted use, including risk of tardive dyskinesia (Findling & Dogin, 1998). Similarly, lithium carbonate has no use in treatment of uncomplicated ADHD.

Other Nonvalidated Treatments

A range of alternative treatments has been advocated for children with ADHD, reflecting the idea that this disorder has diverse symptom manifestations and a generally unknown etiology. Many parents seek other remedies because of concern over the potential risks of treating their children with psychoactive medications (Baumgaertel, 1999). Dietary management has been advocated by many, but there is a great deal of controversy about the utility of such practices. Restriction of ingestion of sugar or aspartame (Wolraich et al., 1994), exposure to food dyes (Rowe & Rowe, 1994), and avoidance of foods containing or contaminated by yeast and molds (Crook, 1986) have had their advocates. Highly restrictive diets, such as the Feingold diet, have been promoted widely, but without convincing evidence (Wender, 1986). Similarly, megavitamin treatment and dietary supplements with such things as iron, magnesium, pyridoxine (vitamin B_6), zinc, and essential fatty acids (EFA's) have been proposed, but to date clear benefit has not been demonstrated for any of these proposed treatments (Baumgaertel, 1999). Other interventions have been proposed, including vision therapy, auditory stimulation, and biofeedback therapy, again without conclusive evidence (Baumgaertel, 1999).

Combined Multimodal Treatment

Because ADHD imparts multiple negative social, academic, and behavioral deficits to the individual child, a multimodal approach to intervention is both advantageous and necessary for most children. The scope and elements of the approach are dependent of the individual needs, which are highlighted by the assessment process. As with other disorders, ADHD must be understood as having a spectrum of severity. For the more moderately and severely handicapped individuals, medications are often used as an adjunctive treatment with parent training, behavioral treatment, cognitive-behavioral treatment, and specialized remediative learning inputs. The behavioral interventions may be thought of as conscious, empirically validated intensifications of the normal process of socialization and enculturation, intended to equip the child for successful participation in the community and society. Together, the combined treatment modes help to address deficiencies and to return the child to a more normal developmental pathway, one that allows for fuller expression of individual capabilities.

Recent evidence from the MTA study suggests that a combination of behavioral and medication therapy is superior to behavioral therapy for children who have oppositional/aggressive symptoms, and those with internalizing symptoms, such as anxiety. Combination of medication and parent training has increased benefit for parent-child relations in cases where the child has a significantly oppositional, obstructive, and dysfunctional behavioral style (MTA Cooperative Group, 1999b). The MTA results also suggest that combined medication/behavioral intervention may lead to lower daily dose needs for methylphenidate use, a finding that, if replicated, would have public health implications for practice (MTA Cooperative Group, 1999a). Overall, the MTA results suggest that for many children, medication therapy alone should be the first line of intervention, and that this approach might obviate the need for more protracted or intensive behavioral interventions.

CASE EXAMPLES OF THE INTEGRATION OF ASSESSMENT AND INTERVENTIONS

ADHD with Oppositional Defiant Disorder

Raydonn was a 9-year-old African American male third-grade student living with his single mother and a 5-year-old half brother. He was referred to the School-Based Services (SBS) team by the school guidance counselor because of inattentiveness, social impulsivity, overactivity, poor classroom organization, defiance of the teacher's and mother's directions, temper outbursts, peer aggression, impatience with others, and expressions of being misunderstood by both peers and adults. According to the mother, these difficulties were first noted when Raydonn was in kindergarten, at which time he was placed in a social-skills group at school. Between that time and the most recent referral, methylphenidate medication was tried briefly on Raydonn, and he was referred for special services. However, because the family moved at least three times to new school districts, there was little follow-up, and the child's behavior deteriorated along with his classroom achievement. Most recently, Raydonn had been suspended from school for defiance and fighting.

The mother was never married and lived with the boy's father for only 1 year. The father was killed in an industrial accident after the separation. The maternal grandparents were both deceased, and there was no extended family. The mother was the sole support of the family; but she had not been able to work because she had to care for her two sons, and she had to manage on Welfare funds and Medicaid.

During the evaluation, the mother appeared overwhelmed in managing her child's needs and behaviors. Raydonn presented as an attractive but impulsive and distractible child who was restless and inattentive during the interview. He appeared sullen and uncooperative in the presence of the mother, but lightened somewhat when seen individually.

The boy's scores on the Child and Adolescent Functional Assessment Scale (CAFAS), DuPaul Teacher Rating Scale, DuPaul Parent Rating Scale, Behavioral Assessment System for Children—Parent Rating Scale (BASC-PRS), and Behavioral Assessment System for Children—Teacher Rating Scale (BASC-TRS) follow.

CAFAS

Role Performance	30
School/Work	(30)
Home	(10)
Community	(0)
Behavior Toward Others	20
Moods	20
Moods/Emotions	(20)
Self-Harm	(0)
Substance Abuse	0
Thinking	0

Total CAFAS Score 70

BASC Scores:

	PRS-C		TRS-C	
	T-Score	Percentile	*T*-Score	Percentile
Clinical Scales:				
Hyperactivity	92	99	64	89
Aggression	92	99	69	94
Conduct Problems	87	99	63	91
Anxiety	48	48	45	37
Depression	77	98	74	97
Somatization	53	68	46	48
Atypicality	97	99	67	94
Withdrawal	57	78	77	98
Attention Problems	79	99	75	99
Learning Problems			67	93
Adaptive Scales:				
Adaptability	30	3	43	27
Social Skills	31	3	36	8
Leadership	41	19	28	1
Study Skills			33	6
Composite:				
Externalizing Problems	97	99	67	92
Internalizing Problems	62	88	56	78
Adaptive Skills	32	4	33	4
Teacher ADHD Rating Scale:	**Parent ADHD Rating Scale:**			

The results of this evaluation were reviewed in a multidisciplinary master treatment planning (MTP) conference and led to diagnoses of:

- 314.01   Attention Deficit Disorder, Combined Type
- 313.01   Oppositional Defiant Disorder

There was discussion about the level of depressive mood, noted both by the teacher and by the parent. It was agreed that this might be secondary to the patient's lack of feelings of security and support in the relationship with the mother, and that this should be addressed in the course of treatment. The lack of consistent parenting skills and application was also noted. This also was to be addressed in treatment. The following interventions were recommended in the MTP Conference:

1. Involvement of Raydonn in a social skills and aggression management group

2. Short-term individual therapy to improve Raydonn's self-esteem and self-efficacy

3. A High Risk Intervention worker for the home on a weekly basis to help improve problem-solving and effective communication between Raydonn and his mother, and to aid the mother in development of more effective parenting skills

4. A trial on a stimulant medication, such as methylphenidate, to address target symptoms of inattentiveness, distractibility, impulsivity, poor personal organization, and overactivity

5. A classroom program of clearly defined behavioral and academic expectations and systematic reinforcements for positive responses

ADHD with Behavioral Disturbance and Learning Disability

James was a 12-year-old African American male living with his 67-year-old maternal grandmother. He had repeated third grade, and at the time of referral was having increasingly significant problems with inattention, overactivity, and impulsivity in the form of disruptive classroom behaviors and excessive talking. James was below grade level in both reading and math, and, according to the teacher, was noted to have problems with short-term memory, following directions, and completion of classwork. The teacher stated that James had a good sense of humor, was generally well-liked by peers, but recently had been challenging adult direction.

For the past 7 years, James had lived with his maternal grandmother and his 9-year-old half sister. Because of emotional instability and recurrent problems with substance abuse, the biological mother was not able to care for the patient or his sister. The mother had her marriage to the student's father annulled, and James did not see him. She also had three other children, none of which were in her care. She had remained an absent figure in James's life until the last year, during which she visited on a more regular basis, expressing the wish to "have a normal family."

James had a long history of attentional, impulsive, and academic problems. He was evaluated by a pediatrician during the third grade because of attentional and impulsive symptoms and was placed on Ritalin, with some improvement. However, there was no follow-through with this treatment and James was not on Ritalin in fourth grade or during the current fifth grade year. The teacher expressed concerns about the student's inability to focus his attention sufficiently to organize and complete his work; and additionally, he had consistent trouble in understanding and following directions.

A school request for mental health assessment by the SBS was made concurrently with the school's evaluation of the boy's learning needs. Results of these assessments follow:

CAFAS

Role Performance	20
School/Work	(20)
Home	(20)
Community	(0)
Behavior Toward Others	10
Moods	10
Moods/Emotions	(10)
Self-Harm	(0)
Substance Abuse	0
Thinking	0
Total CAFAS Score	**40**

BASC Scores

	PRS-C		TRS-C	
	T-Score	Percentile	*T*-Score	Percentile
Clinical Scales:				
Hyperactivity	58	80	79	99
Aggression	64	91	72	96
Conduct Problems	71	96	66	92
Anxiety	47	42	49	53
Depression	44	30	48	51
Somatization	44	32	42	18
Atypicality	51	62	51	70
Withdrawal	42	21	45	35
Attention Problems	66	93	70	97
Learning Problems			72	97
Adaptive Scales:				
Adaptability	42	22	28	1
Social Skills	45	32	37	10
Leadership	39	15	38	11
Study Skills			37	11
Composite:				
Externalizing Problems	67	94	74	97
Internalizing Problems	44	28	45	40
Adaptive Skills	41	18	33	4

Teacher ADHD Rating Scale:

Inattention	27
Overactivity/ Impulsivity	19

Parent ADHD Rating Scale:

Inattention	18
Overactivity/ Impulsivity	9

WISC-3 Scores:

Verbal	Scale Scores	Performance	Scale Scores
Information	10	Picture Completion	6
Similarities	9	Coding	4
Arithmetic	8	Picture Arrangement	5
Vocabulary	9	Block Design	6
Comprehension	10	Object Assembly	(7)
(Digit Span)	(11)		

	IQ/Index
Verbal	95
Performance	73
Full Scale	83
Verbal Comp	98
Perceptual Org	77

Psychomotor Assessment:

	# Errors	Time	SS	Percentile	Age Equivalent
Bender	4	4'44	72	5	8.0–8.5

Educational Assessment: Wechsler Individual Achievement Test (WIAT)

Area	Standard Score	Percentile	Grade Equivalent
Reading	72	3	2.2
Math	70	16	4.0
Writing	71	9	3.6

Adaptive Behavior Assessment:

Vineland Adaptive Behavior Scales (Interview Edition)

Sub-Domain	SS	Percentile	AE
Communication	92 ± 10	30	10.2
Daily Living Skills	89 ± 9	23	9.8
Socialization	83 ± 7	10	7.11
Adaptive Behavior Composite	83 ± 7	13	9.5

The results of this evaluation were reviewed in a multidisciplinary MTP conference and led to the following diagnoses:

- 314.02 Attention Deficit Disorder, Combined Type
- 313.02 Oppositional Defiant Disorder

- 315.0   Reading Disorder
- 315.1   Mathematics Disorder

Based on the identified problems and needs, the following recommendations were made regarding treatment interventions:

1. A trial on a stimulant medication, such as methylphenidate, to address target symptoms of inattentiveness, distractibility, impulsivity, poor personal organization, and overactivity

2. Short-term individual therapy to improve self-monitoring and self-efficacy

3. A High Risk Intervention worker for the home on a weekly basis to help with improving problem-solving and effective communication between James and his grandmother, and to aid the grandmother in development of more effective parenting skills

4. A classroom program of clearly defined behavioral expectations and systematic reinforcements for positive responses

5. On the strength of the findings of learning disability, an Individual Educational Program written by the Learning Assessment Team according to IDEA process and guidelines, to be implemented in the classroom and in pull-out resources, with permission of the guardian

ADHD with Mental Retardation

Jeffrey S. was a 14-year-old Caucasian male who was being served in a ninth-grade self-contained special education classroom of a large metropolitan school district. He was referred to the outpatient child psychiatry clinic of a large medical school for continuing problems with a short attention span and failure to meet academic goals, particularly in reading. He also had social difficulties with adults and peers. His parents were also concerned about his lack of motivation at school, and were concerned about his ability to hold a job in the future.

A problem was first suspected when Jeff was late in meeting early developmental milestones (e.g., sitting, walking, talking). By the time he was 2 years old, he was noted to be more irritable and more "hyper" than other children his age. He was enrolled in an early childhood classroom at age three. Although initially enrolled in a regular kindergarten, he was unable to keep up with the developmental demands of this setting, and his behavior was disruptive to others. His teacher recommended testing, and he was diagnosed with mild mental retardation and ADHD. From that point on, he was placed in special education classrooms with additional speech therapy services.

In addition to his educational intervention, Jeff was seen for medication treatment by a pediatric neurologist who prescribed Cylert. This medication did not work well; James had crying spells, and he was later prescribed Ritalin by a child psychiatrist. Although he experienced loss of appetite on this medication, Jeff's attention span improved, although it was still problematic.

When he was seen in the outpatient clinic, Jeff's parents were very concerned about his lack of friends, which was also starting to bother Jeff. Although the family made consistent efforts to involve Jeff in activities such as the Special Olympics and roller skating, his parents felt that he was unable to "read" others (e.g., he talked "way too much"), and as a result alienated his schoolmates. The family also reported that Jeff's problems were starting to impact the quality of life for the rest of the family significantly, which included both parents and two older sisters (18 and 21 years old). The oldest daughter had moved out the previous year, saying that she could not "stand it" any longer; the middle child was on medication treatment for depression, as was the mother. The family history was also significant for an uncle that was "just like Jeff"—a slow learner who was very inattentive and lived at home with his family all his life. The mother grew very teary-eyed as she related this history, and her husband was overtly supportive to her.

During his psychological testing, Jeff displayed considerable restlessness: He had considerable trouble staying seated, even though he was 14 years old. He was quite talkative, to the point that it occasionally interfered with testing, and he was quite impulsive in his response style (e.g., blurting out the answers to questions before the examiner had finished asking them). It took considerable redirection and breaks from testing, but a neuropsychological test battery was completed in two sessions. This battery included the Stanford-Binet Intelligence Scale–Fourth Edition, the Wide Range Achievement Test—Third Edition (WRAT-III, a screening measure of academic achievement), the Vineland Adaptive Behavior Scales (a measure of everyday living skills), the Child Behavior Checklist (CBCL, a parent-completed multidimensional behavior checklist), the Teacher Report Form (TRF; a teacher-completed multidimensional behavioral rating scale), and the Conners Parent and Teacher Rating Scales, scores for which follow:

Stanford-Binet Intelligence Scale

Standard Area Score (SAS)			SAS
Verbal Reasoning	67	Quantitative Reasoning	68
Abstract/Visual Reasoning	52	Short Term Memory	57
Composite IQ: 56			

Wide Range Achievement Test (WRAT-III)

	Standard Score	Grade Equivalent
Reading	53	1st
Spelling	64	2nd
Arithmetic	<45	1st

Vineland Adaptive Behavior Scales: Interview Edition, Survey Form

	Standard Score	Age Equivalent
Communication Domain	51	7–7
Daily Living Skills Domain	63	9–0
Socialization Domain	53	6–1
Adaptive Behavior Composite	51	7–7

Maladaptive Behavior Score: 8, Intermediate Range

Clinical Scale:	CBCL T-Score (Parent)	TRF T-Score (Teacher)
Withdrawn	65	51
Somatic Complaints	59	50
Anxious/Depressed	63	63
Social Problems	83	68
Thought Problems	70	65
Attention Problems	73	69
Delinquent Behavior	50	61
Aggressive Behavior	54	61

These test results, together with those of a clinical interview with the parents covering developmental history and current behavior, were suggestive of the following diagnoses:

- *DSM-IV* 317.00   Mild Mental Retardation
- *DSM-IV* 314.01   Attention Deficit Hyperactivity Disorder, Combined Type

It was also noted that Jeff's academic achievement in the area of mathematics was below that expected for a child with his cognitive ability. He was referred to the school, where he was given the Woodcock-Johnson–Revised, a more in-depth assessment of academic ability. His standard score on the math section of this test was 30. As such, even though he had mental retardation, he also could be considered to have a learning disorder in the area of mathematics because his scores in this area were significantly less than what would be expected for his age and IQ. He was given additional tutoring in math, both in school and privately. Additional recommendations included the following:

1. Continuing medication treatment regimen
2. Continuing structured special education classroom placement
3. Moving Jeff's seat closer to the teacher
4. Providing respite care through the local MHMRA, to provide "down time" for the family
5. Engaging in family counseling
6. Training Jeff for social skills
7. Participating in activities such as Big Brothers and the Boys Club, which provide more socialization experiences outside the family, but under the supervision of adults
8. Providing contact information for parent support groups and ADHD websites to the family.

OUTCOMES IN ADOLESCENCE

Approximately 50% to 70% of children with symptoms of ADHD will remain symptomatic at age 13, with continued dysfunction in a variety of domains of functioning experienced during adolescence as a result. Outcomes are again affected by the same set of factors already enumerated. These include SES, continued family stress, parental psychopathology, presence of learning difficulties, levels of aggression, and presence of comorbid diagnoses.

Mannuzza et al. (1991) found continuation of symptoms in 40% of 101 of the original ADHD probands at the end of adolescence, but only 3% of controls at 18 years of age, and ongoing antisocial personality disorder in 27% versus 8%. Substance abuse was also found to be higher (16% versus 3%) among the ADHD probands. A replication study by the same group using another cohort (Mannuzza, Klein, Bessler, Malloy, & LaPadula, 1998) yielded similar results during follow-up at 18 years of age that included 94% of the baseline evaluation group of 104 subjects—namely, 43% with continuing ADHD versus 4% of controls, 32% versus 8% with antisocial personality disorder, and 10% compared with 0% with substance abuse.

OUTCOMES IN ADULTHOOD

Persistence of ADHD symptoms, when accompanied by conduct symptoms especially, will predispose to substance abuse and further social deviance in adolescence and into adulthood. Several prospective studies have documented the outcomes of those individuals whose ADHD symptoms persist into adulthood (Weiss, Hechtman, Milroy, & Perlman, 1985; Mannuzza et al., 1991; Mannuzza et al., 1998). Weiss et al. reported a follow-up of 63 hyperactive children and 41 matched controls as adults (with 40% of probands lost of follow-up), with results indicating that 36% versus 2% of the hyperactive group had at least one major symptom of continuing hyperactivity, and that 23% (versus 2% of controls) had antisocial personality disorder. Adult follow-up by Mannuzza et al. (1998) of their original cohort of 104 subjects at the average age of 25 years showed that 33% of the probands (vs. 19% of control subjects) had an ongoing mental disorder, with evidence of high rates of antisocial personality disorder (12% versus 3%), and 12% versus 3% with substance abuse disorder. The substance abuse appeared to be mediated through antisocial personality disorder. There was no increase in current or lifetime (24% versus 23%) mood or anxiety (5% versus 9%) disorders. There was significantly less educational attainment in the ADHD proband group—evidence that ADHD impacts a wide range of competencies beyond symptomatic outcomes, and that it impairs adaptation more generally.

Although there has been an acceleration in the study of ADHD in the past 10 years, much remains to be elucidated, especially regarding interventions to prevent handicapping outcomes. Treatment interventions for most children should be multimodal, and must be individualized for optimal outcomes. Given the prevalence of ADHD among children, and the range of possible adverse outcomes in adolescence and adulthood, these investigations are especially urgent.

REFERENCES

Abikoff, H., Courtney, M., Pelham, W. E., Jr., & Koplowicz, H. S. (1993). Teacher's ratings of disruptive behaviors. The influence of halo effects. *Journal of Abnormal Child Psychology, 21,* 519–533.

Achenbach, T. M. (1991). *Manual for the Child Behavior Checklist 4/18 and 1991 Profile.* Burlington, VT: University of Vermont Department of Psychiatry.

Achenbach, T. M. (1991). *Manual for the Teacher's Report Form and 1991 Profile.* Burlington, VT: University of Vermont Department of Psychiatry.

American Council on Education and Education Commission of the States. (1988). *One-third of a nation. A report by the Commission on Minority Participation in Education and American Life.* Washington, DC.: Author.

American Psychiatric Association. (1968). *Diagnostic and Statistical Manual of Psychiatric Disorders, 2nd Edition.* Washington, DC.

American Psychiatric Association. (1980). *Diagnostic and Statistical Manual of Psychiatric Disorders, 3rd Edition.* Washington, DC.

American Psychiatric Association. (1987). *Diagnostic and Statistical Manual of Psychiatric Disorders, 3rd Edition-Revised.* Washington, DC.

American Psychiatric Association. (1994). *Diagnostic and Statistical Manual of Psychiatric Disorders, 4th Edition.* Washington, DC.

Ando, H., & Yoshimura, I. (1978). Prevalence of maladaptive behavior in retarded children as a function of IQ and age. *Journal of Abnormal Child Psychology, 6,* 345–349.

Angold, A., & Costello, E. J. (1993). Depressive comorbidity in children and adolescents. Empirical, theoretical, and methodological issues. *American Journal Psychiatry, 150,* 1779–1991.

Arnold, L. E. (1996). Sex differences in ADHD: Conference summary. *Journal of Abnormal Child Psychology, 24,* 555–569.

August, G. J., Braswell, L., & Thuras, P. (1998). Diagnostic stability of ADHD in a community sample of school-aged children for disruptive behavior. *Journal of Abnormal Child Psychology, 26,* 345–356.

August, G. L., Realmuto, G. M., MacDonald, A. W., Nugent, S. M., & Crosby, R. (1996). Prevalence of ADHD and comorbid disorders among elementary school children screened for disruptive behavior. *Journal of Abnormal Child Psychology, 24,* 571–595.

Aytaclar, S., Tarter, R. E., Kirisci, L., & Lu, S. (1999). Association between hyperactivity and executive cognitive functioning in childhood and substance abuse in early adolescence. *Journal of the American Academy of Child and Adolescent Psychiatry, 38,* 172–178.

Barkley, R. A. (1996). Specific guidelines for defining hyperactivity in children (Attention Deficit Disorder with Hyperactivity). In B. Lahey & A. Kazdin (Eds.), *Advances in Clinical Child Psychology,* vol. 5 (pp. 137–180). New York: Plenum Press.

Barkley, R. A. (1997). *ADHD and the Nature of Self-Control.* New York: Guilford Press.

Barkley, R. A. (1998). *Attention-Deficit Hyperactivity Disorder. A Handbook for Diagnosis and Treatment* (Second Edition). New York: Guilford Press.

Barkley, R. A. (1990a). *Attention Deficit Hyperactivity Disorder. A Handbook for Diagnosis and Treatment.* New York: Guilford Press.

Barkley, R. A. (1990b). Test and observational measures. In R. A. Barkley (Ed.), *Attention-Deficit Hyperactivity Disorder* (pp. 327–353). New York: Guilford Press.

Barkley, R. A., & Biederman, J. (1997). Toward a broader definition of the age-of-onset criterion for attention-deficit hyperactivity disorder. *Journal of the American Academy of Child and Adolescent Psychiatry, 36,* 1204–1210.

Barrickman, L. L., Perry, P. J., Allen, A. J., Kuperman, S., Arndt, S. V., Herrmann, K. J., & Schumacher, E. (1995). Bupropion versus methylphenidate in the treatment of Attention-Deficit Hyperactivity Disorder. *Journal of the American Academy of Child and Adolescent Psychiatry, 34,* 649–657.

Barrickman, L. L., Noyes, R., Kuperman, S., Schumacher, E., & Verda, M. (1991). Treatment of ADHD with fluoxetine. A preliminary trial. *Journal of the American Academy of Child and Adolescent Psychiatry, 30,* 762–767.

Baumgaertel, A. (1999). Alternative and controversial treatments for attention-deficit/hyperactivity disorder. *Pediatric Clinics of North America, 46,* 977–992.

Biederman, J. (1998). Attention-Deficit/Hyperactivity Disorder. A life-span perspective. *Journal of Clinical Psychiatry, 59(suppl. 7),* 4–16.

Biederman, J., Baldessarini, R., Wright, V., Knee, D., & Harmatz, J. (1989). A double-blind placebo controlled study of desipramine in the treatment of attention deficit disorder. I. Efficacy. *Journal of the American Academy of Child and Adolescent Psychiatry, 28,* 777–784.

Biederman, J., Faraone, S., Mick, E., & Lelon, E. (1995). Psychiatric comorbidity among referred juveniles with major depression fact or artifact? *Journal of the American Academy of Child and Adolescent Psychiatry, 34,* 579–590.

Biederman, J., Faraone, S., Mick, E., Moore, P., & Lelon, E. (1996). Child behavior checklist findings further support comorbidity between ADHD and major depression in a referred sample. *Journal of the American Academy of Child and Adolescent Psychiatry, 35,* 734–742.

Biederman, J., Faraone, S., Milberger, S., Guite, J., Mick, E., Chen, L., Mennin, D., Maris, A., Ouellette, C., Moore, P., Spencer, T., Norman, D., Wilens, T., Kraus, I., & Perrin, J. (1996). A prospective 4-year follow-up study of attention-deficit hyperactivity and related disorders. *Archives of General Psychiatry, 53,* 437–446.

Biederman, J., Faraone, S. V., Weber, W., Russell, R. L., Rater, M., & Park, K. S. (1997). Correspondence between DSM-III-R and DSM-IV attention-deficit/hyperactivity disorder. *Journal of the American Academy of Child and Adolescent Psychiatry, 36,* 1682–1687.

Biederman, J., Milberger, S., Faraone, S. V., Kiely, K., Guite, J., Ablon, S., Warburton, R., & Reed, E. (1995). Family-environment risk factors for attention-deficit hyperactivity disorder. *Archives of General Psychiatry, 52,* 464–470.

Biederman, J., Newcorn, J., & Sprich, S. (1991). Comorbidity of attention deficit hyperactivity disorder with conduct, depressive, anxiety, and other disorders. *American Journal of Psychiatry, 148,* 564–577.

Biederman, J., Wilens, T., Mick, E., Faraone, S. V., Weber, W., Curtis, S., Thornell, A., Pfister, K., Jetton, J. G., & Soriano, J. (1997). Is ADHD a risk factor for psychoactive substance use disorders. Findings from a four-year prospective follow-up study. *Journal of the American Academy of Child and Adolescent Psychiatry, 36,* 21–29.

Birch, H. G. (1964). *Brain Damage in Children. The Biological and Social Aspects.* Baltimore, Williams and Wilkens.

Borcherding, Breck G. Keysor, Cynthia S. Rapoport, Judith L. Elia, & Josephine et al. (1990). Motor/vocal tics and compulsive behaviors on stimulant drugs. Is there a common vulnerability? *Psychiatry Research, 33,* 83–94.

Bowring, M. A., & Kovacs, M. (1992). Difficulties in diagnosing manic disorders among children and adolescents. *Journal Am Acad Child and Adolescent Psychiatry, 31,* 611–614.

Bradley, C. (1937). The behavior of children receiving benzedrine. *American Journal of Psychiatry, 94,* 577–585.

Breier, Joshua I, Simos, P. G., Zouridakis, G., Wheless, J. W., Willmore, L. J., Constantinou, J. E. C., Maggio, W. W., & Papanicolaou, A. C. (1999). Language dominance determined by magnetic source imaging: A comparison with Wada procedure. *Neurology, 53,* 938–945.

Cantwell, D. P. (1972). Psychiatric illness I the families of hyperactive children. *Archives of General Psychiatry, 27,* 414–417.

Cantwell, D. P. (1996). Attention Deficit Disorder: A review of the past 10 years. *Journal of the American Academy of Child and Adolescent Psychiatry, 35,* 978–987.

Cantwell, D. P., & Baker, L. (1991). Association between attention-deficit hyperactivity disorder and learning disorders. *Journal of Learning Disorders, 24,* 88–95.

Carlson, C. L., Tamm, L., & Gaub, M. (1997). Gender differences in children with ADHD, ODD, and co-occurring ADHD/ODD identified in a school population. *Journal of the American Academy of Child and Adolescent Psychiatry, 36,* 1706–1714.

Casat, C. D., Reid, R., Norton, H. J., Anastopoulos, A. D., & Temple, E. P. (2000). Cultural effects and behavioral rating scales: The IOWA Conners. Unpublished data.

Castellanos, F. X., Giedd, J. N., Elia, J., Marsh, W. L., Ritchie, G. F., Hamburger, S. D., & Rapoport, J. L. (1997). Controlled stimulant treatment of ADHD and comorbid Tourette's syndrome. Effects of stimulant and dose. *Journal of the American Academy of Child and Adolescent Psychiatry, 36,* 589–596.

Castellanos, F. X., Giedd, J. N., Marsh, W. L., Hamburger, S. D., Vaituzis, A. C., Dickstein, D. P., Sarfatti, S. E., Vauss, Y. C., Snell, J. W., Kaysen, D. D., Krain, A. L., Rajapakse, J. C., & Rapoport, J. L. (1996). Quantitative brain magnetic resonance imaging in attention-deficit hyperactivity disorder. *Archives of General Psychiatry, 53,* 607–616.

Casey, J. J., Castellanos, F. X., Giedd, J. N., Marsh, W. L., Hamburger, S. D., Schubert, A. B., Vauss, Y. C., Vaituzis, A. C., Dickstein, D. P., Sarfatti, S. E., & Rapoport, J. L. (1997). Implication of right frontostriatal circuitry in response inhibition and attention-deficit/ hyperactivity disorder. *Journal of the American Academy of Child and Adolescent Psychiatry, 36,* 374–383.

Chambless, D. L., Hollon, S. D. (1998). Defining empirically supported therapies. *Journal of Consulting and Clinical Psychology, 66,* 7–18.

Chilcoat, H. D., & Breslau, N. (1999). Pathways from ADHD to early drug use. *Journal of the American Academy of Child and Adolescent Psychiatry, 38,* 1347–1354.

Chandran, K. S. K. (1994). EKG and clonidine (letter). *Journal of the American Academy of Child and Adolescent Psychiatry, 33,* 1351–1352.

Chen, W. J., Faraone, S. V., Biederman, J., & Tsuang, M. T. (1994). Diagnostic accuracy of the Child Behavior Checklist scales for attention-deficit hyperactivity disorder: A receiver-operating characteristic analysis. *Journal of Consulting and Clinical Psychology, 62,* 1017–1025.

Comings, D. E., & Comings, B. G. (1993). Tourette's syndrome and attention deficit disorder with hyperactivity. Are they genetically related? *Journal of the American Academy of Psychiatry, 23,* 138–146.

Conner, D. F., Fletcher, K. E., & Swanson, J. M. (1999). A meta-analysis of clonidine for symptoms of attention-deficit hyperactivity disorder. *Journal of the American Academy of Child and Adolescent Psychiatry, 38,* 1551–1559.

Conners, C. K. (1969). A teacher rating scale for use in drug studies with children. *American Journal of Psychiatry, 126,* 884–888.

Conners, C. K. (1998). Rating scales in attention-deficit/hyperactivity disorder: Use in assessment and treatment monitoring. *Journal of Clinical Psychiatry, 59, (suppl. 7),* 24–30.

Conners, C. K., Casat, C. D., Gualtieri, C. T., Wellen, E., Readen, M., Reiss, A., Wellen, R. A., Khayrallah, M., & Aschen, J. (1996). Bsuprepion hydrochloride in attention deficit disorder with hyperactivity. *Journal of the American Academy of Child and Adolescent Psychiatry, 35,* 1314–1321.

Cook, E. H., Jr., Stein, M. A., & Krasowski, M. D., et al. (1995). Association of attention-deficit hyperactivity disorder and the dopamine transporter gene. *American Journal of Human Genetics, 56,* 993–998.

Corkum, P. V., & Siegel, L. S. (1993). Is the Continuous Performance Task a valuable research tool for use with children with Attention-Deficit-Hyperactivity Disorder? *Journal of Child Psychology and Psychiatry, 36,* 1477–1493.

Crook, W. G. (1986). *The Yeast Connection.* New York, Vintage Books.

Daly, G., Hawi, Z., Fitzgerald, M., & Gill, M. (1999). Mapping susceptibility loci in attention deficit hyperactivity disorder: Preferential transmission of parental alleles at DAT1, DBH and DRD5 to affected children. *Molecular Psychiatry, 4,* 192–196.

Das, J. P., & Melnyk, L. (1989). Attention checklist: A rating scale for mildly mentally handicapped adolescents. *Psychological Reports, 64,* 1267–1274.

Diamond, I. R., Tannock, R., & Schachar, R. J. (1999). Response to methylphenidate in children with ADHD and comorbid anxiety. *Journal of the American Academy of Child and Adolescent Psychiatry, 38,* 402–409.

Dinkmeyer, D., McKay, G. D., & Dinkmeyer, D. (1997). *The Parent's Handbook Systematic Training for Effective Parenting (STEP).* Circle Pines, MN: American Guidance Service.

Dinkmeyer, D. C., McKay, G. D., McKay, J. L., & Dinkmeyer, D., Jr. (1998). *Parenting Teenagers Systematic Training for Effective Parenting of Teens.* Circle Pines, MN: American Guidance Service.

Dinkmeyer, D., McKay, G. D., Dinkmeyer, J. S., Dinkmeyer, D., Jr., & McKay, J. L. (1997). *Parenting Young Children Systematic Training for Effective Parenting of Children Under Six.* Circle Pines, MN: American Guidance Service.

Dishion, T. J., & Patterson, G. R. (1992). Age effects in parent training outcomes. *Behavioral Therapy, 23,* 719–729.

Donnelly, M., Zametkin, A., & Rapoport, J. L., et al. (1986). Treatment of childhood hyperactivity with desipramine plasma drug concentration, cardiovascular effects, plasma and urinary catecholamine levels, and clinical response. *Clinical Pharmacology and Therapeutics, 39,* 72–81.

DuPaul, G. J., Anastopoulos, A. D., Shelton, T. L., Guevremont, D. C., & Metevia, L. (1992). Multimethod assessment of attention-deficit hyperactivity disorder: The diagnostic utility of clinic-based tests. *Journal of Clinical Child Psychology, 21,* 194–202.

DuPaul, G. J., & Stoner, G. (1994). *ADHD in the Schools: Assessment and Intervention Strategies.* New York: Guilford Press.

Dulcan, M., & the American Academy of Child and Adolescent Psychiatry Work Group on Quality Issues. (1997). Practice parameters for the assessment and treatment of children, adolescents, and adults with attention-deficit/hyperactivity disorder. *Journal of the American Academy of Child and Adolescent Psychiatry, 36 10 supplement,* 85S–121S.

Dykman, R. A., Ackerman, P. T., & Holcomb, P. J. (1985). Reading disabled and ADD children. Similarities and differences. In D. B. Gray & J. F. Kavanagh (Eds.). *Behavioral measures of dyslexia* (pp. 47–62). Parkton, MD: Your Press.

Elia, J., Borcherding, B., Rapoport, J., & Keysor, C. (1991). Methylphenidate and dextroamphetamine effects treatments of hyperactivity. Are there true non-responders? *Psychiatry Research, 36,* 141–155.

Emslie, G. J., Walkup, J. T., Pliszka, S. R., & Ernst, M. (1999). Nontricyclic antidepressants, current trends in children and adolescents. *Journal of the American Academy of Child and Adolescent Psychiatry, 38,* 517–528.

Epstein, M. H., Cullinan, D., & Gadow, K. D. (1986). Teacher ratings of hyperactivity in learning-disabled, emotionally disturbed, and mentally retarded children. *Journal of Special Education, 22,* 219–229.

Faraone, S. V., Biederman, J., Lehman, B. K., Spencer, T., Norman, D., Seidman, L. J., Kraus, I., Perrine, J., Chen, W. J., & Tsuang, M. T. (1993). Intellectual performance and school failure in children with attention deficit hyperactivity disorder and in their siblings. *Journal of Abnormal Psychology, 102,* 616–623.

Faraone, S. V., Biederman, J., Weiffenbach, B., Keith, T., Chu, M. P., Weaver, A., Spencer, T. J., Wilens, T. E., Frazier, J., Cleves, M., & Sakai, J. (1999). Dopamine D4 7repeat allele and attention deficit hyperactivity disorder. *American Journal of Psychiatry, 156,* 768–770.

Findling, R. L., & Dogin, J. W. (1998). Psychopharmacology of ADHD: Children and adolescents. *Journal of Clinical Psychiatry, 59(suppl 7),* 42–49.

Fletcher, J. M., Shaywitz, S. E., & Shaywitz, B. A. (1999). Comorbidity of learning and attention disorders. *Pediatric Clinics of North America, 46,* 885–897.

Frick, P. J., Lahey, B. B., Applegate, B., Kerdyck, L., Ollendick, T., Hynd, G. W., Garfinkel, B., Greenhill, L., Biederman, J., & Barkley, R. A., et al. (1994). DSM-IV field trials for the disruptive behavior disorders. Symptom utility estimates. *Journal of the American Academy of Child and Adolescent Psychiatry, 33,* 529–539.

Gadow, K. D., & Poling, A. G. (1988). *Pharmacotherapy and mental retardation.* Boston: Little, Brown, and Company.

Gadow, K. D., Sverd, J., Sprafkin, J., & Nolan, E. E. (1999). Long-term methylphenidate therapy in children with comorbid attention-deficit hyperactivity disorder and chronic multiple tic disorder. *Archivens of General Psychiatry, 56,* 330–336.

Gaub, M., & Carlson, C. L. (1997a). Behavioral characteristics of *DSM-IV:* ADHD subtypes in a school-based population. *Journal of Abnormal Child Psychology, 25,* 103–111.

Gaub, M., & Carlson, C. (1997b). Gender differences in ADHD: A meta-analysis and critical review. *Journal of the American Academy of Child and Adolescent Psychiatry, 36,* 1036–1045.

Geller, B., Reising, D., Leonard, H. L., Riddle, M. A., & Walsh, B. T. (1999). Critical review of tricyclic antidepressant use in children and adolescents. *Journal of the American Academy of Child and Adolescent Psychiatry, 38,* 513–516.

Gillberg, C., Melander, H., & von Knorring, A., et al. (1997). Long-term central stimulant treatment with attention-deficit hyperactivity disorder: A randomized double-blind placebo-controlled trial. *Archives of General Psychiatry, 54,* 857–864.

Golden, G. S. (1988). The relationship between stimulant medication and tics. *Psychiatric Annals, 18,* 409–413.

Goodman, R., & Stevenson, J. (1989). A twin study of hyperactivity: II. The etiological role of genes, family relationships and perinatal adversity. *Journal of Child Psychology and Psychiatry, 30,* 691–709.

Gordon, M. (1986). How is a computerized attention test used in the diagnosis of attention deficit disorder? *Journal of Children in a Contemporary Society, 19,* 53–64.

Goyette, C. H., Conners, C. K., & Ulrich, R. F. (1978). Normative data on Revised Conners Parent and Teacher Rating Scales. *Journal of Abnormal Child Psychology, 6,* 221–236.

Greenhill, L. H. (1998). Diagnosing Attention Deficit/Hyperactivity Disorder in children. *Journal of Clinical Psychiatry, 59, (suppl. 7),* 31–41.

Gualtieri, C. T., & Patterson, D. R. (1986). Neuroleptic-induced tics in two hyperactive children. *American Journal of Psychiatry, 143,* 1176–1177.

Handen, B. L., Feldman, H., Gosling, A., & Breaux, A. M., et al. (1991). Adverse side effects of methylphenidate among mentally retarded children with ADHD. *Journal of the American Academy of Child and Adolescent Psychiatry, 30,* 241–245.

Hedges, D., Reimherr, F. W., Rogers, A., Strong, R., & Wendon, P. H. (1995). An open trial of venlafazine in adult patients with attention deficit hyperactivity disorder. *Psychopharmacology Bulletin, 31,* 779–783.

Hinshaw, S. P. (1991). Stimulant medication and the treatment of aggression in children with attentional deficits. *Journal of Clinical Child Psychology, 20,* 301–309.

Hinshaw, S. P. (1994). Behavior rating scales in the assessment of disruptive behavior disorders in childhood. In J. Richters, & D. Shaffer, (Eds.), *Assessment in Child Psychopathology.* New York: Cambridge Press.

Hunt, R. D., Arnsten, A. F. T., & Asbell, M. D. (1995). An open trial of guanfacine in the treatment of attention-deficit hyperactivity disorder. *Journal of the American Academy of Child and Adolescent Psychiatry, 34,* 50–54.

Hunt, R. D., Capper, L., & O'Connell, P. (1990). Clonidine in child and adolescent psychiatry. *Journal of Child and Adolescent Psychopharmacology, 1,* 350–353.

Hunt, R. D., & Cohen, D. J. (1988). Attentional and neurochemical components of MR: New methods for an old problem. In J. A. Stark, F. J. Menolascino, M. H. Albarelli, & V. C. Gray, (Eds.), *MR and mental health: Classification, diagnosis, treatment, services* (pp. 90–97). New York: Springer-Verlag.

Hunt, R. D., Minderaa, R. B., & Cohen, D. J. (1986). The therapeutic effect of clonadine on attention deficit disorder with hyperactivity: A comparison with placebo and methylphenidate. *Psychopharmacology Bulletin, 22,* 229–236.

Jensen, P. S., Bhatara, V. S., Vitiello, B., Hoagwood, K., Feil, M., & Burke, L. B. (1999). Psychoactive medication prescribing practices for U.S. children: Between research and clinical practice. *Journal of the American Academy of Child and Adolescent Psychiatry, 38,* 557–565.

Johnson, C., Pelham, W. E., Hoaz, J., & Sterges, J. (1988). Psychostimulant rebound in attention deficit disordered boys. *Journal of the American Academy of Child and Adolescent Psychiatry, 27,* 806–810.

Kandel, D. B., Johnson, J. G., Bird, H. R., Canino, G., Goodman, S. H., Lahey, B. B., Regier, D. A., & Schwab-Stone, M. (1997). Psychiatric disorders associated with substance use among children and adolescents. Findings from the Methods for the Epidemiology of Child and Adolescent Mental Disorders (MECA) study. *Journal of Abnormal Child Psychology, 25,* 121–132.

Kazdin, A. E. (1997). Parent management training: Evidence, outcomes, and issues. *Journal of the American Academy of Child and Adolescent Psychiatry, 36,* 1349–1356.

Kazdin, A. E., Crowley, M. (1997). Moderators of treatment outcome in cognitively based treatment of antisocial children. *Cognitive Therapy and Research, 21,* 185–207.

Kazdin, A. E., & Weisz, J. R. (1998). Identifying and developing empirically supported child and adolescent treatments. *Journal of Consulting and Clinical Psychology, 66,* 19–36.

Klorman, R., Hazel-Fernandez, L. A., Shaywitz, S. E., Fletcher, J. M., Marchione, K. E., Holahan, J. M., Stuebing, K. K., & Shaywitz, B. A. (1999). Executive functioning deficits in Attention-Deficit/Hyperactivity Disorder are independent of Oppositional Defiant or Reading Disorder. *Journal of the American Academy of Child and Adolescent Psychiatry, 38,* 1148–1155.

Kuhne, M., Schachar, R., & Tannock, R. (1997). Impact of comorbid oppositional or conduct problems on attention-deficit hyperactivity disorder. *Journal of the American Academy of Child and Adolescent Psychiatry, 36,* 1715–1725.

Lachar, D. (2000). Personality Inventory for Children, Second Edition (PIC-2), Personality Inventory for Youth (PIY), and the Student Behavior Survey (SBS). In M. Maruish (Ed.), *The use of psychological testing for treatment planning and outcome assessment, second edition* (pp. 399–427). Hillsdale, NJ: Erlbaum.

Lahey, B. B., Applegate, B., McBurnett, K., Biederman, J., Greenhill, L., Hynd, G. W., Barkley, R. A., Newcorn, J., Jensen, P., Richters, B. W. (1994). DSM-IV field trials for attention deficit hyperactivity disorder in children and adolescents. *American Journal of Psychiatry, 151,* 1673–1685.

Laufer, M., Denhoff, E., & Solomons, G. (1957). Hyperkinetic impulse disorder in children's behavior problems. *Psychosomatic Medicine, 19,* 38–49.

Law, S. F., & Schachar, R. J. (1999). Do typical clinical doses of methylphenidate cause tics in children treated for attention-deficit hyperactivity disorder? *Journal of the American Academy of Child and Adolescent Psychiatry, 38,* 944–951.

Leckman, J. F., Hardin, M. T., Riddle, M. A., Stevenson, J., Ort, S. I., & Cohen, D. J. (1991). Clonidine treatment of Gilles de la Tourette's syndrome. *Archives of General Psychiatry, 48,* 324–328.

Loney, J. (1983). Research diagnostic criteria for childhood hyperactivity. In S. B. Guze, F. J. Earls, & J. E. Barrett (Eds.), *Childhood psychopathology and development* (pp. 109–137). New York: Raven Press.

Lowe, T. L., Cohen, D. J., Detlor, J., Kremenitzer, M. W., & Shaywitz, B. A. (1982). Stimulant medications precipitate Tourette's Syndrome. *Journal of the American Medical Association, 247,* 1168–1169.

Mannuzza, S., Klein, R. G., Bessler, M. A., Malloy, P., & LaPadula, M. (1998). Adult psychiatric status of hyperactive boys grown up. *American Journal of Psychiatry, 155,* 493–498.

Mannuzza, S., Klein, R. G., Bongura, N., Malloy, P., Giampino, T. L., & Addalli, K. A. (1991). Hyperactive boys almost grown up V: Replication of psychiatric status. *Archives of General Psychiatry, 48,* 77–83.

Margolis, R. L., McInnis, M. G., Rosenblatt, A., & Ross, C. A. (1999). Trinucleotide repeat expansion and neuropsychiatric disease. *Archives of General Psychiatry, 56,* 1019–1031.

Mayes, S. D., Calhoun, S. L., & Crowell, E. W. (1998). WISC-III Freedom from Distractibility as a measure of attention in children with and without attention deficit hyperactivity disorder. *Journal of Attention Disorders, 2,* 217–227.

Mealer, C., Morgan, S., & Luscomb, R. (1996). Cognitive functioning of ADHD and non-ADHD boys on the WISC-III and WRAML: An analysis within a memory model. *Journal of Attention Disorders, 1,* 133–145.

Milberger, S., Biederman, J., Faraone, S. V., Murphy, J., & Tsuang, M. T. (1995). Attention deficit hyperactivity disorder and comorbid disorders: Issues of overlapping symptoms. *American Journal of Psychiatry, 152,* 1793–1799.

Morgan, A. E., Hynd, G. W., Riccio, C. A., & Hall, J. (1996). Validity of DSM-IV predominantly inattentive and combined types: Relationship to previous DSM diagnoses/subtype differences. *Journal of the American Academy of Child and Adolescent Psychiatry, 35,* 325–333.

Morrison, J. R., & Stewart, M. A. (1973). The psychiatric status of the legal families of adopted hyperactive children. *Archives of General Psychiatry, 28,* 888–891.

MTA Cooperative Group. (1999a). A 14-month randomized clinical trial of treatment strategies for Attention-Deficit/Hyperactivity Disorder. *Archives of General Psychiatry, 56,* 1073–1086.

MTA Cooperative Group. (1999b). Moderators and mediators of treatment response of treatment for children with attention-deficit hyperactivity disorder. *Archives of General Psychiatry, 56,* 176–193.

Neuman, R. J., Todd, R. D., Health, A. C., Reich, W., Hudziak, J. J., Bucholz, K. K., Madden, P. A. F., Begleiter, H., Porjesz, B., Kuperman, S., Hesselbrock, V., & Reich, T. (1999). Evaluation of ADHD typology in three contrasting samples. A latent class approach. *J Am Acad Child Adolesc Psychiatry, 38,* 25–33.

Pasamanack, B., Rogers, M., & Lilienfeld, A. M. (1956). Pregnancy experience and the development of behavior disorder in children. *American Journal of Psychiatry, 112,* 613–617.

Pearson, D. A., Norton, A. M., & Farwell, E. C. (1997). ADHD in mental retardation Nature of attention deficits. In J. T. Enns & J. Burack (Eds.), *Attention, development, and psychopathology* (pp. 205–229). New York: Guilford Press.

Pearson, D. A., Lachar, D., Loveland, K. A., Santos, C. W., Faria, L. P., Azzam, P. N., Hentges, B. A., & Cleveland, L. A. (in press). Patterns of behavioral adjustment and maladjustment in mental retardation: A comparison of children with and without ADHD. *American Journal on Mental Retardation.*

Pearson, D. A., Santos, C. W., Roache, J. D., Loveland, K. A., Casat, C. D., Arwell, E. C., Roebuck, T. M., & Lachar, D. (1996). Effects of methylphenidate on behavioral adjustment in children with MR and ADHD. Preliminary findings from a study in progress. *Journal of Developmental Physical Disabilities, 8,* 313–333.

Pelham, W. E., Jr., Bender, M. E., Caddell, J., Booth, S., & Morrer, S. H. (1985). Methylphenidate and children with attention deficit disorder: Dose effects on classroom academic and social behavior. *Archives of General Psychiatry, 42,* 948–952.

Peterson, B. S., & Cohen, D. J. (1998). The treatment of Tourette's syndrome. Multimodal, developmental intervention. *Journal of Clinical Psychiatry, 59(suppl 1),* 62–72.

Pliszka, S. R. (1992). Comorbidity of attention-deficit hyperactivity disorder and overanxious disorder. *Journal of the American Academy of Child and Adolescent Psychiatry, 31,* 197–203.

Pliszka, S. R. (1998). Comorbidity of attention-deficit/hyperactivity disorder with psychiatric disorder An overview. *Journal of Clinical Psychiatry, 59(suppl 7),* 50–58.

Purvis, K. L., & Tannock, R. (1997). Language abilities in children with attention deficit hyperactivity disorder, reading disabilities, and normal controls. *Journal of Abnormal Child Psychology, 25,* 133–144.

Reid, R. (1995). Assessment of ADHD with culturally different groups: The use of behavioral rating scales. *School Psychology Review, 24,* 537–560.

Reid, R., DuPaul, G. J., Power, T. J., Anastopoulos, A. D., Rogers-Adkinson, D., Noll., M-B., & Riccio, C. (1998). Assessing culturally different students for attention deficit hyperactivity disorder using behavior rating scales. *Journal of Abnormal Child Psychology, 26,* 187–198.

Reinecke, M. A., Beebe, D. W., & Stein, M. A. (1999). The third factor of the WISC-III: It's (probably) not Freedom From Distractibility. *Journal of the American Academy of Child and Adolescent Psychiatry, 38,* 322–328.

Reynolds, C. R., & Kamphaus, R. W. (1992). *BASC Behavioral Assessment System for Children Manual.* Circle Pines, MN: American Guidance Service, Inc.

Riccio, C. A., Cohen, M. J., Hall, J., & Ross, C. M. (1997). The third and fourth factors of the WISC-III. What they don't measure. *Journal of Psychoeducational Assessment, 15,* 27–39.

Rispens, J., Swaab, H., van den Oord, E. J. C. G., Coen-Kettenis, P., van Engeland, H., & Yperen, T. (1997). WISC profiles in child psychiatric diagnosis sense or nonsense. *Journal of the American Academy of Child and Adolescent Psychiatry, 36,* 1587–1594.

Rowe, K. J., & Rowe, K. S. (1992). The relationship between inattentiveness in the classroom and reading achievement (Part B): An explanatory study. *Journal of the American Academy of Child and Adolescent Psychiatry, 31,* 357–368.

Rowe, K. S., Rowe, K. J. (1994). Synthetic food coloring and behavior: A dose response effect in a double-blind, placebo-controlled, repeated measures study. *Journal of Pediatrics, 135,* 691–698.

Rubia, K., Overmeyer, S., Taylor, E., Brammer, M., Williams, S. C., Simmons, A., & Bullmore, E. T. (1999). Hypofrontality in attention deficit hyperactivity disorder during higher-order motor control. A study with functional MRI. *American Journal of Psychiatry, 156,* 891–896.

Rutter, M. (1977). Brain damage syndromes in childhood. Concepts and findings. *Journal of Child Psychology and Psychiatry, 18,* 1–21.

Scahill, L., Schwab-Stone, M., Merikangus, K. R., Leckman, J. F., Zhang, H., & Karl, S. (1999). Psychosocial and clinical correlates in a community sample of school-age children. *Journal of the American Academy of Child and Adolescent Psychiatry, 38,* 976–984.

Semrud-Clikeman, M., Steingard, R. J., Filipek, P., Biederman, J., Bekken, K., & Renshaw, P. P. (2000). Using MRI to examine brain-behavior relationships in males with attention deficit disorder with hyperactivity. *Journal of the American Academy of Child and Adolescent Psychiatry, 39,* 477–484.

Sharp, W. S., Walter, J. M., Marsh, W. L., Ritchie, G. F., Hamburger, S. D., & Castellanos, F. X. (1999). ADHD in girls, Clinical comparability of a research sample. *Journal of the American Academy of Child and Adolescent Psychiatry, 38,* 40–47.

Shaywitz, S. (1998). Dyslexia. *New England Journal of Medicine, 338,* 307–312.

Shaywitz, S. E., Shaywitz, B. A., Pugh, K. R., Fulbright, R. K., Constable, R. T., Mencl, W. E., Shankweiler, D. P., Liberman, A. M., Skudlarski, P., Fletcher, J. M., Marchione, K. E., Lacadie, C., Gatenby, C., & Gore, J. C. (1998). Functional disruption in the organization of the brain for reading in dyslexia. *Proceedings of the National Academy of Sciences of the United States of America, 95,* 2636–2641.

Smalley, S. L., Bailey, J. N., Palmer, C. G., Cantwell, D. P., McGough, J. J., Del'Homme, M. A., Asarnow, J. R., Woodward, J. A., Ramsey, C., & Nelson, F. (1998). Evidence that the dopamine D4 receptor is a susceptibility gene in attention deficit hyperactivity disorder. *Molecular Psychiatry, 3,* 427–430.

Spencer, T. J., Biederman, J., Harding, M., O'Donnell, D., Faraone, S. V., Wilens, T. E. (1996). Growth deficits in ADHD children revisited evidence for disorder-associated growth delays? *Journal of the American Academy of Child and Adolescent Psychiatry, 35,* 1460–1469.

Spencer, T. J., Biederman, J., Wilens, T., Harding, M., O'Donnell, D., & Griffin, S. (1996). Pharmacotherapy of attention-deficit hyperactivity disorder across the life cycle. *Journal of the American Academy of Child and Adolescent Psychiatry, 35,* 409–432.

Spencer, T. J., Biederman, J., Wilens, T. (1999). Attention-deficit/hyperactivity disorder and comorbidity. *Pediatric Clinics of North America, 46,* 915–927.

Sprague, R. L., & Sleator, E. K. (1977). Methylphenidate in hyperkinetic children: Differences in dose effects in learning in social behavior. *Science, 198,* 1274–1276.

Steingard, R., Biederman, J., Spencer, T., Wilens, T., & Gonzalez, A. (1993). Comparison of clonidine response in the treatment of attention-deficit hyperactivity disorder with and without comorbid tic disorders. *Journal of the American Academy of Child and Adolescent Psychiatry, 32,* 350–353.

Still, G. F. (1902). Some abnormal psychical conditions in children. *Lancet i.,* 1008–1012.

Tannock, R. (1998). Attention deficit hyperactivity disorder advances in cognitive, neurobiological and genetic research. *Journal of Child Psychology & Psychiatry & Allied Disciplines, 39,* 65–99.

Tannock, R., Schachar, R., & Logan, G. D. (1995). Methylphenidate and cognitive flexibility: Dissociated dose effects in hyperactive children. *Journal of Abnormal Child Psychology, 23,* 235–267.

Tarter, R. E. (1988). Are there indirect behavioral traits which predispose to substance abuse? *Journal of Consulting and Clinical Psychology, 56,* 189–196.

Wechsler, D. (1991). *Wechsler Intelligence Scale for Children—Third Edition Manual.* San Antonio, TX: The Psychological Corporation.

Weiss, G., Hechtman, L., Milroy, T., & Perlman, T. (1985). Psychiatric status of hyperactives as adults a controlled prospective 15-year follow-up of 63 hyperactive children. *Journal of the American Academy of Child and Adolescent Psychiatry, 24,* 211–220.

Wender, E. (1986). The food additive-free diet in the treatment of behavior disorders A review. *Journal of Developmental and Behavioral Pediatrics, 7,* 35–42.

Werry, J. S., & Sprague, R. L. (1970). Hyperactivity. In C. G. Costello (Ed.), *Symptoms of Psychopathology* (pp. 397–417). New York: Wiley.

Whalen, C., Henker, B., Buhrmester, D., Hinshaw, S., Huber, A., & Laski, K. (1989). Does stimulant medication improve the peer status of hyperactive children? *Journal of Consulting and Clinical Psychology, 57,* 545–549.

Wilens, T. E., Biederman, J., Abrantes, A. M., & Spencer, T. J. (1996). A naturalistic assessment of protriptyline for Attention-Deficit Hyperactivity Disorder. *Journal of the American Academy of Child and Adolescent Psychiatry, 35,* 1485–1490.

Wilens, T. E., Biederman, J., Baldessarini, R. J., Geller, B., Schleifer, B. A., Spencer, T. J., Birmaher, B., & Goldblatt, A. (1996). Cardiovascular effects of therapeutic doses of tricyclic antidepressants in children and adolescents. *Journal of the American Academy of Child and Adolescent Psychiatry, 35,* 1491–1501.

Wilens, T. E., Biederman, J., Geist, D. E., Steingard, R., & Spencer, T. (1993). Nortriptyline in the treatment of ADHD a chart review of 58 cases. *Journal of the American Academy of Child and Adolescent Psychiatry, 32,* 343–349.

Wilens, T., Spencer, J. M., Swanson, J. M., Connor, D. F., & Cantwell, D. (1999). Combining methylphenidate and clonidine. A clinically sound medication option.

Wilens, T., & Spencer, T. (2000). The stimulants revisited. *Psychiatric Clinics of North America,* in press.

Winsberg, B. G., & Comings, D. E. (1999). Association of the dopamine transporter gene (DAT1) with methylphenidate response. *Journal of the American Academy of Child and Adolescent Psychiatry, 38,* 1471–1477.

Wolraich, M., Lindgreen, S., Stumbo, P., et al. (1994). Effects of diets high in sucrose or aspartame on the behavior and cognitive performance of children. *New England Journal of Medicine, 330,* 301–307.

Wozniak, J., Biederman, J., Mundy, E., Mennin, D., & Faraone, S. V. (1995). A pilot study of child-onset mania. *Journal of the American Academy of Child and Adolescent Psychiatry, 34,* 1577–1583.

Zametkin, A. J., & Ernst, M. (1999). Problems in the management of attention-deficit-hyperactivity disorder. *New England Journal of Medicine, 340,* 40–46.

Zametkin, A. J., Liebenauer, L. L., Fitzgrald, G. A., et al. (1993). Brain metabolism in teenagers with attention deficit hyperactivity disorder. *Archives of General Psychiatry, 50,* 333–340.

Zametkin, A. J., & Liotta, W. (1997). Neurobiology of Attention-Deficit/Hyperactivity Disorder. *Journal of Clinical Psychiatry, 59*(suppl. 7), 17–23.

Zametkin, A., Rapoport, J. L., Murphy, D. L., Linnoila, M., & Ismond, D. (1985). Treatment of hyperactive children with monoamine oxidase inhibitors: I. Clinical efficacy. *Archives of General Psychiatry, 42,* 962–966.

Zito, J. M., Safer, D. J., dosReis, S., Gardner, J. F., Boles, M., & Lynch, F. (2000). Trends in the prescribing of psychotropic medications to preschoolers. *Journal of the American Medical Association, 283,* 1025–1030.

Chapter 12

EATING DISORDERS: BULIMIA AND ANOREXIA NERVOSA

MERRY N. MILLER AND ANDRES J. PUMARIEGA

INTRODUCTION AND OVERVIEW OF EATING DISORDERS

Eating disorders are possibly the prototypical biopsychosocial behavioral/emotional disorders. They also embody a number of paradoxes in terms of public attitudes about mental illness. Eating disorders affect and are affected by the body and the mind, but they are also greatly influenced by the sociocultural milieu in which young people are raised and develop. Friends, family members, and other individuals who become aware that an individual (usually an adolescent) suffers from an eating disorder usually become highly concerned and distressed by the knowledge of the actual and potential adverse impact of the disorder. At the same time, this is a disorder that has been essentially orphaned by the health and mental health system. This is reflected in practitioners' lack of knowledge and skill in its diagnosis and treatment, the lack of specialized treatment resources available, and the lack of insurance coverage to fund its treatment. Eating disorders are commonly seen among adolescent and young adult women, with a prevalence for anorexia nervosa of 0.5% to 1%, 3% to 5% for bulimia, and up to 10% when subclinical or atypical presentations are included (Walters & Kendler, 1995; Warheit, Langer, Zimmerman, & Biafora, 1993; Kendler et al., 1991). However, eating disorders are still considered rare except among the upper classes; this is a common misconception and a reflection of the denial associated with these disorders. The morbidity and mortality for these disorders are among the highest seen for psychiatric disorders (Harris & Barraclough, 1998): young women with anorexia nervosa have 12 times the mortality of age-matched controls (Sullivan, 1995). In contrast, our society sanctions the glorification and wide dissemination of the images of fashion models and celebrities with bodily proportion which are, at best, naturally unattainable and, at worst, reflective of dangerous levels of weight and nutrition.

This chapter reviews the eating disorders (anorexia nervosa, bulimia, and their variants) from historical, sociocultural, and clinical perspectives. It provides a context for their development among our youth as well as for its identification, diagnosis, treatment, and possible detection and prevention.

HISTORICAL OVERVIEW

Historical Perspectives on Anorexia Nervosa

History shows that disordered eating behaviors have been reported since ancient times in some cultures, but their apparent frequency has varied greatly over time. Ancient Greek and Egyptian cultures have records that indicate ritual fasting for brief periods, but no prolonged fasting (as is seen in anorexia nervosa) is suggested in those records. A spiritually motivated asceticism in ancient Eastern religions led to self-starvation that resembles anorexia nervosa today (Bemporad, 1996). Further examples of asceticism are found at other times in history and in other cultures, such as early Christians and "gnostic cults" (Lacey, 1982), who engaged in severe fasting as a radical reaction against the hedonism and materialism of that age. This spiritual motivation contrasts sharply with the desire for thinness that is believed to be a fundamental characteristic of anorexia in the *Diagnostic and Statistical Manual of Mental Disorders–Fourth Edition* (American Psychiatric Association, 1994).

In contrast, during the Dark Ages, a series of disasters led to a period in which hunger and deprivation were widespread, during this period willful self-starvation appears to have been absent, with a few exceptions (Bemporad, 1996). Later, during the late Middle Ages and the early Renaissance periods, spiritually motivated self-starvation reappeared, and many women who fasted acquired the status of saints in the Roman Catholic church (Bell, 1985).

During the seventeenth and eighteenth centuries, a gradual transformation took place in the interpretations that were made of fasting women. During the Reformation, the belief developed that instead of being holy, such starving women were possessed by the devil. At times self-starvation was seen as a source of entertainment (Bergh & Sodersten, 1998). Later these fasting women were sometimes seen to be frauds. In time they came to be seen as physically or mentally ill, much as they are regarded today (Bemporad, 1996).

Other periods in history have also valued thinness. During the nineteenth century, the "tubercular look" was idealized, and it was considered glamorous to look sickly (Sontag, 1978). During the 1920s flapper era, thinner body forms were again idealized.

Anorexia nervosa became recognized as a medical disorder in the late nineteenth century, and it is noteworthy that these original descriptions did not include a fear of fat, which is considered central to the diagnosis of anorexia nervosa today. The contributions of sociocultural factors have been increasingly prominent in theories about the etiology of anorexia nervosa in recent years. Decreasing prevalence of mass hunger and starvation due to nutritional scarcity and illness have appeared to facilitate the appearance of this disorder.

Historical Perspectives on Bulimia

Bulimia nervosa was only first identified in 1979, and there has been some speculation that it may represent a new disorder rather than one that was previously overlooked (Russell, 1979). This premise, however, is not supported by review of historical precedents, and cultural forces can be observed to play a role in the appearance of bulimic behaviors throughout history.

In contrast to the ascetically motivated self-deprivation described previously, other historical accounts from ancient Egypt, Greece, Rome, and Arabia describe more hedonistically driven behaviors that resemble bulimia (Nassar, 1993). Overeating and induced vomiting in ancient times are well known and do not necessarily represent an ancient equivalent of bulimia nervosa (Russell, 1997). In ancient Rome, vomitoriums were used for the purpose of swallowing an emetic after heavy feasting. Excessive eating followed by habitual vomiting was reportedly practiced by the wealthy elite at that time, which may represent a historical variant of bulimia that was promoted by social forces (Crichton, 1996). In addition, Nassar (1993) has provided accounts of purging that was medically endorsed in ancient Egypt. Again, this self-induced vomiting lacks the desire for thinness as a motivating force, and does not necessarily reflect an ancient form of bulimia. It does suggest an early precedent for bulimic behaviors.

Historical review thus suggests that eating disorders may have been present for thousands of years. Disordered eating behaviors documented throughout most of history raise many questions about whether eating disorders are in fact a product of current social pressures (Bemporad, 1996).

Current Status

The prevalence of eating disorders appears to have increased greatly during the last 50 years (Lucas, Beard, O'Fallon, & Kurland, 1991). Eating disorders were previously thought to be more common in Western industrialized nations and in middle- and upper-class females, but more recent studies demonstrate that there is an increasing diversity of ethnic and socioeconomic groups that are affected by these disorders (Pumariega, Edwards, & Mitchell, 1984; Lacy and Dolan, 1988; Pumariega, 1986; Pate, Pumariega, Hester, & Garner, 1992; Pumariega, Gustavson, Gustavson, Motes, & Ayers, 1994; Miller, Verhegge, Miller, & Pumariega, 1999).

The idealization of the thin body type within Western societies has been identified as a possible factor leading to the development of anorexia nervosa (Bruch, 1962). Garner, Garfinkel, Schwartz, and Thompson (1980) demonstrated an increasing gap between the weights of women in the general population versus the weights of women who serve as role models for attractiveness. The mass media has been blamed by many for playing a possibly pathogenic role in promoting attitudes about body and self that enhance the risk for developing an eating disorder (Stice, Schupak-Neuberg, Shaw, & Stein, 1994; Becker and Hamburg, 1996).

As the image of beauty that is promoted has changed, women in this society show increasing evidence of dissatisfaction with their bodies as well as pressure to conform to this ideal. Increased numbers of diet articles (Garner et al., 1980), and increases in dieting behavior (Nylander, 1971) even among preadolescent girls (Hawkins, Turell & Jackson, 1983; Maloney, McGuire, Daniels, & Specker, 1989) reflect reactions to this dissatisfaction. Such dieting behavior is now believed sometimes to be the precursor to the development of an eating disorder. In addition, certain subpopulations such as ballerinas and models have been associated with particularly high risk for developing eating disorders, due to heightened levels of pressure for thinness (Garner & Garfinkel,

1980; Russell, 1985). Thus, changing sociocultural factors have been identified as the most plausible explanation for rising rates of eating disorders for American and Western women.

Men have been less likely to develop eating disorders (Walsh, 1997), which is consistent with the lower level of social emphasis on male body weight and shape (Rolls, Fedoroff, & Guthrie, 1991). Those men who develop eating disorders closely resemble female eating disorder patients in terms of their dissatisfaction with body image (Olivardia, Pope, Mangweth, & Hudson, 1995). Certain subpopulations of men, such as male wrestlers and jockeys, appear to be at increased risk of developing an eating disorder because their professions require weight restrictions (Mickalide, 1990). A possible association between male homosexuality and the development of eating disorders has also been suggested (Carlat & Camargo, 1991; Silberstein, Mishkind, Striegel-Moore, Timko, & Rodin, 1989; Herzog, Newman, & Warshaw, 1991). The latter association may reflect a male subculture that places males more at risk for disordered eating through its emphasis on appearance and slimness (Silberstein, et al., 1989).

In summary, evidence of eating disorders has been present since ancient times. However, significant changes have occurred in recent times, both in terms of the emphasis on thinness and the apparent increase in prevalence of eating disorders, and also the increased awareness of these illnesses. Disclosure by famous individuals and celebrities, such as Karen Carpenter and Princess Diana, of their own struggles with eating disorders has heightened societal recognition of the existence of these disorders.

PAST AND PRESENT LEADERS IN THE FIELD

Richard Morton is credited with the first medical description of anorexia nervosa in his textbook of medicine published in London in 1689. In this text, he described a "nervous consumption" in which adolescent patients wasted away with no physical illness as the cause of their weight loss (Silverman, 1995). Morton described this starvation process in two of his adolescent patients in painstaking detail.

Despite this and a few other early descriptions of the disorder, anorexia nervosa was not officially named until the late nineteenth century, when it was described almost simultaneously by two prominent physicians, Sir William Gull in England and Charles Lasègue in France. Gull called this condition anorexia nervosa, and Lasègue named it *l'anorexie hystérique* (Walsh, 1997). Their early descriptions are quite similar to the clinical picture of this disorder today. Lasègue emphasized the emotional aspects of this condition, and both recognized the severity of this illness and the role of the mental state in its development (Silverman, 1997).

Within the twentieth century, major advances in understanding of the psychopathology of anorexia nervosa have occurred due to the work of Hilda Bruch. Bruch was a faculty member at Baylor University in Texas, and she spent much time seeking commonalities in the psyches of patients with this condition and writing about her observations. Bruch described three core features that are now considered common signs of anorexia nervosa: disturbance of body image, disturbance of perception, and sense of ineffectiveness (Silverman, 1995). Bruch proposed that this illness represents an attempt to attain autonomy, competence, control, and self-respect. She suggested a psychotherapeutic approach to treatment that emphasizes gradual identification of errors in thinking, aimed at helping patients discover a "genuine self" (Bruch, 1973). Her book, *The Golden Cage,* is considered a classic description of this illness (Bruch, 1978).

David Garner and Paul Garfinkel were two significant figures whose many studies on eating disorders provided an evidence base for many of Bruch's clinical and conceptual insights, as well as advanced systematic approaches to the diagnosis and treatment of these disorders. They were the first to advance the precept that mainstream Western culture's emphasis on thinness was partially responsible for the increasing prevalence of eating disorders, especially among young women. They developed many of the systematic rating measures that are still used today for the clinical and research assessment of eating disorders (the Eating Attitudes Test and the Eating Disorders Inventory). They also contributed to the development of evidence-based treatment approaches, including cognitive-behavioral therapies and pharmacotherapy (Garfinkel & Garner, 1979; Garner & Garfinkel, 1980).

Arthur Crisp also made important contributions to the literature on psychotherapy. Crisp described a developmental model in which anorexia nervosa is conceptualized as a means to cope with fears about physical maturity. By acquiring an anorexic weight level, the patient can regress to a prepubertal shape, hormonal status, and experience. He identified anorexia nervosa as a phobic avoidance disorder, in which the phobic objects are normal adult body weight and shape. He recommended a psychotherapeutic approach that included a focus on dynamic issues that led patients to understand this phobic fear of adult body weight (Crisp, 1997).

In 1979, several centuries after the recognition of anorexia nervosa, Gerald Russell became the first to identify bulimia nervosa. Historical accounts dating back to ancient times describe the occurrence of gross overeating and self-induced vomiting, but these behaviors are not necessarily the equivalent of the disorder now known as bulimia nervosa (Russell, 1997).

ASSESSMENT OF EATING DISORDERS

Detection and Denial

Individuals with eating disorders rarely self-identify and self-refer for treatment. The onsets of these disorders are insidious and are a result of normative behavior (dieting and weight control) carried to an extreme, although the affected individual still believes these are within the range of normality. There are powerful self-reinforcing aspects of either their starvation (positive attention for their new physique or a powerful sense of self-control) or their binge/purge behaviors (relief from distress). These factors as well as shame at being discovered can motivate affected individuals to conceal their deleterious and dangerous behaviors despite their awareness of the risks involved. The detection of eating disorders occurs as a result of the gradual realization by those close to the affected individual of their abnormal behaviors. These include seeing the individual disrobed and suddenly realizing their serious weight loss, catching them in frenetic exercise, realizing their frequent visits to the restroom after meals or noticing traces of vomitus, noticing large quantities of food missing, or multiples of these tell-tale signs.

Physical signs of starvation that can be noted include muscle wasting, fine downy hair over their extremities, loss of hair, and alternating periods of excessive energy and fatigue. Signs of binge-purging include calluses over the dorsum of the hand from stomach acid scarring, swollen cheeks from parotid enlargement, gum irritation and loss of tooth enamel (dentists can often detect early), and frequent gas and gastrointestinal upset (Bunnell et al., 1990).

The process of overcoming the denial of the affected individual is often drawn out and difficult. It frequently requires confrontation of denial at multiple levels. Family members and those close to the individual are often the last to know, due to the gradual onset of symptoms, their idealization of the affected individual, and the concealment and secretiveness associated with the disorders. As in substance abuse, the concepts of denial and enablement are applicable here, with loved ones inadvertently participating in relational patterns that can sustain the disorders. Friends, teachers, and school officials are often placed in the uncomfortable position of confronting these critical relations, but this step is critical. It is only after overcoming the denial of the individuals close to the affected person that an effective intervention can be conducted to confront them about their self-destructive behavior.

With adolescents, it is not uncommon that the initial stages of assessment and treatment are carried out without full cooperation. This is also complicated both by adolescents' natural tendencies to shun greater dependency on authority figures (including treating professionals) and by their use of abnormal eating behaviors as a means of establishing independence and autonomy. A paradoxical and complicating set of family interactions ensues when the family is convinced that, although they see the effect of the disorder on the adolescent, they can take control over the youth's behavior in order to help them overcome it. This often requires a second level of intervention with the family, in which they are helped to see the futility of over-controlling the adolescent's eating behavior as well as the importance of supporting them in assuming control over her or his body, nutrition, and life. This may require specialized interventions by individuals skilled in family therapy. Although individuals with bulimia are likely to recognize their disorder, shame and fear of stigmatization often prevents them from seeking treatment at an early stage (Johnson & Conners, 1987; Rizzuto, 1988).

Psychological/Psychiatric Assessment

Given the degree of denial and mistrust with which individuals with eating disorders approach treatment, the most critical aspect of the assessment process is the development of a therapeutic alliance. The validity of the information collected during the assessment process and the degree of acceptance of treatment depends on the degree of trust, which the evaluating or treating mental health professional establishes with the affected individual and her or his family. The mental health professional needs to be able to communicate respect and support to the affected individual, indicating that the patient has the ultimate control over her or his body and health, while also honestly confronting dangerous or maladaptive behaviors or cognitions. This also involves a balancing act in maintaining both the alliance with the affected individual and her or his family, which may often be at odds with each other (Rizzuto, 1988).

A comprehensive diagnostic evaluation covers a number of areas of information and process. These include information on symptoms and behaviors both from the perspective of the affected individuals and their family or significant others. Multi-informant information allows for the balancing of perspectives or biases of different observers. Information on eating behaviors (including eating rituals or restricted food preferences), attitudes about weight or bodily appearance, and means of restricting or purging food intake (including the use of self-induced vomiting, diuretics, over-exercise or even anorectant medications), and symptoms of comorbid psychiatric disorders are important.

Equally important is information on precipitating stressors or crises (such as losses in relationships, conflicts with peers, or losses in self-esteem), and predisposing or sustaining personality attributes. The individual's level of social and psychological function should be assessed by obtaining information about the quality of her or his peer relations, family relations, involvement in social or community activities, level of withdrawal or engagement with others, and the extent to which the eating disorder interferes in any of these facets of life. Given that food and eating are at the center of much of our socialization, it is not unusual for the affected individual to find it hard to pursue a full social and interpersonal life. Preoccupations with eating rituals, avoidance of food and eating, intense self-consciousness about physical appearance, or scavenging for binge foods may further impair daily function. Psychological testing may be useful to confirm characteristic personality traits and to evaluate personality development. Cognitive assessment is also important to determine the presence of underlying learning disorders producing stress for the youth, or cognitive deficits resulting from nutritional causes. Family history of psychiatric disorders can point to inherited risk factors for psychopathology, whereas family interactional patterns and unresolved conflicts (especially around emotional separation and autonomy) can suggest predisposing or sustaining factors (American Psychiatric Association, 2000; also, see section on diagnostic characteristics of the different eating disorders).

Once the evaluation is completed, the clinician's next task is to present to the affected individual and the family a coherent understanding of the factors contributing to the individual's condition and to engage her or him and the family in the development of a treatment plan resulting from this understanding. Denial may need to be confronted again because the affected individual may try to minimize the severity of the disorder and its resulting functional limitations. The formulation that the clinician achieves from integrating diagnostic information as well as their communication of this formulation to the affected individual and family members guides and supports the rationale for treatment efforts (Rizzuto, 1988).

Medical Evaluation

Individuals affected by eating disorders may find it more acceptable to be evaluated by a nonpsychiatric physician, most commonly a primary care physician, for their initial assessment. The first task is to ensure the medical stability of the individual. However, the findings from such assessment can also be used to help the individual and the family overcome their denial of the disorder and to appreciate the importance of treatment to prevent further morbidity and even mortality.

Eating disorders can lead to various types of medical complications resulting from prolonged starvation, nutritional deficiencies, binging, or purging. The assessment of cardiovascular status is critical, because cardiac function can be weakened either by protein starvation or electrolyte imbalance from purging. In addition, starvation can also affect all organ systems, including renal function, liver function, gastrointestinal function, immune function, reproductive and endocrine function, and musculoskeletal strength and integrity. Laboratory evaluation should include blood tests for serum electrolytes, serum proteins, liver function tests, renal function tests, fasting blood glucose, complete blood cell counts, and endocrine function (thyroid function, gonadal hormones, and gonadal stimulating hormones).

Serious complications from anorexia nervosa and bulimia include sudden cardiac arrest, arrhythmia, congestive heart failure, renal failure, abdominal rupture from binging, esophageal bleeding, and muscle cramping. One critical test that should be performed on any individual with an eating disorder or engaging in long term dieting is a bone scan, which evaluates the risk of osteoporosis. Eating disorders involve the loss of calcium and protein from bones resulting from inadequate nutrition as well as inadequate secretion of estrogen in females, leading to multiple fractures and eventually spinal compression. Such changes, commonly seen in postmenopausal women in their 60s to 80s, can be seen in women with anorexia nervosa in their 20s and 30s. Medical screening assessment for possible underlying medical conditions mimicking eating disorders, such as hypothalamic/pituitary tumors, occult cancer, thyroid disease, or gastrointestinal disease is also indicated, especially in individuals whose psychological presentation is not consistent with common patterns seen with eating disorders (APA, 2000).

DIAGNOSIS AND FORMULATION

Anorexia Nervosa

Anorexia nervosa is characterized by weight loss (or failure to gain weight) to a level over 15 percent below the individual's ideal weight for height resulting from food restriction, purging, or both, overexercise, or other methods of food avoidance. Affected individuals distort their perception of their body, either by thinking they are too fat while continuing to lose weight or by focusing on slimming "out of proportion" body areas while ignoring their overall weight loss. Those areas receiving focus tend to be those characteristic of the feminine form, such as hips, thighs, upper arms, and bust line. These behaviors may start innocently as part of a diet to lose a few excess pounds, but the affected individuals quickly become consumed by the pursuit of thinness and a preoccupation with eating, losing control of their behavior while paradoxically feeling in greater control of their weight. Affected individuals weigh themselves multiple times daily, count calories to great precision, and obsess on planning past or future meals.

Women with anorexia nervosa also experience cessation of menses or menstrual irregularities. These have been thought to be primarily due to weight loss and reduced percentage of body fat resulting in lower levels of gonadal hormones (particularly estrogen). However, menstrual disturbances can be seen prior to weight loss in up to one third of women who later develop anorexia nervosa, which is suggestive of some hormonal and neurotransmitter regulation disturbances that may place some individuals at risk (APA, 1994).

In additional to the physical and behavioral manifestations of this disorder (and the resulting symptoms of starvation previously discussed), there are psychological and emotional characteristics that help distinguish affected individuals. Prior to the onset of overt symptoms of anorexia, these individuals demonstrate perfectionistic and obsessive traits that express themselves in many areas of their lives. They often push themselves to perform and to behave at their best at all times, and they are highly intolerant of flaws or imperfections in themselves (and at times in others). They also measure their performance and their self-worth based on others' opinions or standards, often failing to develop their own views or standards, a characteristic that Bruch termed *other-directedness* (Bruch, 1973). This results in their persistent pursuit to meet others' expectations or to please others while ignoring their needs and wants, leaving them feeling ineffective and emotionally depleted.

Lack of self-awareness is another cardinal feature of individuals with anorexia nervosa. Bruch hypothesized that the individual with anorexia nervosa not only has problems with identity formation as a result of other-directedness, but also fails to develop the internal awareness of hunger or satiety necessary to regulate eating and relies excessively on external cues. Bruch further hypothesized that affected individuals also have difficulty tolerating intense emotions or sensations due to their problems with self-awareness and self-regulation, with a tendency to suppress any such internal experiences. Indeed, individuals with anorexia nervosa are often described as ascetic and avoid sensual experiences of all types and intense emotional experiences, including close relationships, which they find overwhelming. Self-starvation paradoxically becomes a means of controlling these overwhelming experiences and experiencing a greater sense of self-control (Bruch, 1973; Rizutto, 1988). Avoidance of interpersonal conflict is one of the ways in which they achieve others' admiration, which results in their lacking assertiveness and self-advocacy skills. A tendency to cognitive rigidity accompanies their tendency to obsessiveness, where they are unable to think flexibly and to break out of stereotypical solutions or patterns, though not as pervasive as in the developmental disorders (Rizzuto, 1988). The families of affected individuals have been found to reflect many of these traits, including rigidity of beliefs and patterns of behavior, difficulties with problem-solving, avoidance of conflict, difficulties maintaining interpersonal boundaries with over-involvement in the lives of other family members, and a focus on performance and pleasing others to achieve acceptance or affection (Minuchin, Rosman, & Baker, 1978).

Anorexia nervosa affects young women disproportionately, in a proportion of more than 10 to 1 over males. This may reflect the high number of risk factors that affect young women, including hormonal, cultural, and interpersonal. However, when seen in males, it is associated with more serious comorbid psychological disturbance. It has its most frequent onset in early adolescence, immediately after the onset of puberty, when both hormonal factors and weight gain due to growth are significant factors. However, this is the most treatable group with the best prognosis for recovery. Another common onset is in late adolescence, associated with greater peer involvement and separation from the family as precipitating factors. Overall, prognosis is improved if the individual enters treatment shortly after onset, but many do not enter treatment as late as two years after onset. Prognosis is also worse when anorexia nervosa is associated with serious personality disorders. Although mortality has significantly decreased over the years with better treatment and medical management of complications, we are now seeing many individuals who are chronically ill with anorexia nervosa and whose lives are marked with chronic disability as a result (APA, 2000).

Bulimia Nervosa

Bulimia nervosa has a number of similarities and differences with anorexia nervosa. Actually, bulimia has been preceded by anorexia nervosa in a significant percentage of those affected (Bulik, Sullivan, Fear, & Pickering, 1997). Individuals with bulimia engage in preoccupation with thinness, restriction of food, and perceptual distortions of their body. However, they have a greater tendency to impulsivity and less capacity for asceticism and self-denial. Starvation then triggers intense hunger they are unable to control, leading to episodes of binge eating. These can amount to thousands of calories at a time, mostly consisting of carbohydrate foods. The individual feels a transient sense of well-being and tension relief from binging; but great abdominal discomfort and often distension, due to the great quantities of food consumed, quickly follow it. This prompts purging to seek relief, mostly through self-induced vomiting, but also through the use of laxatives, diuretics, or over-exercise. As a result of their frequent binge-purging episodes, they retain a certain amount of food intake, so their weight is maintained at near-normal levels (and even at times overweight levels) despite intermittent food restriction. The minimum frequency of binge-purge episodes necessary for the diagnosis of bulimia is two per week, but affected individuals may secretively engage in binge-purge episodes several times per day. In addition to their compulsive binge-purging, individuals with bulimia may also engage in other compulsive or addictive behaviors, such as substance abuse, shopping, gambling, or reckless sexual activity (APA, 1994).

Psychologically, the individual with bulimia also shares many of the characteristics seen in those with anorexia nervosa, including perfectionism, obsessiveness, cognitive rigidity, other-directedness, and conflict avoidance. They do not engage in the same avoidance of intense emotions or sensual experiences, although they have clear difficulty in regulating their engagement in such. This is reflected in their tendency to mood lability, to intense and stormy relationships, and even to impulsivity and at times violence. They are more socially skilled than individuals with anorexia, but their relationships are either superficial or too intense. The families of individuals with bulimia also reflect these tendencies to greater impulsivity, with a greater tendency to family discord and even family violence. Affected individuals frequently have histories of sexual, physical, or emotional abuse in their families, which appear to be significant risk factors (Rorty, Yager, & Rossotto, 1994). Family histories of mood disorders (depression, bipolar disorder), substance abuse, and other compulsive and addictive behaviors are common (Johnson & Connors, 1987).

The onset of bulimia is most frequently seen in the late adolescent and young adult years. The highest incidence and prevalence is seen in college populations, with separation from the family and difficulties with self-sufficiency and self-regulation (eating, sexuality, time management, etc.) possibly being precipitating factors. However, onset in middle-aged women or younger adolescents are not uncommon. Bulimia is seen most frequently in females in similarly high proportions as with anorexia nervosa, with similar risk factors. The prognosis for recovery is better with early recognition and treatment, as well as treatment of comorbid disorders. Prognosis is worse to the extent that the characteristics of anorexia nervosa are seen coexisting with those of bulimia, or when associated with serious personality disorders. The combination of both disorders, previously termed *bulimarexia* but now classified as anorexia nervosa, binge-purge subtype, has the poorest prognosis of all eating disorders (Johnson & Connors, 1987).

Atypical Forms

The diagnosis of Eating Disorders NOS in the *DSM-IV* (APA, 1994) is used for individuals who have incomplete expression of the symptoms of either bulimia or anorexia nervosa, or who may have combined features, neither of which reach full diagnostic levels. However, individuals who are assigned this diagnosis may have just as severe and incapacitating a disorder as those with either anorexia and bulimia, and may require treatment just as urgently. The diagnosis of Binge Eating Disorder is often used for individuals who engage in compulsive binge episodes without compensatory purging. These individuals may share more behavioral and emotional features with those seen in bulimia, and less with those seen in anorexia. Like the other eating disorders, they have high comorbidity of depression. They are typically overweight, which is reflective of their nonpurging or infrequent purging status, and have the resulting medical complications associated with obesity. However, it is important to distinguish those individuals whose obesity is due primarily to genetic and lifestyle factors from those who engage in compulsive binging, especially in terms of the indication and benefit of psychological and psychiatric treatments (APA, 1994).

Differential Diagnoses

Various psychiatric disorders can mimic eating disorders and need to be ruled out in the process of assessment. Severe major depression should be considered in the differential diagnosis of eating disorders. It can present with either loss of appetite and weight loss or overeating and weight gain, and depression is frequently comorbid with both anorexia nervosa and bulimia. A difference between depression and anorexia is that the patient with depression alone does not have a core disturbance in body image and lack of perception of weight loss, and is not preoccupied with a desire to lose more weight. Another difference is that anorexia nervosa alone does not actually include a loss of appetite (the term "anorexia" is actually a misnomer), whereas decreased appetite is a common symptom of depression.

Bipolar disorder can also mimic anorexia and bulimia if disordered eating or weight loss is part of the symptomatology. Schizophrenia can also mimic anorexia nervosa, presenting with delusions involving food and eating, such as fear of being poisoned, magical beliefs around the avoidance of certain foods, and bodily delusions that can resemble body image distortions. The presence of the full symptomatic and psychological picture of anorexia nervosa or bulimia can serve to rule out these other possible disorders.

Comorbid Conditions

Individuals with eating disorders are frequently diagnosed with other concurrent psychiatric disorders. Major depression or dysthymia is diagnosed in 50% to 75% of individuals with eating disorders, whereas bipolar disorder has been diagnosed in 4% to 13%. Underlying depression may place an individual at risk for an eating disorder beyond the effect of the mood disorder on appetite and eating; some studies have identified that many of the neurotransmitter systems involved in depression are also involved in eating disorders, especially serotonin pathways (Kaye and Weltzin, 1991). Obsessive-compulsive disorder is also seen comorbidly with eating disorders; as high as 25% in individuals with anorexia nervosa, for whom obsessions and compulsions go beyond food and weight. In these instances, an underlying risk for obsessive-compulsive disorder may well place an individual at risk for an eating disorder.

Posttraumatic stress disorder is also commonly seen comorbidly with anorexia nervosa and bulimia. Sexual abuse is a particularly powerful stressor that has been associated with the development of comorbid bulimia and posttraumatic stress disorder (Palmer, Oppenheimer, Dignon, Chaloner, & Howells, 1990; Rorty et al., 1994; Waller, 1991). There has been some debate regarding this issue, and some investigators have found that women with bulimia nervosa are no more likely than women in other psychiatric groups to have been sexually abused as children (Pope & Hudson, 1992). The propensity of individuals with bulimia toward impulsivity and compulsivity, as well as the high comorbidity with depression, places them at risk for substance abuse disorders, most frequently involving alcohol and cocaine. This triple morbidity (bulimia, depression, and substance abuse/dependence) has been reported in the literature with some frequency and is extremely difficult to treat. A similarly problematic comorbidity is that seen with borderline personality disorder. Many of the risk factors for borderline personality disorder are similar to those seen in eating disorders, particularly history of poor relations with parenting figures and recurrent abuse. These factors may also render individuals vulnerable to this serious personality disorder characterized by stormy interpersonal relations perceived in stark black/white extremes, mood lability, and impulsivity (Braun, Sunday, & Halmi, 1994).

Risk Factors and Populations

A number of subpopulations of adolescents and young adults have been found to have an increased prevalence of eating disorders. For most of these, it is still unclear whether the activities they engage in place them at higher risk for developing eating disorders, or whether they attract individuals whose personality traits already place them at some risk that is accentuated by the activities they pursue. Many athlete groups have high prevalence rates for eating disorders; this is especially true for gymnasts, track athletes, male wrestlers, and racehorse jockeys. All of these sports have strict weight limitations and high performance expectations that support the development of eating disorders, particularly anorexia nervosa. Models and dancers also have higher prevalence rates for eating disorders. This is reflective of the unrealistic body size and proportions required for participation, of the high level of dedication and perfectionism expected in the practice, and of the high level of public exposure they receive. The latter has reciprocal negative effects on the general population in terms of representing unrealistic cultural ideals, and on the involved individuals as serving as role models (Powers & Johnson, 1996; Yates, 1996).

Other subpopulations also have increased risk for eating disorders. Immigrant and first-generation youth have been reported to have higher rates of abnormal eating attitudes as they attempt to adapt and be accepted into the mainstream culture. At the same time, the prevalence of eating disorders in most nations and cultures outside the United States is rising (Pumariega, 1986; Pate et al., 1992). Youth suffering from medical illnesses (diabetes mellitus, cystic fibrosis, celiac disease, ulcerative colitis, etc.) that have significant requirements for dietary restriction and have significant effects on body size and weight have also been found to have a higher risk for eating disorders (Rodin, Daneman, & DeGroot, 1993; Pumariega, Pursell, Spock, & Jones, 1986). First degree relatives of individuals with anorexia nervosa have higher rates of anorexia nervosa and bulimia nervosa, but the evidence of inheritable risk in the relatives of individuals with bulimia is mixed (Walters & Kendler, 1995).

CLINICAL CASE STUDIES

The following are case studies based on actual patients. They have been fictionalized in order to conceal the identities of the patients and to demonstrate the common features of these disorders.

Young Athlete with Anorexia Nervosa

Amy is a 16 year old who excels in both school and ballet. She has been taking dance lessons since she was 4 years old, and in recent years has spent much of her free time at dance class. Her mother has become somewhat concerned because Amy has been losing weight, and recently she became very dizzy at a ballet practice and thought she might faint. Her mother has noticed that Amy's eating habits have changed in the last several months as well: she has begun to avoid eating with other family members, and instead sometimes eats alone in her room. When she does eat with the family, she eats very slowly and has begun to cut her food into very small pieces as she eats. Amy is 5 feet 4 inches and now weighs only 88 pounds, yet she has told her mother that she thinks she needs to lose five more pounds. Although Amy reached menarche at age 13, her menses have stopped for the last year.

Amy has also become very moody in the last few months. She is irritable with the family, and sometimes has had crying spells in which she bursts into tears for no clear reason. She reports that she has lost interest in her schoolwork and her social activities, and no longer feels like going out with her friends. Although she has always been a very good student, recently her motivation has been decreasing and she has had to force herself to do her assignments.

Amy is very self-conscious about her weight. She worries constantly about what she has eaten today and is always counting calories. She likes to dress in baggy clothes and often wears several layers of clothes in order to stay warm. She likes the way the baggy clothes hide her stomach.

Amy is the first of three children and is very close to her mother. She has always been an easy child, eager to please and to succeed.

College Student with Bulimia Nervosa

Susan is a sophomore in college who has always worried about her weight and has tried multiple diets. She is 5 foot 6 inches and weighs between 135 and 140 pounds. Since coming to college, she has become progressively more concerned about her weight. She has tried to diet but sometimes "loses control" and eats what she considers to be excessive amounts of food at one sitting. She has eaten a whole large pizza alone, and sometimes she eats large quantities of Twinkies and other sweets. After such a binge, Susan feels miserable, very bloated, and down. She began forcing herself to vomit as a freshman after learning from her roommate that some of the girls in her dorm were doing that to lose weight. As college has progressed, she has found herself binging and purging more and more often, sometimes several times per day. She is embarrassed and ashamed of these behaviors, and has not told anyone about it. Her roommate has become suspicious because Susan often disappears to the bathroom after meals, but Susan has lied when her roommate asked her if she were purging. Susan knows she has a problem but is very concerned about becoming fat.

Susan finally went to her college's mental health center for help after her roommate confronted her. She was very nervous about going and very sheepish to admit what she had been doing. She is also very reluctant for her family to learn about what she has been doing and considers this to be a great secret.

Another motive for finally going to get some help was that Susan has begun to feel physically ill. She has had abdominal pain on several occasions. Her cheeks are swollen. Her teeth have been decaying more rapidly; the last time she went to the dentist she learned that she had three cavities.

Older Female with Chronic Bulimia

Cynthia is a 35-year-old housewife who has been bulimic since she was in college. She began binging and purging during her sophomore year after a breakup with a boyfriend, and at times during college she binged and purged four to five times per day. She realized she had a problem and went to student health center for help when she was a senior. Since then, she has had periods of remission that have lasted as long as a year, but she has relapsed during times of increased stress.

Recently she has been anxious about an upcoming move and is also dreading her daughter's graduation from high school and departure for college next year. She and her husband have been fighting quite frequently for the last few months. She started binging and purging again about three months ago. Her husband is fairly unaware of her behavior, but her daughter has been conscious of her purging and has been encouraging Cynthia to seek help again. Cynthia is also currently quite depressed and has been having crying spells almost daily. She has been trying to cope with her distress by drinking a few glasses of wine every night.

INTERVENTIONS AND REHABILITATION

The treatment and rehabilitation of individuals with eating disorders requires a multi-modal and interdisciplinary approach that is reflective of the multiple precipitating and sustaining factors that impact upon them. We will outline the various components that can be included in a treatment package, though these may be combined and selected in different combinations, at various times, and in various temporal sequences to fit the unique needs of the individual. Ideally these are all found in a coordinated treatment program, or are delivered by a team of professionals with the ability to coordinate care within an organized plan.

Nutritional interventions are an important component of treatment for eating disorders. Almost invariably, patients with eating disorders have a history of dieting prior to the onset of their disorder. Learning to consciously choose a healthy diet can play a key role in helping these patients overcome their disorders. Inclusion of a nutritionist in the treatment team for patients with eating disorders is essential.

Patients with anorexia nervosa need to gain weight to a target level, which is usually determined according to general population weight/height tables that may relate to the age of illness onset (Crisp, 1997). Weight gain by anorexic patients is usually achieved through a prescribed diet combined with reassurance from the nutritionist that the patient will not be led to become overweight. The rate of weight gain should be slow in order to avoid further medical complications. Caloric intake should be gradually increased to achieve an ideal weight gain of 1 to 2 pounds per week (or 2–3 pounds per week for hospitalized patients). In an inpatient setting, a prescription of 3,000 calories per day combined with bedrest leads to a desired weight gain of approximately 1 kg (3 lbs.) per week. As patients progress in treatment, deviation from this rate of weight gain may reflect noncompliance and merits discussion about possible resistant attitudes. It is not unusual for these patients to experience panic or mounting dysphoria as they approach their goal weights.

In the case of bulimia nervosa, patients often attempt to diet only to give in to their hunger and binge impulsively. The experience of binging leads to feelings of guilt and depression and is usually followed by a purge or other compensatory behavior in order to get rid of the excessive intake that was consumed during the binge. Therefore, if a patient with bulimia nervosa can learn to plan meals and avoid excessive hunger, he or she is less likely to succumb to a binge and then to a purge.

Restoration of regular eating patterns for patients with eating disorders includes several components. Meals should occur at set times and with a predetermined plan and should be spaced throughout the day. Patients should be encouraged to include foods that were previously avoided, so that they may become more relaxed about eating. One approach for doing this is to develop a hierarchy of feared foods, and to move up this scale gradually over time. Patients also should be encouraged to monitor their own intake and abnormal eating behaviors, thus allowing them to acquire a greater sense of control (Garner, 1997).

Monitoring of patients with anorexia nervosa and bulimia should be done regularly and is an important indicator of their clinical progress. This can include the monitoring of weight (by clinicians), binge episodes (by the patient), nutritional intake, and emotional triggers for adverse behaviors. Recent evidence shows that weight gain during a hospitalization is the strongest predictor for outcome (Howard et al., 1999). Monitoring can also be integrated into behavioral contracts in which the patient receives reinforcers in exchange for achieving different levels of success in terms of weight gain or other symptom reduction. Such contracts are best developed through active negotiation and participation with the affected individual, in order to enhance their sense of ownership of their recovery and control. Self-monitoring in itself can also be a powerful behavioral technique to motivate the individual to work on symptom reduction. Patients may be quite capable of participating actively in psychotherapy and giving the appearance of progress while still severely restricting their diet and continuing to lose weight or engaging in frequent binge-purging episodes, so it is imperative that the weight itself be monitored.

Medical assessment and intervention may be required at the initial evaluation of eating disorder patients as well as during ongoing treatment. The cardiovascular system should be monitored, especially in patients with anorexia nervosa. Cardiac dysfunction can develop due to electrolyte abnormalities (particularly hypokalemia), especially in patients who vomit or use laxatives or diuretics. Also, the starvation of anorexia can result in bradycardia and low blood pressure. A variety of EKG abnormalities can occur in patients with eating disorders. Repeated medical monitoring is often required to determine electrolyte status, dehydration, and cardiac status (Mitchell, Pomeroy, & Adson, 1997).

Bone health can be damaged by anorexia nervosa these patients may develop delayed maturation of bone, decreased bone density, and pathological fractures. Bone density may not be restored by later weight gain. Bone scans assess for osteoporosis, and treatment with cyclic estrogen or calcium supplementation may be considered. Hormone replacement therapy (e.g., oral contraceptives) are commonly prescribed to treat osteopenia in anorexic females, although there is little evidence at this time to demonstrate its effectiveness (Robinson, Bachrach, & Katzman, 2000).

Malnutrition and vomiting can lead to gastrointestinal bleeding, including esophagitis and erosion. On rare occasions, esophageal rupture can occur; this is a potentially fatal complication that is a medical emergency. Other gastrointestinal problems can develop during the course of eating disorders, including severe constipation and gastrointestinal bleeding due to laxative abuse. Acute pancreatitis can also develop in association with bulimia nervosa (APA, 2000).

In conclusion, due to the multiple medical complications that can develop during the course of eating disorders, it is important that a primary care physician participate actively in the treatment of these patients and follow them regularly.

Medications can be useful in the treatment of bulimia nervosa and to a lesser extent may be helpful in the treatment of anorexia nervosa as well. Antidepressants have been shown to decrease the frequency of binging and purging behaviors in bulimia nervosa. In addition, these medications have been shown to reduce the likelihood of a relapse for anorexic patients who have regained weight. Antidepressants are also useful in the treatment of depression and obsessive-compulsive disorder, both of which often coexist with the eating disorders. The tricyclic antidepressants, especially imipramine, were found to be efficacious in the treatment of bulimia and depression in adults, whereas anafranil was found to be efficacious in the treatment of obsessive-compulsive disorder. However, these older antidepressants were found to have potentially serious side effects, including effects on cardiac conduction and contractility, which compounded the adverse cardiac effects of the eating disorders themselves and led to high overdose toxicity. The advent of the newer classes of antidepressants, especially the selective serotonin reuptake inhibitors, proved both efficacious and much safer in regular use and in overdose. Fluoxetine was found to be efficacious in the treatment of bulimia; fluoxetine and sertraline are efficacious in the treatment of adult and adolescent depression; and both of these as well as fluvoxamine are also efficacious in the treatment of obsessive-compulsive disorder. Lithium carbonate and valproic acid have been used in the treatment of bulimia accompanied by mood lability or bipolar symptoms (APA, 2000).

Psychotherapeutic approaches are the mainstay of treatment for eating disorders. A variety of modalities may be helpful individual therapy, group therapy (with other eating disorder patients), and family therapy (especially for adolescent patients) may all be beneficial. The content of the therapy may include confrontation of distorted thinking processes, emotional support, and learning to identify and express emotions. Confrontation of distorted ideas about weight and shape, rigid rules about dieting, and identification of triggers for binge episodes are primary foci for cognitive therapy. Other common themes addressed in therapy by these patients include struggles around separation from parents and control issues. Cognitive-behavioral therapies and therapeutic techniques that focus on binge prevention and cognitive problem-solving of trigger stresses that lead to binge eating, food restriction, or body image preoccupation have been demonstrated to be quite effective. Some of these are now manualized and have demonstrated efficacy (Wilson, Fairburn, & Agras, 1997; Garner, Vitousek, & Pike, 1997).

Hospitalization is sometimes needed for eating disorder patients. Indications for hospitalization include severe or rapid weight loss, usually to less than 85% of normal weight; failure of outpatient treatment efforts, significant psychiatric comorbidity or risk of self-harm, and significant medical complications (Andersen, Bowers, & Evans, 1997). Within a hospital setting, behavioral programs that reward healthy eating behavior and weight gain for anorexic patients are usually successful; rarely are forced feedings required.

DETECTION AND PREVENTION

Detection and preventative activities in the schools and other community settings have the potential to play a valuable role in reducing the presence of eating disorders. Efforts have been made within the school setting to heighten awareness of these disorders and to diminish the influence of media and peer pressure. An additional focus has been to decrease the amount of dieting that occurs among schoolchildren, because this is a common behavioral antecedent to the development of both anorexia nervosa and bulimia nervosa. Unfortunately, the effectiveness of such primary prevention programs thus far has been disappointing according to several studies (Fairburn, 1997).

Identification of individuals with eating disorders and referral for treatment is important, especially because early recognition can diminish the progression of these illnesses. Education of teachers, coaches, school nurses, and primary care physicians is needed, because these are the individuals most likely to come into contact with individuals who have eating disorders.

Initial detection of these disorders can be difficult. The weight loss of anorexia nervosa is more obvious, although it is not unusual for these patients to hide their appearance with bulky layers of clothing. Bulimic behaviors are often concealed and may be discovered by peers or family members after behavior changes are observed (e.g., repeated disappearances to the bathroom after meals).

One method to aid in detection of individuals at risk for eating disorders is the use of screening surveys, such as the Eating Attitudes Test (EAT; Garfinkel & Garner, 1979). This test is a brief self-administered questionnaire that asks about a variety of attitudes and behaviors regarding eating. A high score on the EAT has been shown to be a reliable indicator of an individual with an increased risk of developing an eating disorder, thus such a test can be used to screen for individuals who warrant further assessment.

The greatest challenge in the early stages of identification of eating disorders is overcoming the strong resistance seen in most patients. These patients are likely to deny that they have a problem and to see any weight loss as a sign of success for themselves rather than as a symptom of an illness. They are also likely to have a strong desire for control and to resist being pressured to change their behaviors. They often hide their unhealthy eating behaviors and may go to great lengths to conceal them. They may be very fearful of treatment, especially if they perceive treatment as leading to weight gain. For these reasons, it is important that an alliance be developed with eating disordered patients. Effort should be made to avoid control battles. Treatment of these disorders is a lengthy process that requires patience and continual reinforcement.

REFERENCES

Agras, W., Schneider, J., Arnow, B., Raeburn, S., & Telch, C. (1989). Cognitive-behavioral and response-prevention treatments for bulimia nervosa. *Journal of Consulting and Clinical Psychology, 57,* 215–221.

American Psychiatric Association. (1994). *Diagnostic and statistical manual of mental disorders* (4th ed.). Washington, DC: Author.

American Psychiatric Association. (2000). Practice guidelines for the treatment of patients with eating disorders [Revision]. *American Journal of Psychiatry, 157(suppl.),* 1–39.

Andersen, A. E., Bowers, W., & Evans, K. (1997). Inpatient treatment of anorexia nervosa. In D. M. Garner & P. E. Garfinkel (Eds.), *Handbook of treatment for eating disorders,* 2nd ed. (pp. 327–353). New York: Guilford Press.

Becker, A. E., & Hamburg, P. (1996). Culture, the media, and eating disorders. *Harvard Review of Psychiatry, 4,* 163–167.

Bell, R. M. (1985). *Holy Anorexia.* Chicago: University of Chicago Press.

Bemporad, J. R. (1996). Self-starvation through the ages: Reflections on the pre-history of anorexia nervosa. *International Journal of Eating Disorders, 19,* 217–237.

Bergh, C., & Sodersten, P. (1998). Anorexia nervosa: Rediscovery of a disorder. *Lancet, 351,* 1427–1429.

Braun, D. L., Sunday, S. R., & Halmi, K. A. (1994). Psychiatric co-morbidity in patients with eating disorders. *Psychological Medicine, 24,* 859–867.

Bruch, H. (1962). Perceptual and conceptual disturbances in anorexia nervosa. *Psychosomatic Medicine, 24,* 287–294.

Bruch, H. (1966). Anorexia nervosa and its differential diagnosis. *Journal of Nervous and Mental Disease, 141,* 555–566.

Bruch, H. (1973). *Eating disorders: Obesity, anorexia nervosa and the person within.* New York: Basic Books.

Bruch, H. (1978). *The golden cage: The enigma of anorexia nervosa.* Cambridge, MA: Harvard University Press.

Bulik, C., Sullivan, P., Fear, J., & Pickering, A. (1997). Predictors of the development of bulimia nervosa in women with anorexia nervosa. *Journal of Nervous and Mental Disorders, 185,* 704–705.

Bunnell, D. W., Shenker, I. R., Nussbaum, M. P., Jacobson, M. S., Cooper, P., & Phil, D. (1990). Subclinical versus formal eating disorders: Differentiating psychological features. *International Journal of Eating Disorders, 9,* 357–362.

Carlat, D. J., & Camargo, C. A. (1991). Review of bulimia nervosa in males. *American Journal of Psychiatry, 148,* 831–843.

Crichton, P. (1996). Were the Roman emperors Claudius and Vitellius bulimic? *International Journal of Eating Disorders, 19,* 203–207.

Crisp, A. H. (1997). Anorexia nervosa as flight from growth Assessment and treatment based on the model. In D. M. Garner & P. E. Garfinkel (Eds.), *Handbook of treatment for eating disorders,* 2nd ed. (pp. 248–277). New York: Guilford Press.

Fairburn, C. G. (1997). The prevention of eating disorders. In D. M. Garner & P. E. Garfinkel (Eds.), *Handbook of Treatment for Eating Disorders,* 2nd ed. (pp. 289–293). New York: Guilford Press.

Garfinkel, P. E., Garner, D. M. (1979). The eating attitudes test: An index of the symptoms of anorexia nervosa. *Psychological Medicine, 9,* 273–279.

Garner, D. M. (1997). Psychoeducational principles in treatment. In D. M. Garner & P. E. Garfinkel (Eds.), *Handbook of treatment for eating disorders,* 2nd ed. (pp. 145–177). New York: Guilford Press.

Garner, D. M., & Garfinkel, P. E. (1980). Socio-cultural factors in the development of anorexia nervosa. *Psychological Medicine, 10,* 647–656.

Garner, D. M., Garfinkel, P. E., Schwartz, D., & Thompson, M. (1980). Cultural expectations of thinness in women. *Psychological Reports, 47,* 483–491.

Garner, D. M., Vitousek, K., & Pike, K. (1997). Cognitive-behavioral therapy for anorexia nervosa. In D. M. Garner & P. E. Garfinkel (Eds.), *Handbook of treatment for eating disorders,* 2nd ed. (pp. 94–144). New York: Guilford Press.

Harris, E., & Barraclough, B. (1998). Excess mortality of mental disorder. *British Journal of Psychiatry, 173,* 11–53.

Hawkins, R. C., Turell, S., & Jackson, L. J. (1983). Desirable and undesirable masculine and feminine traits in relation to students' dietary tendencies and body image dissatisfaction. *Sex Roles, 9,* 705–724.

Herzog, D. B., Newman, K. L., & Warshaw, M. (1991). Body image dissatisfaction in homosexual and heterosexual males. *Journal of Nervous and Mental Disease, 179,* 356–359.

Howard, W. T., Evans, K. K., Quintero-Howard, C. V., Bowers, W. A., & Andersen, A. E. (1999). Predictors of success or failure of transition to day hospital treatment for inpatients with anorexia nervosa. *American Journal of Psychiatry, 156,* 1697–1702.

Johnson, C., & Connors, M. (1987). *The etiology and treatment of bulimia nervosa.* New York: Basic Books.

Kaye, W. H., & Weltzin, T. E. (1991). Serotonin activity in anorexia and bulimia nervosa: Relationship to the modulation of feeding and mood. *J Clin Psychiatry, 52(suppl.),* 41–48.

Kendler, K., MacLean, C., Neale, M., Kessler, R., Heath, A., & Eaves, L. (1991). The genetic epidemiology of bulimia nervosa. *American Journal of Psychiatry, 148,* 1627–1637.

Lacey, J. H. (1982). Anorexia nervosa and a bearded female saint. *British Medical Journal, 285,* 1816–1817.

Lacy, H., & Dolan, B. (1988). Bulimia in British blacks and Asians. *British Journal of Psychiatry, 152,* 73–79.

Lucas, A. R., Beard, C. M., O'Fallon, W. M., & Kurland, L. T. (1991). Fifty-year trends in the incidence of anorexia nervosa in Rochester, Minnesota: A population-based study. *American Journal of Psychiatry, 148,* 917–922.

Maloney, M. J., McGuire, J., Daniels, S. R., & Specker, B. (1989). Dieting behavior and eating attitudes in children. *Pediatrics, 84,* 482–489.

Mickalide, A. D. (1990). Sociocultural factors influencing weight among males. In A. Andersen (Ed.), *Males with eating disorders* (pp. 30–39). New York: Brunner/Mazel.

Miller, M. N., Verhegge, R., Miller, B., & Pumariega, A. J. (1999). Assessment of risk of eating disorders among adolescents in Appalachia. *Journal of the American Academy of Child and Adolescent Psychiatry, 38*(4), 437–443.

Minuchin, S., Rosman, B., & Baker, L. (1978). *Psychosomatic families: Anorexia nervosa in context.* Cambridge, MA: Harvard University Press.

Mitchell, J. E., Pomeroy, C., & Adson, D. E. (1997). Managing medical complications. In D. M. Garner & P. E. Garfinkel (Eds.), *Handbook of treatment for eating disorders,* 2nd ed. (pp. 383–393). New York: Guilford Press.

Nassar, M. (1993). A prescription of vomiting: Historical footnotes. *International Journal of Eating Disorders, 13,* 129–131.

Nylander, J. (1971). The feeling of being fat and dieting in a school population. *Acta Sociomedica Scandinavica, 1,* 17–26.

Olivardia, R., Pope, H. G., Jr., Mangweth, B., & Hudson, J. I. (1995). Eating disorders in college men. *American Journal of Psychiatry, 152,* 1279–1285.

Palmer, R., Oppenheimer, R., Dignon, A., Chaloner, D., & Howells, K. (1990). Childhood sexual experiences with adults reported by women with eating disorders: An extended series. *British Journal of Psychiatry, 156,* 699–703.

Pate, J. E., Pumariega, A. J., Hester, C., & Garner, D. (1992). Cross-cultural patterns in eating disorders: A review. *Journal of the American Academy of Child and Adolescent Psychiatry, 31,* 802–809.

Pope, H. G., & Hudson, J. I. (1992). Is childhood sexual abuse a risk factor for bulimia nervosa? *American Journal of Psychiatry, 149,* 455–463.

Powers, P., & Johnson, C. (1996). Small victories: Prevention of eating disorders among athletes. *Eating Disorders. Journal of Treatment and Prevention, 4,* 364–377.

Pumariega, A. J. (1986). Acculturation and eating attitudes in adolescent girls: A comparative and correlational study. *Journal of the American Academy of Child and Adolescent Psychiatry, 25,* 276–279.

Pumariega, A. J., Edwards, P., & Mitchell, C. B. (1984). Anorexia nervosa in black adolescents. *Journal of the American Academy of Child Psychiatry, 23,* 111–114.

Pumariega, A. J., Gustavson, C. R., Gustavson, J. C., Motes, P. S., & Ayers, S. (1994). Eating attitudes in African-American women: The Essence eating disorders survey. *Eating Disorders, 2,* 5–16.

Pumariega, A. J., Pursell, J., Spock, A., & Jones, J. (1986). Eating disorders in adolescents with cystic fibrosis. *Journal of the American Academy of Child and Adolescent Psychiatry, 25,* 269–275.

Rizzuto, M. (1988). Transference, language, and affect in the treatment of bulimarexia. *International Journal of Psychoanalysis, 69,* 369–387.

Robinson, E., Bachrach, L. K., & Katzman, D. K. (2000). Use of hormone replacement therapy to reduce the risk of osteopenia in adolescent girls with anorexia nervosa. *Journal of Adolescent Health, 26,* 343–348.

Rodin, G., Daneman, D., & DeGroot, J. (1993). The interaction of chronic medical illness and eating disorders. In A. Kaplan & P. Garfinkel (Eds.), *Medical issues and the eating disorders: The interface.* New York: Brunner/Mazel.

Rolls, B. J., Fedoroff, I. C., & Guthrie, J. F. (1991). Gender differences in eating behavior and body weight regulation. *Health Psychology, 10,* 133–142.

Rorty, M., Yager, J., & Rossotto, E. (1994). Childhood sexual, physical, and psychological abuse in bulimia nervosa. *American Journal of Psychiatry, 151,* 1122–1126.

Russell, G. F. M. (1979). Bulimia nervosa: An ominous variant of anorexia nervosa. *Psychological Medicine, 9,* 429–448.

Russell, G. F. M. (1985). The changing nature of anorexia nervosa: An introduction to the conference. *Journal of Psychiatric Research, 19,* 101–109.

Russell, G. F. M. (1997). The history of bulimia nervosa. In D. M. Garner & P. E. Garfinkel (Eds.), *Handbook of treatment for eating disorders* (pp. 11–24). New York: Guilford Press.

Silberstein, L. R., Mishkind, M. E., Striegel-Moore, R. H., Timko, C., & Rodin, J. (1989). Men and their bodies: A comparison of homosexual and heterosexual men. *Psychosomatic Medicine, 51,* 337–346.

Silverman, J. A. (1995). History of anorexia nervosa. In K. D. Brownell & C. G. Fairburn (Eds.), *Eating disorders and obesity: A comprehensive handbook.* New York: Guilford Press.

Silverman, J. A. (1997). Anorexia nervosa. Historical perspective on treatment. In D. M. Garner & P. E. Garfinkel (Eds.), *Handbook of treatment for eating disorders,* 2nd ed. (pp. 3–10). New York: Guilford Press.

Sontag, S. (1978). *Illness as metaphor.* New York: Farrar, Straus and Giroux.

Stice, E., Schupak-Neuberg, K., Shaw, H. E., & Stein, R. I. (1994). Relation of media exposure to eating disorder symptomatology: An examination of mediating mechanisms. *Journal of Abnormal Psychology, 103,* 836–840.

Sullivan, P. (1995). Mortality in anorexia nervosa. *American Journal of Psychiatry, 152,* 1073–1074.

Waller, G. (1991). Sexual abuse as a factor in eating disorders. *British Journal of Psychiatry, 159,* 664–671.

Walsh, B. T. (1997). Eating disorders. In A. Tasman, J. Kay, & J. A. Lieberman (Eds.), *Psychiatry* (Vol. 2). Philadelphia: Saunders.

Walters, E., & Kendler, K. (1995). Anorexia nervosa and anorexic-like syndromes in a population-based female twin sample. *American Journal of Psychiatry, 152,* 64–71.

Warheit, G., Langer, L., Zimmerman, R., & Biafora, F. (1993). Prevalence of bulimic behaviors and bulimia among a sample of the general population. *American Journal of Epidemiology, 137,* 569–576.

Wilson, G., Fairburn, C., & Agras, W. (1997). Cognitive-behavioral therapy for bulimia nervosa. In D. M. Garner & P. E. Garfinkel (Eds.), *Handbook of treatment for eating disorders,* 2nd ed. (pp. 67–93). New York: Guilford Press.

Yates, A. (1996). Athletes, eating disorders, and the overtraining syndrome. In W. Epling & W. Pierce (Eds.), *Activity anorexia: Theory, research, treatment* (pp. 179–188). Hillsdale, NJ: Earlbaum.

Chapter 13

CHILD ABUSE AND PSYCHIC TRAUMA IN CHILDREN

STEVEN P. CUFFE AND MARGARET SHUGART

If one looks only at the clinical manifestations of trauma in a given day in the life of the traumatized child, one could diagnose conduct disorder, borderline personality, major affective disorder, attention deficit hyperactivity disorder, phobic disorder, dissociative disorder, obsessive compulsive disorder, panic disorder, adjustment disorder, and even such conditions, as yet unofficial in the nomenclature, as precursors of multiple personality or acute dissociative disorder and not be wrong.

—Lenore Terr, 1991

Infanticide and violence against children have been part of the human social experience from the time of antiquity to the current day. Children in most societies today receive unprecedented protection under the law, but the epidemic of violence against our children continues unabated. Child abuse, infanticide, sexual abuse and other forms of child maltreatment have been present in all societies throughout recorded history. Although the maltreatment of children has been recognized since ancient times, the full recognition of the tragedy is only a recent phenomenon. Child abuse has been so pervasive, and the response so subdued and ineffectual, that we must consider the possibility that the capacity to abuse children is part and parcel of being human. The motives and underlying causes of child murder and maltreatment are complex and multiple. In this chapter we begin with a historical review of child maltreatment. We then discuss the scope of the problem in the United States today and the impact traumatic events have on children. Finally, we discuss issues of assessment, diagnosis, and treatment of traumatized children and adolescents.

HISTORY OF CHILDHOOD TRAUMA AND MALTREATMENT

In some ancient societies infanticide was used as a method of birth control (Smith, 1975). In regions of China and Padua a mother was likened to an animal if she had too many children. In some cultures a limit of three children per family was set. If the mother had more than three, the babies were killed. The shame and embarrassment of bearing a child out of wedlock was and is another primary cause of infanticide throughout the world. In ancient Greece, Rome, China, India, and throughout the orient deformed children were usually destroyed at birth (Radbill, 1968). Religious ritual sacrifice also accounted for countless infant deaths. Infanticide was important with regard to fertility rights in China, India, Mexico, and Peru. Children were cast into rivers as offerings to the gods in hopes of a good harvest (Smith, 1975).

Infanticide was also extremely common in Europe. Selwyn Smith (1975, p. 7) quotes Werner from his 1917 book *The Unmarried Mother in German Literature:* "The fact is that infanticide was so common in the last half of the 18th Century that no one could be looked upon as a sole source of any particular literary production." Werner also reports that in 1781 in Europe a contest was held for the best essay as to how to prevent infanticide: "the prize question, how infanticide might be checked, has alarmed so many scholars in all of the faculty that one is amazed at the large number of essays submitted" (p. 112). Further, Frederick the Great, King of Prussia between 1740 and 1786, was so upset by the prevalence of infanticide that he abolished church penance for unmarried mothers because the punishment caused such embarrassment and disgrace that it propelled many mothers to kill their neonates to hide their shame. Infanticide is virtually ubiquitous in all cultures, and references to the killing of children can be found from such diverse sources as Greek and Roman mythology, the Bible, English fairy tales, and Shakespeare.

Physical abuse has also been widespread throughout the centuries and is felt in some ways to be an expression of infanticidal wishes. Maltreatment has been justified for centuries by the persistent belief that severe physical punishment is necessary to maintain discipline and transmit educational and moral ideas. Parents and teachers alike have quoted the Bible: "he that spareth the rod hateth his son" (Proverbs 13:24). Until recent times it was a given that parents and guardians had a right to do what they pleased with their children even if it meant "beating the devil out of them." In fact, possession by the devil was a common reason given by parents for their children's misbehavior from medieval times to the dawn of the twentieth century. Unfortunately, many epileptics were mistakenly thought to be possessed by the devil and after an epileptic seizure were beaten to rid them of the demonic possession (Radbill, 1968).

In addition to physical abuse and child murder, abandonment of children has been a form of abuse. Child abandonment, also known as exposure, almost invariably resulted in death in ancient times (Radbill, 1987), although parents frequently hoped their exposed children would be saved. Ancient Rome and Athens developed orphan homes for such children. In medieval Europe, churches provided for foundlings. The first foundling hospital was established by the Arch Priest of Milan Datheus in 787 (Radbill, 1987). The Foundling Family Hospital of St. Petersburg, Russia, was the largest, caring for approximately 25,000 children. Institutional care, however, was not beneficial for these children. About one in four died, and the foundling hospitals did not prevent exposure and infanticide (Radbill, 1987). They suffered from deprivation and starvation and were frequently beaten and forced to work long hours. In fact, children from orphanages and foundling hospitals were a cheap source of labor.

With the rise of industrial society in the eighteenth century, another form of child abuse began to take shape. Although child labor was common in the Middle Ages under the apprenticeship system, the rise of factories during the industrial revolution in the eighteenth century created a site for the systematic exploitation of large numbers of children. Children as young as four years old were employed in cotton mills where they were mercilessly beaten and overworked. The practice continued until child labor laws initiated reforms during the nineteenth century.

HISTORY OF LEGAL PROTECTION OF CHILDREN

The history of legal protection of children goes back 4,000 years to the Code of Hammurabi which provided sanctions related to child murder. Infanticide was also illegal in ancient Egypt, and it was a capital offense in Thebes (Radbill, 1987). In ancient Rome the father's authority was sacrosanct. The Patria Potestas gave a father the supreme right to sell, mutilate or even kill his offspring, although infanticide was relatively uncommon in ancient Rome (Bakan, 1971). The Bible and the Koran both prohibit infanticide. Early Christian church fathers equated infanticide with murder and described it as a sin against the commandment not to kill. Both Constantine in A.D. 315 and Valentinian III in A.D. 451 issued edicts against infanticide and the sale of children into slavery (Smith, 1975, p. 18).

The first child labor laws were enacted in England in 1802. Child labor reform was initiated by Robert Owen and Sir Robert Peel and led to the breakup of the pauper/apprentice system (Smith, 1975). However, the absolute right of parents over their children continued unabated as the act did not apply to children under the supervision of their parents. Is was not until 1871 in New York City that there was a legal challenge to the absolute right of parents over their children. In that year a group of church workers took an interest in a young child named Mary Ellen. She lived with her adopted parents in New York City. Mary Ellen was physically abused and at times chained to her bed (Kempe & Helfer, 1972). The church workers were aghast and brought the family into court. The court, however, took no action because child abuse was not technically against the law. The church workers were persistent and requested the assistance of the Society for the Prevention of Cruelty to Animals (because Mary Ellen was a member of the animal kingdom). The case was subsequently heard, and the child was removed from the parents. As a direct result, the National Society for the Prevention of Cruelty to Children was formed in the United States and many other countries. The societies were instrumental in passing child protective laws. It is mystifying to realize that the American Society for the Prevention of Cruelty to Animals (founded in 1866) antedated the child protection societies by almost a decade (Kempe & Helfer, 1972, p. ix).

The recognition of child abuse, and therefore the uncovering of the hidden epidemic, was yet another societal difficulty. Humans have a tendency to deny that parents could be the instrument of such brutality to their children. In 1925 John Caffey, a radiologist and pediatrician in New York, reported X-ray findings of multiple fractures due to trauma. He was unable to convince his colleagues that the parents should be implicated (Radbill, 1987). Over 20 years later, in 1946, Caffey finally published his paper titled "Multiple Fractures in the Long Bones of Infants Suffering from Chronic Subdural Hematoma" (Caffey, 1946). This ushered in the age of medicine in the diagnosis of child abuse. C. Henry Kempe and his staff of radiologists and pediatricians studied child abuse from 1951 to 1958 and were the first group to link child abuse systematically to pediatric practice. In 1961 Kempe became Chairman of the Program Committee of the

American Academy of Pediatrics and organized a multidisciplinary conference with the provocative title of Battered Child Syndrome (Kempe et al., 1962). Thus began the modern era both of the study of child abuse and neglect and of society's acknowledgment that child abuse is a serious public health problem affecting uncounted numbers of children.

The study of childhood trauma in its broader sense—that is, any traumatic event affecting children—did not begin in earnest until the 1970s, when Lenore Terr performed her initial clinical research project on the children of Chowchilla (Terr, 1979). In July 1976 these children were kidnapped on a school bus and driven to a pit where the bus and its children were buried. After they escaped, Terr studied each of the children and their response to this traumatic incident. She continued studying children that were traumatized throughout the next 25 years and has become the preeminent theorist on the impact of psychic trauma on children. Her 1991 paper titled "Childhood Traumas: An Outline and Overview" is essential reading for all professionals working with abused and traumatized children (Terr, 1991). In this paper she detailed the results of her research and presented a theoretical model for how children respond to traumas. This model is discussed thoroughly later.

During the 1980s research into the effects of violence on children expanded dramatically Robert Pynoos and his group at UCLA studied the impact on children of witnessing violence. They reported the traumatic responses of the children who witnessed sexual assaults on their mothers (Pynoos & Nader, 1988) and the impact of a sniper attack on the children playing on an elementary school playground (Pynoos et al., 1987). In their 1986 paper "Witness to Violence: The Child Interview," Pynoos and Eth presented a widely applicable technique of interviewing traumatized children (Pynoos & Eth, 1986). Also at UCLA, Rowland Summitt studied child victims of sexual abuse and wrote the now classic article titled "The Child Sexual Abuse Accommodation Syndrome" (Summit, 1983). In this article he describes a syndrome composed of five categories that characterize the response of children to sexual abuse. These categories include (a) secrecy, (b) helplessness, (c) entrapment and accommodation to the abuser, (d) delayed and unconvincing disclosure of the abuse, and (e) retraction of the allegations. This article led to a dramatic improvement of the understanding of how children respond to the trauma of child sexual abuse.

In the 1980s the study of child sexual abuse blossomed. Researchers such as Finkelhor and Baron (1986), and MacFarlene et al. (1986) and her group wrote books describing the problem of sexual abuse. Gail Wyatt performed a community prevalence study of child sexual abuse and describes the impact child sexual abuse has on the functioning of adults (Wyatt & Powell, 1988). Kendall-Tackett, Williams, and Finkelhor (1993) presented a review and synthesis of the significant research on the impact of sexual abuse on children. Over the past two decades there has been a marked increase in research and knowledge of the extent, variety, and impact of traumas in childhood.

DEFINITIONAL ISSUES

Definitions of physical abuse vary with the cultural practices of a society and with the needs for which they have been devised. There is a different emphasis between definitions intended for legal purposes and those intended for clinical or research purposes.

Cultural differences may be a significant issue because behaviors that are viewed as abusive by some cultures or subcultures may not be considered abusive by others. For example, corporal punishment of children is outlawed in many Scandinavian countries, whereas it is viewed as an essential practice in child rearing by much of the population in the United States.

The two primary kinds of definitions are legal versus research. The Child Abuse, Prevention, Adoption, and Family Services Act of 1988 (as quoted in Kaplan, 1996, p. 1034) defined physical abuse of children as "the physical injury of a child under the age of 18 years of age by a person who is responsible for the child's welfare, under circumstances which indicate that the child's health or welfare is harmed or threatened thereby as determined in accordance with regulations prescribed by the Secretary of Health and Human Services." Mirroring most other legal definitions, this legal definition is vaguely defined. On the other hand, the Third National Incidence Study of Child Abuse and Neglect defines physical abuse as present when a child under the age of 18 has experienced an injury or risk of injury as the result of having been hit with a hand or other object, or having been kicked, shaken, thrown, burned, stabbed, or choked by a parent or parent substitute (Sedlack & Broadhurst, 1996).

EPIDEMIOLOGY OF CHILD ABUSE AND CHILDHOOD TRAUMA

Each year the U.S. Department of Health and Human Services surveys all states regarding child protective services statistics. In a most recent report, the 1997 survey, child protective service agencies investigated two million reports alleging the maltreatment of almost three million children (U.S. Department of Health and Human Services [DHHS], 1999). Of the three million children reported for suspected abuse, approximately one million children were documented as victims by child protective services throughout the country. This represents a slight decrease from the 1996 statistics. The national rate of victimization was 13.9 children per 1,000 population of children. Fifty-four percent were judged to have suffered neglect, and 24% percent physical abuse. Caucasians constituted 67% of the children; African Americans, 29.5%; Hispanics, 13%; American Indian or Alaskan Native children, 2.5%; and Asian or Pacific Islander children, 1%. The proportion of African American or American Indian/Alaskan Native victims was two times greater than the proportion of these children in the general population.

These data further estimate that 1,196 child fatalities attributed to maltreatment occurred in 1997. Children age 3 and younger accounted for 77% of these fatalities. Overall, 75% of the perpetrators of child maltreatment were parents or legal guardians. An additional 10% were other relatives of the victims. The majority of the perpetrators (66%) were females. The data on child fatalities were estimated from reports from 41 states reporting a total of 967 fatalities. Determining the actual number of children who died from abuse each year is very difficult. It is believed that many child abuse deaths may be labeled as accidents, child homicides, or sudden infant death syndrome. The actual number of child fatalities due to maltreatment is believed to be significantly higher than the estimate given above (U.S. Advisory Board on Child Abuse and Neglect, 1995).

Another source of epidemiological data on child maltreatment comes from the three National Incidence Studies (NIS) that have been conducted (1980, 1986 and 1993). The

Table 13.1   National Incidence Study (NIS) Data: Estimated Incidence of Child Maltreatment Using the Harm Standard

Type of Maltreatment	NIS-3 (1993)	NIS-2 (1986)	NIS-1 (1980)
Abuse			
Physical	5.7	4.3	3.1
Emotional	3.0	2.5	2.1
Neglect			
Physical	5.0	2.7	1.6
Emotional	3.2	0.8	0.9

Note: Incidence of maltreatment per 1,000 children
Source: Table adapted from Kaplan et al. (1999)

most recent survey, the NIS-3, sampled child protective services, law enforcement, juvenile probation, public health, hospitals, school, day care, mental health, and social service agencies for a three-month period during 1993 (Sedlack & Broadhurst, 1996). The incidence of all types of maltreatment has increased significantly over the 13 years covered by the three studies (Kaplan, Pelcovitz, & Labruna, 1999; see Table 13.1). The incidence of physical abuse increased from 3.1 per 1000 children in 1980 to 5.7 in 1993. Emotional abuse increased from 2.1 per thousand in 1980 to 3.0 per thousand in 1993; physical neglect increased from 1.6 to 5; and emotional neglect from 0.9 to 3.2. In 1993 there were an estimated 16.9 per thousand children maltreated in the United States. This is 18% higher than the Child Protective Services survey of the states and still does not address the problem of cases not identified. The actual number of cases is probably much higher.

The type of abuse suffered by children varies as a function of age and gender. A greater proportion of neglect victims are children under the age of 8, whereas physical and sexual abuse victims were more often 8 years or older (DHHS, 1999). Girls are approximately twice as likely to be sexually abused than boys, and there is little gender difference with physical and emotional maltreatment (Kaplan et al., 1999).

The prevalence of other types of traumas in childhood is likewise significant. Recent studies have reported the prevalence of trauma in childhood to be between 15% and 69% (Breslau, Davis, Andreski, & Peterson, 1991; Cuffe et al., 1998; Giaconia et al., 1995; Norris, 1992; Resnick et al., 1993). The variation in prevalence may well result from different methodological approaches used in the studies. It has been suggested that the sensitive nature of many traumas may cause an individual to be reluctant to report to an interviewer, particularly during a face-to-face interview (Vrana & Lauterbach, 1994; Resnick, et al., 1993). Females are more likely to have experienced sexual abuse, while African Americans appear to be more likely to experiencing or witnessing crime with a threat to their physical safety (Cuffe et al., 1998).

CAUSES OF CHILD ABUSE AND NEGLECT

In 1980 Belsky proposed an ecological model for the cause of child maltreatment (Belsky, 1980). This model integrates the complex and multiple causes of child abuse and neglect into one theoretical framework. The contributing factors include parental vulnerabilities (affective instability, mental illness, substance abuse), child vulnerabilities (temperament, medical or psychiatric problems), and social stressors. Risks for child abuse may be increased when there is excessive stress (financial, marital, family, health and illness, etc.) or when parental vulnerabilities are combined with an especially difficult temperament in a child (Belsky, 1984). The model is just as applicable today as it was 20 years ago.

THE IMPACT OF ABUSE AND PSYCHIC TRAUMA IN CHILDHOOD

The consequences of child maltreatment and psychic trauma in childhood are extremely varied. There is no single psychiatric diagnosis or syndrome consistently found in children who have experienced abuse and trauma. Children react to such traumas in their own unique ways and as a result of the complex interplay of biological, psychological, and social factors. Genetic vulnerabilities for psychiatric illnesses; pretrauma levels of self-esteem; psychosocial adjustment; and family, peer, and community support systems all play a role in the variability of responses by children to severe traumas. Children can manifest many different psychiatric diagnoses, behavioral problems, cognitive deficits, and personality characteristics (Terr, 1991; Kendall-Tackett, et al., 1993; Kaplan et al., 1999). Psychic trauma is environmentally determined by a traumatic event. There must be a stressful, traumatic event in which death, serious injury, or a threat to the physical integrity of self or others occurs for the diagnosis of Posttraumatic Stress Disorder (PTSD; American Psychiatric Association, 1994). Not all trauma leads to psychological symptoms or psychic trauma (Terr, 1996). There is no one psychiatric disorder resulting from being traumatized, although PTSD is the most common response. If the traumatic event is intense enough, any child will be traumatized (Pynoos et al., 1987; Terr, 1979). The response to the trauma must have involved intense fear or helplessness, or in children the response may involve disorganized or agitated behavior. For the "experience" to be traumatic, certain mental processes must include understanding the danger or horror, sensing helplessness, and registering and storing the traumatic memory (Terr, 1996). Once these thought processes have occurred, there is usually one or more posttraumatic symptom (Terr, 1996).

Kaplan (1999) reviewed the recent literature on the effects of physical and emotional abuse and neglect. The review showed significant problems in children who had suffered physical maltreatment. Deficits in social functioning were found in analyses of studies based on the reports of parents, teachers, and peers. Abused children tend to show an insecure pattern of attachment and are found to be more disliked and rejected by their peers than are nonabused children. These difficulties are present even when variables such as socioeconomic status and negative life events have been controlled. Adolescents who have been abused in childhood exhibit more aggression in their peer relationships and more abusive and coercive behaviors in dating relationships. This pattern of aggressive and delinquent behaviors is highly associated with a history of physical abuse.

Cognitive and academic impairment have also been consistently correlated with a history of maltreatment. Carrey et al. (1995) reported that abused children had lower verbal and full-scale IQ scores. In fact, IQ scores were inversely related to the severity of abuse that had been experienced. They hypothesized that abuse delays cognitive development and inhibits physiological responsiveness to the environment. Other authors have reported deficits in receptive and expressive language and in mathematics skills. Interestingly, there is some evidence that neglect actually results in greater cognitive deficits than does physical abuse (Kaplan et al., 1999).

Abused adolescents are at particularly high risk for depression and suicide and other risk-taking behaviors. Livingston et al. (1993) reported that 10 of 41 children who had been repeatedly physically or sexually abused had significant suicidal ideation, and 46.3% of the 41 were diagnosed with major depression. Sexual abuse was more highly associated with suicidal ideation in this study. Abused youth are also more likely than their nonabused counterparts to engage in other health risk behaviors, such as cigarette smoking, substance abuse, and risky sexual behaviors (Riggs et al., 1990). This behavior may also explain why physical abuse and neglect are correlated with teenage parenthood for both males and females (Herringkohl et al., 1998).

A broad array of psychiatric diagnoses is found in victims of child abuse and childhood trauma. Approximately 50% of these children have a lifetime diagnosis of PTSD; 40% have major depressive disorder; and at least 30% have lifetime diagnosis of some disruptive behavior disorder, such as conduct disorder, oppositional defiant disorder, or attention deficit disorder (Kaplan et al., 1999; McLeer et al., 1998; March et al., 1997b; Cuffe et al., 1994). Young children frequently have separation anxiety, withdrawal, and regression (bedwetting, clingyness, etc.).

The effects of emotional maltreatment have only recently begun to be studied. According to Kaplan et al. (1999), the existing research indicates a stronger relationship between emotional maltreatment and long-term psychological problems than any other form of maltreatment. Emotional abuse is a stronger predictor than physical maltreatment of a wide variety of problems, including internalizing and externalizing behaviors, social impairment, low self-esteem, and suicidal behaviors, as well as current and previous psychiatric diagnoses and hospitalizations.

Sexual abuse can affect different children in different ways (Spaccarelli, 1994). There is no single symptom that is characteristic of sexually abused children (Kendall-Tackett et al., 1993). Kendall-Tackett, Williams, and Finkelhor (1993) reviewed 45 studies of sexually abused children. These authors found that fears, posttraumatic stress disorder, behavior problems, sexualized behaviors, depression, anxiety, and poor self-esteem were common in sexually abused children. The severity of psychological problems was related to the severity of the abuse (i.e., the invasiveness, coerciveness, and use of threats or violence), the number of abuse episodes, and the closeness of the relationship of the perpetrator to the child. However, roughly 30% of children who had experienced sexual abuse were not symptomatic at the initial evaluation (Kendall-Tackett et al., 1993; Knutson, 1995). These children may not be truly clinically affected, or the defenses of avoiding and numbing may be so effective that the children appear not to be affected (Arroyo & Eth, 1995). There is a correlation between long-standing sexual abuse and sexualized behavior. Being sexually abused puts a child at risk for anxiety, depression, and somatization (Yates, 1997). Posttraumatic Stress Disorder is a frequent sequella of sexual abuse (Kendall-Tackett et al., 1993, McLeer et al., 1988). Adults who were molested as children also exhibit a plethora of mental health problems, including low self-esteem, self-destructive behavior, anxiety, substance abuse, difficulty trusting others, sexual maladjustment, and other psychological problems (Wyatt et al., 1988).

PTSD is the single most common diagnosis. The *Diagnostic and Statistical Manual of Mental Disorders–Fourth Edition* (*DSM-IV*) criteria for PTSD include symptoms from three categories: (a) persistently reexperiencing the traumatic event, (b) persistent avoidance of stimuli associated with the trauma and numbing of general responsiveness, and (c) persistent symptoms of increased arousal, such as difficulty falling asleep, irritability, difficulty concentration, and hypervigilance (APA, 1994). Additional information on the PTSD diagnosis is presented in the assessment section.

Lenore Terr, the foremost clinical researcher in the field of childhood trauma, takes our understanding of the disorder in children to a more advanced level. In her 1991 paper Terr presents a new model for understanding the impact of psychic trauma on children and adolescents. This model represents a significant improvement in our clinical understanding of these children, and will be presented here in detail.

Terr posits that childhood psychic trauma leads to a number of mental changes that account for behavioral and psychiatric problems in children and adolescents, and in adults who experienced trauma in childhood. She divides all traumas into two types. Type 1, the results of one sudden, shocking, terrifying event; and Type 2, the result of longstanding, repeated traumas with concomitant sickening anticipation of the events. There are four characteristics she describes as common to both types of childhood trauma. The first characteristic is repeatedly perceived memories of the trauma. Reseeing the trauma is the most common repeatedly perceived memory for most people; however, tactile, positional, and smell memories may also follow severe traumas. These memories are stimulated by reminders of the traumatic event, but they may come "out of the blue." These repeatedly perceived memories tend to come during times of boredom (for instance in classes at school), or at night before falling asleep. One of us (Cuffe) has a patient whose visualizations of her trauma come whenever she assumes the position in bed in which she was sexually abused by her father. These memories are vivid and frightening for her. Another patient, when reminded of the sexual abuse that she experienced, has memories of the smell of the cologne her abuser wore.

Repetitive play behaviors and behavioral reenactments are common manifestations of psychic trauma in childhood. Young children characteristically play out elements of the terrifying events that they have experienced. This posttraumatic play, as it is frequently called, may be described as fun by the child; observing adults, however, note no elements of fun. The repetitions appear grim, and in the play the terrible result of the trauma is inescapable. Behavioral reenactments also occur frequently. Sexually abused children frequently playact the sexual acts that were perpetrated against them. The traumatic events also frequently inspire trauma-specific fears in their victims. They are related to the specific events that occurred and may cause panic and extreme avoidance in children and adolescents. One child who suffered a severe dog bite was unable to approach closely the neighbors house in which the event occurred, even with the relative protection of being inside an automobile. This caused her parents to change their driving patterns to avoid the street where the event occurred.

The final characteristic common to all traumas is a drastically changed attitude about people, life, and the future. These children, and later the adults they become, have a severely limited sense of the future. They have a tendency to live "one day at a time" and frequently make comments such as "you never know what will happen." The child's basic trust in the goodness of life and people becomes shattered. For example, a 38-year-old patient who had been abused in her childhood reported the long-lasting sense that she would die at some point in the near future. She described feelings in her teenage years that she would "not live to be 20 years old." She always had a sense of impending doom and never made plans for the future. At the age of 38 she was asked how she currently felt. Her response was, "I don't think I will make it alive until my fortieth birthday." Although she was able to understand intellectually that she probably would survive long after her fortieth birthday, she was unable to shake the feeling that her life would be short, and she continually expected that she would die in the near future.

Other characteristics associated with childhood traumas are more specific for Type 1 or Type 2 disorders. Type 1 disorders generally present with the children able to describe full, detailed memories of the events. The facts and details may contain some errors due to misperceptions or mistiming of the sequencing of what happened, but most children have a remarkable capacity for detailing the event that occurred to them. In contrast, Type 2 traumas (longstanding physical or sexual abuse in particular) cause spotty memories of events. Frequently these children have amnesias for major parts of their childhood and for the traumatic events that occurred to them.

Children suffering single terrifying events also frequently use defense mechanisms that change the causal attribution of the trauma. This allows them to gain a sense of control over random, uncontrolled events. Children frequently find omens or reasons to explain why they suffered the traumatic event. One child witnessed his father become severely burned trying to remove a burning Christmas tree from their house. He then watched the entire house and all of its contents burn to the ground as his father and mother were taken to the hospital in an ambulance. Later he described himself starting the tree on fire. Investigators determined that the fire was caused by a short circuit in the lights at the top of the tree. The child could not have set the tree on fire; however, his belief that he had done this gave him a sense of control over the events, and the ability to believe that he could prevent it in the future.

Other features characteristic of multiple or long-standing traumas include denial and psychic numbing in addition to the amnesias. These children avoid talking about themselves or their abuse and may go for years, even a lifetime, without saying a word to anyone. Whereas a child victim of a Type 1 single trauma may speak inappropriately about their trauma (e.g., in situations where the child should be doing something else, such as in school), children experiencing Type 2 traumas rarely speak of the events. When they do report the events, they frequently retract their allegations. They may forget whole segments of their childhood and are described as forgetful children. They frequently feel numb and invisible. One 13-year-old girl drew a self portrait. This self portrait consisted of a blouse and a skirt with no body. She described herself as invisible, "I feel like no one can see me."

Children experiencing Type 2 traumas frequently use self-hypnosis and dissociation as defense mechanisms. These techniques enable the child mentally to escape the traumatic events that occur to them. They are in their way extremely adaptive. The point at which they become nonadaptive is when the children cannot prevent themselves from dissociating even in situations long after the traumas have ceased. Although it occurs rarely, some of these children may go on to develop adult multiple personality disorders. Children having experienced Type 2 traumas frequently have intense rage (which may be turned against themselves) alternating with passivity. They frequently self-mutilate or attempt suicide. These children also have intensely low self-esteem and chronic depression.

ASSESSMENT OF CHILD ABUSE AND TRAUMA

Trauma should be considered in any child or adolescent when there is a significant change in the child's behavior. Sexual or aggressive play, suicidal behavior, and self-mutilation may represent traumatic reenactments or maladaptive expressions of fear or anger in children or adolescents who have been abused (Albach et al., 1992; Goodwin, 1985). Possible traumatic experiences should be considered in such cases. The possibility of physical abuse should be considered in every child who presents with an injury. A history and physical exam should be completed. If there are physical findings such as multiple bruises, lab work should include blood tests for an abnormal bleeding or clotting disorder. When suspicions arise of physical abuse in a child under 5 years of age, an X-ray survey is frequently performed to assess for fractured or healing bones. Signs of injury that may be suggestive of physical abuse include bruises or burns of specific shapes, such as an iron or cigarette burns; bruises at different stages of healing; repeated, suspicious injuries; a history not compatible with the physical findings; a delay in getting treatment for the child; a lack of concern about the injury by the caregiver; the caregiver's blaming the child or a sibling for the injury; or the child's accusing the caregiver of causing the injury (Green, 1997). A parent who was abused as a child is at higher risk for becoming an abuser, but one must be mindful that only 30% of abused children develop into abusive parents. Parents who have unreasonable expectations of their children are also at risk of abusing their children. As noted earlier, some characteristics of physically abused children include anxiety disorders, particularly PTSD, attachment disorders, low self-esteem, depression, mistrust of others, suicidal behavior, poor impulse control, Attention Deficit Hyperactivity Disorder (ADHD), and poor peer relationships (Green, 1997). Therefore, a thorough mental health assessment should be performed. Clinicians must also be aware of and follow guidelines for their states' reporting requirements for child abuse.

The assessment of trauma and abuse involves direct clinical interviews of the child and parents or primary caregivers. The clinician must ask the child and caregiver directly about the trauma. This is essential in the assessment and treatment of trauma-induced psychological difficulties. The child and caregiver should be asked directly about PTSD symptoms as well. Assessment of PTSD continues to rely primarily on the clinical interview of the child and caregiver (Cohen et al., 1998). Caregivers will frequently underreport or minimize the symptomatology of the child (Malmquist, 1986; Sack et al., 1986). Children must be questioned about their internal experiences because the parent will often not be aware of these experiences and feelings. Interviews of the child and play sessions are probably the most useful techniques for assessing PTSD in children. Repetitive play themes can be very informative about possible trauma. For example, John, a 9-year-old boy hospitalized for Bipolar Disorder who had also been traumatized, drowned the boy doll in the dollhouse tub in every session for several months. Drawing and story telling are also useful techniques. One must be cautious and not ask leading or suggestive questions. This is particularly important if legal charges and court testimony are involved. The roles of treating clinician and forensic evaluator should remain separate (Cohen et al., 1998).

Parents are better at reporting children's externalizing symptoms as well as giving timelines of symptoms. For example, Marie, a 12 year old, was referred for evaluation of depression. Marie's parents described her irritability and anger outbursts, which affected the entire family. They noted that the symptoms began 6 months prior to evaluation. Her parents described a constricted range of emotion as well as a decreased frequency of activities with friends. Marie was more aware of her difficulties with insomnia, frequent nightmares, poor concentration in school, and feeling "bad." When directly asked about abuse, she disclosed being sexually abused by an adult male family friend. She further reported intrusive memories of the abuse, attempts to avoid reminders of the abuse, and hypervigilence. Marie understood the horror of being molested by the family friend as well as the danger involved in disclosing the abuse, as he had threatened to kill her father if she "told." She did feel helpless about the situation, and clearly stored memories of the abuse that were intrusive.

The parental response is an important factor affecting how the child will react to the traumatic event. The level of family support should be assessed in all traumatized children. Symptoms can be decreased by having a stable, supportive, cohesive family. This was the case with Marie, whose parents were supportive of her, believed her disclosure, sought charges against the perpetrator and treatment for Marie, and continued their support throughout the legal investigation, court hearing, and after the incarceration of the offender.

Diagnostic Interviews and Symptom Checklists

There must be an assessment of the stressors responsible for the symptomatology. There is no gold standard of diagnostic instruments or interviews for the assessment of PTSD in children and adolescents (Cohen et al., 1998). McLeer (1992) studied standardized instruments to assess PTSD symptoms in children. She found three instruments that distinguished PTSD from non-PTSD children, the Child Behavior Checklist (CBCL; Achenbach & Edelbrook, 1983), the PTSD Reaction Index (Frederick, 1985a, 1985b), and the Schedule for Affective Disorders and Schizophrenia in School-age Children–Epidemiologic Version (K-SADS-E) (Orvaschel et al., 1981; Orvaschel et al., 1982). Three semistructured interviews have been modified to meet *DSM-IV* criteria (Cohen et al., 1998). One is the Schedule for Affective Disorders and Schizophrenia in School Age Children–Present and Lifetime Version–PTSD Scale (K-SADS-PL; Kaufman et al., 1997), which has high interrater reliability and good test-retest reliability. A second semistructured interview is the Childhood PTSD Interview–Child Form (Fletcher, 1997), which has high interrater reliability and strong construct and convergent validity. The third semistructured interview is the Clinician-Administered PTSD Scale–Child and Adolescent Version (CAPS-C), *DSM-IV* version developed by Nader et al. (1996). It does capture *DSM-IV* criteria and is used in diagnostic and treatment outcome studies (March et al., 1997a). Its reliability and validity are being evaluated. There are several self- and parent-report instruments that measure PTSD symptoms in children (Cohen et al., 1998). None of these gives a single score that indicates the presence or absence of PTSD (Cohen et al., 1998).

One instrument that is frequently used is the Childhood PTSD Reaction Index (CPTSRI). The CPTSRI is an interview that assesses PTSD symptoms in children and adolescents using *DSM-IV* criteria. It is the most commonly used instrument in published research studies (Cohen et al., 1998; see also Goenjian et al., 1995; Pynoos et al., 1987). This semistructured interview or self-report measure of 20 items was developed by Frederick et al. (1992). The CPTSRI does not determine if *DSM-IV* diagnosis criteria are met, but the composite score does indicate severity of PTSD symptoms. The PTSD Reaction Index is useful in documenting symptom severity and monitoring symptoms over time.

There is a new series of self-report instruments to assess for *DSM-IV* PTSD symptoms in children and adolescents developed at the UCLA Trauma Psychiatry Service, the UCLA PTSD Index for *DSM-IV,* Child Version, Parent Version, and Adolescent Version (Pynoos et al., 1998). Parents report on their children's symptoms of PTSD for the child version. The Children's PTSD Inventory (Saigh, 1988; Saigh, 1989; March, 1998) is a self-report instrument with 5 subscales: exposure, reexperiencing, avoidance, hyperarousal, and degree of distress. It has high interrater reliability, sensitivity and specificity of diagnosis, and a high correlation with clinical diagnosis. It is the only instrument that provides a discrete diagnosis of no PTSD, or acute, chronic, or delayed-onset PTSD (Cohen et al., 1998).

The Child PTSD Symptom Scale (Johnson et al., 1996) is a 17-item self-report specifically designed for research as well as clinical use. It is based on *DSM-IV* criteria and has high internal consistency and test-retest reliability. The Impact of Event Scale (IES) has sound psychometric properties, correlates well with other PTSD measures (Allen, 1994), and has been reported by some to be the best questionnaire available for evaluating childhood PTSD (McNally, 1991). The Children's Impact of Event Scale (Wolfe et al., 1989) is a 52-item self-report instrument based on *DSM-III* criteria and is especially applicable to sexually abused children. Other instruments are briefly reviewed in the Practice Parameters for the Assessment and Treatment of Children and Adolescents with Posttraumatic Stress Disorder (Cohen et al., 1998).

Comorbidity with Other Psychiatric Disorders

Several studies have supported the prevalence of significant comorbidity of PTSD with other psychiatric disorders. Depressive conditions are the most common comorbidities in PTSD (Yule, 1992; Yule & Canterbury, 1994). There is overlap between symptoms of PTSD and Major Depression and/or Dysthymia (Brent et al., 1995; Goenjian et al., 1994; Green, 1985; Hubbard et al., 1995; Kinzie et al., 1986; Kiser et al., 1991; Looff et al., 1995; Singer et al., 1995; Weine et al., 1995; Yehuda & McFarlane, 1995; Yule & Udwin, 1991). Insomnia inattention and depressed mood are common symptoms found with PTSD. Clinicians may mistake these for depression, even when a diagnosis of depression is not present. In the clinical example discussed above, Marie presented with depressive symptoms of irritability, insomnia, and decreased concentration, but criteria of Major Depression or Dysthymia were not met. Instead, direct questioning led to the diagnosis of PTSD.

There is also comorbidity with other anxiety disorders, such as Generalized Anxiety Disorder and Separation Anxiety Disorder (Arroyo & Eth, 1985; Brent et al., 1995; Clark et al., 1995; Looff et al., 1995; Sullivan, 1994). Increased behaviors of attachment, especially concerns about the safety of family members, frequently occur. Marie described fears that her father or mother would be killed by the perpetrator, or that they might die accidentally. Some children develop somatic symptoms of anxiety, such as stomachaches, headaches, or panic attacks.

Comorbidity of PTSD with substance abuse disorders also occurs commonly (Arroyo et al., 1985; Brent et al., 1995; Clark et al., 1995; Looff et al., 1995; Sullivan, 1994). This is especially true in adolescents, who at times drink alcohol or use other substances in order to decrease intrusive thoughts and memories of the trauma.

Due to the variety of symptoms seen in children who have been traumatized, including those who meet diagnostic criteria for PTSD, clinicians often desire to track these other symptoms (such as anxiety, depression, and hyperactivity) over time. Due to the number of comorbid symptoms found in PTSD, outcome studies should include these other symptoms or diagnoses as part of the assessment of treatment outcomes. For anxiety symptoms, the Multidimensional Anxiety Scale for Children (MASC) developed by March et al. (1997) is frequently used. The MASC is a self-report scale for assessing anxiety in children and adolescents. For depressive symptoms, the Children's Depression Inventory–Short Form (CDI-S) is a standard measure of symptomatology in Major Depressive Disorder and is a well-validated self-report measure (Kovacs, 1985).

PTSD often coexists with ADHD (McLeer et al., 1988; McLeer, 1992), or ADHD symptoms such as hyperactivity, impulsivity, and distractibility may represent anxiety or PTSD in young children (Cuffe et al., 1994; Looff et al., 1995; McLeer et al., 1994; Glod & Teicher, 1996; DeBellis et al., 1994). Parent and teacher measures of externalizing symptoms, such as the Conners' Parent and Teacher Rating Scales (Conners et al., 1995) are frequently used to assess and follow these symptoms over time. Symptoms of anger and aggression may occur in traumatized children and adolescents. At times the youth's presentation may appear to be Oppositional Defiant Disorder or Conduct Disorder due to these symptoms of anger and aggression.

DIAGNOSIS

The diagnosis of PTSD is made using the *DSM-IV* criteria (APA, 1994). These criteria were developed using adult presentations of PTSD. There is concern among many child clinicians that these criteria are not optimal for use in children due to the different developmental levels and cognitive and verbal abilities of children. Thus, presentations vary in younger children due to developmental factors (Amaya-Jackson & March, 1995; Pynoos et al., 1995), whereas adolescents' symptoms are more like adults'. Children traumatized before 3 years of age appear to store memories of the trauma not as verbal memory but instead as "pictorial" or "feel" memories (Terr, 1988). Thus, traumatized toddlers can exhibit fears, reenactments, and dreams of the trauma even in the absence of the ability to talk about them (Terr, 1988). Younger children may not be able to express feeling numb. Instead, they may exhibit behaviors that keep them from feeling emotions. Numbing and avoidance may present in young children as restlessness, behavior problems, or poor concentration (Malmquist, 1986).

To meet the criteria for PTSD, one must have experienced a trauma involving the threat of death or serious injury. In addition, there must have been a response of intense fear, horror, or helplessness. The trauma can be chronic, as in repeated physical or sexual abuse, or acute, such as an episode of rape, fire, bombing, or hurricane. The trauma can be experienced directly, by observation, or by learning of a trauma to a relative or close friend. The degree of exposure to the trauma is directly related to the severity of PTSD (Pynoos et al., 1987).

The traumatic event is reexperienced in one or more ways in PTSD. This can involve recurrent, intrusive, distressing memories of the trauma, which may be expressed as repetitive play in young children in which themes or portions of the trauma are enacted. There may be recurrent, distressing dreams or daydreams of the trauma, or more nonspecific frightening dreams in young children. A reliving of the experience may occur that again can involve play in a young child. Psychological or physiological distress at exposure to cues or reminders of the traumatic event may occur. This distress may be exhibited in young children through disorganized or agitated behavior. Children may lose skills that they had previously attained (such as the return of bed wetting or thumb sucking), or may regress to behaviors exhibited at a younger developmental age. Jacob, an 8-year-old boy who was sexually abused, began bed wetting after the abuse. Adolescents are more likely to experience flashbacks than are young children.

Avoidance of stimuli associated with the trauma and psychic numbing of general responsiveness are the second area of symptomatology in the *DSM-IV* criteria for PTSD. There must be at least three such symptoms for the *DSM-IV* criteria. These symptoms include efforts to avoid thoughts, feelings, or conversations about the trauma, or activities, places, or people that trigger recollections of the trauma. This may extend to a decrease in any feeling, such as a decreased ability to feel pleasure in activities, to be interested in previously pursued activities, or to show tender feelings towards others. In addition, there may be an inability to recall an important aspect of the trauma, a decreased interest or participation in certain activities, a feeling of detachment or estrangement from others, a restricted range of affect, or a sense of foreshortened future. Children may withdraw from new experiences. They may express hopelessness about the future and show decreased motivation in different areas of functioning. Due to difficulties with understanding time in general and future time especially, a sense of foreshortened future may not occur in young children (Cohen et al., 1998). As mentioned, numbness and avoidance may present in children as restlessness, poor concentration, hyperalertness, and behavioral problems (Malmquist, 1986). Thus, evaluation involves consideration of an ADHD diagnosis.

The third area of symptomatology involves at least two symptoms of arousal. These include difficulty falling asleep or staying asleep, irritability or outbursts of anger, difficulty concentrating, hypervigilence, and exaggerated startle response. Difficulties with sleep are also common in younger children (Benedek, 1985; Drell et al., 1993). A new onset of aggression is often seen in young children who have been traumatized (Scheeringa et al., 1995). These symptoms must be new in onset after the traumatic event occurred to be included in the PTSD criteria.

Survivor guilt can occur in children as well as adults. Survivor guilt can be more intense in children due to the normal presence of magical thinking and the egocentricity of young children, thus enabling them to believe that they caused the traumatic event. Acute stress disorder is diagnosed when symptoms are less than 1 month in duration. Also, if the stressor is not extreme, a diagnosis of an Adjustment Disorder could be made.

As discussed, comorbidity is the rule rather than the exception in childhood psychopathology. Those children who experience PTSD may also have other conditions, such as Major Depression, Dysthymia, Generalized Anxiety Disorder, or Separation Anxiety Disorder Trauma and PTSD can exacerbate or cause disruptive behavior disorders (Famularo et al., 1992; Lonigan et al., 1994; March & Amaya-Jackson, 1995; Shannon et al., 1994). Impulsivity and decreased concentration may be secondary to the trauma or comorbid ADHD. Impulsivity and decreased control of aggression may result in Oppositional Defiant Disorder or Conduct Disorder (Arroyo & Eth, 1985; Steiner et al., 1997). Substance abuse is a common problem occurring subsequent to PTSD symptoms. Occasionally someone will develop dissociative episodes or panic attacks following trauma. Differential diagnoses should also include organic disorders due to trauma, such as concussions, delirium, and intoxication. Assessment and diagnosis of traumatized children are complicated tasks. A thorough history, physical exam, and assessment for the full range of possible diagnoses is in order.

TREATMENT INTERVENTIONS FOR CHILDREN EXPERIENCING SEVERE TRAUMAS

The treatment of abused or otherwise traumatized children is a complex undertaking that can intimidate therapists. There are many variables that mediate the effects of the trauma on children and many ways in which these children respond to the traumas. As noted earlier, there is no single diagnosis or syndrome. Each child responds to the traumas based on the biological/psychological/social matrix in which he or she lives. Thus, treatment must be appropriate for the child's developmental level and individual history. Diagnostic considerations run the gamut of psychiatric disorders and are further complicated by the fact that the child may look very different in varying settings or time periods (Terr, 1991).

Most research studies on the treatment of traumatized children are uncontrolled and provide little scientific evidence on which to base interventions. The best-designed studies have tended to use cognitive behavioral approaches. Cohen and Mannarino (1997) described cognitive behavioral therapy with preschool children and compared this treatment with nondirective supportive therapy. The cognitive behavioral interventions targeted many of the common symptoms experienced by these children (Cohen & Mannarino, 1993). Cognitive behavioral treatment was found to be superior to nondirective supportive therapy in this group. Fantuzzo et al. (1996) used play sessions with socially adept peers to increase interactive play and decrease solitary play in maltreated children (Fantuzzo et al., 2000). O'Donohue and Elliot (1992) reviewed the literature on sexual abuse treatments and found only 11 treatment outcome studies. Similarly Oates & Bross (1995) cited only 13 empirical studies between 1983 and 1992 meeting even minimal research standards for the treatment of physical abuse and neglect. Although O'Donohue and Elliot conclude that there is no evidence that definitively demonstrates the efficacy of any treatment method, the children studied all showed improvements in symptoms and behaviors after treatment. Behavioral and cognitive interventions, in particular, are fairly well supported, however, some studies include psychodynamic interventions that also appear successful. The clinical significance of the improvements were sometimes unclear, and the long-term benefits are not known at this time.

Phases of Treatment

When treating abused or traumatized children, therapists should conceive of the treatment in three phases: (a) crisis intervention, (b) trauma-specific treatment, and (c) long-term treatment. The crisis intervention phase is generally the shortest and consists of stabilizing the child and family, evaluating their psychological needs, and supporting them through the process of evaluations, medical exams, and court appearances, if applicable.

The immediate posttrauma phase is extremely important, even critical, for the child. His or her emotional response to the trauma may be shaped at this time. The child's views of the trauma, of himself or herself, and of the world are vulnerable during this time. First and foremost, the child should be protected from continuing trauma. In the case of child abuse, this means creating a safe, nurturing environment in which the child can live. Whenever possible the child should remain within the family or with nonabusing family members. These family members, however, must be supportive of the child. The research to date is clear about the consequences of an unsupportive environment: the child suffers greatly (Everson et al., 1989; Green, 1993). Green goes so far as to recommend that children be removed from the care of a nonoffending parent who denies that abuse has occurred. Cohen and Mannarino (1993) found that maternal support became an increasingly strong predictor of positive outcome at 6- and 12-month follow-up points to their treatment program. The needs of the family during this time should not be overlooked. Following traumatic events families may become extremely stressed and sometimes dysfunctional (Terr, 1989). Individual or group work with parents can be extremely helpful.

During the crisis intervention phase the child should be allowed to process the traumatic events either through verbal interactions or through play, art, or journal writing. If the child's parents or guardians are sufficiently supportive and the child is relatively asymptomatic at the time of presentation, a time-limited crisis intervention treatment may be all that is required. It is interesting to note that children who have experienced traumas are frequently asymptomatic at the time of their assessment. For example, Kendall-Tackett et al., reported that between 31% and 49% of children who had been sexually abused were asymptomatic at the time of their assessment. They further report, however, that the asymptomatic children were the ones most likely to worsen by the time of the 18-month follow-up. Thirty percent of asymptomatic children developed symptoms during that time period. Parents of asymptomatic children should be educated concerning the typical problems seen in children who have been traumatized so they can watch for symptom development over time. The asymptomatic child may well require treatment at a later date. Parent education should also include instruction about talking to their children about their traumas. Dumas (1992) presents guidelines for such education for parents.

If psychiatric disorders are found during the assessment of the child, then specific treatments should be addressed for those disorders. For example, if a child shows symptoms of major depressive disorder, then antidepressant medication may be valuable, and further psychotherapeutic interventions should take place as is appropriate for any child with major depressive disorder. Medication should only be used with clear target symptoms so that response can be readily assessed. Many of the instruments mentioned in the assessment section are useful for this purpose. Selective serotinin reuptake inhibitors (SSRIs) such as sertraline, paroxetine, or fluoxetine treat depression effectively. They also show promise in the treatment of PTSD symptoms. Clonidine and quanfacine have been used for PTSD, as have mood stabilizers such as valpoate, depakote, and carbamozepine. There is little scientific evidence thus far for any but the SSRIs. Sertraline was recently the first to receive an indication for PTSD from the FDA.

Trauma-specific treatment is probably required for most children. The trauma-specific phase may last a variable length of time but typically is from 6 to 12 months. This phase of treatment should focus on the traumatic aspects of the abuse or trauma, allowing expression of affects and working through of traumatic memories. Symptomatic children with relatively stable and supportive homes, and who are not multiply traumatized over long periods of time (i.e., Type 2 traumas), may be effectively treated with short-term therapy. Children who have been victims of Type 2 traumas will most often require long-term treatment to deal with the major symptoms and characterological problems that frequently develop in these children.

Psychological issues are an important aspect of any treatment of these children. The sense of a lack of trust, feeling betrayed, feeling guilty (particularly with sexual and physical abuse), and issues of self-mastery are particularly difficult and require interventions. Frequently children experiencing massive trauma feel a loss of control and powerlessness over events. They may be overly passive and compliant, showing little initiative or assertiveness. They also tend to repress feelings of anger and hostility, although these may be expressed in tantrums, fights, and other aggressive behaviors.

The importance of the family cannot be over emphasized. The support of family members, particularly the mother, is vital for successful treatment. Therefore, families should be included in the treatment. Although it is beyond the scope of this chapter to describe, many treatment programs for sexual abuse recommend a multimodal approach involving individual therapy for the child and both parents, parent-child dyads (first with the mother, then with the father), and finally family therapy when treatment has reached the point that reintegration of the family seems possible (Giarretto, 1989; Kolko, 1987; Orenchuk-Tomiuk et al., 1990; Sgroi, 1982). Orenchuk-Tomiuk et al. (1990) conceptualized incest families as following a continuum of acceptance versus denial of the abuse. They describe three treatment stages, consisting of (a) the noncommittal or oppositional stage (denial), (b) the middle stage (beginning acceptance), and (c) the resolution stage (full acceptance and acknowledgment of guilt/blame by the perpetrator, nonoffending parent, and child). Characteristically, each family member moves along this continuum independently, and at times fluidly. Issues involve conflict resolution, roles, boundaries, and the awareness and management of perceived responsibility for the abuse. Such programs typically utilize a combination of individual, group, and family therapies in the treatment.

Specific Treatment Techniques

Play therapy is probably the single most common treatment technique used in treating children. Pretend play gives the child perspective and enhances problem solving by encouraging flexibility in thinking and by providing children with symbolic ways of coping (Rubin, 1988; Matthews et al., 1980). Play allows children to experience feelings, fears, and conflicts in a relatively safe and socially acceptable manner. Traumatic life events can be reenacted in play, allowing the child to remember the event and express feelings about it that may have been too painful or too frightening to handle at the time of the experience. Play also allows children to reverse the roles of actors in a remembered situation. Through play, a child can become the perpetrator and the perpetrator become the victim. This role reversal empowers the child by giving him or her a sense a mastery and control that was not present in the original situation. Therapists should remember, however, that following the child's play and "staying within the metaphor" (or not connecting the play themes with reality too directly) will encourage the child to express feelings regarding the trauma. Connecting play themes too directly or too soon with the child's traumatic experiences may result in an interruption of the play and a setback in the therapy.

Children do have a natural tendency to repeat their traumas in play. Terr (1983) described a repetitive, compulsive, unsatisfying reiteration of play involving traumatic themes called posttraumatic play. Unfortunately, children often become stuck in these highly negative play themes, having no chance of resolving the traumatic situation. Terr (1981) warns that play in and of itself may not resolve the child's dilemma of powerlessness. Therapist may need to interrupt such repetitions with possible solutions for the child. This caution is echoed by James (1989), who suggested that the child be shown in play how to "restructure the traumatizing event as a victorious survivor" (p. 18). For example, one 5-year-old girl named Anna constantly reenacted her trauma by having "the bad man" come out of nowhere to abduct the girl doll. No one was ever there to help her. She was asked who might be able to help the poor little girl and she said, "the police but they aren't here." After multiple reenactments over weeks of therapy, her cue was taken and the police car was taken out of the cabinet in an effort to help the little girl doll. Anna resisted this intervention at first and would not allow the police to find "the bad man" or the girl. However, over time she did allow the police to help, and eventually the little girl doll was able to deal with "the bad man" by herself. Please see the case example of Allan for another example of using play therapy in treatment.

Art therapy is another highly effective technique for affective expression. It has been used successfully with sexually abused and physically abused children (Johnson, 1989; Kelley, 1985; Allan, 1988; James, 1989). All describe the unique uses of art materials and art therapy for abused children. Art can be used to explore the details of the abuse, feelings about the abuse and the perpetrator, and the child's self-esteem (through the use of self-portraits). Indeed, art can be helpful with any age group, including adults.

Older children and adolescents may be much more verbal and therefore amenable to more traditional psychotherapy. Time is often required to allow the development of therapeutic alliance and feelings of safety and security in the therapeutic relationship before traumatic themes can be approached successfully. In our experience it is sometimes easier to engage children in this task in a group setting.

Cognitive behavioral interventions have been successful in treating abused and traumatized children. Lipovsky (1992) described the range of cognitive behavioral interventions appropriate for use with sexually abused children. These techniques may also be used with children traumatized in other ways. Generally this treatment approach combines coping skills training with behavioral and cognitive techniques. Relaxation training can be very useful to reduce tension and anxiety. Many techniques are available, including deep muscle relaxation, deep breathing, and guided imagery. We have found guided imagery to be especially helpful for children. They are taught to imagine their personal safe place where they are free from any possible harm and can let the tension drain from them. Combining this technique with deep breathing exercises has also been helpful. These techniques should be explored in the treatment when the child shows evidence of becoming overwhelmed by the memories and the affect on which he or she is working. The use of these techniques in the treatment session will not only titrate the level of affect the child experiences in the treatment process but will also reinforce the utility of the relaxation techniques he or she has been taught. This kind of practice will allow the child to transfer the skill outside the treatment setting.

Self-talk is another useful cognitive behavioral technique that can be used with children who are old enough to comprehend the instructions and significance of the technique. For instance, Rachel was a 9-year-old girl who felt afraid whenever she entered a strange bathroom. She had been abused in a bathroom, and anxiety frequently prevented her from using available facilities when she was away from home. She was instructed to talk to herself each time she felt afraid in this way, saying, "I am safe, and nothing will happen. I can remain calm." By focusing on this self-dialogue and using the deep-breathing technique, Rachel gradually improved her ability to use bathrooms away from home. Her therapist also employed another useful cognitive technique in treating this symptom: desensitization.

Desensitization is a core cognitive technique that has been highly effective in treating anxiety symptoms. Patients are asked to make a list of all the situations that produce anxiety in them and prioritize them from the least frightening to the most frightening. Therapists then systematically treat each situation in turn, beginning with the mildest situation. The patient is first instructed in relaxation techniques and is totally relaxed at the onset of the desensitization therapy. The patient is then instructed to imagine themselves in the frightening situation until they become unable to tolerate the feelings and anxiety is felt. Relaxation techniques are used when the anxiety occurs, and tolerance of the anxious feelings increases over time. This routine is repeated until the patient is able to tolerate the imagined experience without anxiety. Next, the patient begins to confront the actual situation in real life. Similar repetitions of the experience occur during this in vivo treatment. Each fearful situation is handled in turn, until the most frightening situation is encountered without anxiety. The case presentation of Betsy provides an example of this modality.

Communication and problem-solving skills can be very helpful and are usually taught well in group settings. Assertiveness training (how to say no without anger or aggression), games, stories, and role playing can be used to teach communication and trust-building skills. Board games, such as Communicate and Communicate Junior are fun for children and set up various situations to role-play (Mayo & Gajewski, 1991). Group activities such as Lighthouse, where a blindfolded child is verbally led through a room full of other group members by the child playing the lighthouse, can teach both communication skills and the ability to trust other people. One group program has been designed to have children in the group produce a drama about the abuse that occurred to them (Powell & Faherty, 1990). The children then act out the drama, including the roles of the perpetrator, victim, family, and so on. Social skills training is also an important part of this treatment process.

CASE EXAMPLES

Allan

Allan was a 4-year-old white male who presented with his mother for treatment of aggressive, out-of-control behaviors in addition to clinginess and problems with separation. His early life was characterized by physical abuse from his father and chaotic family functioning. His mother and father frequently had verbal arguments, and chronic fear and anxiety were in the home. His parents separated when Allan was 2 years old due to the father's sexual abuse of Allan's then 10-year-old sister. At the time of the evaluation Allan showed delays in both speech and motor development, in addition to his anxious, clingy, and oppositional behaviors. During the assessment, Allan showed a good ability to interact in play with the therapist. He was placed in weekly play therapy where themes of aggression and fear predominated. The primary metaphor through which Allan worked was the three little pigs fairy tale. He would take the role of the big bad wolf, and in his version of the fairy tale the three little pigs were always consumed by the big bad wolf. During the course of therapy, the therapist encouraged Allan to take on different roles in this play theme. He was highly resistant at first and would not allow the therapist to take the role of the wolf while he took the role of the three little pigs. Alternate endings to the story were suggested, but Allan rejected any resolution that included the survival of the three little pigs. During the course of one year in treatment, Allan's behavior at home and in his preschool gradually improved.

Work was also done with Allan's mother regarding her response to both Allan's physical abuse and her daughter's sexual abuse. She was quite depressed and irritable initially, having a good deal of anger at both her ex-husband and her children. She was highly intelligent and had insight into her feelings, including understanding that her anger at her children was misplaced. She was able to also understand that she could not get away from those feelings toward her children. At one point during the course of her treatment, she tearfully stated, "I can't help feeling angry at my daughter sometimes. I look at her and see the woman who slept with my husband." As her treatment progressed, family functioning improved, and there was more stability and cohesion in the family.

Finally, after approximately 1 year in treatment, Allan was able to allow the therapist to take the role of the big bad wolf. He was quite anxious during the initial phases of play, with hypervigilence and an exaggerated startle response to any movement that the big bad wolf would make. He became quite obviously pleased and excited when during the course of this play therapy session the therapist allowed the three little pigs to defeat the big bad wolf. He seemed to develop an increased sense of control, empowerment, and improved self-esteem during the course of the next several weeks and months. The treatment was ended after approximately 2 years with improved functioning by both Allan and his mother. Interestingly, his then 13-year-old sister presented herself as asymptomatic and well put together. She refused any individual treatment sessions but did participate twice in family sessions.

Betsy

Betsy was a 12-year-old white female who was referred after a severe attack by the dog of a close neighbor and friend. The dog attacked for no apparent reason, jumping on Betsy, knocking her to the floor, and causing severe lacerations over and around her left eye. She presented with her mother approximately 4 months after her incident. She had always been an excellent student, with strong peer relationships and multiple extracurricular activities. She had become extremely withdrawn, staying home with her mother after school and on weekends. She did not like to leave the house alone and never went by the house where the traumatic event occurred. Her sleep was disturbed, and she reported nightmares concerning the attack approximately three times per week. She wore her hair falling over her left eye, trying to cover the scars from two previous surgeries to repair the damage. She was noted on evaluation to be anxious and mildly depressed. She was very concerned about her self-image and the impact the rather significant scarring would have on her future life. She was quite bright but unable to verbalize her feelings or memories about the abuse. She continued to do extremely well academically. Because most of her symptoms consisted of anxiety, and because she had great difficulty verbalizing her feelings, it was recommended that she pursue a cognitive behavioral desensitization therapy. Relaxation techniques were first taught. A hierarchy of stimuli that produced anxiety was then developed. She had a facility with drawing, and this became the medium through which she was able to express herself. She began by drawing pictures of things that reminded her of the dog attack but were not part of the attack itself. For instance, she drew a picture of a generic dog. She also drew pictures of her friend and her friend's mother. She proceeded to draw a picture of her friend's house where the attack occurred, and then a picture of the dog that attacked her. Finally she was able to draw a picture of the attack itself in full detail. Work on self-image was also done through art. She was asked to draw a portrait of herself both prior to and after the dog attack. She was able to discuss her drawings after they were completed. During the latter part of treatment, she was given homework to begin to desensitize herself to going outdoors, and to traveling past the house where the attack occurred. She initially approached her friend's house in an automobile, close enough to see it but not to go by it. She gradually worked herself to the point where she was able to ride by the house in an automobile. A similar exercise was begun with her riding a bicycle, and finally walking up to and past her friend's house. During the course of this treatment, her anxiety symptoms improved; she began to do more activities with her friends; and her separation anxiety diminished. The length of treatment was approximately four months of weekly sessions.

Katie

Katie was a 13-year-old seventh-grade student who presented with her foster mother with distressing symptoms after being sexually molested by her stepfather over a period of time. She was subsequently removed from her mother's custody. Her mother continues to call Katie a "liar" about the abuse, despite an investigation with substantiation of the abuse and charges filed against the perpetrator. Not being believed by her mother and being removed from her home have been traumatic for Katie. Other trauma reported included family violence with fighting, shooting, and assaults among family members. Katie reported going over and over the sexual abuse in her mind, feeling like other people don't understand what she went through, feeling so upset that she doesn't want to know how she feels, avoiding things that remind her of the abuse, experiencing intrusive thoughts of the abuse, trying to avoid thoughts of the abuse, feeling numb, having bad dreams about the abuse, worrying that the sexual abuse will happen again, feeling irritable and jumpy, having insomnia, and getting upset when reminded of the abuse. She met *DSM-IV* criteria for PTSD. She scored 37 on the Child Post-Traumatic Stress Reaction Index, indicating a moderate degree of disorder. Her Clinical Global Impression severity of illness on admission to the clinic was rated moderately ill. Her Multidimensional Anxiety Scale for Children score was in the clinically significant range for total score, as well as for physical symptoms of anxiety, perfectionism, and separation and panic. The CDI-S was clinically significant for depression as well. Initial score on the ASQ-P was clinically significant with labile mood, easy frustration, and impulsivity being frequent. She began individual psychotherapy and took 25 mg Sertraline daily, with decreases in her PTSD symptoms as well as in depression and anxiety. These improvements were sustained despite a change in foster home and her mother's continuing disbelief about the sexual abuse. Her grades improved to honor roll status, and she experienced an increase in age-appropriate friendships.

Mary

Mary was a 9-year-old third-grade student who presented for treatment at her mother's request due to recent sexual abuse by an adult male neighbor over a period of 6 months. The perpetrator was arrested but died prior to his court trial, which was another trauma for Mary and her family. A significant presenting problem for Mary was difficulty paying attention at school, resulting in poor school performance. She reported feeling upset when thinking about the abuse; feeling like other people did not understand how she feels; startling easily; avoiding thoughts, places, and things that reminded her of the abuse; and having intrusive thoughts of the abuse, irritability, and nervousness. She met *DSM-IV* criteria for PTSD. The Conners ASQ-P was clinically significant for total score with frequent symptoms of crying easily, being frustrated easily, labile mood, distractibility, restlessness, and decreased attention span. She scored in the moderate range on the PTSRI. Depression (CDI-S) and anxiety (MASC) instrument were not clinically significant. The PTSD and ADHD symptoms decreased with individual psychotherapy for Mary and 25 mg Sertraline daily. Mary felt "smarter" due to an increased ability to focus and pay attention because her intrusive thoughts and feelings about the abuse decreased significantly.

REFERENCES

American Psychiatric Association. (1994). *Diagnostic and statistical manual of mental disorders* (4th ed.). Washington, DC: Author.

Achenbach, T. M., & Edelbrock, C. (1983). *Manual for the Child Behavior Checklist and Revised Child Behavior Profile.* Burlington: University of Vermont Press.

Albach, F., & Everaerd, W. (1992). Posttraumatic stress symptoms in victims of childhood incest. *Psychotherapy and Psychosomatics, 57,* 143–151.

Allan, J. (1988). *Inscapes of the child's world.* Dallas, TX: Spring.

Allen, S. N. (1994). Psychological assessment of post-traumatic stress disorder: Psychometrics, current trends, and future directions. *Psychiatric Clinics of North America, 17,* 327–349.

Amaya-Jackson, L., & March, J. S. (1995). Posttraumatic stress disorder. In J. S. March (Ed.), *Anxiety disorders in children and adolescents* (pp. 276–300). New York: Guilford Press.

Arroyo, W., & Eth, S. (1985). Children traumatized by Central American warfare. In S. Eth & R. S. Pynoos (Eds.), *Posttraumatic stress disorder in children* (pp. 101–120). Washington, DC: American Psychiatric Press.

Arroyo, W., & Eth, S. (1995). Assessment following violence-witnessing trauma. In E. Peled, P. J. Jaffe, & J. L. Edleson (Eds.), *Ending the cycle of violence: Community responses to children of battered women.* Thousand Oaks, CA: Sage.

Bakan, D. (1971). *Slaughter of innocence: A study of the battered child phenomenon.* San Francisco: Jossey-Bass.

Belsky, J. (1980). Child maltreatment: An ecological integration. *Journal of American Psychology, 35,* 320–335.

Belsky, J. (1984). The determinants of parenting: A process model. *Child Development, 55,* 83–96.

Benedek, E. (1985). Children and psychic trauma: A brief review of contemporary thinking. In S. Eth & R. S. Pynoos (Eds.), *Posttraumatic stress disorder in children* (pp. 1–16). Washington, DC: American Psychiatric Press.

Brent, D. A., Perper, J. A., Moritz, G., Liotus, L., Richardson, D., & Canobbio, R. (1995). Posttraumatic stress disorder in peers of adolescent suicide victims: Predisposing factors and phenomenology. *Journal of the American Academy of Child and Adolescent Psychiatry, 34*(2), 209–215.

Breslau, N., Davis, G. C., Andreski, P., & Peterson, E. (1991). Traumatic events and posttraumatic stress disorder in an urban population of young adults. *Archives of General Psychiatry, 48,* 216–222.

Caffey, J. (1946). Multiple fractures in the long bones of infants suffering from chronic subdural hematoma. *American Journal of Roentgenology, 56,* 163–173.

Carrey, N. J., Butter, H. J., Personger, M. A., & Bialik, R. J. (1995). Physiological and cognitive correlates of child abuse. *Journal of the American Academy of Child and Adolescent Psychiatry, 34,* 1067–1075.

Clark, D. B., Bukstein, O. G., Smith, M. G., Kaczynski, N. A., Mezzich, A. C., & Donovan, J. E. (1995). Identifying anxiety disorders in adolescents hospitalized for alcohol abuse or dependence. *Psychiatric Services, 46,* 620.

Cohen, J., Bernet, W., Adair, M., Arnold, V., Beitchman, J. H., Benson, R. S., Bukstein, O. G., Kinlan, J., McClellan, J., & Rue, D. (1998). Practice parameters for the assessment and treatment of children and adolescents with posttraumatic stress disorder. *Journal of the American Academy of Child and Adolescent Psychiatry, 37,* 4S–83S.

Cohen, J. A., & Mannarino, A. P. (1997). A treatment study for sexually abused preschool children: Outcome during a one-year follow-up. *Journal of the American Academy of Child and Adolescent Psychiatry, 36,* 1228–1235.

Cohen, J. A., & Mannarino, A. P. (1993). A treatment model for sexually abused preschoolers. *Journal of Interpersonal Violence, 8,* 115–131.

Cohen, J. A., & Mannarino, A. P. (1998). Factors that mediate treatment outcome of sexually abused preschool children: Six- and 12-month follow-up. *Journal of the American Academy of Child and Adolescent Psychiatry, 37,* 44–51.

Conners, C., March, J., & Erhardt, D. (1995). Assessment of attention-deficit disorders. *Journal of Psychoeducational Assessment, 28,* 186–205.

Cuffe, S. P., Addy, C. L., Garrison, C. Z., Waller, J. L., Jackson, K. L., McKeown, R. E., & Chilappagari, S. (1998). Prevalence of PTSD in a community sample of older adolescents. *Journal of the American Academy of Child and Adolescent Psychiatry, 37,* 147–154.

Cuffe, S. P., McCullough, E. L., & Pumariega, A. J. (1994). Comorbidity of attention deficit hyperactivity disorder and post-traumatic stress disorder. *Journal of Child and Family Studies, 3,* 327–336.

DeBellis, M. D., Chrousos, G. P., & Dorn, L. D. (1994). H-P-A axis dysregulation in sexually abused girls. *Journal of Clinical Endocrinology and Metabolism, 78,* 249–255.

Drell, M. J., Siegel, C. H., & Gaensbauer, T. J. (1993). Posttraumatic stress disorder. In C. H. Zeanah (Ed.), *Handbook of infant mental health* (pp. 226–250). New York: Guilford Press.

Dumas, L. S. (1992). *Talking with your child about a troubled world.* New York: Fawcett Columbine.

Everson, M. D., Hunter, W. M., Runyon, D. K., Edelsohn, G. A., & Coulter, M. L. (1989). Maternal support following disclosure of incest. *American Journal of Orthopsychiatry, 59,* 197–207.

Famularo, R., Kinscherff, R., & Fenton, T. (1992). Psychiatric diagnoses of maltreated children: Preliminary findings. *Journal of the American Academy of Child and Adolescent Psychiatry, 31,* 863–867.

Fantuzzo, J., Sutton-Smith, B., & Atkins, M. (2000). Community-based resilient peer treatment of withdrawn maltreated preschool children. *Journal of Consulting and Clinical Psychology, 64,* 1377–1386.

Finkelhor, D., & Baron, L. (1986). Risk factors for child sexual abuse. *Journal of Interpersonal Violence, 1,* 43–71.

Fletcher, K. (1997). Childhood PTSD interview–child form. In E. Carlson (Ed.), *Trauma assessments: A clinician's guide* (pp. 248–250). New York: Guilford Press.

Frederick, C. J., Pynoos, R. S., & Nader, K. (1992). *Child post traumatic stress reaction index.* Unpublished manuscript.

Frederick, C. J. (1985b). Selected foci in the spectrum of posttraumatic stress disorders. In L. J. Murphy (Ed.), *Perspectives on disaster recovery.* East Norwalk, CT: Appleton-Century-Crofts.

Frederick, C. J. (1985a). Children traumatized by catastrophic situations. In S. Eth & R. Pynoos (Eds.), *Posttraumatic stress disorders in children.* Washington, DC: American Psychiatric Press.

Giaconia, R. M., Reinherz, H. Z., Silverman, A. B., Pakiz, B., Frost, A. K., & Cohen, E. (1995). Traumas and posttraumatic stress disorder in a community population of older adolescents. *Journal of the American Academy of Child and Adolescent Psychiatry, 34,* 1380.

Giarretto, H. (1989). Community-based treatment of the incest family. *Pediatric Clinics of North America, 12,* 351–361.

Glod, C. A., & Teicher, M. H. (1996). Relationship between early abuse, PTSD, an activity levels in prepubertal children. *Journal of the American Academy of Child and Adolescent Psychiatry, 35,* 1384–1393.

Goenjian, A. K., Najarian, L. M., Pynoos, R. S., Steinberg, A. M., Manoukian, G., Tavosian, A., & Fairbanks, L. A. (1994). Posttraumatic stress disorder in elderly and younger adults after the 1988 earthquake in Armenia. *American Journal of Psychiatry, 151,* 895–901.

Goenjian, A. K., Pynoos, R. S., Steinberg, A. M., Najarian, L. M., Asarnow, J. R., Karayan, I., Ghuabi, M., & Fairbanks, L. A. (1995). Psychiatric comorbidity in children after the 1988 earthquake in Armenia. *Journal of the American Academy of Child and Adolescent Psychiatry, 34,* 1174–1184.

Goodwin, J. (1985). Post-traumatic symptoms in incest victims. In S. Eth & R. S. Pynoos (Eds.), *Posttraumatic stress disorder in children* (pp. 155–168). Washington, DC: American Psychiatric Association.

Green, A. H. (1985). Children traumatized by physical abuse. In S. Eth & R. S. Pynoos (Eds.), *Posttraumatic stress disorder in children.* Washington, DC: American Psychiatric Association.

Green, A. H. (1993). Child sexual abuse: Immediate and long-term effects and intervention. *Journal of the American Academy of Child and Adolescent Psychiatry, 32,* 890–902.

Green, A. H. (1997). Physical abuse of children. In J. M. Weiner (Ed.), *Textbook of child and adolescent psychiatry.* Washington, DC: American Psychiatric Association.

Herringkohl, E. C., Herringkohl, R. C., Egolf, B. P., & Russo, M. J. (1998). The relationship between early maltreatment and teenage parenthood. *Journal of Adolescence, 21,* 291–303.

Hubbard, J., Realmuto, G. M., Northwood, A. K., & Masten, A. S. (1995). Comorbidity of psychiatric diagnoses with posttraumatic stress disorder in survivors of childhood trauma. *Journal of the American Academy of Child and Adolescent Psychiatry, 34,* 1167–1173.

James, B. (1989). *Treating traumatized children.* Lexington, MA: Lexington.

Johnson, K. (1989). *Trauma in the lives of children.* Claremont, CA: Hunter House.

Johnson, K. M., Foa, E. B., & Jaycox, L. H. (1996). A self-report diagnostic instrument for children with PTSD. In *Proceedings of the International Society for Traumatic Stress Studies.* San Francisco, CA: International Society for Traumatic Stress Studies.

Kaplan, S. J. (1996). Physical abuse and neglect. In M. Lewis (Ed.), *Child and adolescent psychiatry: A comprehensive text* (pp. 1033–1041). Baltimore, MD: Williams & Wilkens.

Kaplan, S. J., Pelcovitz, D., & Labruna, V. (1999). Child and adolescent abuse and neglect research: A review of the past 10 years. Part I: Physical and emotional abuse and neglect. *Journal of the American Academy of Child and Adolescent Psychiatry, 38,* 1214–1222.

Kaufman, J., Birmaher, B., Brent, D., Rao, U., Flynn, C., Moveci, P., Williamson, D., & Ryan, N. (1997). Schedule for affective disorders and schizophrenia for school-age children–present and lifetime version (K-SADS-PL): Initial reliability and validity data. *Journal of the American Academy of Child and Adolescent Psychiatry, 36,* 980–988.

Kelley, S. J. (1985). Drawings: Critical communications for sexually abused children. *Pediatric Nursing, 11,* 421–426.

Kempe, C. H., & Helfer, R. E. (1972). *Helping the battered child and his family.* Philadelphia: Lippincott.

Kempe, C. H., Silverman, F. M., Steele, B. F., Droegemueller, W., & Silver, H. K. (1962). The battered child syndrome. *Journal of the American Medical Association, 181,* 17–24.

Kendall-Tackett, K. A., Williams, L. M., & Finkelhor, D. (1993). Impact of sexual abuse on children: A review and synthesis of recent empirical studies. *Psychological Bulletin, 113,* 164–180.

Kinzie, J. D., Sack, W. H., Angell, R. H., Manson, S., & Rath, B. (1986). The psychiatric effects of massive trauma. *Journal of the American Academy of Child and Adolescent Psychiatry, 24,* 370–376.

Kiser, L. J., Heston, J., Milsap, P. A., & Pruitt, D. B. (1991). Physical and sexual abuse in childhood: Relationship with post-traumatic stress disorder. *Journal of the American Academy of Child and Adolescent Psychiatry, 30,* 776–783.

Knutson, J. F. (1995). Psychological characteristics of maltreated children: Putative risk factors and consequences. *Annual Review of Psychology, 46,* 401–431.

Kolko, D. J. (1987). Treatment of child sexual abuse: Programs, progress and prospects. *Journal of Family Violence, 2*, 303–318.

Kovacs, M. (1985). The children's depression inventory (CDI). *Psychopharmacological Bulletin, 21*, 995–998.

Lipovsky, J. S. (1992). Assessment and treatment of post-traumatic stress disorder in child survivors of sexual assault. In D. W. Foy (Ed.), *Cognitive-behavioral strategies* (pp. 127–164). Baltimore: Williams & Wilkens.

Livingston, R., Lawson, L., & Jones, J. G. (1993). Predictors of self-reported psychopathology in children abused repeatedly by a parent. *Journal of the American Academy of Child and Adolescent Psychiatry, 32*, 948–953.

Lonigan, C. J., Shannon, M. P., Taylor, C. M., Finch, A. J., & Sallec, F. R. (1994). Children exposed to disaster. II: Risk factors for the development of posttraumatic symptomatology. *Journal of the American Academy of Child and Adolescent Psychiatry, 33*, 94–105.

Looff, D., Grimley, P., Kuiler, F., Martin, A., & Shunfield, L. (1995). Carbamazepine for posttraumatic stress disorder [letter]. *Journal of the American Academy of Child and Adolescent Psychiatry, 34*, 703–704.

MacFarlene, K., Waterman, J., Conerly, S., Damon, L., Durfee, M., & Long, S. (1986). *Sexual abuse of young children.* New York: Guilford Press.

Malmquist, C. P. (1986). Children who witness parental murder: Posttraumatic aspects. *Journal of the American Academy of Child and Adolescent Psychiatry, 25*, 320–325.

March, J. S. (1998). Assessment of pediatric posttraumatic stress disorder. In P. Saigh & J. Bremner (Eds.), *Posttraumatic stress disorder: A comprehensive approach to assessment and treatment.* Needham Heights, MA: Allyn & Bacon.

March, J. S., Amaya-Jackson, L., & Pynoos, R. S. (1997a). Pediatric posttraumatic stress disorder. In J. M. Weiner (Ed.), *Textbook of child and adolescent psychiatry* (pp. 103–119). Washington, DC: American Psychiatric Association.

March, J. S., Parker, J. D. A., & Sullivan, K. (1997b). Posttraumatic symptomatology in children and adolescents after an industrial fire. *Journal of the American Academy of Child and Adolescent Psychiatry, 36*, 554–565.

March, J. S., Parker, J. D. A., Sullivan, K., Stallings, P., & Conners, K. (1997). The multidimensional anxiety scale for children (MASC). *Journal of the American Academy of Child and Adolescent Psychiatry, 36*, 554–565.

Matthews, W. S., Beebe, S., & Bopp, M. (1980). Spatial perspective taking and pretend play. *Perceptual and Motor Skills, 5*, 49–50.

Mayo, P., & Gajewski, N. (1991). *Communicate, Jr.* Eau Claire, WI: Thinking.

McLeer, S. V. (1992). Post-traumatic stress disorder in children. In G. Burrows, M. Roth, & R. Noyes Jr. (Eds.), *Handbook of anxiety: Contemporary issues and prospects for research in anxiety disorders.* New York: Elsevier.

McLeer, S. V., Callaghan, C., Henry, D., & Wallen, J. (1994). Psychiatric disorders in sexually abused children. *Journal of the American Academy of Child and Adolescent Psychiatry, 33*, 313–319.

McLeer, S. V., Deblinger, E., Atkins, M. S., Foa, E. B., & Ralphe, D. L. (1988). Post-traumatic stress disorder in sexually abused children. *Journal of the American Academy of Child and Adolescent Psychiatry, 27*, 650–654.

McNally, R. J. (1991). Assessment of posttraumatic stress disorder in children. *Psychological Assessment, 3*, 531–537.

Nader, K. O., Kriegler, J. S., & Blake, D. D. (1996). *Clinician administered PTSD scale for children and adolescent for DSM-IV.* Los Angeles, National Center for PTSD and UCLA Trauma Psychiatry Program, Department of Psychiatry, UCLA School of Medicine.

Norris, F. H. (1992). Epidemiology of trauma. Frequency and impact of different potentially traumatic events on different demographic groups. *Journal of Consulting and Clinical Psychology, 60,* 409–418.

Oates, R. K., & Bross, D. C. (1995). What have we learned about treating child physical abuse? A literature review of the last decade. *Child Abuse and Neglect, 19,* 463–473.

O'Donohue, W. T., & Elliot, A. N. (1992). Treatment of sexually abused children: A review. *Journal of Clinical Child Psychology, 21,* 218–228.

Orenchuk-Tomiuk, N., Matthey, G., & Christensen, C. P. (1990). The resolution model: A comprehensive treatment framework in sexual abuse. *Child Welfare, 69,* 417–431.

Orvaschel, H., Puig-Antich, J., Chambers, W., Tabriz, M. A., & Johnson, R. (1982). Retrospective assessment of prepubertal major depression with the Kiddie-Sads-E. *Journal of the American Academy of Child and Adolescent Psychiatry, 21,* 392–397.

Orvaschel, H., Weissman, M. M., Padian, N., & Lowe, T. L. (1981). Assessing psychopathology in children of psychiatrically disturbed parents: A pilot study. *Journal of the American Academy of Child and Adolescent Psychiatry, 20,* 112–122.

Powell, L., & Faherty, S. L. (1990). Treating sexually abused latency age girls. *Arts Psychotherapy, 17,* 35–47.

Pynoos, R. S., & Eth, S. (1986). Witness to violence: The child interview. *Journal of the American Academy of Child and Adolescent Psychiatry, 25,* 306–319.

Pynoos, R. S., Frederick, C., Nader, K., Arroyo, W., Steinberg, A., Eth, S., Nunez, F., & Fairbanks, L. (1987). Life threat and posttraumatic stress in school-age children. *Archives of General Psychiatry, 44,* 1057–1063.

Pynoos, R. S., & Nader, K. (1988). Children who witness the sexual assaults of their mothers. *Journal of the American Academy of Child and Adolescent Psychiatry, 27,* 567–572.

Pynoos, R. S., Rodriquez, N., & Steinberg, A. (1998). *UCLA PTSD Index for DSM-IV.* Unpublished manuscript.

Pynoos, R. S., Steinberg, A. M., & Wraith, R. (1995). A developmental model of childhood traumatic stress. In D. Cicchetti & D. Cohen (Eds.), *Manual of developmental psychology: Vol. 2. Risk, disorder, and adaptation* (pp. 72–95). New York: Wiley.

Radbill, S. X. (1968). A history of child abuse and infanticide. In S. M. Smith (Ed.), *The battered child syndrome* (pp. 83–101). London: Butterworths.

Radbill, S. X. (1987). Children in a world of violence: A history of child abuse. In R. E. Helfer & R. S. Kempe (Eds.), *The battered child* (pp. 3–22). Chicago: University of Chicago Press.

Resnick, H. S., Kilpatrick, D. G., Dansky, B. S., Saunders, B. E., & Best, C. L. (1993). Prevalence of civilian trauma and posttraumatic stress disorder in a representative national sample of women. *Journal of Consulting and Clinical Psychology, 61,* 984–991.

Riggs, S., Alario, A. J., & McHorney, C. (1990). Health risk behaviors and attempted suicide in adolescents who report prior maltreatment. *Journal of Pediatrics, 116,* 815–821.

Rubin, K. H. (1988). Some "good news" and some "not-so-good" news about dramatic play. In D. Bergen (Ed.), *Play as a medium for learning and development* (pp. 67–71). Portsmouth, NH: Heinemann.

Sack, W. H., Angell, R. H., Kinzie, J. D., & Rath, B. (1986). The psychiatric effects of massive trauma on Cambodian children: II. The family, the home and the school. *Journal of the American Academy of Child and Adolescent Psychiatry, 25,* 377–383.

Saigh, P. (1988). The validity of the *DSM-III* posttraumatic stress disorder classification as applied to adolescents. *Professional School of Psychology, 3,* 283–290.

Saigh, P. (1989). The development and validation of the children's posttraumatic stress disorder inventory. *International Journal of Special Education, 4,* 75–84.

Scheeringa, M., Zeanah, C., Drell, M., & Larrieu, J. (1995). Two approaches to the diagnosis of posttraumatic stress disorder in infancy and early childhood. *Journal of the American Academy of Child and Adolescent Psychiatry, 34,* 191–200.

Sedlack, A. J., & Broadhurst, D. D. (1996). *The third national incidence study of child abuse and neglect.* Washington, DC: U.S. Department of Health and Human Services.

Sgroi, S. M. (1982). *Handbook of clinical intervention in child sexual abuse.* Lexington, MA: Lexington.

Shannon, M. P., Lonigan, C. J., Finch, A. J., Jr., & Taylor, C. M. (1994). Children exposed to disaster: I. Epidemiology of post-traumatic symptoms and symptom profiles. *Journal of the American Academy of Child and Adolescent Psychiatry, 33,* 80–93.

Singer, M. I., Anglin, R., & Song, L. (1995). Adolescents' exposure to violence and associated symptoms of psychological trauma. *Journal of the American Medical Association, 273,* 477–482.

Smith, S. M. (1975). *The battered child syndrome.* London: Butterworths.

Spaccarelli, S. (1994). Stress, appraisal, and coping in child sexual abuse: A theoretical and empirical review. *Psychological Bulletin, 116,* 340–362.

Steiner, H., Garvia, I. G., & Matthews, Z. (1997). Posttraumatic stress disorder in incarcerated juvenile delinquents. *Journal of the American Academy of Child and Adolescent Psychiatry, 36,* 357–365.

Sullivan, J. M. (1994). Integrated treatment for the survivor of childhood trauma who is chemically dependent. *Journal of Psychoactive Drugs, 26,* 369–378.

Summit, R. C. (1983). The child sexual abuse accommodation syndrome. *Child Abuse and Neglect, 7,* 177–193.

Terr, L. C. (1979). Children of Chowchilla. *Journal of Psychoanalytic Study of the Child, 34,* 547–623.

Terr, L. C. (1981). Forbidden games. Post-traumatic child's play. *Journal of the American Academy of Child Psychiatry, 20,* 741–760.

Terr, L. C. (1988). What happens to the early memories of trauma? A study of twenty children under age five at the time of documented traumatic events. *Journal of the American Academy of Child and Adolescent Psychiatry, 27,* 96–104.

Terr, L. C. (1989). Family anxiety after traumatic events. *Journal of Clinical Psychiatry, 50,* 15–19.

Terr, L. C. (1991). Childhood traumas: An outline and overview. *American Journal of Psychiatry, 148,* 10–20.

Terr, L. C. (1983). Life attitudes, dreams, and psychic trauma in a group of "normal" children. *Journal of the American Academy of Child and Adolescent Psychiatry, 22,* 221–230.

Terr, L. C. (1996). Acute responses to external events and posttraumatic stress disorder. In M. Lewis (Ed.), *Child and adolescent psychiatry: A comprehensive textbook* (pp. 753–763). Baltimore, MD: Williams & Wilkins.

U.S. Advisory Board on Child Abuse and Neglect. (1995). *A nation's shame: Fatal child abuse and neglect in the United States.* U.S. Department of Health and Human Services. Washington, DC: U.S. Government Printing Office.

U.S. Department of Health and Human Services. (1999). *Child maltreatment 1997: Reports from the states to the national child abuse and neglect data system.* U.S. Department of Health and Human Services. Washington, DC: U.S. Government Printing Office.

Vrana, S., & Lauterbach, D. (1994). Prevalence of traumatic events and posttraumatic psychological symptoms in a nonclinical sample of college students. *Journal of Traumatic Stress, 7,* 289–302.

Weine, S., Becker, D. F., McGlashan, T. H., Vojvoda, D., Hartman, S., & Robbins, J. P. (1995). Adolescent survivors of "ethnic cleansing": Observations of the first year in America. *Journal of the American Academy of Child and Adolescent Psychiatry, 34,* 1153–1159.

Wolfe, V. V., Gentile, C., & Wolfe, D. A. (1989). The impact of sexual abuse on children: A posttraumatic stress disorder formulation. *Behavioral Therapy, 20,* 215–228.

Wyatt, G. C., & Powell, G. C. (1988). Identifying the lasting effects of child sexual abuse. In G. C. Wyatt & G. J. Powell (Eds.), *Lasting effects of child sexual abuse* (pp. 11–18). Newbury Park: Sage.

Yates, A. (1997). Sexual abuse of children. In J. M. Weiner (Ed.), *Textbook of child and adolescent psychiatry* (pp. 699–710). Washington, DC: American Psychiatric Association.

Yehuda, R., & McFarlane, A. C. (1995). Conflict between current knowledge about posttraumatic stress disorder and its original conceptual basis. *American Journal of Psychiatry, 152,* 1705–1713.

Yule, W. (1992). Post-traumatic stress disorder in child survivors of shipping disasters: The sinking of the "Jupiter." *Psychotherapy and Psychosomatics, 57,* 200–205.

Yule, W., & Canterbury, R. (1994). The treatment of posttraumatic stress disorder in children and adolescents. *International Review of Psychiatry, 6,* 141–151.

Yule, W., & Udwin, O. (1991). Screening child survivors for posttraumatic stress disorder: Experiences from the "Jupiter" sighting. *British Journal of Clinical Psychology, 30,* 131–138.

Chapter 14

DISORDERS OF INFANCY AND EARLY CHILDHOOD

TAMI V. LEONHARDT AND HARRY H. WRIGHT

INTRODUCTION

As we enter the twenty-first century, families, communities, clinicians, researchers, and policy makers are recognizing the importance of ensuring the biopsychosocial-cultural health and well-being of infants and young children. Most institutions have now accepted the principle that *all* young children need protection, care, and nurturance in an environment that supports their physical and emotional development. Families and communities have also adopted these principles as they pay greater attention to the mental health of infants and young children. However, policy makers continue to be slow in embracing these principles as matters of policy.

Infant mental health, the subspecialty area that focuses on the mental health needs of infants and young children, is a relatively new field, but it has had a significant impact on thinking about emotions and behavior in young children. Although the basic science of this field has been developing for the last 50 years, its empirical basis and clinical applications have expanded greatly in the last two decades. There has also been a significant increase in clinical referrals of infants and young children for mental health assessment and intervention in the last 5 to 10 years. As a result of this increased activity, the discipline of clinical infant mental health emerged as a new subspecialty focus in the 1990s. Professional organizations interested in infant mental health services, such as the World Association of Infant Mental Health (WAIMH) and Zero to Three/National Center for Infants, Toddlers, and Families (ZTT) have matured in the last decade, and new clinical organizations have developed at the local level (Wright & Leonhardt, 1998).

Currently, there is no national- or state-level infant mental health policy, but there are numerous public policies that affect the mental health and well-being of infants and young children. These policies have been, and continue to be, influenced by a number of historical, cultural, biological, economic, and political factors. If these policies are to be effective for young children, however, they must be child-focused and family-centered regardless of the range of influences. Additionally, the importance of the care-giving context must be considered an integral part of any assessment and intervention process. Unfortunately, national- and state-level policy focused on child and family has developed slowly despite the enormous volume of comprehensive and currently available information about young children's well-being. Since assessment and diagnostic procedures tend to follow well-developed policy or, at least, significant interest in a population, the absence of consensus regarding assessment procedures is not unexpected.

The broad diversity of needs for this population must be addressed with a range of assessment, intervention, and support options. This chapter attempts to summarize the range of clinical mental health assessment issues involving infants and young children and describes diagnostic concepts, assessment processes, and intervention options currently in use with this population.

HISTORICAL OVERVIEW

The field of clinical infant mental health has roots that can be traced at least as far back as the first International Congress of the World Association of Infant Mental Health (then the World Association of Infant Psychiatry), which was held in Portugal in 1980 and, at the time, was considered the beginning of clinical infant mental health. This congress of clinicians and researchers from several countries represented one of the first efforts to recognize the importance of infant mental health. This congress also had a significant influence on the development of standard mental health practices, including assessment, diagnosis, and intervention with infants and young children around the world.

Many disciplines and theories have contributed to the development of infant mental health. These include attachment theory, family systems theory, parenting research, and, more recently, early brain development research. Infant characteristics, the caregiver-infant relationship, and broader aspects of the environmental context have emerged as extremely important elements for infant well-being. Clearly, contextual factors like poverty, living situations, and violence may also greatly influence the developmental process of infants and young children.

Knowledge about young children has increased greatly over the last few decades, but policy makers and society in general have been relatively slow to respond to new information about the needs of our youngest citizens. If one reviews the history of childhood, the relative unresponsiveness to new findings is not that surprising, given past practices and customs that continued long after they were proven to be detrimental, like harsh physical treatment and early separation of very young children from their primary caretakers. For example, severe practices, such as killing one's infant, usually by drowning or suffocation, were considered to be acceptable solutions to dealing with unwanted offspring three centuries ago (Langer, 1974). Infanticide was not considered criminal or defined as child abuse. In fact, child abuse and neglect only came to the attention of public policy in the 1970s with the passage of the Childhood Abuse Prevention and Treatment Act of 1974. Early separation of infants from their mothers to be cared for by a nurse was a common practice by the well-to-do and less privileged in parts of Europe in the seventeenth and eighteenth centuries (deMaise, 1974). It was not until Robertson and colleagues produced movies documenting the responses of young children to early and prolonged separation from their mothers that mental health problems related to separation from caregivers were recognized as serious concerns (Robertson & Bowlby, 1952).

By contrast, parenting has been recognized as an important issue when working with infants and young children since as early as Locke in the fifteenth century (Minde & Minde, 1986). Infant-parent psychotherapy was one of the earlier mental health interventions developed for treating infants. Infant-parent psychotherapy was based on the premise that disorders of attachment originate in the parents' reenactment of their own unresolved childhood conflicts. Current writing on infant-parent psychotherapy indicates that it is the treatment of choice when the child's mental health issues are rooted in a distorted parent-child relationship (Lieberman, VanHorn, Grandison, & Pekarsky, 1997). Many other interventions for infants, young children, and their families have evolved since the 1970s. Some examples include infant massage therapy (Field, Schandberg, Davalos, & Malphus, 1997), parent training, developmental stimulation programs, home visiting, and the application of a variety of behavioral therapy techniques in use for nearly 80 years and recently adapted for application with infants and young children. Early leaders in the emerging infant mental health field recognized the importance of preventive interventions with infants and their parents. They also recognized that the effectiveness of prevention-oriented interventions is likely to vary based on knowledge of risk and protective factors affecting this population, as well as in a case-by-case basis.

The first clinics developed to treat mental disorders in infants and young children were started in the 1960s. Some of the early clinical leaders in the infant mental health field include Selma Fraiberg in Ann Arbor; Stanley Greenspan in Washington, DC; and Sally Providence in New Haven. Each of these early leaders developed clinical infant mental health programs and wrote extensively about mental health issues affecting infants and young children from their own theoretical perspectives.

One of the first descriptions of an infant treatment clinic was presented in a book titled *Clinical Studies in Infant Mental Health* by Selma Fraiberg (1980). This book outlined the progress of the clinical and developmental research of infancy for the previous two decades (1960–1980). Dr. Fraiberg described the Child Development Project at the University of Michigan, which began in 1965 and represented one of the earliest infant mental health clinics. The Child Development Project involved direct patient care, clinical training, and research activities. Dr. Fraiberg describes in detail the clinical assessment process used in this early clinic. More recently, the experiences of other infant mental health programs have been described (Harmon & Frankel, 1997; Luby & Morgan, 1997; Minde & Tidmarsh, 1997; Thomas Goskin, & Klass, 1997). Like the Child Development Project, all of the clinical programs described in the recent literature provide clinical training and engage in clinical research in addition to direct patient care. Early programs recognized the importance of training clinicians for work with infants, young children, and their families, as well as the need for disseminating new knowledge based on empirical research.

Few epidemiological studies have focused on the mental health needs of infants and young children. The needs of this group, however, are not trivial. Most studies of preschool children, for example, suggest that between 5% and 15% of the population would benefit from at least a mental health evaluation (Mayes, 1999). Clinicians working with infants and young children are called on to deal with a variety of developmental, emotional, and behavioral problems commonly seen in this age group. They treat the less severe, as well as the most complex and severe problems. Issues related to the clinical assessment and diagnosis of infants and young children are discussed in the following section. Components of a comprehensive assessment are also described.

ASSESSMENT OF DISORDERS IN INFANCY AND EARLY CHILDHOOD

Infants and young children are referred to mental health professionals for a variety of reasons. These include specific behavioral or emotional concerns, regulatory disturbances, developmental questions or concerns about possible delays or disabilities, and both general and specific parenting concerns. For example, one young child might be referred due to questions regarding the "goodness of fit" between the young child's constitutional temperament and the parental expectations impacting the parent-child relationship, whereas another child might be referred due to concerns about failure to meet expected developmental milestones. The most frequent referral concerns involving infants center around regulatory disturbances, including fussiness, excessive crying, or colicky behavior; feeding and sleeping problems; and failure to thrive. Toddlers are most often referred for concerns related to behavioral disturbances, including aggression, defiance, impulsivity, and overactivity (American Academy of Child & Adolescent Psychiatry, 1997).

Referral sources include concerned parents or caregivers, the child's pediatrician or teacher, or a mental health professional or social service provider who is involved with one or more family members. In general, referrals typically stem from what McConaugy and Achenbach have described as "a mismatch between environmental challenges and stresses versus the developmental skills necessary to negotiate or master those challenges" (McConaugy & Achenbach, 1990; in Gilliam, 1996, p. 26).

The evaluation and treatment of infants, young children, and their families is both challenging and complex. It requires working with a number of interrelationships between different influences and aspects of development (Greenspan, 1992) and teamwork and collaboration between family members and professionals, as well as among professionals from different disciplines. A variety of professional disciplines are involved in infant mental health. The most common ones are listed in Table 14.1.

Working with infants and young children also requires a broad knowledge base and special skills. Assessment of infants and young children requires specialized training and experience in the principles and practice of teamwork and family work, as well as in the principles and techniques of assessment with this age group. Some of the most important skills needed to work with infants and young children and their families include the following:

- Clinical assessment of young children across several domains (i.e., psychiatric, psychological/developmental, parenting, etc.)
- Collaboration with other disciplines
- Summarizing and synthesizing information

Table 14.1 Disciplines Involved in Infant and Early Childhood Mental Health Work

Psychiatry	Speech and Language
Psychology	Occupational Therapy
Social Work	Physical Therapy
Nursing	Early Childhood Education
Pediatrics	Child Care
Neurology	Child Protection/Social Services
Nutrition	The Court System
Genetics	Law Enforcement Officers
Child Development	

- Diagnosing problems according to specific criteria
- Treatment planning
- Application of intervention practices

In 1997 the American Academy of Child and Adolescent Psychiatry published practice parameters for the psychiatric assessment of infants and toddlers 0 to 36 months of age (AACAP, 1997). According to its authors, these practice parameters

> suggest structure and content for the family interview; guide observations of interactions and relationships; present the Infant and Toddler Mental Status Exam (ITMSE); describe the Diagnostic Classification: 0–3 (DC: 0–3) (Zero to Three/National Center for Clinical Infant Programs, 1994); discuss adjunctive, helpful standardized instruments; suggest interdisciplinary team and referral strategies for integrating complex multidimensional information; and guide the diagnostic formulation process and development of a treatment plan. (AACAP, 1998, p. 127; AACAP, 1997).

Table 14.2 outlines the major components, purposes, and processes of a comprehensive infant/toddler psychiatric assessment as recommended by and adapted from the AACAP practice parameters (AACAP 1998; AACAP 1997).

Developmental Assessment

Developmental assessment is considered the foundation of a comprehensive mental health evaluation of infants and young children (Gilliam, 1999; AACAP, 1997; Clark, Paulson, & Conlin, 1993). Developmental assessment is used to assist with diagnosis, to guide treatment interventions, and to qualify a child for early intervention services (Gilliam, 1999). In some cases, developmental issues or concerns may be the primary reason for referral, such as in the examples of autism, mental retardation, or developmental disabilities or delays. In other cases, the primary goal of assessment is to develop a comprehensive understanding of a child's current developmental functioning across different domains (e.g., physical-motor, sensory-perceptual, cognitive, language, social-emotional, and play), primary relationships (e.g., parents and caregivers, family members, teachers, service providers, evaluators), and contexts (e.g., home, school, clinic).

Table 14.2   AACAP Recommended Components of a Comprehensive Assessment of Infants and Toddlers (0–36 months)

Component	Purpose	Assessment Process
Family Interview	Exploration of families concerns and impact on child and family functioning; developmental history; assessment of family biopsychosocial-cultural functioning; assessment of parent-child relationships.	Interview. History taking. Data gathering. Observations of parent-child interactions during structured activity and free play.
Reason for Referral	Parents' perceptions and concerns seen as primary, but other referring parties' perceptions also explored. Emphasis not only on problems or concerns but also on identification of child and family strengths and positive attributes.	Data gathering from parents and other referral sources.
Developmental History	Assessment of past concerns as related to current, presenting concerns. Identification of past and current child and family strengths, resources, and positive attributes as well as vulnerabilities. Focus on strengths helps to build hope for families and is important in guiding interventions.	Detailed history taking regarding child's physical, cognitive, emotional, and early behavioral organization, and adaptation to stress. Eliciting parents' perceptions of child's strengths and adaptive abilities as well as sharing others' observations of child and family strengths.
Clinical Observation	Focus on parent and child's capacity for and interest in interpersonal relatedness.	Observation of parent-child interactions during history taking and interactive play situations (structured and unstructured). Generally, 15–20 min recommended. May include specific activities, such as planned brief separation-reunion or limit setting, depending on age of child and presenting problem or concern. Video taping or use of standardized measure of parent-child interaction sometimes used as adjunct to clinical observation.

(continued)

Table 14.2 Continued

Component	Purpose	Assessment Process
Infant/Toddler Mental Status Exam (Benham, 2000)	Helps organize observations of young children in play situations and is an adaptation of traditional mental status examinations to met assessment needs of infants and toddlers.	Includes observations of child, parent-child interactions, and child's reaction to an unfamiliar adult. Clinician at times may interact directly with child to elicit information. Observations are compared with parental perceptions of what is typical of child's behavior at home. Instrument provides examples of normal and abnormal findings.
Standardized Instruments	May augment clinician's understanding of child's functioning and allow for data gathering in short period of time. Should never be used as sole basis for decision-making due to problems with reliability and validity.	Examples might include parental report measures, child behavior or symptom checklists, parenting stress or style inventories, standardized developmental assessment batteries, or observational measures. See AACAP (1997), Table 2, and Nuttall, Romero, and Kalesnik (1992) for more detailed information regarding specific assessment measures.
Interdisciplinary Assessment and Referral	To put together comprehensive picture of infant/young child with input from various disciplines, such as pediatrics, neurology, OT, PT, speech and language, psychiatry, psychology, and educational services.	This can sometimes be accomplished within an established multidisciplinary team setting. Adjunctive referrals can also be used to accomplish this purpose.
Diagnostic Formulation	Represents synthesis of biopsychosocial influences that contribute to, help maintain, or help resolve the child's presenting difficulties.	Use of classification systems such as DC: 0–3 (Zero to Three/National Center for Clinical Infant Programs, 1994) and DSM-IV.
Treatment Planning	Development of treatment recommendations that are individualized and build upon child, family, and other environmental strengths and resources.	Discussion over one or more sessions of relevant findings, diagnostic formulation, diagnostic formulation and treatment recommendations, and additional referrals.

Source: AACAP Summary of the Practice Parameters for the Psychiatric Assessment of Infants and Toddlers (0–36 Months), AACAP, 1998.

The mental health clinician aims not only to understand the child's overall development and behavior, but also his or her current functioning in relation to normative standards and common developmental processes (Bergen, Thomas, & Rubin, 1994). From the information presented, the clinician formulates a picture of the individual child's behavioral style and unique pattern of skill strengths and deficits (Clark et al., 1993). This process requires an understanding of basic developmental principles and typical developmental milestones. An awareness of biological and environmental factors that affect development is also necessary in order to tailor the assessment process, interpret the results, plan interventions, and evaluate progress accordingly (Bergen, 1994; Clark et al., 1993).

When assessing infants and toddlers, it is important that the evaluator look for patterns of behavior rather than discrete behavioral incidents. The reason is that the behavior of typically developing infants and young children is constantly changing to meet developmental and situational demands. Therefore, when patterns of behavior that are observed that appear to lie outside expected norms given the child's age and situational demands, there is greater likelihood that there is a more significant problem or concern for which intervention may be needed. In contrast, discrete behaviors are more likely to indicate individual differences within the normal range of development (Kalmanson, 1989). It is always important to inquire whether observed behavior is typical for the infant or toddler in other similar situations and to assess how his or her behavior may differ in other environments, contexts, or situations. Behavioral observations across time and situations (e.g., home, clinic, with parents, with other caregivers, with the evaluator) are often necessary to elicit a valid picture of the young child's behavior repertoire and competencies. Context and knowledge of relevant environmental and cultural issues also need to be considered throughout the assessment process and when planning interventions (Wright & Leonhardt, 1998). Determining the frequency, intensity, duration, and situations in which problem behaviors occur is an essential feature of the assessment process. Identifying child and family strengths is another crucial aspect of the assessment process, because it helps to guide interventions and build on existing child and family strengths.

A number of special considerations must be taken into account when assessing infants and young children. One is the need for flexibility in scheduling the time of day and length of assessment sessions. The behavior of very young children, in particular, is very state dependent and influenced by biological needs such as hunger and sleep. An infant or toddler cannot be expected to delay gratification of these needs in order to meet assessment demands. Instead, the evaluator must be cognizant of these issues as well as sensitive and flexible in meeting such demands. Cultural influences must also be taken into account when assessing a culturally diverse population of infants and toddlers, as they may impact the young child's ability to demonstrate competencies in the context of an assessment situation (Bergen & Mosley-Howard, 1994). Thus, the clinician must strive to distinguish through culturally sensitive inquiry the degree to which observation findings and assessment results are reflective of culturally diverse but normal variations in parenting practices or child development versus evidence of more significant problems or impairments (Wright & Leonhardt, 1998).

The developmental assessment of infants and toddlers is also influenced by legal considerations. General guidelines for the developmental assessment of young children have been provided in Public Law 99-457 (1986). More specifically, PL 99-457 and its amendments require states to plan for a coordinated approach to the provision of assessment and planning of intervention services for young children with suspected difficulties. It requires a multifactorial, multidisciplinary, family-centered approach to assessment (Bergen, 1994). The law mandates the provision of special education for preschoolers with significant developmental delays and disabilities (including psychiatric problems) and authorizes states to provide optional early intervention services for infants and toddlers (Gilliam, 1993).

Formal and Informal Assessment Measures

A variety of assessment measures is currently available for assessing developmental and psychological functioning of infants and young children and screening for potential developmental problems. Screening and assessment strategies are also diverse and range from the collection and review of relevant child and family history to structured and unstructured observations of infant behavior and infant-caregiver interactions, to standardized testing to determine levels of functioning across various developmental domains. Selection of appropriate assessment tools depends on a number of factors, including the purpose of assessment (e.g., screening, diagnosis, intervention planning), sources of data (e.g., direct assessment, observation, or informant report), standardization (prescribed method of administration), and reliability and validity of the instruments themselves. These considerations are briefly summarized later. See Gilliam (1999) and Gilliam and Mayes (1999) for more detailed discussions of these factors.

In general, developmental tests are used for the purposes of screening, diagnosis, and intervention planning. Screening instruments are typically administered to large groups of children to identify those children at risk for problems and refer them for more comprehensive diagnostic assessment. Some tests are designed to assess a specific area of functioning; others are more broad-based and cover several developmental domains. Tests also vary in terms of the amount of time and level of training required for administration and interpretation.

Although there are standardized assessment tools for infants and toddlers, their usefulness and suitability in routine clinical practice have not been clearly defined (AACAP, 1997). When selecting an assessment instrument, it is important to note how a test was normed to be sure that the reference group is appropriate and representative of a population that is similar in background to the children being assessed. It is also important to make sure that the norms are not outdated and that the test includes prescribed accommodations that are appropriate in situations when it is used for testing children with known disabilities (Gilliam, 1999). Finally, although while standardized instruments may be helpful as part of a comprehensive assessment, they should never be used as the sole bases for diagnosis or treatment planning. Doing so would violate the principle that infants and toddlers must be understood in the context of the relationships within which they are developing (AACAP, 1997).

Assessment measures should also be chosen based on evidence of adequate reliability and validity. *Test-retest reliability* refers to the likelihood that similar results will be obtained when the test is administered at two different points of time. *Interrater relia-*

Table 14.3   Examples of Standardized Measures

Measure	Age	Purpose
Bayley Scale of Infant Development	1–42 mo	Used to measure infant/toddler development
Child Behavioral Checklist	2–3 yr	Parent reported behavioral problems
Vineland Adaptive Behavioral Scale	0–18 yr	Parent reported performance on daily living activities
Parenting Stress Index	0–10 yr	Parent report of parent-child system under stress

bility refers to consistency in results when tests are administered by different evaluators. Test-retest reliability at young ages, particularly for ages 2 and younger, is typically quite poor. Validity is basically concerned with whether a test actually measures what it was intended to measure. *Content validity* is demonstrated by evidence that a test has items that sample the range of important skills associated with the area of functioning the test is designed to assess. *Concurrent validity* is concerned with the relationship between tests that purport to measure the same construct. *Predictive validity* is based on evidence that a test is able to predict future performance with some degree of accuracy. Information regarding reliability and validity is typically included in a technical manual that is provided with standardized assessment tools. The *Mental Measurements Yearbook* is an excellent source for evaluating the reliability and validity of assessment tools and for assisting evaluators in the selection of appropriate assessment measures (Gilliam, 1999).

Standardized instruments may be an important component of a comprehensive assessment, although as previously mentioned, due to problems in reliability at younger ages and the need to consider broader contextual issues, they should never be used in isolation. In general, test results should be interpreted cautiously at young ages and used primarily as estimates of current functioning and not as predictions of future functioning. Selected measures of individually administered assessment tools for infants and young children are also reviewed in Clark et al. (1993) and Bergen (1994; see appendix B for an overview of selected assessment instruments). Examples of standardized instruments for infant and toddler development currently in use are included in Table 14.3.

Observations and Mental Status Examination

The systematic observation of infants and toddlers is a critical source of information for diagnosis and treatment planning. Good observational systems not only look at individual child and parent-child interaction behaviors but also focus on developmental and emotional processes. One tool recommended for this purpose is the Infant and Toddler Mental Status Exam (ITMSE; AACAP, 1997). The ITMSE is an adaptation of traditional mental status examination dimensions that includes new categories such as sensory and state regulation that make the system more compatible with important areas of infant and toddler development and functioning. Areas of function assessed by the ITMSE include the following:

- Appearance
- Apparent reaction to situation
- Motor
- Speech and language
- Thought
- Affect and mood
- Play
- Cognition
- Relatedness
- Self-regulation

SPECIAL ISSUES IN ASSESSMENT OF AT-RISK POPULATIONS

The field of early development and infant mental health has been significantly influenced by the discipline of developmental psychopathology. The major concerns in developmental psychopathology are predicting maladaptive development patterns and identifying the process by which biological and psychosocial factors influence them (Fonagy & Higgit, 2000). Research has shown that risk and protective factors are quite complex, and many of the factors occur simultaneously. For example, Rutter has shown that the number, rather than the type, of risk factor is predictive of outcome (Rutter, 1990).

Biological compromises such as premature birth, low birth weight, and major medical illness can greatly influence infant outcome. Social class variables, especially poverty, influence developmental outcomes. Poverty has a significant negative effect on the child's home environment. Other family risk factors commonly associated with child outcome include marital problems, adolescent parenting, and family violence. Child maltreatment clearly impacts child outcome. The quality of parenting and the quality of attachment between parent and child have powerful effects on child development.

Risk and protective factors influence the process of assessment and subsequent interventions. There are special assessment issues with certain at risk-populations. Such populations that have been studied include infants and toddlers in the following situations:

- Exposure to alcohol and other drug use
- Maltreatment
- Pre-term birth or low birth weight
- Adolescent mothers
- Mentally ill mothers
- Medical conditions

The fourth volume of the *WAIMH Handbook of Infant Mental Health* is devoted to groups of young children at high risk and includes chapters on each of the above populations (Osofsky & Fitzgerald, 2000).

DIAGNOSING DISORDERS IN INFANCY AND EARLY CHILDHOOD

The classification and diagnosis of disorders of infancy and early childhood do not fit into the traditional medical model. Yet, because of the significant developmental risk associated with many disorders that begin in the first few years of life, accurate diagnosis is an essential prerequisite of any early intervention and treatment (Dunitz, Scheer, Kvas, & Macari, 1996). Emde, Bingham, and Harmon (1993) have reviewed features of the infant mental health diagnostic process that challenge the medical tradition of diagnosis. These include its multidisciplinary focus, developmental perspective, multigenerational focus, and prevention orientation, as summarized in Table 14.4.

The purpose of assessment is to identify distinguishing features of an individual infant, family, and context, whereas the goal of diagnosis is to identify features common to a disorder. Thus, the primary focus of assessment is on the individual, not the disorder, whereas the primary focus of diagnostic classification is on the disorder, not the individual (Zero to Three, 1994). Diagnosis of developmental problems must be done with the knowledge of typical developmental processes (Bergen, 1994). The schemes for classifying mental disorders in infants and toddlers are still evolving. Frequent changes in diagnostic classification systems reflect an effort to incorporate new findings from recent research and clinical experience.

Diagnostic classification systems of mental and developmental disorders manifested in infants and young children serve a wide range of purposes. These include organizing observations; assisting in assessment and intervention planning; and further modifying and changing diagnostic criteria in an attempt to provide a common language for communicating information about a disorder in terms of its symptoms, expected course, and effectiveness of interventions.

At present there are two classification systems in use for the 0- to 3-year-old population: *The Diagnostic and Statistical Manual of Mental Disorders–Fourth Edition* (DSM-IV; American Psychiatric Association, 1994) and *The Diagnostic Classification of Mental Health and Developmental Disorders of Infancy and Early Childhood* (DC:0–3; Zero to Three, 1994).

The *DC:0–3* attempts to integrate psychodynamic, developmental, interactional, neurological, and psychiatric aspects of mental health and developmental problems af-

Table 14.4   Challenges of Infant Mental Health Diagnosis/Classification

Infant Mental Health Model	Traditional Medical Model
Developmental perspective	Focus seems to be on fixed symptom clusters
Multigenerational focus	Individual focus
Prevention orientation	Treatment orientation
Multiple etiological factors and interactions	Single etiological factor
Problems viewed along a continuum	Problems conceptualized as categorically present or absent
Disorder often seen as residing in caregiving relationship	Disorder presumed to reside in individual

Table 14.5 *DSM-IV* and *DC: 0–3* Multiaxial Categories

AXIS	*DSM-IV*	*DC: 0–3*
Axis I	Clinical Disorder	Primary Diagnosis
Axis II	Personality Disorder/MR	Relationship Classification
Axis III	General Medical Condition	Physical, Neurological, and Developmental Conditions
Axis IV	Psychosocial and Environmental Problems	Psychosocial Stress
Axis V	Global Assessment of Functioning	Functional Emotional Developmental Level

fecting the 0- to 3-year-old population into a new diagnostic system. The use of this assessment tool requires a comprehensive pediatric exam or records, an interview with the child's primary caregivers, and observation of parent-child interactions (Dunitz et al., 1996). The *DSM-IV* is the standard diagnostic classification system of mental disorders in use today in America. It includes new diagnostic categories that are relevant to the 0 to 3 age group.

Both of these systems use a multiaxial (domain) scheme as illustrated in Table 14.5. Multiaxial systems involve an assessment on several axes, each related to a domain of information, that may help the provider develop an intervention plan and predict outcomes. Multiaxial systems offer an organized approach for considering various important aspects of the infant or toddler's situation, for example

- Presenting symptoms
- Symptom pattern and possible specificity
- Personality traits of the infant or young child
- Temperament and goodness of fit between temperamental characteristics of the infant or young child and his/her caretaker
- Regulatory patterns
- Psychosocial and environmental influences
- General medical conditions
- Infant or toddler's level of functioning and relating
- Role of the immediate caregivers with respect to the mutual relationship between infant and caregiver and between the caregivers themselves

Additionally, multiaxial diagnostic systems promote the application of a biopsychosocial-cultural model for conceptualizing individual cases because they focus not only on symptoms but also on biological, psychosocial, and cultural influences that contribute to, maintain, or ameliorate the infant's or toddler's difficulties (AACAP, 1998). Finally, the application of standardized diagnostic classification systems helps the provider learn to think in organized and systematic ways on different levels and from various perspectives (Dunitz et al., 1996; Long, Leonhardt, & Wright, 1998).

Table 14.6   *DSM-IV* Diagnostic Categories Applicable to Infants and Toddlers

Motor Skills Disorders	Reaction Attachment Disorder
Communication Disorders	Stereotypic Movement Disorder
Pervasive Developmental Disorder	Selective Mutism
Attention-Deficit and Disruptive Behavior Disorders	Mood Disorder
	Anxiety Disorder
Feeding and Eating Disorder of Infancy and Early Childhood	Sleep Disorders
	Trichotillomania (hair pulling)
Tic Disorders	Adjustment Disorders
Elimination Disorders	
Separation Anxiety Disorder	

Table 14.7   *DC:0–3*: Zero to Three Classification for Infants and Toddlers

Disorders of Social Development and Communication	Regulatory-Based Sleep Disorder
	Regulatory-Based Eating Disorder
Autism	Disorders of Affect
Atypical Pervasive Developmental Disorder	Anxiety Disorder
Traumatic Stress Disorders	Mood Disorders
Acute, Single Event	Prolonged Bereavement
Chronic, Repeated	Depression
Regulatory Disorders	Labile Mood Disorder
Hypersensitive Type	Mixed Disorder of Emotional Expressiveness
Underreactive Type	Deprivation Syndrome
Active-Aggressive Type	Adjustment Reaction Difficulties
Mixed Type	

Table 14.6 lists *DSM-IV* diagnoses (excluding Mental Retardation) that are generally thought to be relevant to the 0- to 3-year-old population. Table 14.7 lists the DC:0–3 diagnostic categories.

Behavioral difficulties are probably the most common reason for mental health referrals involving infants and toddlers. Of course, practitioners must understand typical behavior for infants and toddler before they can effectively assess and intervene with atypical behavior. Infants and toddlers are vulnerable to a range of mental, behavioral, and developmental problems that affect older children and adults. Common behavioral problems found in the 0 to 3 population include the following:

- Excessive crying
- Excessive fearfulness
- Feeding Problems
- Habit Disorders
- Separation/attachment difficulties
- Sleeping Difficulties

One must assess each problem in detail in order to reach an appropriate diagnosis. For example, an infant who is referred with the presenting problem of excessive crying may eventually be diagnosed under *DSM-IV* as meeting criteria for one or more of the following diagnoses: Pervasive Developmental Disorder, Attention-Deficit/ Hyperactivity Disorder or another Disruptive Disorder, Feeding Disorder, Reactive Attachment Disorder, Mood Disorder, Anxiety Disorder, Sleep Disorder, or Adjustment Disorder. Similarly, under *DC:0–3*, this presenting problem may eventually result in one or more diagnoses across the diagnostic spectrum. Only after a detailed assessment across domains and from within a developmental framework will an appropriate diagnosis emerge.

Although most systems of care use the *DSM-IV*, some are beginning to use *DC:0–3*. For infants and toddlers, the *DC:0–3* system provides a classification scheme that is conceptually easier to understand and apply than is that of the *DSM-IV*. *DC:0–3* includes 10 specific guidelines for selecting the most appropriate diagnosis. These are outlined in Appendix 3 of the *DC:0–3 Classification System Manual* (pp. 74–83). The guidelines specify, for example, that traumatic stress disorder should be considered as a first option in cases in which there is an identifiable stressor. The underlying assumption is that the disorder would not be present without that stress. Another guideline specifies that regulatory disorders should be considered when there is "a clear constitutionally or maturational-based sensory, motor, processing, organizational, or integration difficulty" (p. 74). Another indicates that on rare occasions a child may meet criteria for two primary conditions (e.g., a sleep disorder and a separation anxiety disorder).

Dunitz et al., (1986) compared the specificity of symptom patterns using two diagnostic classification schemes: *DSM-IV* and *DC:0–3*. Both systems were used to classify a sample of infants (0 to 2 years old) presenting with a variety of functional behavioral concerns (i.e., feeding difficulties, sleep disturbances, excessive screaming or crying). Pattern specificity was found to be reliable and significant for nearly all groups. The authors found that *DC:0–3* offered some new categories that were well matched for very young infants for whom a diagnosis in *DSM-IV* was not assignable. The authors point out, however, that their study design did not allow for evaluation of other important issues that should be studied in the future, such as which classification system does a better job at predicting etiology, outcome, or response to treatment. In addition, Dunitz and colleagues outlined some of the scientific limitations that must be considered when comparing these two systems, including the following (Dunitz et al., 1986, pp. 20–21):

1. Both systems deal with psychological problems in infants and young children, but they use different approaches. Comparison between the two is based only on observations.

2. Classification items are different in each system, as are their manuals. In order to compare systems, one must first examine the relationship between diagnosable versus undiagnosable children and then compare the pattern of symptoms of a child with a diagnosable disorder in each system.

3. A comparison of diagnostic systems usually refers to questions of internal validity, such as construct validity and sensitivity. However, this study focused on the

clinical practicality of using each system and the impact on scientific communication of the tools, rather than on issues of internal validity.

4. A control group of healthy children is necessary in order to rule out the possibility of diagnosing pathology in a "healthy" population.

More recently, there have been attempts to develop structured assessment/diagnostic measures for young children. The Infant-Toddler Social and Emotional Assessment (ITSEA) uses symptoms that map onto the *DC:0–3* and *DSM-IV* diagnostic systems for infants and toddlers to make diagnoses (Carter, Little, Briggs-Gown, & Kogan, 1999). Two other measures designed for this purpose include an adaptation of the Diagnostic Interview Schedule for Children (DISC) for children aged 3 to 8 years and the Preschool Age Psychiatric Assessment (PAPA), an adaptation of the Child and Adolescent Psychiatric Assessment (CAPA) for children aged 2 to 5 years. All three measures are structured parental interviews and are subject to the limitation of parent report.

Clinical Case Study ·

Brenda, an African American female aged 2 years 9 months was referred to an outpatient infant mental health clinic for evaluation by her maternal uncle, a psychiatric nurse who lives and works near the clinic, which is located approximately 30 miles from where Brenda resides with her mother and grandmother. Presenting problems included frequent screaming in response to loud noises, hitting herself when someone takes something away from her, and pulling out her hair when she is upset. Additionally, the uncle reported that Brenda often pulls her hair when she is not in close proximity to her mother or when a stranger enters her environment.

Brenda lives with her 24-year-old biological mother and her 70-year-old maternal grandmother in the grandmother's home in a rural area outside of a major city. The mother stays at home and serves as Brenda's primary caretaker. The family has been relatively isolated because the mother lacks transportation. Brenda's mother is a high school graduate and the youngest of six children. All of her siblings are reportedly functioning well at present. Brenda's mother has never worked outside of the home, and Brenda has never been to day care. However, Brenda's mother is considering going back to school to study nursing.

Brenda was brought to the initial family interview by her mother and uncle. Her grandmother was unable to attend due to health issues. Brenda's mother served as the primary informant. She expressed that her major concern was Brenda's self-abusive behaviors, namely hitting herself and pulling out her hair when upset. Brenda's uncle noted that Brenda typically gets along well with other family members and seems happy much of the time. However, he expressed concern that she seems to have a difficult time separating from her mother and will often scream intensely or cry persistently when her mother leaves the room or an unfamiliar person tries to engage her. Brenda's mother agreed with these observations and stated she was very worried about whether or not she could ever leave Brenda in order to resume her education.

Brenda's father lives out of state. He left Brenda's mother when she was 5 months pregnant. Brenda's mother was initially ambivalent about the pregnancy but chose to continue

(continued)

it. The pregnancy itself was uneventful and the birth was without difficulty. Brenda's mother reported that all developmental milestones were met at appropriate times. However, she described Brenda as very active from the early months of life. Brenda's biological father reportedly has a high school education and works in the construction industry. According to both Brenda's mother and uncle, he has a short temper. Brenda's mother reported that he frequently was verbally and sometimes physically abusive toward her during their 3-year relationship, which was punctuated by frequent separations and reunions. According to Brenda's mother, he only had a few contacts with Brenda during her first year of life.

Information regarding the father's health history was unavailable. Brenda's mother reported a positive maternal family history of anxiety disorders—more specifically, separation anxiety and obsessive compulsive disorder.

Brenda was evaluated by several members of the multidisciplinary infant clinic assessment team, including a pediatrician who screened her for potential health problems, a nurse who evaluated her developmental status using a standardized instrument (the Denver Developmental), and a speech and language pathologist who assessed her speech and language functioning during free and structured play situations. The mother and uncle were interviewed by a social worker while other team members, including a child psychiatry resident, a clinical psychology intern, and the director of the infant clinic observed the assessment process through a one-way mirror.

Brenda is an attractive African American toddler with large brown eyes and an engaging smile. She was casually but neatly dressed in play clothes. Brenda was carried into the assessment situation on her mother's hip but did not fuss when her mother put her down on the floor and directed her toward the toys in one corner of the room. Brenda initially stayed close to her mother but with some encouragement from her mother and her uncle began exploring the room, making eye contact with various treatment team members, and exploring the room's contents. Assessment of her physical stature and overall health indicated that she is in the average range for height, weight, and head circumference, compared to other toddlers her age and in good health. Brenda's fine and gross motor coordination were assessed to be within normal limits for her age.

Brenda demonstrated a range of affect, from smiling to crying. Her mood during the assessment was predominantly positive. Her mother indicated that her behavior in the session was better than she expected, given her typical difficulty with novel situations. Brenda started to cry several times during the course of the evaluation, usually in response to a newcomer entering the room or during transitions from one activity to another. She also cried on one occasion, during free play, seemingly out of frustration. In this instance, she had attempted to perform a specific task, depositing shapes in a shape sorter, but had difficulty doing so. Typically, her crying jags were short-lived and ended quickly with redirection back toward play activities either by her mother or one of the clinic staff. Brenda played with toys throughout the session and did not whine or cling to her mother at any time. Her activity level was within normal limits for a child her age. She impressed the team as being a bit "slow to warm up" in terms of her reactions to new situations and somewhat cautious in her interactions with unfamiliar adults.

Brenda's speech was characterized by several two-word utterances and a great deal of jargon-like speech, which was difficult to understand. Her receptive language, or ability to comprehend others' speech and follow simple two-step commands was better than her expressive communication skills. Her cognitive abilities were assessed to be roughly average given age expectations. Brenda demonstrated an interest and capacity for engaging in pretend play.

During a planned situation designed to evaluate Brenda's response to separation, her mother was asked to leave the room, informing Brenda that she would be back shortly. Brenda started to protest by telling her mother, "No!" Her mother started to reach out as if to pick up Brenda, but instead offered verbal reassurance that she would soon return. Brenda calmed down fairly quickly, and she returned to the play area and continued to explore the toys until her mother's return. Upon reunion, Brenda ran over to her mother and tried to engage her with a toy.

In another planned assessment situation, Brenda and her mother were left alone with the instructions to play for a few minutes and then for the mother to instruct Brenda to help pick up the toys. The assessment team observed their interactions through the one-way mirror. Brenda and her mother played with blocks during this part of the assessment. At times, Brenda's mother dominated the play situation, giving her daughter too many directives instead of building on presented themes. Overall, however, she seemed interested in Brenda's activities and seemed to derive enjoyment from their interactions. Similarly, Brenda seemed to enjoy her mother's attention and tried to include her in her play. Brenda's mother had difficulty setting appropriate limits during the clean-up phase of this exercise. She asked Brenda if she would like to help pick up toys. Brenda initially ignored her request and instead continued to play, and the mother started cleaning up herself, never insisting that Brenda assist her. However, when she asked Brenda for the final toy that needed to be put away, Brenda gave the toy up without protest.

Brenda exhibited several episodes of hair pulling during her clinic appointment. She twisted and pulled her hair while engaged in free play, and also when sitting quietly in her mother's lap while the adults exchanged information. Brenda's mother appeared to be very attuned to these episodes and responded by telling her child to stop whenever she observed her pulling her hair. In contrast, Brenda at times seemed to pull her hair with great intent, and at other times seemed relatively unaware of what she was doing. She was consistently compliant with her mother's requests to stop pulling her hair but after a time required reminding to discontinue this behavior.

Discussion of Case

The approach to the assessment and diagnosis of the problems presented by Brenda and her family involves many features of the infant mental health assessment and diagnostic processes outlined earlier in this chapter.

Reason for Referral

The purpose of the assessment is to define the problem and to find out its cause, if possible. Brenda's mother was primarily concerned about her child's self-abusive behavior, but also had concerns regarding Brenda's tantrums and difficulty with separation problems. Her uncle was particularly concerned about Brenda's difficulties with separation. Brenda demonstrated difficulties with change in routines, separations, and mood regulations by screaming or self-abuse.

Assessment Process

The assessment was carried out by an interdisciplinary team and included a family interview with Brenda's available caretakers, her mother and uncle. Ideally, information should be obtained from the grandmother, but she was not available. A detailed developmental history was obtained from the caretakers, and a standard screening measure (the Denver) was used to gather current information about Brenda's developmental functioning. Clinical observation focused on the parent-child interactions and included a brief separation and reunion. Areas assessed included Brenda's reaction to various situations, her motor skills, her speech and language, her play skills, her self-regulation, and her affect and mood.

Findings from the Assessment

Many factors likely contributed to the problems presented in this case. From a biological perspective, Brenda's family history suggests that Brenda is at higher risk for anxiety disorders. Environmental factors that may have contributed to Brenda's difficulties include father absence, the family's social isolation, and Brenda's relative lack of experience with adapting to new situations outside the immediate family context. The mother's own anxiety and ambivalence about leaving Brenda with alternate caretakers in order to pursue her own career interests may have contributed to overprotectiveness in her parenting style. Her own anxiety may have also contributed to ineffectiveness in setting appropriate limits. Developmental screening indicated that Brenda was functioning near her age expectations except for delays in expressive language and difficulties with affective self-regulation. The interaction between Brenda and her mother was characterized by anxious ambivalence on the mother's part and anxious frightened behavior by Brenda.

Diagnosis

Based on the information presented, several *DSM-IV* and *DC:0–3* diagnoses were considered including *DSM-IV* Anxiety Disorder Not Otherwise Specified, Separation Anxiety Disorder, and Trichotillomania; and *DC:0–3* Anxiety Disorder of Early Childhood. Table 14.8 summarizes the *DSM-IV* and *DC:0–3* multiaxial diagnoses for the clinical case.

Recommendations for Interventions

Based on the information obtained from the assessment and initial formulation of problems, the following recommendations were made:

Table 14.8   *DSM-IV* and *DC: 0–3* Multiaxial Diagnoses for Clinical Case

	DSM-IV	*DC:0–3*
Axis I	Trichotillomania (hair pulling) [conceptualized as an anxiety variant]	Anxiety Disorder of Early Childhood [includes excessive separation anxiety, excessive inhibition and uncontrollable crying]
Axis II	None	Mixed Relationship Disorder characterized by anxious/tense relationship
Axis III	None	None
Axis IV	Family Social Isolation Father Absence	Family Social Isolation Father Absence
Axis V	GAF = 60	PIR – GAS = 50 (distressed)

1. Brenda and her mother should be involved in child-parent therapy directed at decreasing the anxiety within that relationship.

2. Make a home visit to obtain more observation information about the child-parent relationship and obtain additional information from the grandmother.

3. Refer Brenda and the family for consultation with a speech and language therapist to address the issue of delayed expressive language.

4. Offer Brenda's mother the opportunity to work individually on her worries and other anxieties about Brenda.

This case illustrates the value of comprehensive assessment in diagnosing disorders of infancy and early childhood and planning treatment interventions.

INTERVENTIONS AND REHABILITATION: GENERAL COMMENTS

No two families are alike. What works for one child and family may not work for another. Different infants and families will respond differently to the same intervention. Treatment planning should therefore be tailored to an individual child and family and should be based on assessment findings, diagnostic formulations, and available resources. Treatment recommendations should always be developed in consultation with the family.

Interventions are difficult to evaluate. Implementation of intervention strategies is likely to vary across interventionists, families, and contexts. Professionals must have a working knowledge about community resources available and accessible to children and families so that they can make appropriate referrals. Many health systems now have systems in place to refer and/or initiate contacts with various community resources. Interdisciplinary teamwork is also an important part of assessment and treatment planning when working with infants and young children. Sometimes this work is done by an established interdisciplinary team. At other times a solo practitioner may rely on adjunctive referrals for the purpose of putting together a comprehensive assessment or carrying out treatment recommendations.

INTERVENTIONS AND REHABILITATION: SPECIFIC STRATEGIES AND APPROACHES

Early intervention encompasses a broad range of programs and services designed to promote development during the first 3 years of life. Early intervention can be home-based, hospital-based, center- or clinic-based, or some combination of the above. Interventions can be child-focused, parent-focused, both child- and parent-focused, or neither as in the case of simply providing screening and follow-up for certain groups designated to be at risk due to some factor such as prematurity (Meisels et al., 1994).

Child-focused programs provide direct services to the infant or young child. For example, a child-focused program might provide direct stimulation to a premature infant, aim to reduce stress in the infant's environment, or focus on regulating infant behaviors and facilitating positive parent-child interactions. Some of the goals of child-focused programs include improved scores on measures of cognitive, sensory, social, or adaptive functioning.

In *parent-focused programs,* the primary targets of intervention are the parents. An assumption of parent-focused programs is that parents are in need of support or specific training in order to improve parenting skills needed to their meet child's general or particular needs. The ultimate goal of these programs is to support optimal child development, and it is assumed that this goal can be reached by modifying parent-child interactions. Specific strategies include increasing social support, decreasing family stress, teaching parents about aspects of development or available community resources, and improving parental confidence and skills in caring for or teaching their child.

Jointly focused programs focus on both parent and child. Many emphasize a teaching role for the parent and the use of parent-child activities to achieve the goal of increasing the child's rate of development in cognitive, social, communication, motor, and self-help skills. Some jointly focused programs view the parent's role more comprehensively than instruction and therefore offer other components, such as parent support and guidance.

Infant-parent psychotherapy is a particular type of intervention that jointly focuses on both parent and child. Infant-parent psychotherapy was one of the first infant mental health interventions and was originated by Selma Fraiberg and colleagues at the University of Michigan in the 1970s. The goal of infant-parent psychotherapy is to support optimum social-emotional functioning in the infant or young child (birth to 3 years) by improving the infant-parent relationship (Lieberman & Pawl, 1993). Typically, both the parent and the preverbal infant are seen together for therapy sessions. However, with toddlers and young preschool-aged children, the format may alternate between conjoint sessions with parent and child and parent alone. An underlying assumption of this approach is that having both parent and child together in the session allows for a wider range of observations, experiences, and reflections of parent-child interactions. In this model, the parent is considered a full partner in the assessment and treatment process. The relationship between the parent and the provider is seen as a critical component of the intervention because it is intended to be a catalyst for improvement in the parent-child relationship. The therapist strives to create a therapeutic relationship with the parent characterized by mutual respect, flexibility, and receptiveness to the needs of both parent and child. Infant-parent psychotherapy uses a variety of therapeutic modalities, including insight-oriented approaches, developmental guidance, emotional support, parent skill building, and concrete assistance.

Developmental guidance, also sometimes referred to as *anticipatory guidance,* offers parents and other caregivers ideas regarding what to expect given a child's current and emerging developmental stages. This is an important part of any consultation or therapeutic work involving infants and toddlers. Anticipatory guidance can be helpful in addressing both general and specific questions or concerns. For example, one question that anticipatory guidance might address is the types of fears developing young children are typically likely to experience at various ages. Anticipatory guidance can also be helpful in establishing reasonable treatment goals for a young child with a known developmental disability, such as cerebral palsy. In this case, anticipatory guidance is used to communicate expectations given what is known about that particular child's developmental functioning, the family situation, and the expected impact of the disability on developmental functioning.

Family resource and support programs are quite diverse but share the goal of enhancing the competence of parents by providing community resources that are responsive to their needs. Some family resource and support programs provide direct services to parents, whereas others provide indirect support such as informational materials. Some provide a comprehensive array of services over time, and others provide a more limited number of services at times of crisis or during specific life events, such as teenage pregnancy, divorce, or family crisis (Weissbourd, 1993).

Clinical work with infants and toddlers typically involves family work and shares many of the principles that are the foundations of family therapy. From a family therapy perspective, the infant or young child's presenting problems are considered symptomatic of problems in the family system. The family system, rather than the individual, is therefore the focus of interventions. When family therapy first emerged, psychoanalysis was still the dominant treatment modality. Theoretical shifts that constitute some of the principles of family therapy were made in response to perceived shortcomings of the psychoanalytic approach. For example, in contrast to psychoanalysis, which involves a focus on reexamining past events and early influences in an attempt to foster personal growth through insight, family therapy is a brief, action-oriented approach designed to resolve symptoms by changing behavior in the present. Another shift is from a focus on *content* to a focus on *process*. Thus, rather than focusing on a sequence of historical events, for example, when trying to understand the determinants of some presenting problem, family therapy focuses on process variables such as patterns of communication within the family system (Nichols, 1984). A common goal of family therapy is to help family members gain a better understanding of family structure, roles, beliefs, expectations, and interaction patterns, and of the relative impact of these variables on child and family functioning for the purpose of discovering new, healthier ways of relating.

Behavior therapy is frequently used as an intervention strategy in clinical work with infants and young children. Behavior therapy includes any of a large number of specific techniques that employ psychological (especially learning) principles to change human behavior constructively. Behavior therapy tends to concentrate on behavior itself rather than on some presumed underlying cause. Behavior therapy rejects classical trait theory, which suggests that behavioral consistency is to be expected based on an individual's predispositions or traits. Behavior therapy assumes that maladaptive behaviors are, to a considerable degree, acquired through learning, the same way that any behavior is learned. Behavior therapy assumes that learning principles can be extremely effective in modifying maladaptive behaviors. Behavior therapy involves setting specific, clearly defined treatment goals. The behavioral therapist adapts his treatment methods to fit the client's problems. Behavior therapy focuses on the here and now. Finally, behavior therapists place great value on obtaining empirical support for their various techniques (Rimm & Masters, 1979).

More recently, there has been great concern about the increased use of psychoactive medicine in childhood populations including toddlers and preschoolers (Zito et al., 2000). At this point, *psychopharmacology* should be a rare intervention with toddlers and young children, given the little data supporting the effectiveness of this intervention for this population.

Prevention-oriented interventions focus on "promoting and maintaining health and minimizing illness, disability, and suffering" (Barnard et al., 1994, p. 386). *Primary pre-*

vention aims to prevent problems before they begin or to reduce the risk of new cases of disability or disease by reducing known risk factors. Primary prevention programs emphasize universal access to interventions designed to reduce risk. Examples of primary prevention interventions include making prenatal care accessible for all pregnant women and immunizations available and accessible to all children to reduce the risk of potentially serious illnesses or diseases.

Secondary prevention targets individuals who have characteristics that place them at risk for future conditions or problems. In secondary prevention, services are provided to individuals or groups identified as at risk before any actual problem is identified. An example of secondary prevention would include offering early intervention services to families of young children identified as at risk for developmental problems or delays based on results of a developmental screening.

Tertiary prevention efforts target individuals who have a known disorder or problem. Tertiary prevention is treatment oriented. However, it is also prevention oriented in its aim to reduce the risk of greater problems occurring in the target group in the future. An example of tertiary prevention might include the provision of early intervention services for infants and toddlers with diagnosed developmental disorders. In this case, the goal of prevention would be to minimize the negative impact of those disorders on developmental functioning and instead build on identified competencies and strengths of the target group.

FUTURE DIRECTIONS

In the past 20 years there have been considerable advances in the recognition and understanding of mental disorders of infancy and early childhood. However, there are many issues that need to be addressed if all young children are to have the protection, care, and nurturance that they need. First, all policies that affect the mental health and well-being of infants and young children should be reviewed to assure that they are child focused and family centered. Researchers and clinicians should work to translate infant mental health research into practice. An effective diagnostic system for infants and young children should be developed and used to guide intervention for young children and their families. The range of interventions from infant-parent psychotherapy to psychopharmacology should be examined to determine the circumstances and characteristics where these interventions are effective. Finally, a major task is the training of competent infant mental health clinicians. The next 20 years are likely to see an explosion of research findings and innovations in clinical care for infants and young children.

REFERENCES

American Academy of Child and Adolescent Psychiatry. (1997). Practice parameters for the psychiatric assessment of infants and toddlers (0–36 months). *Journal of the American Academy of Child and Adolescent Psychiatry, 36*(10, Suppl.), 21S–34S.

American Academy of Child and Adolescent Psychiatry. (1998). Summary of the practice parameters for the psychiatric assessment of infants and toddlers (0–36 months). *Journal of the American Academy of Child and Adolescent Psychiatry, 37*(1), 127–132.

American Psychiatric Association. (1994). *Diagnostic and statistical manual of mental disorders* (4th ed.). Washington, DC: Author.

Barnard, K., Morisset, C., & Spieker, S. (1993). Preventive Interventions: Enhancing parent-infant relationships. In C. H. Zeanah (Ed.), *Handbook of infant mental health* (pp. 386–401). New York: Guilford Press.

Benham, A. L. (2000). The observation and assessment of young children including those of the Infant-Toddler Mental Status Exam. In C. H. Zeanah (Ed.) *Handbook of infant mental health,* 2nd ed. (pp. 249–270). New York: Guilford Press.

Bergen, D. (1994). *Assessment methods for infants and toddlers: Transdisciplinary team approaches.* New York: Teachers College Press.

Bergen, D., & Mosley-Howard, S. (1994). Assessment perspectives for culturally diverse young children. In D. Bergen (Ed.), *Assessment methods for infants and toddlers: Transdisciplinary team approaches* (pp. 190–206). New York: Teachers College Press.

Bergen, D., Thomas, A., & Rubin, J. (1994). Psychological assessment perspectives. *Assessment methods for infants and toddlers: Transdisciplinary team approaches* (pp. 165–179). New York: Teachers College Press.

Carter, A., Little, C., Briggs-Gown, M. J., & Kogan, N. (1999). The Infant-Toddler Social and Emotional Assessment (ITSEA): Comparing parent ratings to laboratory observations of task mastery, emotion regulation, coping behaviors and attachment status. *Infant Mental Health Journal, 20,* 375–392.

Clark, R., Paulson, A., & Conlin, S. (1993). Assessment of developmental status and parent-infant relationships: The therapeutic process of evaluation. In C. H. Zeanah (Ed.), *Handbook of infant mental health* (pp. 191–209). New York: Guilford Press.

Cox, C. (1999). Obtaining and formulating a developmental history. *Child and Adolescent Psychiatric Clinics of North America, 8*(2), pp. 271–279.

DeMaise, L. (1994). *The history of childhood.* New York: Psychohistory Press.

Dunitz, M., Scheer, P., Kvas, E., & Macari, S. (1996). Psychiatric diagnoses in infancy: A comparison. *Infant Mental Health Journal, 17*(1), pp. 12–23.

Emde, R. N., Bingham, R., & Harmon, R. (1993). Classification and diagnostic process. In Zeanah (Ed.), *Handbook of infant mental health* (pp. 225–235). New York: Guilford Press.

Fraiberg, S. (1980). *Clinical studies in infant mental health: The first year of life.* New York: Basic Books.

Field, T., Schanberg, S., Davalos, M. & Malphus, J. (1997). Massage therapy effects on infants. *Pre- and Perinatal Psychology Journal, 12,* 73–78.

Fonagy, P., & Higgitt, A. (2000). An attachment theory perspective on early influences on development and social inequalities in health. In Osofsky & Fitzgerald, *WAIMH handbook of infant mental health* (Vol. 4, pp. 521–578). New York: Wiley.

Gilliam, W. (1999). Developmental assessment: Its role in comprehensive psychiatric assessment of young children. *Child and Adolescent Psychiatric Clinics of North America, 8*(2), 225–238.

Gilliam, W., & Mayes, L. (1999). Developmental assessment of infants and toddlers. In C. Zeanah (Ed.), *Handbook of infant mental health* (2nd ed., pp. 236–248). New York: Guilford Press.

Greenspan, S. (1992). *Infancy and early childhood: The practice of clinical assessment and intervention with emotional and developmental challenges.* Madison, WI: International University Press.

Harmon, R. J., & Frankel, K. A. (1997). The growth and development of an infant mental health program: An integrated perspective. *Infant Mental Health Journal, 18,* 126–134.

Hirshberg, L. M. (1993). Clinical interviews with infants and their families. In C. H. Zeanah (Ed.), *Handbook of infant mental health* (pp. 171–190). New York: Guilford Press.

Kalmanson, B. (1989). Assessment considerations: Developmental vulnerabilities. *Early Childhood Update, 5*(4), 6–7.

Langer, W. (1974). Infanticide: A historical survey. *History of Childhood Quarterly, 1,* 354–365.

Lieberman, A., VanHorn, P., Grandison, C., & Pekarsky, J. (1997). Mental health assessment of infants, toddlers and preschoolers in a service program on treatment outcome research program. *Infant Mental Health Journal, 18*(2), 158–170.

Lieberman, A., & Pawl, J. (1993). Infant-parent psychotherapy. In C. H. Zeanah (Ed.), *Handbook of infant mental health* (pp. 427–442). New York: Guilford Press.

Long, K., Leonhardt, T., & Wright, H. (1998). *Mental health in birth to six year old children.* Columbia, SC: Department of Disabilities and Special Needs.

Luby, J. L., & Morgan, K. (1997). Characteristics of an infant/preschool psychiatric clinic sample: Implications for clinical assessment and nosology. *Infant Mental Health Journal, 18,* 209–220.

Mayes, L. (1999). Addressing mental health needs of infants and young children. *Child and Adolescent Psychiatric Clinics of North America, 8*(2), 209–220.

McConaughy, S., & Achenbach, T. (1990). Contributions of developmental psychopathology to school services. In T. Gutkin, & C. Reynolds (Eds.), *The handbook of school psychology,* 2nd ed. (pp. 244–268). New York: Wiley.

Meisels, S., Dichtemiller, M., & Liaw, F. (1993). A multidimensional analysis of early childhood intervention programs. In C. H. Zeanah (Ed.), *Handbook of infant mental health* (pp. 361–386). New York: Guilford Press.

Minde, K., & Minde, R. (1986). *Infant psychiatry: An introductory textbook.* Beverly Hills: Sage.

Minde, K., & Tidmarsh, L. (1997). The changing practices of an infant psychiatry program: The McGill experience. *Infant Mental Health Journal, 18,* 135–144.

Nichols, M. (1984). *Family therapy: Concepts and methods.* New York: Gardner Press.

Nuttall, E., Romero, I., & Kalesnik, J. (1992). *Assessing and screening preschoolers: Psychological and educational dimensions.* Needham Heights, MA: Allyn & Bacon.

Osofsky, J. D., & Fitzgerald, H. E. (Eds.). (2000). Infant mental health in groups at high risk (Vol. 4). In *WAIMH handbook of infant mental health.* New York: Wiley.

Rimm, D., & Masters, J. (1979). *Behavior therapy: Techniques and empirical findings* (2nd ed.). Orlando, FL: Academic Press.

Robertson, J., & Bowlby, Jr. (1952). Responses of young children to separation from their mothers. *Counier: Centre internationale de l'enfants, 2,* 131–142.

Rutter, M. (1990). Psychosocial resilience and projection mechanisms. In J. Rolf, D. Johnson, & D. Peoples (Eds.), *Risk and protective factors in the development of psychopathology* (pp. 181–214). New York: Cambridge University Press.

Thomas, J. M., Goskin, K. A., & Klass, C. S. (1997). Early development program: Collaborative structures and processes. *Infant Mental Health Journal, 18,* 198–208.

Weissbourd, B. (1993). Family support programs. In C. H. Zeanah (Ed.), *Handbook of infant mental health* (pp. 402–413). New York: Guilford Press.

Wright, H., & Leonhardt, T. (1998). Service approaches for infants, toddlers, and preschoolers: Implications for systems of care. In M. Hernandez & M. Isaacs (Eds.), *Promoting cultural competence in children's mental health services* (pp. 229–249). Baltimore: Brookes.

Zero to Three. (1994). Diagnostic classification: 0–3. *Diagnostic classification of mental health and developmental disorders of infancy and early childhood.* Arlington, VA: Author.

Zito, J. M., Safer, D. J., dos Reis, S., Gardner, J. F., Boles, M., & Lynch, F. (2000). Trends in the prescribing of psychotropic medications to preschoolers. *Journal of the American Medical Association, 283,* 1025–1030.

Chapter 15

ANXIETY DISORDERS IN CHILDREN AND ADOLESCENTS

EUGENIO M. ROTHE AND DANIEL CASTELLANOS

INTRODUCTION

The presence of anxiety is common in children and adolescents. The entire spectrum of anxiety symptoms—from typical, developmentally appropriate anxiety, to clinical anxiety syndromes that may cause impairment and severe subjective suffering—is encountered by most mental health professionals who work with children and adolescents. Because anxiety can interfere with concentration and may affect school performance and socialization, it is frequently the teacher or the school psychologist who is the first to sound an alarm indicating that something is wrong with the child. The relatively high prevalence rates of anxiety disorders in children and adolescents are comparable to the rates of many physical disorders, such as asthma (Yunginger, 1994; Selzak, Persky, & Kviz, 1998). Thus, it is also not uncommon for anxiety disorders to be first identified in the medical doctor's office by pediatricians or family physicians. Because anxiety is a typical, developmentally appropriate reaction during certain periods of life, the importance of differentiating developmentally normal anxiety from clinical (pathological) anxiety requiring treatment is of crucial importance.

DEFINITION

Anxiety (from the Latin *anxietas,* "troubled mind"; Ayd, 1993) may be broadly defined as the emotional uneasiness associated with the anticipation of danger. It is usually distinguished from fear, which is regarded as the emotional response to objective danger; the physical manifestations, however, are the same (Livingston, 1996).

Anxiety is characterized by a subjective feeling of apprehension, dread, or foreboding, ranging from excessive concern about the present or future to feelings of panic, accompanied by a variety of physical symptoms mediated by the autonomic nervous system (palpitations, shortness of breath, trembling, sweating, skin pallor, and dry mouth). Traditionally, anxiety has been divided into two broad categories according to its etiology: (a) exogenous, when anxiety arises as a result of external events and is psychological, rather than biological, in nature; and (b) endogenous, when it occurs as a result of an underlying biological cause and can have a predictable developmental path, such as the clinical syndrome of anxiety with panic attacks. There is usually some overlap between these two categories because both follow the same physiological mechanisms, and endogenous anxiety can also be triggered by external events (Ayd, 1993). Not only is anxiety a common human experience, but it is also presents or may coexist with many medical or psychiatric disorders, such as depression. A quarter of a century ago, the presence of anxiety disorders in children and adolescents was practically unknown and virtually ignored. The last two decades have brought a mushrooming of investigations and knowledge on anxiety disorders in the child and adolescent population. This progress, in turn, has produced an improvement in research methodologies and in the diagnosis and treatment of anxiety disorders in this particular population (Bernstein et al., 1996).

HISTORICAL PERSPECTIVE

From the time of Aristotle and up to the theories of Darwin in mid-nineteenth century, emotions were more often viewed—when considered at all—as biologically derived and functioning separately from the concepts of mind and soul. It was recognized that emotions followed events or perceptions, but it was not until the late nineteenth century that issues of causality and attribution began to be widely debated (Livingston, 1996).

Psychoanalytic Perspective

In 1926, Sigmund Freud published "Inhibitions, Symptoms, and Anxiety," the first of 15 manuscripts dealing with the subject of anxiety (Freud, 1926). In this first manuscript Freud questioned the origin of anxiety: "Where does this energy come from, which is employed for giving the signal of unpleasure?" (p. 92). He went on to elaborate a psychoanalytic explanation of the phenomenon. This psychoanalytic view of anxiety predominated in Europe and in the United States until the early 1960s. According to Freud, instinctual forces demanding satisfaction arose from an intrapsychic structure that he called the Id. These demands could not always be met, so it became the function of the Ego (the seat of common sense) to curb these demands by the mechanism of repression. Along with the Ego in repressing the instinctual forces came the Superego (the person's internalized set of social and moral rules), which also contributed in forbidding the Id's expressing these instinctual forces. Freud suggested that anxiety broke into consciousness only when repression failed to completely block the conflict from conscious awareness. He theorized that anxiety functions as a signal that forewarns of a dangerous situation and that it appears in response to the emergence of specific thoughts, as these threaten to break into conscious awareness (Freud, 1926; Shapiro & Hertzig, 1988).

Freud presented as an example of anxiety the case of Little Hans (Freud, 1909), the boy who experienced both loving and hateful feelings towards his father. Little Hans developed a fear that a horse would bite him (an unconscious displacement of his fear that his father would hurt Hans for having angry feelings toward him). Freud saw the little boy's fear of horses as representative of the anxiety that arose from experiencing conflicting internal feelings that could only be repressed partially (in this partial compromise, the role of the aggressor is displaced to the horse and away from the father). Freud went on to elaborate a theory about age-appropriate fears (a hierarchy of threats) that he deemed universal to all human beings. He explained that the first threat in early childhood was (a) the fear of loss of or separation from the loved person (caretaker), which would render the infant truly helpless. Next came what he called (b) the fear of castration, a concern over bodily integrity or a fear of being physically hurt by the loved person due to some real or imagined transgression. This was followed by (c) the loss of the love from the loved person (judgment or disapproval), and finally (d) a fear of disapproval by the person's own Superego prohibitions (which embody the internalized value system that the child learns from the influential figures of his childhood and which constitute his conscience and are responsible for feelings of guilt).

Carl Jung (1924), a disciple of Freud, believed that aside from the conflict model, innate temperamental factors also contributed to the development of social anxiety and avoidance as well as panic symptoms associated with hysteria. Freud disagreed with this view. Interestingly, it was perhaps Jung (1924), half a century ahead of his time, who was the first to herald what was to be a more empirically based and broader biopsychosocial understanding of the phenomenon of anxiety.

TEMPERAMENT AND ANXIETY

The emergence and persistence of temperamental differences among children has been the focus of research in developmental psychology. Temperament refers to stable, presumably inherited response dispositions that are evident in early life, are observable in a variety of situations, and probably influence personality development (Biederman, 1990).

The New York Longitudinal Study of Child Development (Chess et al., 1960, 1984) was the first prospective study undertaken to determine the presence and persistence of characteristics of reactivity in children starting in the 3rd month of life. The authors quantified and scored nine categories of reactivity in 110 children, reporting serial observations over a period of several years. The nine categories were (a) activity-passivity, measuring the diurnal proportion of active versus inactive periods; (b) regular-irregular, which refers to elimination, appetite, and demand cycles; (c) intense-mild, referring to the quality of response and its vigor; (d) approach-withdrawal, representing the child's response to new things; (e) adaptive-nonadaptive, referring to the child's response in altered situations and how the child modified the responses in desired directions; (f) high threshold–low threshold, a complex category involving sensory threshold, response to environmental objects, and social responsiveness; (g) positive mood–negative mood, referring to the expression of pleasure-pain and joy-crying; (h) selectivity-nonselectivity, referring to the difficulty with which an established direction of functioning can be altered; and (i) distractibility-nondistractibility, referring to the ease with which new peripheral stimuli can divert the child from ongoing activity. Chess et al. (1960) found that in each category there was consistency and stability over a period of several years. They concluded that initial primary reactivity is a crucial variable, together with environmental influences, in shaping both personality structure and temperament.

Kagan and colleagues (1987; 1988a,b; 1989) at the Harvard Infant Study Laboratory in Cambridge, Massachusetts, have conducted the most extensive research on behaviorally inhibited children. Their work suggests that approximately 10% to 15% of American white children are born predisposed to be irritable as infants; shy and fearful as toddlers; and cautious, quiet, and introverted when they reach school age. In contrast, about 15% of the population shows the opposite profile, and the rest fall somewhere in between (Reznick et al., 1986; Kagan et al., 1987; 1988a,b; 1989). The literature suggests that temperamental profiles in infancy may be associated with later difficulties. For example, Chess and Thomas (1977; 1984; 1986) found that infants with preponderant withdrawal tendencies were at risk for developing avoidant or overanxious disorders in childhood. Carey et al. (1977) reported that infant temperament is a significant factor in predicting school adjustment in early grades Biederman et al. (1990) examined a cohort of children whose parents suffered from panic disorder and agoraphobia and compared them with a cohort of children already being studied by Kagan and collaborators (Rosenbaum et al., 1988), as well as with a third group of normal controls. They found that both groups of vulnerable children (the ones whose parents suffered anxiety disorders and the ones identified by the Kagan group as temperamentally shy) had a higher rate of multiple anxiety disorders (two or more anxiety disorders per child), accounting for more overanxious disorders in the children with affected parents and more phobic disorders in Kagan's cohort of temperamentally shy children.

BEHAVIORAL INHIBITION

A different construct for looking at the same problem consists of analyzing behavioral inhibition, which some investigators believe predisposes to development of anxiety. For example, Turner et al. (1996) proposed that behavioral inhibition could be a genetically transmitted trait that culminates in the development of anxiety; however, they noted that the research suggests that the full emergence of anxiety disorders is dependent on environmental factors, thus accounting for the fact that not all children who are behaviorally inhibited develop anxiety disorders. Biederman et al. (1990) found that close to 70% of inhibited children are free of anxiety disorders (Craske, 1997). Turner et al. (1996) also proposed that behavioral inhibition may be a genetically transmitted predisposition resulting in a proneness to respond intensely to anxiety-producing events, perhaps due to physiological and behavioral regulatory systems. Suomi et al. (1981), in studying Rhesus monkeys, have found that 20% of their subjects are behaviorally inhibited. This pattern of behavior continues through the monkeys' development. In the same way that Kagan has found this to be true in humans (1987; 1988a,b; Reznick et al., 1986), Suomi et al. (1981) found elevated hypothalamic-pituitary axis reactivity in his behaviorally inhibited Rhesus monkeys. An increasing body of longitudinal data from Suomi's investigations (1981) indicate that certain early experiences can alter both behavioral and physiological developmental trajectories. Gray (1982) proposed that individuals who are anxious have an overly active behavioral inhibition system. The behavioral inhibition system is believed to be located in the septo-hippocampal area of the limbic system and to respond to specific conditions of punishment, novelty, or frustrative nonreward conditions by suppressing ongoing behaviors and redirecting behavior toward the relevant stimulus. Likewise, Quay (1993) suggested that an overactive behavioral inhibition system underlies anxiety disorders, whereas an underactive system may be responsible for Attention-Deficit/Hyperactivity Disorder. However, empirical support for these models is lacking. Eysenck (1967), using a similar model, proposed that behavior is determined largely by two sets of traits: introversion-extroversion and neuroticism-stability. Introversion and neuroticism are believed to predispose to neuroses (or anxiety) and depression and to have a biological substrate. Specifically, neuroticism (anxiety) is believed to be associated with the limbic system and elevated autonomic arousal, whereas introversion is believed to be associated with high levels of cortical arousal controlled by the reticular formation (Eysenck, 1987). Research has shown that the dimensions of introversion-extroversion and neuroticism-stability are highly heritable. Eysenck (1967) proposed that introversion and neuroticism predispose toward strong emotional responding and may cause a vulnerability toward the development of fears and anxiety disorders.

All of these findings suggest an association between behavioral inhibition and childhood anxiety disorders. Also, children with behavioral inhibition may be at a higher risk for school maladjustment, social dysfunction, and distress. Furthermore, Caspi et al. (1988, 1995) examined the adult outcomes, 30 years later, of children who were found to be shy and reserved in late childhood. Although shyness did not relate to extreme pathology in childhood, males who were shy as children showed delayed marriage, fatherhood, and entrance into stable careers relative to males who were not shy. On the other hand, shyness did not affect adult development of women, most likely due to the compatibility of shy behavior with female sex role expectations (Caspi et al., 1988).

Turner et al. (1987), in a review of the literature of the relationship between anxiety disorders and behavioral inhibition, suggested that most research studies in this area are beset by methodological limitations—specially, differing criteria in defining behavioral inhibition. Nevertheless, Craske (1997) concluded that the findings are generally robust. The best methodological studies, she concluded, reveal the following: (a) Children with behavioral inhibition are more likely to have a significant anxiety syndrome and are more likely to have phobias than uninhibited children; (b) this result is particularly true for stably inhibited children; (c) inhibited children are more prone to fears that have a social-evaluative basis, such as crowds, strangers, and public speaking; and (d) parents of children with behavioral inhibition are more likely to have anxiety disorders during childhood and as adults, particularly disorders with social-evaluative basis.

ETHOLOGICAL DEVELOPMENT

Ethology is the study of the characteristic behavior patterns of animals (Ayd, 1993). Bowlby (1969) was the first to build a human development psychology by combining psychoanalytic and ethological concepts. He developed his early work by studying children who were separated from their parents in England during and immediately after World War II. His work paralleled that of Spitz (1945). Bowlby reviewed the nature of the mother-infant tie, which was mediated by what he called the component instinctual response system. The infant is described as having five instincts that make up attachment behavior: (a) sucking, (b) clinging, (c) following, which are also present in other species; and (d) crying and (e) smiling, which achieve their goal in humans by bringing the mother to the infant. Bowlby speculated that attachment had an important survival value in the human species. He proceeded to systematize the infant response to the separation from mother into three phases: (a) protest, (b) grief, and (c) despair. His research indicated that children who were poorly attached to their mothers had later untoward consequences. Bowlby's work on the consequences of attachment and separation served as the foundation for many of the works of later investigators.

GENETIC FIELD THEORY

Rene Spitz (1945) developed this theory by direct (in-the-field) observation of infants. He described early human behavior as mediated by an intrinsic biological-maturational thrust, which had the purpose of allowing the infant to interact with his environment. He described three maturational milestones or organizers: (a) the smiling response (at 6 weeks); (b) the stranger response (at about 7 months); and (c) the "no" response, which signalled the child's individuation (at 15 months). According to this model, the infant's development progresses in the direction of engaging in more complex social interactions and discriminating his or her level of attachment to different people. At 16 weeks the infant begins to show interest in the father, and around 4 to 6 months he begins to enjoy being handed over to different people. Around 7 months he becomes cautious in the presence of strangers, and outright fear in the presence of a stranger first appears between 7 and 10 months (expressions of fear are less likely to occur if a stranger approaches the child slowly in the presence of the parent and more likely to occur when the stranger intrudes rapidly to pick up the infant). Also, around this time, the infant has developed selective attachments to a small number of people—not only to mothers but also to fathers, siblings, or babysitters. There is usually a marked hierarchy between these attachments, the mother being at the top. The term *separation anxiety* has been used to describe the distress exhibited by the baby when the mother is unavailable. It has been attributed to biological causes as well as to disturbed parent-infant bonds. Bowlby (1969) explained that the distress that the child experiences at separation is a sign of not only anxiety but also of depression resulting from the loss of the loved person.

Strange Situation Test

Ainsworth et al. (1978) developed a research method to assess the quality of attachment in 12- to 18-month-old children. The strange situation test involves a series of three-minute separations and reunions that alternate between the caregiver and an unfamiliar stranger in another room. According to the results, children are classified in three categories: (a) securely attached children, who show mild protest at the separation but are easily placated when the mother returns and who constitute about 2/3 of the sample of 1-year-old middle-class American children; (b) avoidant children, who become markedly upset at departure and who resist mother's efforts to comfort them when she returns; and (c) resistant or anxiously attached children, who respond with chaotic fluctuations or by seeking and avoiding the caretaker. Babies showing secure attachment grow up to exhibit greater social competence and better peer relationships (Shapiro & Hertzig, 1988).

PSYCHOLOGICAL FACTORS AND ANXIETY

There is a significant scientific literature supporting the effects of environmental events and parental influences on the development of anxiety disorders in children and adolescents. For example, Barlow (1988) has demonstrated that early experiences of uncontrollability may contribute to the later development of an anxious temperament in the child. Also, certain parenting behaviors contribute to a state of anxiousness and neuroticism in the child. Barret et al. (1996) showed that parents of anxious children tend to focus selectively on future negative outcomes for their children's present activities, and Krohne et al. (1991) showed that high anxiety in a child is closely related to frequent negative feedback and parental restriction. Siqueland et al. (1996) suggested that parents who become overinvolved, overindulgent, and overprotective of their children contribute to these children's developing a concept of themselves as "fragile and incompetent." Several studies show that anxious children exhibit a cognitive processing information bias toward threat (Martin et al., 1992) and tend to interpret ambiguous situations as more threatening, when compared to controls (Barrett et al., 1996). Ollendick and King (1991) studied informational transmission of fears from parents to children. In their sample, the majority of children attributed fears to "modeling" of their parents behavior (65%) and "informational" transmission (89%). In reviewing this literature, the origin of anxiety disorders in children points to a combination of biological, genetic, temperamental, and environmental factors, many of which are based in early life experiences (Barlow, 1988; Craske, 1997).

EPIDEMIOLOGY

Over the past 10 years, several studies have examined the rates of anxiety disorders in children and adolescents. The prevalence rates for the different anxiety disorders vary according to the study. However, there is general agreement among investigators that anxiety disorders are one of the most prevalent categories of child and adolescent psychopathology (Practice Parameters, 1997). Costello (1989) found that in a general pediatric sample of 800 patients 7 to 11 years old, 8.9% met criteria for at least one anxiety disorder.

Some controversy exists about what constitutes a clinical and diagnosable anxiety disorder. The classic Methods for the Epidemiology of Children and Adolescent Mental Disorders (MECA) (Shoffer et al., 1996) data were collected on 1,285 children and adolescents ages 9 through 17 years and their parents or caretakers using a large battery of measures. The investigators concluded that a "substantial proportion of individuals who meet symptomatic criteria for diagnosis appear to be functioning normally." (p. 876) This suggests that a more accurate definition of anxiety disorder should include both symptoms and impairment, rather than symptoms alone (Shaffer et al., 1996). Taking these criteria into account, Kashani and Orvaschel (1988) studied a representative sample of 150 adolescents and found that 8.7% had at least one anxiety disorder that was causing a clinical dysfunction requiring treatment. Bowen et al. (1990) studied a nonreferred sample of children and adolescents and found that 2.4% met criteria for Separation Anxiety Disorder. In a similar study, Bird et al. (1988) found a prevalence rate of 4.7% of the same disorder. Anderson et al. (1987) studied the prevalence rates of Overanxious Disorder and found that 2.9% met criteria for the disorder; a similar study by Costello (1989) found a prevalence rate of 4.6%. Kashani and Orvaschel (1990) studied the prevalence rate of Social Phobia in American children ages 8, 12, and 17 years and found that 1% met criteria for the disorder. Anderson et al. (1987) undertook a large epidemiological study of 11-year-old children in New Zealand and found a 0.9% prevalence of Social Phobia in this population. McGee et al. (1990) reevaluated the same subjects fifteen years later and found that 1.1% had the disorder. More studies are needed to determine the gender distribution of anxiety disorders in children and adolescents. Werry (1991) determined that Overanxious Disorder had an equal gender distribution until adolescence, after which the disorder appeared to predominate in girls. Last et al. (1992) studied 188 children in an anxiety disorders clinic. They determined that the children with Separation Anxiety Disorder had an equal gender distribution and an earlier age of onset (mean = 7.5 years) than other anxiety disorders and that these children were more likely to come from low socioeconomic status and single parent homes. Other studies also report sociodemographic findings associated to particular anxiety disorders. However, these findings appear to be influenced by specific referral patterns.

COMORBIDITY

Comorbidity refers to the overlap of two or more psychiatric disorders on the same patient (Ayd, 1995). At least one third of the children with anxiety disorders meets criteria for two or more anxiety disorders (Kashani & Orvaschel, 1990; Strauss & Last, 1993). Children with anxiety disorders also commonly have major depression. The rates of depression range from 28% (Strauss et al., 1988) to 69% (Kashani & Orvaschel, 1988). Children who have a combination of anxiety and depression are older and have more severe symptoms than those with anxiety alone (Bernstein & Broschardt, 1991; Strauss et al., 1988).

Several investigators have found an association between anxiety disorders and Attention-Deficit/Hyperactivity Disorder (ADHD; Anderson et al., 1987; Biederman et al., 1991; Bird et al., 1988). For example, Last et al. (1987) found that between 15% to 24% of the children with Separation Anxiety or Overanxious Disorder also met criteria for ADHD. Identification of comorbidity is of extreme importance when determining the particular treatment modality—for example, if only one of the conditions is addressed therapeutically, and the other is ignored. Only partial success can be accomplished with this treatment.

ASSESSMENT

In order to make the correct diagnosis of anxiety disorders in children and adolescents, the clinician should be familiar with the *Diagnostic and Statistical Manual of Mental Disorders–Fourth Edition* (*DSM-IV;* American Psychiatric Association, 1994) diagnostic criteria for each particular anxiety disorder (Table 15.1). The DSM-III-R (APA, 1987) included three disorders of anxiety in childhood and adolescence: (a) Separation Anxiety, (b) Avoidant Disorder, and (c) Overanxious Disorders. In the passage on to the *DSM-IV,*

Table 15.1   *DSM-IV* Criteria for Anxiety Disorders in Children and Adolescents

Separation Anxiety Disorder (309.21)

A. Developmentally inappropriate and excessive anxiety concerning separation from home or from those to whom the individual is attached, as evidenced by three (or more) of the following:

1. Recurrent or excessive distress when separation from home or major attachment figures occurs or is anticipated.

2. Persistent or excessive worry about losing, or about possible harm befalling, major attachment figures.

3. Persistent or excessive worry that an untoward event will lead to separation from a major attachment figure (e.g., getting lost or being kidnapped).

4. Persistent reluctance or refusal to go to school or elsewhere because of fear of separation.

5. Persistently or excessively fearful or reluctant to be alone or without major attachment figures at home or without significant adults in other settings.

6. Persistent reluctance or refusal to go to sleep without being near a major attachment figure or to sleep away from home.

7. Repeated nightmares involving themes of separation.

8. Repeated complaints of physical symptoms (such as, headaches, stomachaches, nausea, vomiting, etc.) when separation form major attachment figures occurs or is anticipated.

B. The duration of the disturbance is a least 4 weeks.

C. The onset is before age 18 years.

D. The disturbance causes clinically significant distress or impairment in social, academic (occupational), or other important areas of functioning.

E. The disturbance does not occur exclusively during the course of a Pervasive Developmental Disorder, Schizophrenia, or other Psychotic Disorder and, in adolescents and adults, is not better accounted for by Panic Disorder With Agoraphobia.

Generalized Anxiety Disorder (300.02)

A. Excessive anxiety and worry (apprehensive expectation) occurring more days than not for at least 6 months, about a number of events or activities (such as work or school performance).

B. The person finds it difficult to control the worry.

C. The anxiety and worry are associated with one (or more) of the following six symptoms (with at least some symptoms present for more days than not for the past 6 months):

1. restlessness or feeling keyed up on edge

2. being easily fatigued

3. difficulty concentrating or mind going blank

4. irritability

5. muscular tension

6. sleep disturbance (difficulty falling or staying asleep, or restless unsatisfying sleep)

D. The focus of the anxiety and worry is not confined to features of an Axis I disorder, e.g., the anxiety or worry is not about having a Panic Attack (as in Panic Disorder), being embarrassed in public (as in Social Phobia), being contaminated (as in Obsessive-Compulsive Disorder), being away from home or close relatives (as in Separation Anxiety Disorder), gaining weight (as in Anorexia Nervosa), having multiple physical complaints (as in Somatization Disorder), or having a serious illness (as in Hypochondriasis), and the anxiety and worry do not occur exclusively during Posttraumatic Stress Disorder.

(continued)

Table 15.1 Continued

E. The anxiety worry, or physical symptoms cause clinically significant distress or impairment in social, occupational, or other important areas of functioning.

F. The disturbance is not due to the direct physiological effects of a substance (e.g., a drug of abuse, a medication) or a general medical condition (e.g., hyperthyroidism) and does not occur exclusively during a Mood Disorder, a Psychotic Disorder, or a Pervasive Developmental Disorder.

Panic Attack

A. A discrete period of intense fear or discomfort, in which four (or more) of the following symptoms developed abruptly and reached a peak within 10 minutes:

   1. palpitations, pounding heart, or accelerated heart rate
   2. sweating
   3. trembling or shaking
   4. sensations of shortness of breath or smothering
   5. feeling of choking
   6. chest pain or discomfort
   7. nausea or abdominal distress
   8. feeling dizzy, unsteady, lightheaded or faint
   9. derealization (feelings of unreality) or depersonalization (feeling detached from oneself)
   10. fear of losing control or going crazy
   11. fear of dying
   12. paresthesias (numbness or tingling sensation)
   13. chills or hot flushes

Panic Disorder without Agoraphobia (300.01)

A. Both 1 and 2:

   1. recurrent unexpected panic attacks
   2. at least one of the attacks has been followed by:
      a. 1 month (or more) of one (or more) of the following:
         i. persistent concern about having additional attacks
         ii. worry about the implications of the attack or it consequences (e.g., losing control, having a heart attack, "going crazy")

Absence of Agoraphobia

B. The panic attacks are not due to the direct physiological effects of a substance (e.g., drug of abuse, a medication) or a general medical condition (e.g., hyperthyroidism).

C. The panic attacks are not better accounted for by another mental disorder, such as social phobia (e.g., occurring on exposure to feared social situations), specific phobia (e.g., on exposure to a specific phobic situation), obsessive-disorder (e.g., on exposure to dirt in someone with an obsession about contamination), Post-Traumatic Stress Disorder (e.g., in response to stimuli associated with a severe stressor), or separation anxiety disorder (e.g., in response to being away from home or close relative).

Table 15.1   Continued

Panic Disorder with Agoraphobia (300.21)

D. Both 1 and 2:

1. recurrent unexpected panic attacks

2. at least one of the attacks has been followed by one month (or more) of one (or more) of the following:

    a. worry about the implications of the attack or its consequences (e.g., losing control, having a heart attack, "going crazy")

E. The presence of agoraphobia.

F. The panic attacks are not due to the direct physiological effects of a substance (e.g., drug of abuse, a medication) or a general medical condition (e.g., hyperthyroidism).

G. The panic attacks are not better accounted for by another mental disorder, such as social phobia (e.g., occurring on exposure to feared social situations), specific phobia (e.g., on exposure to a specific phobic situation), Obsessive-Compulsive Disorder (e.g., on exposure to dirt in someone with an obsession about contamination), Post-Traumatic Stress Disorder (e.g., in response to stimuli associated with a severe stressor), or separation anxiety disorder (e.g., in response to being away from home or close relatives).

Agoraphobia

Note: Agoraphobia is not a codable disorder.

A. Anxiety about being in places or situations from which escape might be difficult (or embarrassing) or in which help may not be available in the event of having an unexpected or situationally predisposed. Panic Attack or panic-like symptoms. Agoraphobic fears typically involve characteristic clusters of situations that include: being outside the home alone; being in a crowd or standing in line; being on a bridge; and traveling in a bus, train or automobile.

The situations are avoided (e.g., travel is restricted) or else are endured with marked distress or with anxiety about having a panic attack or panic-like symptoms, or require the presence of a companion. The anxiety or phobic avoidance is not better accounted for by another mental disorder, such as Social Phobia (e.g., occurring on exposure to feared social situations), specific phobia (e.g., on exposure to a specific phobic situation), obsessive-compulsive disorder (e.g., on exposure to dirt in someone with an obsession with contamination), Post-Traumatic Stress Disorder (e.g., in response to stimuli associated with a severe stressor), or Separation Anxiety Disorder (e.g., in response to being away from home or close relatives).

Specific Phobia (300.29)

A. Marked and persistent fear that is excessive or unreasonable, cued by the presence or anticipation of a specific object or situation (e.g., flying, heights, animals, receiving an injection, seeing blood).

B. Exposure to the phobic stimulus almost invariably provokes an immediate anxiety response, which may take the form of a situationally bound or situationally predisposed panic attack. In children, the anxiety may be expressed by crying, tantrums, freezing or clinging.

C. The person recognized that the fear is excessive or unreasonable. This may be absent in children.

D. The phobic situation(s) is avoided or else is endured with intense anxiety or distress.

(continued)

Table 15.1 Continued

E. The avoidance, anxious anticipation, or distress in the feared situation(s) interferes significantly with the person's normal routine, occupational (or academic) functioning, or social activities or relationships), or there is marked distress about having the phobia.

F. In individuals under age 18 years, the duration is at least 6 months.

G. The anxiety, panic attacks or phobic avoidance associated with the specific object or situation are not better accounted for by another mental disorder, such as obsessive-compulsive disorder (e.g., fear of dirt in someone with an obsession about contamination), Post-Traumatic Stress Disorder (e.g., avoidance of stimuli associated with a severe stressor), Separation Anxiety Disorder (e.g., avoidance of school), social phobia (e.g., avoidance of social situations because of fear of embarrassment), panic disorder with agoraphobia, or agoraphobia without history of panic disorder.

Social Phobia (300.23)

A. A marked and persistent fear of one or more social or performance situations in which the person is exposed to unfamiliar people or to possible scrutiny by others. The individual fears that he or she will act in a way (or show anxiety symptoms) that will be humiliating or embarrassing. In children, there must be evidence of the capacity for age-appropriate social relationships with familiar people and the anxiety must occur in peer settings, not just in interactions with adults.

B. Exposure to the feared social situation almost invariably provokes an immediate anxiety response, which may take the form of a situationally bound or situationally predisposed panic attack. In children, the anxiety may be expressed by crying, tantrums, freezing or shrinking form situations with unfamiliar people.

C. The person recognized that the fear is excessive or unreasonable. This may be absent in children.

D. The feared or performance situations are avoided or else are endured with intensive anxiety or distress.

E. The avoidance, anxious anticipation, or distress in the feared social or performance situation(s) interferes significantly with the person's normal routine, occupational (or academic) functioning, or social activities or relationships, or there is marked distress about having the phobia.

F. In individuals under age 18 years, the duration is at least 6 months.

G. The disturbance is not due to the direct physiological effects of a substance (e.g., a drug of abuse, a medication) or a general medical condition and is not better accounted for by another mental disorder (e.g., panic disorder with or without agoraphobia, separation anxiety disorder, body dysmorphic disorder, a pervasive developmental disorder, or schizoid personality disorder).

H. If a general medical condition or another mental disorder is present, the fear in Criterion A is unrelated to it, e.g., the fear is not of stuttering, trembling in Parkinson's disease, or exhibiting abnormal eating behavior in anorexia nervosa or bulimia nervosa.

Obsessive-Compulsive Disorder (300.3)

A. Either obsessions or compulsions:
Obsessions as defined by 1, 2, 3, and 4:

1. recurrent and persistent thoughts, impulses or images that are experienced, at some time during the disturbance, as intrusive and inappropriate and that cause marked anxiety or distress.

Table 15.1   Continued

2. the thoughts, impulses or images are not simply excessive worries about real life problems.

3. the person attempts to ignore or suppress such thoughts, impulses or images, or to neutralize them with some other thought or action.

4. the person recognizes that the obsessional thoughts, impulses, or images are a product
   of his or her mind (not imposed from without as in thought insertion).

Compulsions, such as:

1. repetitive behaviors (e.g., hand washing, ordering, checking) or mental acts (e.g., pray-
   ing, counting, repeating words silently) that the person feels compelled to perform in response to an obsession, or according to rules that must be applied rigidly.

2. the behaviors or mental acts are aimed at preventing or reducing distress or preventing
   some dreaded event or situation, however, these behaviors or mental acts either are not
   connected in a realistic way with what they are designed to neutralize or prevent or are
   clearly excessive.

B. At some point during the course of the disorder, the person has recognized that the obsessions or compulsions are excessive or unreasonable. This does not apply to children.

C. The obsessions or compulsions cause marked distress, are time consuming (take more than
   1 hour a day), or significantly interfere with the person's normal routine, occupational (academic) functioning, or usual social activities or relationships.

D. If another Axis I disorder is present, the continents of the obsessions or compulsions is not
   restricted to it (e.g., preoccupation with food in the presence of an eating disorder; hair
   pulling in the presence of trichotillomania; concern with appearance in the presence of
   body dysmorphic disorder; preoccupation with drugs in the presence of substance use disorder; preoccupation with having a serious illness in the presence of hypochondriasis;
   preoccupation with sexual urges or fantasies in the presence of paraphilia; or guilty ruminations in the presence of major depressive disorder).

E. The disturbance is not due to the direct physiological effects of a substance (e.g., a drug of
   abuse, a medication) or a general medical condition.

Post-Traumatic Stress Disorder (309.81)

A. The person has been exposed to a traumatic event in which both of the following were present:

1. the person experienced, witnessed, or was confronted with an event or events that involved actual or threatened death or serious injury, or a threat to the physical integrity
   of self or others

2. the person's response involved intense fear, helplessness or horror. In children, this may
   be expressed by disorganized or agitated behavior

B. The traumatic event is persistently re-experienced in one (or more) of the following ways:

1. recurrent and intrusive distressing recollections of the event, including images, thoughts,
   or perceptions. In young children, repetitive play may occur in which themes or aspects
   of the trauma are expressed.

2. recurrent distressing dreams of the event. In children, there may be frightening dreams
   without recognizable content.

(continued)

Table 15.1   Continued

3. acting or feeling as if the traumatic event were recurring (includes a sense of reliving the experience, illusions, hallucinations, and dissociative flashback episodes, including those that occur on awakening or when intoxicated). In young children, trauma-specific re-enactment may occur.

4. intense psychological distress at exposure to internal or external cues that symbolize or resemble an aspect of the traumatic event.

5. physiologic reactivity on exposure to internal or external cues that symbolizes or resembles an aspect of the traumatic event.

C. Persistent avoidance of stimuli associated with the trauma and numbing of general responsiveness (not present before the trauma), as indicated by three (or more) of the following:

1. efforts to avoid thoughts, feelings, or conversations associated with the trauma

2. efforts to avoid activities, places, or people that arouse recollections of the trauma

3. inability to recall an important aspect of the trauma

4. markedly diminished interest or participation in significant activities

5. feeling detached or estrangement from others

6. restricted range of affect (e.g., unable to have loving feelings)

7. sense of foreshortened future (e.g., does not expect to have a career, marriage, children or a normal life span)

D. Persistent symptoms of increased arousal (not present before the trauma), as indicated by two (or more) of the following:

1. difficulty falling or staying asleep

2. irritability or outbursts of anger

3. difficulty concentrating

4. hypervigilance

5. exaggerated startle response

E. During of the disturbance (symptoms in Criteria B, C, and D) is more than 1 month.

F. The disturbance causes clinically significant distress or important in social, occupational, or other important areas of functioning.

Reprinted with permission from the Diagnostic and Statistical Manual of Mental Disorders, Fourth Edition. Copyright 1994 American Psychiatric Association.

only Separation Anxiety Disorder remains. Most cases of Overanxious Disorder will now be subsumed under Generalized Anxiety Disorder, and Avoidant Disorder has been conceptualized as Social Phobia (Bernstein et al., 1996). However, the most important tool in making the correct diagnosis is always a comprehensive clinical interview. This should include a history of the onset and development of anxiety symptoms and associated stressors, as well as a medical history, school history, family psychiatric history, and mental status examination (Practice Parameters for the Assessment and Treatment of Anxiety Disorders; AACAP, 1993). Because there is often low concordance between child and parent reports of anxiety (Klein, 1991), and because mothers sometimes tend to over-report anxiety symptoms in their children due to their own maternal anxiety (Frick et al., 1994), it is also important to assess anxiety using a structured questionnaire. Clinician rating scales are useful because they integrate the clinician's expertise with the child or adolescent's self-report of anxiety symptoms, which can sometimes be subjective and difficult to detect by the untrained observer (Bernstein et al., 1996). Table 15.2 offers a com-

Table 15.2 Instruments for Assessment of Anxiety in Children and Adolescents

Measure	Type of Measure	Informant
Schedule for Affective Disorders and Schizophrenia for School-Age Children (Chambers et al., 1985)	Semi structured psychiatric interview, information from all available sources used to derive a summary score	Parent and child, epidemiological version available (K-SADS-E) (Orvaschel et al., 1982)
Anxiety Disorders Interview Schedule for Children (Silverman & Nelles, 1988)	Semistructured psychiatric interview includes other disorders but focuses on anxiety disorders	Parent and child versions
Diagnostic Interview for Children and Adolescents-Revised (Welner et al., 1987)	Structured psychiatric interview	Parent, Child and adolescent versions
NMH Diagnostic Interview Schedule for Children (Schaffer et al., 1996)	Highly structured psychiatric interview, designed for lay interviewers	Parent and child versions
State-Trait Anxiety Inventory for Children (Spielberger, 1973)	Severity measure assess state and trait anxiety	Self-report
Revised Children's Manifest Anxiety Scale (Reynolds and Richmond, 1978)	Severity measure with three anxiety subscales and a Life subscale	Self-report
Revised Fear Survey Schedule for Children (Ollendick, 1983)	Severity measures examines fears	Self-report
Visual Analogue Scale for Anxiety–Revised (Bernstein and Garfinkel, 1992)	Visual analogues to quantify anxiety related to anxiety-producing situations	Self-report
Social Anxiety Scale for Children–Revised (La Greca & Stone, 1993)	Severity measure of social anxiety	Self-report
Multidimensional Anxiety Scale for Children (March, 1996)	Severity measure with four main anxiety factors	Self-report
Hamilton Anxiety Rating Scale (Hamilton, 1959)	Clinician rating scale for adults that has been validated for adolescents (Clark and Donovan, 1994)	Clinician rating using adolescent report
Anxiety Rating for Children–Revised (Bernstein et al., 1996)	Clinician rating scale assesses severity; has Anxiety subscale and Physiological subscale	Clinician rating using child or adolescent report
Personality Inventory for children (Wirt et al., 1996)	Multiple scales including Anxiety scale	Parent report
Child Behavior Checklist (Achenbach, 1991)	Multiple scales including Anxious/Depressed scale	Parent report

Note: NIMH = National Institute of Mental Health.

prehensive listing of diagnostic instruments used in assessing anxiety in children and adolescents. These rating scales are also useful because they provide a measurement of the
severity of the different anxiety symptoms. Also, some of the briefer ones, such as the
Hamilton Anxiety Rating Scale (Hamilton, 1959), can be easily administered by the clinician in a sequential manner at different points throughout the treatment to measure improvements of symptoms and treatment responses.

CLINICAL SYNDROMES

Separation Anxiety Disorder

Separation Anxiety Disorder is probably the most common anxiety disorder in children
(Anderson, Williams, & McGee et al., 1987; Costello, Angold, & Burns et al., 1996).
Separation Anxiety Disorder can occur at any age but is seen most often in prepubertal children (Bernstein & Borschardt, 1991; Francis, Last, & Strauss, 1987; Kashani &
Orvaschel, 1988). The gender ratio for Separation Anxiety Disorder is poorly understood. Clinic or referred samples are comprised of an equal number of girls and boys
(Last, Perrin, & Hersen et al., 1992), whereas epidemiologic studies report more females with this disorder (Costello, Angold, & Burns, 1996; Last, Perrin, & Hersen et
al., 1992).

The essential feature of Separation Anxiety Disorder is excessive anxiety about separation from home or parents or other attachment figures (Table 15.1). The child's reactions to separation are extreme and beyond what would be expected for his or her developmental age. Other symptoms include unrealistic worry about harm to self or
parents, repeated nightmares with themes of separation, reluctance to sleep alone or
away from parents, school refusal and physical complaints (such as stomach aches,
vomiting, headaches, etc.) at times of separation or anticipation of separation. The
manifestations and disturbances should be enduring and not limited to a single
episode. Also, significant distress or impairment in functioning secondary to the anxiety disorder must be present. Children with Separation Anxiety Disorder present difficulties carrying out various aspects of their normal daily activities, such as attending
school and sustaining regular sleep habits. Mere symptoms of separation anxiety alone
are not sufficient to meet the criteria or threshold for a diagnosis. It should be remembered that separation anxiety is a normal developmental phenomenon from approximately 10 months to the early preschool years. Diagnosis of clinical Separation Anxiety Disorder during this period is made with caution.

Developmental differences in the expression of Separation Anxiety Disorder symptoms in children and adolescents exist. Children younger than 8 years old are more
likely to report school refusal and worries about unrealistic harm to a parent (Kashani
& Orvaschel, 1988; Last, Perrin, & Hersen et al., 1992). Children ages 9 to 12 more frequently endure excessive distress at time of separation. Adolescents ages 13 to 16 will
frequently report school refusal and physical symptoms. Nightmares with themes of
separation are frequently described by the younger children but rarely by older youngsters (Kashani & Orvaschel, 1988; Last, Perrin, & Hersen, 1992).

An association between Separation Anxiety Disorder and Panic Disorder in children has been reported. Although the subject of continued debate, some authors suggest that Separation Anxiety Disorder and Panic Disorder may be different clinical presentations of a common underlying disorder (Klein, 1981; Black & Robbins, 1990).

Clinical Vignette

Angela is a 7-year-old girl who presents with her mother because of school refusal for the past three weeks. Her mother reports that she becomes extremely apprehensive on school mornings, cries excessively, and has vomited on several occasions. The few times that Angela's mother has succeeded in getting her to school, she has been called by school personnel with complaints that Angela has been feeling sick. In the evenings Angela has refused to sleep alone and has been sleeping in her parent's bed. She has been complaining of nightmares and fears that someone would break into her house and kidnap her.

Generalized Anxiety Disorder

Children with Generalized Anxiety Disorder represent different demographic characteristics than do children with Separation Anxiety Disorder. In contrast to Separation Anxiety Disorder, children referred for treatment with Generalized Anxiety Disorder are older at the time of initial intervention. In addition, whereas the frequency of Separation Anxiety Disorder decreases with increasing age, Generalized Anxiety Disorder is observed more frequently in older, rather than younger, children and adolescents (Kashani & Orvaschel, 1988).

In contrast to Separation Anxiety Disorder, which is characterized by a fear of separation, Generalized Anxiety Disorder involves a worry of a more general nature. Children with Generalized Anxiety Disorder display excessive anxiety and worry about various aspects of their lives. They may worry excessively about their own competence, how they will do on an examination, what they will wear the next day, what major they will choose in college, and so forth. Concerns about competence often have a perfectionistic quality: children with Generalized Anxiety Disorder want to excel in school, athletics, social relations, physical appearance, and so on. Possibly as a result of this excessive worry and self-focus, these children often show marked self-consciousness (Martini, 1995). Somatic complaints, such as fatigue, difficulties concentrating, restlessness, sleep difficulties, and muscle tension, are common. The child or adolescent frequently finds it difficult to control the worrying or to be able to attenuate the anxiety symptoms. As has been previously mentioned, the anxiety produces significant distress for the child or interferes with some aspect of daily functioning (APA, 1994).

Clinical Vignette

Robert is a 16-year-old boy who has been presenting changes in behavior over the past several months. He is noted to be preoccupied nearly daily with many areas of his life. His parents report that he worries that he will not get A's in all his subjects at school. He has difficulties falling asleep several days per week. Friends note that he has become increasingly anxious in social situations and appears overly preoccupied with his appearance. All who know him describe him as more tense and irritable. Robert's reality testing is intact, and he acknowledges that he is having difficulties controlling his worrying.

Panic Disorder

The age of onset of the first panic attack in patients with Panic Disorder peaks between 15 and 19 years of age (Bernstein, Borschardt, & Perwien, 1996; Ollendick, Mattis, & King, 1994). Spontaneous panic attacks appear to be rare before puberty. The essential feature in Panic Disorder is the presentation of a panic attack. A panic attack is characterized by a discrete period of intense fear or discomfort that develops acutely. It is associated with multiple physiological symptoms, such as palpitations, sweating, trembling, sensations of choking, shortness of breath, dizziness, and so forth. Fears of losing control, dying, or going crazy are also common during the attack. Anticipatory anxiety or persistent apprehension about experiencing a future attack, worries about the consequences of the attack, and changes in behaviors related to the attack are also typical (Albano & Chorpita, 1995). At least some of the panic attacks are not precipitated by events and occur unexpectedly. Panic attacks that result solely from drug abuse, medications or medical illnesses are excluded in Panic Disorder. In general, the manifestations of Panic Disorder in youngsters and in adults are similar. As in adults, panic attacks in children and adolescents can have debilitating consequences.

In the *DSM-IV*, two diagnostic criteria for Panic Disorder are included, one with and one without agoraphobia (see Table 15.1). Children and adolescents with agoraphobia manifest anxiety and fear about being in situations in which they may be embarrassed or incapacitated. They typically fear they will find it difficult to escape or leave a particular situation. They avoid situations in which they would find it difficult to obtain help. Interpersonal conflicts can arise as children with agoraphobia insist on being accompanied by family and friends when they leave the house.

Clinical Vignette

Agnes reports that her panic attack occurred at age 16. She was waiting in line at a movie theater and began feeling acutely anxious, as if she could not stand still. Her heart was racing; she experienced feelings that she could not get air into her lungs, and thought she was having a heart attack. Twenty minutes later this episode spontaneously remitted. She has experienced more than 15 similar episodes throughout the past 3 months. Agnes admits to daily worries about experiencing another panic attack. She has refused to drive alone and avoids going to the same movie theater where she experienced her first panic attack.

Specific Phobias

Compared to normal fears, which are developmentally appropriate, specific phobias (also referred to as phobias) are excessive and out of proportion to the demands of the situation, are beyond voluntary control, cannot be reasoned away, lead to avoidance, persist over time, and are maladaptive (Albano & Chorpita, 1995). Children with specific phobias exhibit these marked and persistent fears when they are prompted by the presence or anticipation of circumscribed stimuli. These stimuli include a variety of specific situations or objects, such as blood, injections, animals, or heights. Phobias are differentiated from Separation Anxiety Disorder when the fear is not separation specifically. With social phobias (or social anxiety disorders) the fear of humiliation and embarrassment is specific to a social setting.

Mild fears are common throughout childhood (Muris, Meesters & Merkelbach, 1998; Albano & Chorpita, 1995; Bernstein, Borschardt, & Perwien, 1996). In general, girls report fears more than boys. Several themes are consistently reported among children of different age groups. These fears are not only consistent among age groups but also among different cultural groups (Kashani & Orvaschel, 1988). Common fears and themes include falling from a high place, getting poor grades, having a burglar break into a house, and being exposed to snakes. A phobia should therefore be considered and differentiated from nonclinical anxiety only when the fears are excessive, persistent to a specific situation or object, and result in impairment in some aspect of the child's functioning.

Clinical Vignette

Maria, a 10-year-old sixth-grade student, has a long-standing fear of having her blood drawn at doctor's visits. When she was 7 she sustained a superficial laceration to her forehead that bled profusely. Her mother became lightheaded and fainted when she discovered Maria covered in blood. Since this incident Maria has displayed tantrums, uncontrollable crying, and clinging behavior when blood needs to be drawn. The mere mention of having blood drawn produces anxiety with increased respiration and heart rate. Over the past several months she has resisted going to the pediatrician's office because she was restrained for blood drawing approximately one year ago. On the last scheduled pediatric appointment. Maria's mother had to turn back due to the severity of Maria's response in the car. Maria has not allowed her immunizations to be updated.

Obsessive-Compulsive Disorder

Obsessive-Compulsive Disorder (OCD) can be a severe and debilitating disorder in children and adolescents. Approximately 33% to 50% of adults with OCD report onset in childhood or adolescence (Martini, 1995). In psychiatrically referred populations the average age of onset is between 10 to 12 years old (Kashani & Orvaschel, 1988).

OCD is characterized by recurring obsessions or compulsions that produce significant distress or impairment. Obsessions are recurrent, persistent thoughts that are experienced as senseless and intrusive. Compulsions are repetitive, purposeful behaviors or rituals. The symptoms of Obsessive-Compulsive Disorder in children and adults are typically similar. In children and adolescents the most frequently reported obsessions are fear of contamination (35%) and thoughts of harming oneself and familiar figures (30%). The most common compulsions are washing and cleaning rituals (75%), checking behavior (40%), and straightening (35%). Obsessions without rituals are usually rare. In teenagers, multiple obsessions and compulsions are frequent (Kashani & Orvaschel, 1988).

A relationship exists between a subgroup of children with OCD and tic disorders.

Children with tic-related OCD typically present with a family history of tics, higher rates among males, prepubertal onset, a broader spectrum of obsessive compulsive symptoms, and a poorer response to selective serotonin reuptake inhibitors (Tucker, Leckman, & Scahill et al., 1996). Neuroimaging studies have also identified specific anatomical areas associated with OCD. The areas of the brain most frequently identified are the caudate nucleus, anterior cingulate area, and the orbitofrontal cortex (Insel, 1992).

An association between autoimmune processes and OCD has also been identified. Some cases of pediatric OCD may be associated with viral and group A B-hemolytic streptococcus infection in children (Tucker, Leckman, & Scahill et al., 1996; Kiessling, Marcotte, & Culpepper, 1994; Swedo, Leonard, & Kiessling, 1994; Allen, Leonard, & Swedo, 1995). Children with onset of OCD prior to puberty and with evidence of an antecedent or concomitant upper respiratory infection (such as positive streptococcal serological findings, positive cultures, etc.), who have responded poorly to typical treatment strategies, suggest that this subtype of OCD should be considered.

Clinical Vignette

Thomas has always been described as neat and as a perfectionist. As a youngster he always adhered to a bedtime ritual in which he counted the slats in the window blinds three times and then proceeded to fold down his bed covers in a specific pattern. Attempts by his parents to stop him were met with resistance and difficulties with sleep that night. Throughout the past two years he has also become increasingly preoccupied with keeping clean and avoiding dirt. He has refused to shower at school due to fears that he would contract an infection. On one occasion six months ago, when his coach did not allow him to skip his postbasketball shower, Thomas spent nearly 3 hours bathing at home. He subsequently quit the team to avoid being forced to shower after games. His hands are chafed due to his washing his hands about 13 to 15 times per day.

Posttraumatic Stress Disorder

Posttraumatic Stress Disorder (PTSD) has been increasingly recognized in children and adolescents over the past several years. Onset can occur at any age. Gender differences in the development of PTSD symptoms following the exposure to trauma are unclear (Cohen et al., 1998). PTSD is characterized by the development of characteristic symptoms that follow exposure to a traumatic event or severe stressor. The stressful event involves the threat of death or physical injury of the physical or emotional integrity of the person. The traumatic stressor may present as a single event or may be prolonged or chronic in nature (as in cases of physical or sexual abuse). In children and adolescents, a variety of stressors can lead to the development of PTSD, and it can present with a wide variety of clinical features.

In general, the older the child, the more likely the presentation will approximate that in adults. The clinical presentation can vary according to the developmental age of the child. For example, very young children may present with very few classical *DSM-IV* PTSD symptoms. Since many of the symptoms require verbal endorsement and report, it appears that the less-developed language skills in young children may account for this

(Scheeringa et al., 1995). Loss of acquired skills (regression) may also present differently according to the age of the child.

Children and adolescents typically reexperience the traumatic event with intrusive thoughts, dreams, and play. Classical flashbacks are less common in children than in adults (March, Amaya-Jackson, & Pynoos, 1997; Cohen et al., 1998). Avoidance of factors related to the trauma are typical. Younger children may not experience amnesia for certain parts of the trauma (Cohen et al., 1998). The child usually responds with extreme fear or helplessness. Increased physiological arousal can be manifested by exaggerated startle responses, irritability, sleep disturbances, and aggressive outbursts (March, Amaya-Jackson, & Pynoos, 1997; Kashani & Orvaschel, 1988; Albano & Chorpita, 1995).

Clinical Vignette

Timmy is a 7-year-old boy who was sexually victimized by his uncle on several occasions. Last year prior to disclosure, he exhibited frequent nightmares involving themes of being attacked and killed. He presented with bed wetting for over 6 months and frequently refused to sleep alone. Timmy described feeling anxious and fearful at home. He was described as clinging to his mother and would not want to leave her side. For several months he was more irritable. The mothers of his peers complained that he was aggressive in his play their children. Recently he has engaged in sexually inappropriate behaviors, such as masturbating in front of others, attempting to touch the genitals of his siblings, and so on. The mother now brings him for treatment due to complaints from friends and school.

Comprehensive Case Vignette

Jimmy presents for evaluation at the urging of his pediatrician. He is a 13-year-old boy who has had acute anxiety attacks over the past 2 to 3 months. He has begun to refuse to leave the house without his parents. Jimmy specifically avoids going to the grocery store with his mother. Upon elaboration of the history, this was where his first panic attack occurred. Jimmy's panic attacks have increased in frequency to about 3 to 4 per week. They are characterized by acute rushes of anxiety, worrying that he will experience a stroke, and are associated with choking sensations, nausea, racing heart beats, and restlessness. He was sent home from school twice last week due to these episodes. Jimmy's parents have resisted bringing him for evaluation and only did so because the pediatrician insisted.

The pediatrician was contacted and reported that the presentation was not explained by known pathophysiologic mechanisms. He describes Jimmy as a good student who appears to always be concerned with everything's being neat and organized. The Child Behavior Checklist (CBCL) was completed by Jimmy's mother and his main teacher (Teacher's Report Form). The T score for the Internalizing factor was 75 and 81 for the Anxious scale. On the Obsessive-Compulsive scale the average of the two was a T score of 69.

When Jimmy was interviewed, he endorsed all the classic symptoms of Panic Disorder. He notes that most of his panic attacks are spontaneous. During these attacks he feels he

---

(*continued*)

will be "out of control" and fears he may even die. He admits to being more fearful of leaving the house because he may experience one of these attacks while away from home.

Jimmy also reports that he has always been neat, perfectionistic, and highly organized. Over the past 3 years he has been making several lists everyday (e.g., books to bring home, subjects with homework due, T.V. shows to watch that day, etc.). He has become increasingly preoccupied with dirt and keeping clean. Jimmy admits that he will shower for over 1 hour a day. When he brushes his teeth he has to do so in a specified sequence and must repeat this procedure again after rinsing. He also wipes down his desk every morning and evening. Jimmy must dress in a ritualistic manner that includes putting on part of his clothes in the bathroom and part in his bedroom. He admits to being unable to sleep over at friends' houses because he cannot complete these rituals there. When Jimmy is not able to complete some of these rituals at home, he becomes irritable and ruminates about this until he is able to do so later. The Child version of the Yale-Brown Obsessive Compulsive Scale (CY-BOCS) was administered and confirmed the presence of these moderately severe obsessions and compulsions. Jimmy admits that he has hidden these behaviors from his parents for some time.

The treatment plan began with education of Jimmy and his parents regarding his Panic Disorder and OCD. His parents were given literature on each of these disorders. They were referred to the local chapter of a national Obsessive-Compulsive Disorder foundation for support. Since the Panic Disorder was more acute and created more short term impairment, a behavioral management protocol was initiated. Pharmacologic consultation with a child and adolescent psychiatrist was to be considered if he did not improve or if his symptoms worsened over the next 3 to 4 weeks. As Jimmy's panic symptoms improved, a cognitive behavioral approach was undertaken. Jimmy began keeping a weekly log of his maladaptive thoughts and behaviors. Treatment focussed on decreasing his obsessions and compulsions as well as improving his overall level of functioning. Six months after initiating treatment, Jimmy no longer experiences panic attacks. He remains preoccupied with cleanliness but has dramatically decreased the number and frequency of his rituals. He is now able to participate in more social activities with his friends.

COURSE AND OUTCOME

Several longitudinal studies have examined the persistence of anxiety disorders in children and adolescents. A paucity of studies has utilized standardized diagnostic assessment instruments, and few have been prospective in nature. Cantwell and Baker (1989) studied young children with speech and language disorders. For those children with anxiety disorders, the remission rate of comorbid anxiety disorders at 4- to 5-year follow-ups was 77%.

Last et al. (1996) followed 84 children with blind interviews for 3 to 4 years after the initial diagnosis of an anxiety disorder. Eighty-two percent of the cohort no longer met criteria for the initial anxiety disorder at follow-up. Separation anxiety disorder had the highest rate of remission at 96%; panic disorder had the lowest rate at 70%. During the follow-up period, approximately one third of the children with anxiety disorders developed new comorbid psychiatric disorders. Half of these children developed new (additional) anxiety disorders (Last, Perrin, & Hersen et al., 1996). In their 8-year follow-up of anxiety disordered children, Last, Hansen, & Franco (1997) suggested that the children are relatively well adjusted in young adulthood. Social impairment for these young adults did persist, though. In addition, the presence of comorbid depression predicted a more negative outcome (Last, Hansen, & Franco, 1997).

Referral biases may limit the generalizability of clinic-based samples. In a naturalistic study assessing the psychiatric histories of 275 children, Keller and colleagues (1992) examined the course of 38 (14%) of those youngsters with an anxiety disorder. The most salient finding was the prolonged course of the anxiety. Using lifetime estimates of the duration of illness, 46% of the anxiety disordered children would still be ill 8 years after the onset of the disorder. The fact that 75% of these children were untreated appears to have contributed to the chronicity (Keller et al., 1992).

Using longitudinal data, Pine et al. (1998) prospectively examined the relationship between adolescent and early adulthood anxiety. Over the 9-year study period, they discovered that adolescent anxiety disorders predicted an approximate two-fold increase in risk for adult anxiety disorders. Their results suggest that although most adolescent anxiety disorders do not persist into adulthood, most adult disorders are preceded by an anxiety disorder in adolescence (Pine et al., 1998).

With other epidemiologic studies also supporting the stability and chronicity of anxiety in children over time (Verhulst & Verluis-den Bieman, 1995), it appears that many anxious children and adolescents remain at risk for continuing anxiety in adulthood.

TREATMENT

In general, a multimodal treatment approach is recommended in the treatment of children and adolescents with an anxiety disorder. Components can include feedback and education to the child and parents about the anxiety disorder, behavioral interventions, psychotherapy, and pharmacologic treatment. The specific treatment modality will vary according to the type of anxiety disorder. The two mainstays of treatment, behavioral therapy and pharmacologic treatment, are discussed here.

Behavioral Treatment

A variety of psychotherapeutic techniques has been used in the different anxiety disorders. Behavioral interventions have been the most widely used in the management of anxiety disorders. Of these, cognitive-behavioral therapy has been the most widely used. Cognitive-behavioral therapy focuses on changing maladaptive thoughts and assumptions and learning new ways of changing overt behaviors. It emphasizes how children may use cognitive processes to restructure, reframe, and solve problems and change maladaptive behaviors (Ollendick & King, 1998). Randomized clinical trials have suggested that cognitive-behavioral therapy is probably efficacious in the treatment of childhood anxiety disorders (Kendall, 1994; Barrett, Dadds, & Rapee, 1996). Last, Hansen, and Franco (1997) also provided evidence to support the use of psychosocial interventions in managing anxiety disorders in children. In contrast to previous studies, their findings suggest that traditional supportive and educational treatments (which were used as a control for the nonspecific effects of therapy) may be as beneficial for anxious children as are highly structured cognitive-behavioral interventions. The use of cognitive-behavioral therapy should be considered in children and adolescents who suffer from Separation Anxiety Disorder, OCD, Social Phobia, and Panic Disorder. A comprehensive review on the status of behavioral interventions in the treatment of anxiety disorders in children is found in the overview by Ollendick and King (1998).

The most successful treatment approach for specific phobias continues to be desensitization behavioral techniques. Systematic desensitization involves teaching a child relaxation techniques and then exposing the child to progressively more distressful stimuli. As the child experiences anxiety after exposure to the phobic object, the relaxation technique is invoked.

Limited empirical evidence exists for various treatment interventions of PTSD. At least three studies provide empirical support for the use of cognitive-behavioral therapy in children with PTSD. Although extensive empirical support is lacking, clinical consensus suggests the following essential components of treatment for children with PTSD: "direct exploration of the trauma, use of specific stress management techniques, exploration and correction of inaccurate attributions regarding the trauma, and inclusion of the parents" (Cohen et al., 1998).

In summary, the evidence supporting the effectiveness of cognitive-behavioral therapy for anxiety disorders in youth remains promising but only suggestive. More methodologically sophisticated research is needed to address this issue.

Pharmacologic Treatment

The therapeutic efficacy of antianxiety medications in adults has been clearly demonstrated, but far fewer studies in children and adolescents exist (Castellanos & Hunter, 1999). The medications used fall into two broad categories, the benzodiazepines (BZDs) and the antidepressants, along with a unique antianxiety compound, buspirone.

The antianxiety properties of BZDs are caused by their effects on the gamma-aminobutyric acid (GABA) receptor/chloride ion channel complex. Results of studies examining the efficacy of benzodiazepines in treating school refusal have been mixed. Some studies have reported increased school attendance (D'Amato, 1962; Kraft, Ardali, & Duffy et al., 1965; Biederman, 1987), whereas others have not observed statistically significant differences over placebo (Bernstein, Garfinkle, & Borschardt, 1990). The other studies were not placebo controlled. Studies examining the use of benzodiazepines for overanxious disorder (Simeon, Ferguson, & Knott et al., 1992) and panic disorder (Kutcher & MacKenzie, 1988; Ballenger, Carey, & Steele, 1989) have been promising but do not provide robust evidence of their efficacy. In sum, the use of benzodiazepines in the management of childhood anxiety remains poorly studied and understood.

Antidepressant medications used to treat child and adolescent anxiety disorders include the tricyclic antidepressants (TCAs), the selective serotonin reuptake inhibitors (SSRIs), and several unique compounds. Not all antidepressants are effective for the same conditions. Choice of antidepressant is based on efficacy for the particular condition and on side-effect profiles.

TCAs are believed to exert their action by blocking the reuptake of norepinephrine and serotonin from the synaptic cleft. Caution should be exercised in the use of TCAs in children with anxiety disorders because of their limited usefulness and several case reports of sudden death associated (although not unequivocally proven to be directly related) with their use (Riddle, Nelson, Kleinman et al., 1991; Varley & McClellan, 1997). SSRIs are named for their serotonin selectivity in reuptake inhibition. As a group, they are better tolerated and have fewer side effects than the tricyclic antidepressants. Anecdotal reports suggest that SSRIs may be effective in treating separation anxiety disorder, but empirical support is lacking.

OCD is the best studied of all the childhood anxiety disorders, but there are only a few controlled trials of medications. Both clomipramine (Leonard, Swedo, & Lenane et al., 1991; DeVaugh, Geiss, Moroz, & Biederman et al., 1992), a tricyclic in structure but more like SSRIs in function, and fluoxetine (Riddle, Schahill, & King et al., 1992) have proven effective versus placebo in treating OCD.

Buspirone is an antianxiety agent not related to the benzodiazepines. It has a favorable side effect profile in that it is nonsedating and nondisinhibiting. It does not have an immediate onset of action like the benzodiazepines, does not appear to be habit forming, and is ineffective on a PRN ("as needed") basis. Though there have been several studies of buspirone treating Generalized Anxiety Disorder successfully in adults, there are no controlled studies with children or adolescents.

In summary, the knowledge base concerning medications to treat anxiety disorders in children is limited. In moderate to severe cases, pharmacologic treatment should be instituted cautiously and judiciously along with appropriate psychosocial interventions.

CONCLUSIONS

Any professional who deals with children will likely encounter a child with an anxiety disorder at some point. Each clinical disorder presents a unique challenge in evaluation and management. This is especially true in children. Knowledge of child development is essential for a true understanding of these disorders in children and adolescents. Our knowledge base of the management and treatment of anxiety disordered children and adolescents remains relatively limited. Empirically based, methodologically sophisticated research is still needed. Research examining appropriate thresholds for diagnosis, effectiveness of different psychotherapeutic interventions, and clinical medication trials is greatly needed.

REFERENCES

Ainsworth, M. D. S., Blehar, M. D., & Waters, E. (1978). *Patterns of attachment: A psychological study of the strange situation.* Hillsdale, NJ: Erlbaum.

Albano, A. M., & Chorpita, A. B. (1995). Treatment of anxiety disorders of childhood. *Psychiatric Clinics of North America, 18,* 767–784.

Allen, A. J., Leonard, H. L., & Swedo, S. E. (1995). Case study: A new infection-triggered, autoimmune subtype of pediatric OCD and Tourette's Syndrome. *Journal of the American Academy Child and Adolescent Psychiatry, 34,* 307–311.

American Academy of Child and Adolescent Psychiatry. (1997). AACAP Official Action: Practice parameter for the assessment and treatment of Anxiety Disorders. *Journal of the American Academy of Child and Adolescent Psychiatry, 36*(10, Suppl.), 69–84.

American Psychiatric Association. (1987). *Diagnostic and statistical manual of mental disorders* (3rd ed., revised). Washington, DC: Author.

American Psychiatric Association. (1994). *Diagnostic and statistical manual of mental disorders* (4th ed.). Washington, DC: Author.

Anderson, J. C., Williams, S., McGee, R., & Silva, P. A. (1987). *DSM III* Disorders in preadolescent children: Prevalence in a large sample from the general population. *Archives General Psychiatry, 44,* 69–76.

Ayd, F. J. (1995). *Lexicon of psychiatry, neurology and neurosciences.* Baltimore: Williams & Wilkins.

Ballenger, J. C., Carey, D. J., & Steele, J. J. (1989). Three cases of panic disorder with agoraphobia in children. *American Journal of Psychiatry, 146,* 922–925.

Barlow, D. H. (1988). *Anxiety and its disorders: The nature and treatment of anxiety and panic.* New York: Guilford Press.

Barlow, D. H., Craske, M. D., Cerny, J. A., & Klosko, J. S. (1989). Behavioral treatment of panic disorder. *Behavior Therapy, 20,* 261–282.

Barrett, P. M., Dadds, M. R., & Rapee, R. M. (1996). Family treatment of childhood anxiety: A controlled trial. *Journal of Consulting Clinical Psychology, 64,* 333–342.

Bernstein, G. A., Garfinkel, B. D., & Borchardt, C. M. (1990). Comparative studies of pharmacotherapy for school refusal. *Journal of the American Academy of Child and Adolescent Psychiatry, 29,* 773–781.

Bernstein, G. A., & Borchardt, C. M. (1981). Anxiety disorders of childhood and adolescence: A critical review. *Journal of the American Academy of Child and Adolescent Psychiatry, 30,* 519–532.

Bernstein, G. A., Borchardt, C. M., & Perwien, B. A. (1986). Anxiety disorders in children and adolescents: A review of the past 10 years. *Journal of the American Academy of Child and Adolescent Psychiatry, 35,* 1110–1119.

Biederman, J. (1987). Clonazepam in the treatment of prepubertal children with panic-like symptoms. *Journal of Clinical Psychiatry, 48*(10, Suppl.), 38–41.

Biederman, J., Faraone, S. V., Keenan, K., Steingard, R., & Tsuang, M. T. (1991). Familial association between attention deficit disorder and anxiety disorders. *Journal of American Psychiatry, 148,* 251–256.

Biederman, J., Rosenbaum, J. F., & Bolduc-Murphy, E. A. (1993). A 3-year follow-up of children with and without behavioral inhibition. *Journal of the American Academy of Child and Adolescent Psychiatry, 32,* 814–821.

Biederman, J. (1990). The diagnosis and treatment of adolescent anxiety disorders. *Journal of Clinical Psychiatry, 51* (Suppl.), 20–26.

Biederman, J., Rosenbaum, J. F., Hirshfeld, D. R., Faraone, S. V., Bolduc, E. A., Gersten, M., Meninger, S. R., Kagan, J., Snidman, N., & Reznick, J. S. (1990). Psychiatric correlates of behavioral inhibition in young children of parents with and without psychiatric disorders. *Archives of General Psychiatry, 47,* 21–26.

Bird, H. R., Canino, G., & Rubio-Stipec, M. (1988). Estimates of prevalence of childhood adjustment in a community survey in Puerto Rico. *Archives of General Psychiatry, 45,* 1120–1126.

Black, B., & Robbins, D. R. (1996). Panic disorder in children and adolescents. *Journal of the American Academy of Child and Adolescent Psychiatry, 29,* 36–44.

Bowen, R. C., Offord, D. R., & Boyle, M. H. (1997). The prevalence of overanxious disorder and separation anxiety disorder: Results from the Ontario child health study. *Journal of the American Academy of Child and Adolescent Psychiatry, 29,* 753–758.

Bowlby, J. (1969). *Attachment and loss.* New York: Basic Books.

Cantwell, D. P., & Baker, L. (1989). Stability and natural history of DSM-III childhood diagnoses. *Journal of the American Academy of Child and Adolescent Psychiatry, 28,* 691–700.

Carey, W. B., Fox, M., & McDevitt, S. C. (1977). Temperament as a factor in early school adjustment. *Pediatrics, 60,* 621–624.

Caspi, A., Elder, G. M., & Bern, D. L. (1988). Moving away from the world: Life-course patterns of shy children. *Developmental Psychology, 24,* 824–831.

Caspi, A., Henry, B., McGee, R. O., Moffitt, T. E., & Silva, P. A. (1995). Temperamental origins of child and adolescent behavior: From age three to age fifteen. *Child Development, 66,* 55–68.

Castellanos, D., & Hunter, T. (1999). Anxiety disorders in children and adolescents. *Southern Medical Journal, 92,* 946–954.

Chess, S., Thomas, A., Birch, H. G., & Hertzig, M. (1960). Implications of a longitural study of child development for child psychiatry. *American Journal of Psychiatry, 117,* 434–441.

Chess, S., & Thomas, A. (1984). *Origins and evolution of behavior disorders: From infancy to early adult life.* New York: Brunner/Mazel.

Chess, S., & Thomas, A. (1977). Temperamental individuality from childhood to adolescence. *Child and Adolescent Psychiatry, 16,* 218–226.

Cohen, J. A. (1988). Practice parameters for the assessment and treatment of children and adolescents with posttraumatic stress disorder. *Journal of the American Academy of Child and Adolescent Psychiatry, 37*(Suppl.), 4S–26S.

Costello, E. J. (1989). Child psychiatric disorders and their correlates: A primary care pediatric sample. *Journal of the American Academy of Child and Adolescent Psychiatry, 28,* 851–855.

Costello, E. J., Angold, A., & Burns, B. J. (1996). The great smoky mountains study of youth. *Archives of General Psychiatry, 53,* 1129–1136.

Costello, E. J. (1989). Child psychiatric disorders and their correlates: A primary care pediatric sample. *Journal of the American Academy of Child and Adolescent Psychiatry, 28,* 851–855.

Craske, M. G. (1997). Fear and anxiety in children and adolescents. *Bulletin of the Meninger Clinic, 61*(2), 11–14.

D'Amato, G. (1962). Chlordiazepoxide in management of school phobia. *Diseases of the Nervous System, 23,* 292–295.

DeVaugh-Geiss, J., Moroz, G., & Biederman, J. (1992). Clomipramine hydrochloride in childhood and adolescent obsessive-compulsive disorder: A multicenter trial. *Journal of the American Academy of Child and Adolescent Psychiatry, 31,* 45–49.

Eisenck, H. J. (1967). *The biological basis of personality.* Springfield, IL: Thomas.

Eisenck, H. J. (1987). The role of heredity, environment, and preparedness in the genesis of neurosis. In H. J. Eisenck & I. Martin (Eds.), *Theoretical foundations of behavior therapy,* (pp. 379–402). New York: Plenum Press.

Francis, G., Last, C. G., & Strauss, C. C. (1987). Expression of separation anxiety disorder: The roles of age and gender. *Child Psychiatry Human Development, 18,* 82–89.

Freud, S. (1926). *Inhibitions symptoms and anxiety* (Vol. 10). London: Hogarth Press.

Freud, S. (1909). *The Case of "Little Hans" and the "Rat Man"* (Vol. 10). London: Hogarth Press.

Frick, P. J., Silverthorn, P., & Evans, C. (1994). Assessment of childhood anxiety using structured interviews: Patterns of agreements among informants and association with maternal anxiety. *Psychological Assessment, 6,* 372–379.

Gray, J. A. (1982). The neuropsychology of anxiety: A inquiry into the functions of the septo-hippocampal system. New York: Oxford University Press.

Hamilton, J. (1959). The assessment of anxiety states by rating. *British Journal of Medical Psychology, 32,* 50–55.

Insel, T. R. (1992). Toward a neuroanatomy of obsessive-compulsive disorder. *Archives of General Psychiatry, 49,* 739–744.

Jung, C. J. (1924). *Psychological types.* New York: Harcourt-Brace.

Kagan, J., Reznick, J. S., & Snidman, N. (1988). Biological basis of childhood shyness. *Science, 240,* 167–171.

Kagan, J., Reznick, J. S., & Snidman, N. et al. (1989). Childhood derivatives of inhibition and lack of inhibition to the unfamiliar. *Child Development, 59,* 1580–1589.

Kagan, J. (1989). Temperamental contributions to social behavior. *American Psychologist, 44,* 668–674.

Kagan, J., Reznick, J. S., & Snidman, N. (1987). The physiology and psychology of behavioral inhibitions in children. *Child Development, 58,* 1459–1473.

Kashani, J. H., & Orvaschel, H. (1988). Anxiety disorders in mid-adolescence: A community sample. *American Journal of Psychiatry, 145,* 960–964.

Kashani, J. H., & Orvaschel, H. (1990). A community study of anxiety in children and adolescents. *American Journal of Psychiatry, 147,* 313–318.

Keller, M. B., Lavori, P. W., & Wunder, J. (1992). Chronic course of anxiety disorders in children and adolescents. *Journal of the American Academy of Child and Adolescent Psychiatry, 31,* 595–599.

Kendall, P. C. (1994). Treating anxiety disorders in children: Results of a randomized clinical trial. *Journal of Consulting Clinical Psychology, 62,* 100–110.

Khrohne, H. W., & Hock, M. (1991). Relationships between restrictive mother-child interactions and anxiety disorder in the child. *Anxiety Research, 4,* 109–124.

Kiessling, L. S., Marcotte, A. C., & Culpepper, L. (1994). Antineuronal antibodies: Tics and obsessive-compulsive symptoms. *Journal of Developmental Behavioral Pediatrics, 15,* 421–425.

Klein, D. F. (1981). Anxiety reconceptualized. In J. Rabkin & D. F. Klein (Eds.), *Anxiety: New research and changing concepts* (pp. 235–263). New York: Raven Press.

Kraft, I. A., Ardali, C., & Duffy, J. H. (1965). A clinical study of chlordiazepoxide used in psychiatric disorders in children. *International Journal of Neuropsychiatry, 1,* 433–437.

Kutcher, S. P., & MacKenzie, S. (1988). Successful clonazepam treatment of adolescents with panic disorder. *Journal of Clinical Psychopharmacology, 8,* 299–301.

Last, C. G., Perrin, S., Hersen, M., & Kazdin, A. E. (1992). *DSM-III-*R anxiety disorders in children: Sociodemographic and clinical characteristics. *Journal of the American Academy of Child and Adolescent Psychiatry, 31,* 1070–1076.

Last, C. G., Perrin, S., & Hersen, M. (1996). A prospective study of childhood anxiety disorders. *Journal of the American Academy of Child and Adolescent Psychiatry, 35,* 1502–1510.

Last, C. G., Hansen, C., & Franco, N. (1997). Anxious children in adulthood: A prospective study of adjustment. *Journal of the American Academy of Child and Adolescent Psychiatry, 36,* 645–652.

Last, C. G., Hansen, C., & Franco, N. (1998). Cognitive-behavioral treatment of school phobia. *Journal of the American Academy of Child and Adolescent Psychiatry, 37,* 404–411.

Last, C. G., Hersen, M., Kazdin, A. E., Finkelstein, R., & Strauss, C. (1987). Comparison of DSM-III. Separation Anxiety Disorder and Overanxious Disorders: Demographic characteristics and patterns or comorbidity. *Journal of the American Academy of Child and Adolescent Psychiatry, 26,* 527–531.

Leonard, H. L., Swedo, S. E., & Lenane, M. C. (1991). A double blind desipramine substitution during long-term clomipramine treatment in children and adolescents with obsessive compulsive disorder. *Archives of General Psychiatry, 48,* 922–927.

Livingston, R. (1996). Anxiety disorders. In M. Lewis (Ed.), *Child and adolescent psychiatry: A comprehensive textbook,* 2nd ed. (pp. 674–684). Baltimore: Williams & Wilkins.

March, J. S., Amaya-Jackson, L., & Pynoos, R. S. (1997). Pediatric posttraumatic stress disorder. In J. Weiner (Ed.), *Textbook of child and adolescent psychiatry* (pp. 507–527). Washington, DC: American Psychiatric Press.

Martin, M., Horder, P., & Jones, G. V. (1992). Integral bias in naming phobia-related words. *Cognition and Emotion, 6,* 479–486.

Martini, D. R. (1995). Common anxiety disorders in children and adolescents. *Current Problems in Pediatrics, 25,* 271–280.

McGee, R., Feehan, M., & Williams, S. (1990). *DSM-III* disorders in a large sample of adolescents. *Journal of the American Academy of Child and Adolescent Psychiatry, 29,* 611–619.

Muris, P., Meesters, C., & Merkelbach, H. (1998). Worry in normal children. *Journal of the American Academy of Child and Adolescent Psychiatry, 37,* 703–710.

Ollendick, T. H., & King, N. J. (1998). Empirically supported treatments for children with phobic and anxiety disorders: Current status. *Journal of Clinical Child Psychology, 27,* 156–167.

Ollendick, T. H., Mattis, G., & King, N. J. (1994). Panic in children and adolescents. *Journal of Child Psychology and Psychiatry, 35,* 113–134.

Pine, D. S., Cohen, P., & Gurley, D. (1998). The risk for early-adulthood anxiety and depressive disorders in adolescents with anxiety and depressive disorders. *Archives of General Psychiatry, 55,* 56–64.

Quay, H. C. (1993). The psychobiology of undersocialized aggressive conduct disorders: A theoretical perspective. *Development and Psychopathology, 5,* 165–180.

Reznick, J. S., Kagan, J., & Snidman, N. (1986). Inhibited and uninhibited children: A follow-up study. *Child Development, 51,* 660–680.

Riddle, M. A., Nelson, J. C., & Kleinman, C. S. (1991). Sudden death in children receiving Norpramine: A review of three reported cases and commentary. *Journal of the American Academy of Child and Adolescent Psychiatry, 30,* 104–108.

Riddle, M. A., Schahill, L., & King, R. A. (1992). Double-blind, crossover of fluoxetine and placebo in children and adolescents with obsessive-compulsive disorder. *Journal of the American Academy of Child and Adolescent Psychiatry, 31,* 1062–1069.

Rosenbaum, J. F., Biederman, J., Gersten, M., Hirshfeld, D. R., Meninger, S. R., Herman, J. B., Kagan, J., Reznick, J. S., & Snidman, N. (1988). Behavioral inhibition in children of parents with panic disorder and agoraphobia. *Archives of General Psychiatry, 45,* 463–470.

Scheeringa, M. S., Zeanah, C. H., Drell, M. J., & Larrieu, J. A. (1995). Two approaches to diagnosing posttraumatic stress disorder in infancy and early childhood. *Journal of the American Academy of Child and Adolescent Psychiatry, 34,* 191–200.

Shaffer, D., Fisher, P., & Dulcan, M. (1996). The NIMH diagnostic interview schedule for children version 2.3 (DISC-2.3): Description, acceptability, prevalence rates and performance in the MECA study. *Journal of the American Academy of Child and Adolescent Psychiatry, 35,* 865–877.

Shapiro, T., & Hertzig, M. E. (1988). Normal growth and development. In J. Talbott, R. E. Haleo, & S. Yudofsky (Eds.), *Textbook of psychiatry* (pp. 91–121). Washington, DC: American Psychiatric Press.

Simeon, J. G., Ferguson, H. B., & Knott, V. (1992). Clinical, cognitive and neuropsychological effects of alprazolam in children and adolescents with overanxious and avoidant disorders. *Journal of the American Academy of Child and Adolescent Psychiatry, 31,* 29–33.

Simonoff, E., Pickles, A., & Meyer, J. M. (1997). The Virginia twin study of adolescent behavioral development. *Archives of General Psychiatry, 54,* 801–808.

Siqueland, L., Kendall, P. C., & Steinberg, L. (1966). Anxiety in children: Perceived family environments and observed family interaction. *Journal of Consulting and Clinical Psychology, 25,* 225–237.

Selzak, J. A., Persky, V. W., & Kviz, F. J. (1998). Asthma prevalence and risk factors in selected Head Start sites in Chicago. *Journal of Asthma, 35,* 203–212.

Spitz, R. (1965). *The first year of life: A psychoanalytic study of normal and deviant development of object relationships.* Connecticut: International University Press.

Strauss, C. C., & Last, C. G. (1993). Social and Simple Phobias in Children. *Journal of Anxiety Disorders, 7,* 141–152.

Strauss, C. C., Last, C. G., Hersen, M., & Kadin, A. E. (1988). Association between anxiety and depression in children and adolescents with anxiety disorders. *Journal of Abnormal Child Psychology, 16,* 57–68.

Suomi, S. J., Kraemer, G. W., Baysinger, C. M., & DeLizio, R. D. (1981). Inherited and experimental factors associated with individual differences in anxious behavior displayed by Rhesus monkeys. In D. F. Klein & J. Rabkin (Eds.), *Anxiety: Research and changing concepts* (pp. 179–200). New York: Raven.

Swedo, S. E., Leonard, H. L., & Kiessling, L. S. (1994). Speculations on antineuronal antibody mediated neuropsychiatric disorders of childhood. *Pediatrics, 93,* 323–326.

Tucker, D. M., Leckman, J. F., & Scahill, L. (1996). A putative poststreptococcal case of OCD with chronic tic disorder, not otherwise specified. *Journal of the American Academy of Child and Adolescent Psychiatry, 35,* 1684–1691.

Turner, S. M., Beidel, D. C., & Costello, A. (1987). Psychopathology in the offspring of anxiety disorders patients. *Journal of Consulting and Clinical Psychology and Psychiatry, 36,* 439–447.

Turner, S. M., Beidel, D. C., & Wolff, P. L. (1996). Is behavioral inhibition related to anxiety disorders? *Clinical Psychology Review, 16,* 157–172.

Varley, C. K., & McClellan, J. (1997). Case study: Two additional sudden deaths with tricyclic antidepressants. *Journal of the American Academy of Child and Adolescent Psychiatry, 36,* 390–394.

Verhulst, F. C., & Versluis-den Bieman, H. (1995). Developmental course of problem behaviors in adolescent adoptees. *Journal of the American Academy of Child and Adolescent Psychiatry, 34,* 151–159.

Werry, J. S. (1991). Overanxious Disorder: A review of its taxonomic properties. *Journal of the American Academy of Child and Adolescent Psychiatry, 30,* 533–544.

Yunginger, J. W. (1994). Immunologic Diseases. In R. E. Behrman & R. M. Keligman (Eds.), *Nelson essentials of pediatrics,* 2nd ed. (p. 263). Philadelphia: Saunders.

Chapter 16

CHILDHOOD MOOD DISORDERS: HISTORY, CHARACTERISTICS, DIAGNOSIS, AND TREATMENT

DAVID A. SABATINO, BONNIE G. WEBSTER, AND H. BOONEY VANCE

In 1990, 11 million people in the United States reportedly suffered from major depression. Seven to fourteen percent of those were children experiencing at least one episode of major depression before the age of 15 (Brandenburg, Friedman, & Silver, 1989). The incidence of clinically significant depression in children has been estimated from 1% to 5% of the general population. Twenty to thirty percent of adult bipolar patients report experiencing their first depressive episode before the age of 20 (Robins & Regier, 1991). Out of 100,000 adolescents, 2 to 3 thousand will have mood disorders, from which 8 to 10 will commit suicide (National Center for Health Statistics, 1992). Twenty percent of the adolescents in the general population suffer from a mental disorder, and one third of those adolescents are diagnosed with depression (Clarke, Lewinsohn, & Hops, 1990). The World Health Organization reports that depression will be the leading cause of disability and death by the year 2020 (Knitzer, 1993).

INTRODUCTION

Depression in children is a major cause of an overwhelming sense of failure in relationships, in social and academic aspects of school, and in most aspects of developing responsibility for self and others (Hoagwood & Rupp, 1995). It occurs as both a primary (familial-genetic disorder) and secondary (symptomatic depression) relation to social and physical stressors such as the threat of school failure or loss, such as fear of abandonment in the primary social care system (family). Depression is feeling sad, lonely, unloved, dumb, and worthless, along with feelings of guilt, shame and being overwhelmed.

The symptoms of depression are evident in difficulty falling to sleep (initial insomnia), restless sleep with recurrent awakening (interval insomnia), or early morning waking with an inability to fall back to sleep (terminal insomnia). Depression manifests as feelings of anxiousness, fatigue, anger, limited attachments (i.e., friendships), unusual and overwhelming fears, loss of interest, poor concentration, limited memory, and inat-

The authors greatfully acknowledge the editorial comments of Christine A. Oetjen, MSW.

tentiveness. Clinically these symptoms must persist for 3 weeks or longer and cause significant behavioral change (usually observable) in school, home, and play.

Childhood is considered a period of security, happiness, and growing up amidst pleasant surroundings filled with the dreams of tomorrow. For many of us it is somewhat difficult to imagine that children do experience prolonged hopelessness, despair, or despondency, caused by the loss or death of family member or friend, human or animal, or by betrayal or abandonment in family systems. Thirty years ago the mental health community believed that prepubertal children did not experience depression (Pfeiffer & Strzelecki, 1990). It was thought that although adolescents may experience episodic aspects of depression due to overwhelming problems in their life, those emotions would quickly fade away.

Until the 1970s it was the belief of the mental health community that although children experienced sadness, even severe unhappiness, they did not fall into a "psychopathological state." It was not until 1972 that Cytryn and McKnew (1996) first proposed a diagnostic classification of childhood depression. The full extent of such a diagnosis in childhood is outlined by Harrington, Fudge, Rutter, Pickles, and Hill (1990), who reported that children experiencing depression have a higher risk for psychiatric problems, including depression, in their adult life. Depressive disorders in children do carry over into adulthood. Weissman, Leaf, and Tischler (1988) have confirmed that a high prevalence of anxiety and depressive disorders exists in the general population and has symptoms traceable into childhood. Childhood depression shows up as both a cause and a response to school failure, conduct disorders, attention-deficit/hyperactivity disorders, delinquency, anorexia and bulimia, school phobia, and panic disorders. It is often related to the antecedents associated with childhood and adolescent suicidal ideation.

Although far less is known about childhood depression than adult depression, there is growing recent literature (Sondheimer, Schoenwald, & Rowland, 1994) that childhood depression differs from that of teenagers, and both childhood and adolescent depression is different from that of adults. Children are assumed to respond more readily to short-term critical (acute) stressors and are at risk for depressive responses to longer-term chronic behaviors such as attentional problems, learning disorders, and conduct disorders. Children are more prone to display agitation when depressed and are thought to have shorter cycles, especially in adolescence. Kovacs (1996) reported that childhood depression manifests a number of unique aspects, such as social withdrawal in the primary social group, aggressiveness and assaultativeness, conduct problems, and school refusal. Behavioral characteristics vary widely from child to child but often include at least one of the following: persistent sadness, an inability to enjoy favorite activities, increased irritability, frequent complaints of physical illnesses, frequent absences from school or poor performance in school, persistent complaints of boredom, low energy, poor concentration, observable changes in eating or sleeping patterns, overwhelming feelings of worthlessness, hopelessness, and exhaustion. Weinberg, Rutman, Sullivan, Penick, and Dietz (1973) stated that the symptoms must differ from the child's usual behavior, and these symptoms must continue for a least one month. The Weinberg criteria for depression in young people (Reynolds & Johnston, 1994) were first published in 1973 and isolated 10 major symptoms associated with this mental disorder. These 10 criteria are generally regarded as diagnostic descriptors of childhood depression:

1. Dysphoric mood
2. Self-deprecatory ideation
3. Agitation
4. Sleep disturbance
5. Changes in school performance
6. Diminished socialization
7. Change in attitude toward school
8. Somatic complaints
9. Unusual loss of energy
10. Unusual change in appetite or weight

The child must present with both (a) dysphoric moods and affect and (b) self-deprecatory ideation and any four of the remaining eight symptoms displayed above.

Practically any factor that threatens the security of the child's relationship in the family or to his or her care providers can be related to the onset of depression. Some of these factors include the following:

- Parental rejection
- Family or school depreciation
- A depressed parent
- A loss of a parent or close family member
- Emotional, physical, or sexual abuse
- Abandonment
- Parental or family betrayal
- Circumstances triggering psychological threat to nurturance
- Inability to meet ones performance expectations or those of others in obtaining approval from a valued source
- Separation from a loved person or place
- Loss of strong attachment

HISTORICAL PERSPECTIVE

Historically, depression in adults is reported in the Old Testament of the Bible and by Hippocrates and Galen in ancient Greek and Roman times. Depression has and continues to affect highly successful persons in the world order: prime ministers, presidents, statesman, scientists, scholars, poets, and artists. No ethnic, religious, or cultural group is free of depression; however, it does appear more prevalent in some societies than in others.

The initial scientific description of depression and manic depressive disease for adults was first offered by Emil Kraepelin in the early 1900s. It was not until the 1940s and 1950s that research was produced on conditions related to childhood depression. Spitz and Wolf (1946) described the mixed emotions of forced dependency and isolation observed in "anaclitic depression."

Bowlby (1969) described the sequence of protest, despair, and detachment following cutting children off emotionally from the caregivers and isolating them into a world of sterile whiteness during hospitalization. It is apparent in children that the flow of emotional comfort and support known as nurturance is an absolute necessity to the maintenance of normal regulatory mood. The connection between being aware of mood status apparently limits the range of mood swings in adults and children. The term *mood* is used to describe the child's emotional feeling status. The term *affect* is used to describe the child's appearance in relation to his or her mood.

There are five major schools of thought on childhood depressive disorders. The oldest emulated the psychoanalytic theorists and held that children were incapable of producing a state of depression because of immature personality structure incapable of a defensive response, producing what was then termed an *affective disorder.* This view dominated the field of childhood psychopathology until the mid 1960s and created the conditions for ignoring childhood depression clinically and empirically.

By the 1960s a different view (Glasser, 1968) was advanced: Depression in childhood is masked and is expressed in the form of other behaviors. The data that supported this position were based on the observation that childhood depression appears in the form of conduct disorders, behavioral disorders, somatic complaints, delinquency, and acting out aggressiveness, or sharp social and personal withdrawal. It is now believed that what was held to be a masking of depression was more likely comorbid mental disorders, and that depression and other comorbid mental disorders often have common antecedents and etiologies. The concept of masked depression has very limited use.

Both the next two schools of thought on childhood depression accept the existence of childhood depression as a clinical phenomenon. By the early 1980s the prevailing belief was that childhood depression was much like adult depression but with some additional features. Just like its adult counterpart, childhood depression includes such symptoms as sadness, fatigue, low self-esteem, loss of purpose and pleasure seeking, hopelessness, helplessness, and loss of control. Childhood depression manifests a number of unique aspects, such as social withdrawal, aggressiveness, assaultiveness, conduct problems, and school refusal. The fourth school of thought on childhood depression is that childhood and adult depression are mirror images of each other with the one exception being the developmental aspect of childhood and how it affects and is in turn affected by the symptoms of depression. Hence, in a span of 30 years the field had gone from denying the existence of depression in children to disagreeing over which clinical features are shared between children and adults.

The fifth clinical view of childhood depression, and a more research-oriented one, represents a cognitive-developmental position. The position taken is that it is unrealistic to expect behavioral isomorphism in observed symptoms of depression across the life span. In fact, children of various ages may produce variations in their behavioral responses to depression that will require classification and diagnostic consideration and recognition at each age level (McMahon, 1994). A three-year-old does not manifest the same symptoms of depression as does a 15-year-old. The developmental differences in cognition, linguistics, socioemotional capacities, and affective development will demonstrate chronological age and developmental variances in symptoms of depression, both in how they are displayed and in the impact they have on self and others.

In adults the percentage of persons in the general population with major depressive disorders are 8.7% for women and 3.6% for men (Robins & Regier, 1991). It is estimated that major childhood depression affects hundreds of thousands of children, or about 1.7% of the U.S. population. However, depression in children most often presents as a Dysthymic Disorder. This lower-grade, clingy depressiveness producing fatigue and feelings of hopelessness and helplessness has often been considered a minor form of depression, and it affects about 3.6% of the childhood population.

FACTORS AND CHANGES WITHIN CHILDHOOD DEPRESSION

In the *Diagnostic and Statistical Manual of Mental Disorders–Third Edition–Revised* (*DSM-III-R;* American Psychiatric Association, 1987), depression was considered an affective disorder. In the *DSM-IV* (APA, 1994), depression is classified as a mood disorder. Research continues into the multiple and varied genetic and psychosocial causes of childhood depression, and many scholars propose a strong family-genetic relationship (Rohde, Lewinsohn, & Seeley, 1994). In twins born to bipolar mothers and then reared apart, the prevalence of depression is greater than chance. In many case studies there is often evidence of genetically based affective disorders that could remain either active or dormant throughout the life span depending upon the presence of environmental, task, or relationship stressors. Episodes of Major Depressive Disorder often follow a severe psychosocial stressor, such as the death or divorce. Research (Lewinsohn, Clarke, & Rohde, 1994) findings suggest that psychosocial stressors are more significant factors in first or second episodes of Major Depressive Disorder than in subsequent episodes. Chronic general medical conditions and Substance Dependence (particularly Alcohol or Cocaine Dependence) may also contribute to the onset or exacerbation of Major Depressive Disorder (APA, 1994).

It should be noted that the literature (Kovacs, Akiskal, Gatsonis, & Parrone, 1994) is in agreement that most family problems do not produce recurrent chronic depression, but rather dysthymic disorders (Rutter, 1990). The two parental factors that have received the most attention are (a) interference of the disorder with the ability to parent and (b) the presence of severe marital discord and divorce (Wallerstein, 1991). It should also be noted that children with unipolar depression often develop bipolar disorders later in life (Geller, Fox, & Clark, 1994). Only rarely do young children display bipolar disorders.

Age is an important variable of risk to depression in children. Infants, toddlers, and preschool children of affectively ill parents rarely develop depression and usually do so only under the most adverse circumstances. The risk increases with age; the rate of depression in the offspring of a parent with mood disorder reaches as high as 30% by the end of adolescence (Downey & Coyne, 1990).

It is difficult to predict whether the first episode of a Major Depressive Disorder in a child will ultimately evolve into a more severe pattern of depression. Some data suggest that the acute onset of severe depression, especially with psychotic features and psychomotor retardation, in a young person without prepubertal psychopathology is more likely to predict a bipolar course. A family history of Bipolar Disorder may also be suggestive of subsequent development of Bipolar Disorder. Major Depressive Disorder is 1.5 to 3 times more common among first-degree biological relatives of persons with this disorder than among the general population. There is evidence for an increased risk of Alcohol Dependence in adult first-degree biological relatives, and there may be an increased incidence of Attention-Deficit/Hyperactivity Disorder in the children of adults with this disorder (APA, 1994).

As early as 1951, studies reporting problem school behavior showed that unless the child acts out aggressively in school and is socially withdrawn, he or she rarely comes to the attention of teachers. Their poor self-image and deep-seated conflict over handling of hostile and angry feelings tend to make children with moods disorders shy, quiet, and reserved. It is not uncommon for teachers and even parents to describe them as uncomplaining, helpful to others, thoughtful, and hard working. All the while they feel that their worlds are coming apart, and they cannot control their sadness and discomfort (Weinberg et al., 1973).

Another behavioral aspect of childhood depression that should be watched is a pattern of fatigue and loss of interest in things that at one time were considered very important. Both of these symptoms frequently accompany dysthymia and depression. Other critical behaviors are changes in sleep patterns and eating habits, loss of interest in favorite foods, the appearance or sadness of expression, immobility, and inconsolable crying. In adolescents, self-deprecating statements, negativistic or frankly antisocial behaviors, restlessness, grouchiness, and aggressiveness are common, as are sulkiness, a reluctance to cooperate in family, school, and community ventures, and withdrawal from social activities. Another very common behavior associated with depression in adolescence is inattention to personal appearance and increased emotional lability, with heightened sensitivity to feelings of rejection, the absence of peer acceptance and feelings of peer and even parental rejection, worthlessness, and an ominous fear of failure and loss.

One common early sign of depression in preadolescents and adolescents is school truancy, absenteeism, and tardiness. School problems in general can be expected in both academic and social areas, but tardiness and absenteeism are indicators of academic and social withdrawal.

ACUTE, CHRONIC, AND MASKED CHILDHOOD DEPRESSION

Cytryn and McKnew (1996) classified childhood depression as acute, chronic, and masked. Acute and chronic depression have similar features. The difference between chronic (recurrent) and acute (episodic) depression occurs in the child's adjustment before illness, the length of illness, and the family history. Children with recurrent depression usually have no immediate cause; the onset is sudden; and the depression has a short duration. They frequently do not have a family history of depressive illness, particularly in the mother. The overpowering feelings of inadequacy and ineptness frequently promote the consideration of other options: self destructiveness, suicide, social withdrawal from loved ones.

Masked depression results from psychological threat, such as academic noncompetitiveness, peer or parent rejection, absence of approval (peer, parent, or teacher), unpleasant or abusive conditions in the home, emotional abandonment, emotional neglect, physical abuse or threat, and sexual abuse or threat. Masked depression is often comorbid with other mental disorders, such as conduct disorders, anxiety disorders, disruptive behavioral disorders—that is, with disruptive school behavior and delinquency.

DEGREES OF DEPRESSIVENESS

Depression occurs in degrees of severity or amount of depressiveness. All depression does not produce the same limitations and incapacitations. Some persons are more depressed than others, and some depressive cycles are worse than others in the same person. The *DSM-IV* (APA, 1994) lists the degrees of depressiveness as mild, moderate, and severe.

Mild depression results in only minor disturbances in school functioning or in usual activities and relationships with family and friends. It is sometimes difficult to realize that children with mild depression is experiencing depressiveness at all. They seldom appear different from others and seem to blend in and manage their daily activities well unless the clinician looks deeper, or unless they are stressed. They do not tolerate stressors or anxiety well and seem to have a very narrow tolerance band.

Moderate impairment, on the other hand, does show up in facial expressions, mannerisms, social interactiveness, and alertness. Children with moderate depression appear to be have difficulty tolerating even the most minimal stressors, and their behavior suggests that they are ready to withdraw at any time from the requirements that a task, environment, or relationship may place upon them. Children in moderate depression may be tearful for little or no reason, and they may withdraw and appear isolated from interaction even when nothing in the interpersonal relationship or immediate environment appears to be threatening.

Severe depression presents with marked symptoms and interferes in all usual activities, such as social, school, and interpersonal relationships.

DEPRESSION, AFFECT, AND MOOD

When affective disorder is (or was) used as a synonym for depression or mood disorders, it is used to cover anxiety disorders as well, including separation anxiety, agoraphobia, avoidant disorder, and overanxious disorder. In most children, the term affective disorder is highly justified because it denotes all those factors (anxiety and depression) that interfere with attachment, beauty, and joy of relationships and life. There is a strong link between anxiety and depressive disorders in childhood. It is possible that precursors of anxiety disorders may be manifest in the temperament of some children (Weisman et al., Tischler, 1988). Kagan (1984) offered support for the classic studies on temperament by Chess and Thomas (1977), which established that 10% to 15% of children "appear predisposed to be irritable as infants, shy, or fearful as toddlers, and cautious and introverted when they reach school age" (p. 29) Kagan's observation certainly has been upheld by previous beliefs on childhood temperament, which reported that 15% of young children have difficulty with human interaction and relationships and do feel cut off, isolated, and alone. There is an impressive stability over time of temperament characteristics from childhood to adulthood.

Most adult mood disorders follow a chronic and intermittent course, despite continuing improvements in psychotherapeutic and psychopharmacologic treatment interventions. It is now clear that many adults with depressive or anxiety disorders report histories that suggest depressiveness and anxiety disorder as early as the preschool years. During the intake procedure, adults with depressive and anxiety disorders report a significantly higher incidence of mood-related problems than does the same age group in the general population (Weissman, Leckman, Merikangas, Jammon, & Prusoff, 1984).

CHILDHOOD SUICIDE AND DEPRESSION

The adolescent suicide rate has increased more than 200% over the last decade and is now responsible for more deaths in youths aged 15 to 19 than is cardiovascular disease or cancer (Frank & Dewa, 1992). The age-specific suicide rate for children under 14 was 0.5 per 100,000 in 1991 (Andrus et al., 1991). The latest information from the Center for Disease Control and Prevention reports that children aged 10 to 14 are committing suicide twice as often as in 1980, and are increasingly using guns to kill themselves (National Center for Health Statistics, 1992).

This same study reports a high rate of nonfatal suicidal behaviors among children aged 6 to 12. There are feeling and thought differences between suicidal and nonsuicidal children. Suicidal children are preoccupied with thoughts of dying. In the 6 months before the study began, the group containing the suicide children reported that those children in were becoming increasingly more depressed and hopeless. The mothers of suicidal children were more frequently depressed than were the mothers of nonsuicidal children. The belief that death is a pleasant state was related significantly to the degree of seriousness of the child's suicidal behavior. Also, significantly more of the suicidal children worried about doing poorly in school. Pfeffer et al. (1993) studied 133 children aged 6 to 8 who were diagnosed with mood disorders. Forty percent reported suicidal ideation, whereas 36% reported suicidal attempts. In a 6- to 8-year follow-up on these same children, 15% had attempted suicide, and half of those reported multiple attempts.

Kovacs, Goldston, and Gatsonis (1993) followed 60 children aged 8 to 13 who were in outpatient treatment for mood disorders. Sixty-six percent had suicidal ideation, while 9% had made attempts. There were no differences in rates of suicidal thought or attempts between boys and girls. In a 12-year follow-up the rate of suicidal ideation was unchanged, whereas the rate of suicide attempts climbed steadily. As the children entered middle to late adolescence, a much larger proportion of girls than boys had suicidal ideation and had made suicidal attempts. For all of these children, comorbidity of depression with conduct disorders and substance abuse also continued to increase; and the more prevalent these other diagnoses were with depression, the higher the risk was for suicidal attempts. Other predictive suicidal behaviors were:

1. Changes in eating and sleeping habits

2. Withdrawal from friends, family, and social activities

3. Violent actions, rebellious behavior, or running away

4. Drug and alcohol use

5. Unusual neglect of personal appearance

6. Marked personality change

7. Persistent boredom, difficulty concentrating, or a decline in the quality of school-work

8. Loss of interest in pleasurable activities

9. Intolerance for praise or rewards

10. Preoccupation with death and suicide

DEPRESSION AND SUICIDAL THREATS

Patros and Shamoo (1989) concluded from existing literature that approximately 8 to 10 percent of the children admitted for hospitalization are referred for suicidal threat. Cohen-Sandler, Berman, and King (1982) found that about 12,000 children aged 5 to 14 have been admitted annually to psychiatric hospitals for suicidal behaviors. In the past 20 years the rate of suicide has drastically increased. Over 1,300 teenagers per day, or fifty-seven per hour, attempt suicide. Estimates are that nearly 20 adolescents per day succeed with their suicide attempts. There is speculation that suicidal attempts have risen as much as 3,000% a year (Patros & Shamoo, 1989).

Suicidal behavior of children is a complex symptom that is influenced by the interactive effects of environmental, developmental, and intrapsychic factors: (a) Children younger than 10 years of age do not have the concept of the finality of death (Patros and Shamoo, 1989); (b) completed suicide among children is rare (Shaffer, 1974); (c) children do not have the physical prowess to effect a fatal self-injury (Gould, 1965); and (d) there is a lack of standard diagnostic techniques for suicide assessment.

There is confusion about the age at which suicide threats should be taken seriously. Garfinkel, Froese, and Hood (1982) implied that children use suicidal threats to draw attention to their conflicts, and they lack the size, strength, motor coordination, and access to life threatening material to succeed. Turkington's (1983) data reveal that it is not uncommon for children to "attempt suicide without intending to complete it, but than have succeed" (p. 13).

Clinical studies highlight a variety of techniques that children use for their self-destructive acts. Cohen-Sandler et al. (1982) indicated that children over the age of 9 are more likely to take medications, toxic substances (i.e. herbicides and insecticides), rubbing alcohol, and turtle food, whereas younger children are prone to death from falls, jumps, and vehicles.

Suicide is thought to occur across four dimensions (Orbach, Gross, & Glaubman, 1981): (a) the attractiveness and enjoyment of life; (b) the repulsiveness of life, often measured by failure, fear of failure, or overwhelming feelings of inadequacy; (c) the attractiveness of death, which is usually based on cultural and religious beliefs; and

(d) the repulsiveness of death, referring to the degree to which death arouses fear and anxiety (Clarke et al., 1995). Suicidal behavior is rarely a response to a single factor and more often to a combination of factors. Alcohol and drugs are often related to suicidal behaviors. The dependency, fears, isolation, and depression that in part cause suicide will also in part produce alcohol and drug abuse and dependency. These addictions reduce inhibitions, which allows the adolescent to express more easily his or her anger and unhappiness through suicidal behavior. Alcohol and drugs also allow suicidal impulses to be magnified, thus increasing risk (Pfeffer, 1986). Other family system factors that affect adolescent suicide are the loss of stable family roots in a mobile society, role relationship failure and confusion, and loss of family support systems across generational lines (Pfeiffer & Strezelecki, 1990).

DEPRESSION AND LEARNING DISABILITIES/ADHD

Rappley (1999) summarized a 4-year study on preschool-aged children and reported that ADHD exists in about 2% of the general population. Her findings over a 14-month period indicated that some children as young as 1 year old were diagnosed with ADHD and treated with a variety of medications, including Ritalin, Clonidine, and Prozac; in all, 22 different psychotropic medications were used. The use of psychotropic medication between 1991 and 1995 increased 180 percent.

Patros and Shamoo (1989) advanced the clinical hypothesis that some children, after initial school histories of academic success, will develop symptoms similar to those displayed by learning disabled children or children with ADHD. Depression in adults is often manifested in the inability to concentrate, to focus on factual information, and to organize information for retention. These same symptoms, when manifested in school-aged children in the academic environment, would appear to be those of a child with a concentration or attention problem, or a cognitive dysfunction in a short- or long-term component of memory. It is not uncommon for depressed children to lose focus to the degree that they appear hyperkinetic and impulsive and to have limited attentional sets (Friedman, 1990). Of course, all of the behaviors normally associated with a learning disability or ADHD, or a combination of the two, mask depression. The critical diagnostic factor is the onset of the academic problem. Depression in children can have a sudden onset or a gradual build up. There may be records of successful academic performance and periods when ADHD behaviors were not being reported. School records and parental observations are very important in making the diagnosis of depression and ruling out a learning disability or ADHD (Knitzer, Steinberg, & Fleisch, 1990).

Stress is defined as a result of the frustration, conflict, and pressure a child or adolescent feels, and school is often a very real cause of stress. School may be thought of as having two major aspects contributing many pieces to its whole: (a) social and (b) academic. Peer acceptance and recognition and meeting the expectations of teachers and other school officials all generate stressful conditions. Body image, establishing attributional information of self, self-esteem, and self-concept are all psychological constructs that give us hope or further reduce it (Kutash & Rivera, 1995).

Children enter the educational environment to be academically successful. Children want to be successful in basic subjects, and they strive to be competitive. When that success does not follow, their perceptions are altered. School is a very large proportion of a child's life during the growing-up period. It is in this period that adjustment skills are learned and that the child should learn to cope with a full range of academic and social stressors. When children are affectively intact, these social and academic requirements provide an excellent learning opportunity by opening gateways to new adjustment skills that elevate the responsibility for self and others. When children are affectively challenged, these requirements seem overwhelming to them and threaten their control of self in relationship to others, to tasks, and to environments (McMahon, 1994).

DEPRESSION AND AGGRESSIVE ACTING-OUT BEHAVIORS

Historically, depressiveness in children is associated with social isolation, withdrawal, and nonassaultive and compliant behaviors rather than oppositionality or conduct disorders. However, that is not always the case. Children have but two choices when they are challenged by depression. They can withdraw further, seeking a more comfortable world, or they can act out by aggressively expressing their feelings through anger and discomfort. Pfeffer (1986) examined the relationship between suicidal and assaultive behaviors in 100 hospitalized children with conduct disorders and found that one fourth of them were depressed. The aggressive children's behavior was marked with anger, lying, stealing, truancy, and by bad experiences such as parental violence.

Marttunen, Aro, Henriksson, and Lonnqvist (1994) speculated that suicidal behavior and assaultiveness were two independent patterns of behavior produced by different factors. Cytryn and McKnew (1996) disagreed and offered their own research supporting common antecedents in defining the relationship between depression and anger. Many depressed children showed feelings of anger toward their parents. These feelings were more predominant in children from homes where there was no depressive illness. Puig-Antich, Blau, Marx, Breengill, and Chambers (1978) reported that 40% of the children seen with depressive disorders also had conduct disorders. The conclusion reached from research on the comorbidity of depression and conduct disorders concluded that both inward- and outward-directed aggression can occur in the same individual. Of those children who require and receive initial treatment in outpatient facilities, children who were comorbid were more likely to access services (Armbruster and Schwab-Stone, 1994).

PROBLEMS AND PRACTICES IN DIAGNOSIS

Diagnosis of any psychopathology depends on a clear definition of that disorder and the observable or measurable distinctions in the classifications of that disorder. In the absence of a defining process and classification structure, the establishment of reliable and valid diagnostic procedures cannot be achieved. However, three certainties exist: (a) The incidence of children and adolescents with mental disorders is increasing, as is the cost, although little is known about whether the quality of service is increasing as well (National Mental Health Association, 1989); (b) more children are being diagnosed with severe mental disorders, and the assumption is that more severe problems require more extensive treatment efforts, and hence that treatment will be costlier (Cheung & Zinn, 1991); and (c) the amount of available agency monies appears to be less than it was in the past, and most of it goes to residential facilities (Knitzer, Steinberg, & Fleisch, 1990). Mental health services for children cost more than such services for adults. Pecora and Conroyd stated (1982) that the amount of time the agency allows for an intake evaluation should not be based on the adult treatment model, which is inadequate and inappropriate for children.

Weissman and Markowitz (1994), in a study on the increased prevalence of major depression as well as a variety of other psychiatric problems in children of depressed parents, believed that mood disorders in children and adolescents represent one of most under-diagnosed groups of illnesses in psychiatry. This is due to several factors:

1. Children are not always able to express their feelings.
2. The symptoms of mood disorders take on different forms in children and adults.
3. Mood disorders are often accompanied by other psychiatric disorders that can mask depressive symptoms.
4. Many physicians tend to think of depression and bipolar disorders as illnesses in adulthood only.

A child's assessment must include a detailed developmental history of the child, a mental health status exam, separate interviews with the parent and child, and significant collateral contacts, such as public schools, child protective services, and juvenile court services (Rutter, 1986, p. 12). In clinical practice 50 percent more staff time is required to treat a single child than a single adult (Burns, 1994).

The principle issue in the diagnosis of children with depression is the differentiation of the "quantitative variations from normality which represent qualitatively distinct disease entities" (Rutter, 1986, p. 9). What is normal sadness, and what is the psychopathological state of depression? The diagnosis of childhood affective disorders must distinguish between the effects of developmental features on psychopathology and conversely the effects of psychopathology on development. The diagnostic process must therefore evaluate a number of factors:

1. Age-dependant susceptibilities to stress
2. Age-differentiated forms of responses to adversity
3. Age-determined patterns of psychopathology
4. Presence of varied types of psychopathology
5. Presence of comorbid psychopathology
6. Effects of psychopathology on psychosocial development

DSM CRITERIA USED IN DIAGNOSING VARIOUS MOOD DISORDERS

In the following sections, some of the diagnostic criteria used in diagnosing mood disorders have been taken from the *DSM-IV* (APA, 1994). These criteria are provided for selected major depressive disorders, bipolar disorders, dysthymia, and cyclothymia. Although the *DSM-IV* is written for adults and children, clearly more is known about mood disorders in adults. The reader is encouraged to read these materials fully in the original source.

Major Depressive Disorder, Single Episode

Diagnostic criteria for Major Depressive Disorder, Single Episode, include presence of a single Major Depressive Episode that is not better accounted for by other psychotic disorders. There must never have been a Manic Episode, a Mixed Episode, or a Hypomanic Episode. Psychosocial stressors often play a more significant role in first or second episodes and play less of a role in the onset of subsequent episodes. It is difficult to predict whether the first episode of a major depressive disorder in a young person will ultimately evolve into a bipolar disorder. Some data suggest that the acute onset of severe depression—especially with psychotic features and psychomotor retardation—in a child without prepubertal psychopathology is predictive of a bipolarity. A family history of bipolar disorder may also be suggestive of subsequent development of bipolar disorder.

Major Depressive Disorder, Recurrent

A Major Depressive Episode, Recurrent, is characterized by two separate depressive episodes in an interval of at least 2 consecutive months in which criteria are not met for a Single Major Depressive Episode. In addition, there must never have been a Manic Episode, a Mixed Episode, or a Hypomanic Episode, and depressive episodes must not be due to the direct physiological effects of a general medical condition. Major Depressive, Manic, Mixed, and Hypomanic Episodes must be distinguished from episodes of either a Mood Disorder Due to a General Medical Condition or a Substance-Induced Mood Disorder, or a bipolar disorder.

Bipolar I Disorder

Bipolar I Disorder is distinguished from Major Depressive Disorder and Dysthymic Disorder by the lifetime history of at least one Manic or Mixed Episode. When an individual previously diagnosed with Bipolar II Disorder develops a Manic or Mixed Episode, the diagnosis is changed to Bipolar I Disorder. Bipolar I Disorder is distinguished from Cyclothymic Disorder by the presence of one or more Manic or Mixed Episodes. If a Manic or Mixed Episode occurs after the first 2 years of Cyclothymic Disorder, then Cyclothymic Disorder and Bipolar I Disorder may both be diagnosed. If there is a very rapid alternation (over days) between manic symptoms and depressive symptoms (e.g., several days of purely manic symptoms followed by several days of purely depressive symptoms) that do not meet minimal duration criteria for a Manic Episode or Major Depressive Episode, the diagnosis is Bipolar Disorder Not Otherwise Specified.

Bipolar II Disorder

Bipolar II Disorder is distinguished from Bipolar I Disorder by the presence of one or more Manic or Mixed Episodes. Diagnostic criteria tend to be higher for Bipolar II

Disorder than for Major Depressive Disorder, Recurrent. Bipolar II Disorder is distinguished from Major Depressive Disorder and Dysthymic Disorder by the lifetime history of at least one Hypomanic Episode.

When an individual previously diagnosed with Bipolar II Disorder develops a Manic or Mixed Episode, the diagnosis is changed to Bipolar I disorder. Bipolar II Disorder is distinguished from Cyclothymic Disorder by the presence of one or more Major Depressive Episodes. If a Major Depressive Episode occurs after the first 2 years of Cyclothymic Disorder, the additional diagnosis of Bipolar II Disorder is given. Bipolar II Disorder must be distinguished from Psychotic Disorders.

Diagnostic criteria for Bipolar II Disorder are the presence (or history) of one or more Major Depressive Episodes and a history of at least one Hypomanic Episode, a Manic Episode, or a Mixed Episode. The mood symptoms must not be better accounted for by other psychotic disorders. There must be clinically significant distress or impairment in social, occupational, or other important areas of functioning as a result of the mood disturbance. The impairment may develop as a result of prolonged periods of cyclical, often unpredictable, mood changes. The symptoms cause clinically significant distress or impairment in social, occupational, or other important areas of functioning. The interval between episodes tends to decrease as the individual ages.

Approximately 50% of individuals with Bipolar II Disorder have multiple (four or more) mood episodes (Hypomanic or Major Depressive) within a given year. If this pattern is present, it is noted by rapid cycling moods. A rapid cycling mood pattern is associated with a poorer prognosis. Although the majority of individuals with Bipolar II Disorder return to a fully functional level between episodes, approximately 15% continue to display mood liability and interpersonal or occupational difficulties.

Dysthymic Disorder

The essential feature of Dysthymic Disorder is a chronically depressed mood that occurs for most of the day, more days than not, for at least 2 years. Individuals with Dysthymic Disorder describe their mood as sad or "down in the dumps." In children, the mood may be irritable rather than depressed, and the required minimum duration is only 1 year. During periods of depressed mood, at least two of the following additional symptoms are present: poor appetite or overeating, insomnia or hypersomnia, low energy or fatigue, low self-esteem, poor concentration or difficulty making decisions, and feelings of hopelessness. Individuals may note the prominent presence of low interest and self-criticism, often seeing themselves as uninteresting or incapable. The diagnosis of Dysthymic Disorder can be made following Major Depressive Disorder only if the Dysthymic Disorder was established prior to the first Major Depressive Episode.

Cyclothymic Disorder

The essential feature of Cyclothymic Disorder is a chronic, fluctuating mood disturbance involving numerous periods of hypomanic symptoms and numerous periods of depressive symptoms. The hypomanic symptoms are of insufficient number, severity, pervasiveness, or duration to meet full criteria for a Manic Episode; and the depressive symptoms are of insufficient number, severity, pervasiveness, or duration to meet full criteria for a Major Depressive Episode. The diagnosis of Cyclothymic Disorder is made only if the initial 2-year period of cyclothymic symptoms is free of Major Depressive, Manic, and Mixed Episodes. The diagnosis is not made if the pattern of mood swings is better accounted for by psychotic disorder.

Cyclothymic Disorder often begins in adolescence or early adult life and must be differentiated from other Mood Disorders. Borderline Personality Disorder is associated with marked shifts in mood that may suggest Cyclothymic Disorder. If the criteria are met for each disorder, both Borderline Personality Disorder and Cyclothymic Disorder may be diagnosed.

DIAGNOSTIC PROCEDURES

Typically, there are three diagnostic procedures involved in the diagnosis of children with mental disorders. These three procedural aspects attempt to ascertain the child's current psychological status through (a) interview procedures, (b) direct observations, and (c) personality and behavioral descriptive measurement procedures.

The purpose of obtaining the child's history and interview data is to obtain a continuous pattern of the child's development from conception to his current level through the eyes of a number of different observers (e.g., parents, guardians, teachers, case workers). There are structured history forms and interview procedures to assist the clinician with these activities. Using the Weinberg criteria described earlier, the interview process with a primary caretaker must establish that the two primary symptoms of dysphoric moods and self-deprecation are present along with four of eight other symptoms. A symptom is accepted as positive when at least one of the characteristic behaviors listed for that symptom category is present. The criteria symptoms for depression must represent a change from the individual's usual self or a worsening of the usual self, must be present for more than 3 weeks, and must be associated with poor performance and guarded behavior in at least one of three environments: home, school, or play.

Direct observational data is obtained from the child's play, his social interaction with caregivers and treatment providers, and how he responds to developmentally appropriate tasks and strange and familiar environments. Consistency of behavioral interaction is sought; however, adjustment capabilities are also examined as the child interacts with persons, places, and things. Direct observation data is often augmented by oral-vocal dialogue between the clinician and the child to the degree that is possible. Often the data from direct verbal interaction is quite useful even in children of 2 to 3 years of age. More formal measurements using observer and self-report rating scales, subjective personality measures, and objective personality test instruments are also used.

The formal diagnostic instruments most commonly used to determine the risk of depressive behaviors in children are self-reporting instruments. The strengths of these instruments are in the economy of test-taking time, their ease of scoring, their straightforward interpretation, and their simplicity of test administration. Most of the self-report instruments require at least a fourth-grade reading or language comprehension level. The utility of most self report instruments for children under 10 years of age is somewhat limited. To offset that problem and extend the age range down, the self-report format is altered to an observer's descriptive format for use by teachers and parents.

Teachers are often the first group of professionals to suspect that a student has a behavioral or emotional problem. Research (Cannon, Mednick, & Parnas, 1990) has indicated that teachers are often accurate predictors of mental health problems. One of the major strengths of the self-report and behavioral observer instruments and reporting devices is that objectivity can be established for these devices. Reliability data establish instrument stability over time and across various groups of observers. Agreement between self-reported data and observer-reported data can also be obtained.

Some of the more common self-report and observer report instruments are the Bellevue Index of Depression (BID; Reynolds & Johnston, 1994) which offers a systematic interview approach to both the young child and the caretaker; the Children's Depression Rating Scale–Revised (Poznanski et al., 1984); the Beck Depression Inventory (BDI; Beck, Ward, Mendelson, Mock, & Erbaugh, 1961) and the Children's Depression Inventory (CDI; Kovacs, 1981) for children and adolescence ages 7 to 17.

Two relatively new and highly regarded objective self-report instruments that have utility with children are the Minnesota Multiphasic Personality Inventory–Adolescent (MMPI-A; Butcher et al., 1992) and the Behavior Assessment System for Chil-dren–Self Report Form A (BASC; Reynolds & Kamphaus, 1992). Both of these tests measure a number of Axis I (clinical disorders) and Axis II (personality disorders) features including depression.

MMPI-A

The MMPI-A (Butcher et al., 1992) is a 478-item true/false objective personality test for adolescents ages 14 to 18. The MMPI-A maintains ten clinical scales: Hypochondriasis (*1*), Depression (*2*), Conversion Hysteria (*3*), Psychopathic Deviance (*4*), Masculinity/Femininity (*5*), Paranoia (*6*), Psychasthenia (*7*), Schizophrenia (*8*), Hypomania (*9*), and Social Introversion (*0*). The validity indices of *L* (lie), and *K* (question) and three *F* (faking) scales (*F, F1, F2*) assess odd thoughts, sensations and experiences, and antisocial attitudes and behaviors. The MMPI-A has two validity scales (*VRIN* and *TRIN*) that are used to offset adolescents' "faking good" responses.

The MMPI-A also has 22 content scales. Six of those content scales assess drug/alcohol or psychological problems frequently associated with adolescence: (a) MacAndrew Alcoholism–Revised (*MAC-R*), (b) Alcohol/Drug Acknowledgement (*ACK*), (c) Alcohol/Drug Proneness (*PRO*), (d) Immaturity (*IMM*), (e) Anxiety (*A*), and (f) Repression (*R*). The MAC-R scale distinguishes an increased likelihood of alcohol/drug abuse, self-indulgence, impulsivity, a conduct disorder diagnosis, and violation of social norms. In addition the MMPI-A has two unique school content scales that assess the student's attitude toward school and teachers.

The Behavioral Assessment System for Children (BASC) is also contains a self-Report (Form-A; Reynolds & Kamphaus, 1992), which is a 186-item true/false objective personality test for adolescents ages 12 to 18. The BASC is composed of Clinical and Adaptive Scales that factor into three Composites (Clinical, School, Personal). Clinical scales include Anxiety, Atypicality, Depression, and Somatization. Adaptive scales include Interpersonal Relations, Relations with Parents, and Self-Esteem. This test has three validity indices: *F, L,* and *V.*

The BASC self-rating forms provide four composite scales and one emotional symptom index. The four composites are (a) clinical maladjustment (comprised of anxiety, atypicality, locus of control, social stress, and somatization), (b) school maladjustment (comprised of attitudes toward school, attitudes toward teachers, and sensation seeking), (c) other problems (comprised of depression and sense of inadequacy), and (d) personal adjustment (comprised of relations with parents, interpersonal relations, self-esteem and self-reliance). An Emotional Symptoms Index provides a global measure of serious emotional disturbance based on anxiety, social stress, interpersonal relations, self-esteem, and sense of inadequacy. Students with emotional and behavioral disorders were included in the normative sampling. The BASC as a system also contains stand-alone teacher-report and parent-report instruments that may be used in combination with the child's self-report depending upon the child's age.

A positive correlation was found between the BASC-Depression and MMPI-A A-depression subtests ($R = .60$; Sabatino & Vance, 1999). These two same-name subtests on the two different instrument measure a somewhat but not completely similar emotional/behavioral traits.

Other Instruments: Brief Descriptions

Instrument: **Personality Inventory for Youth (PIC)**

Test Authors: Robert D. Wirt, David Lackar, James, E. Klinedinst, Phillip D. Seat, and William E. Broen

Description: The PIC is a widely used multidimensional diagnostic instrument for children. It has been researched and developed on more than a million children. The PIC ascertains behavior, affect, and cognitive status in children ages 3 to 16 years. The instrument is designed to provide clinical information, intake data, and screening information. It is used primarily as in the differential diagnosis and educational placement of children.

Administration: The parent or other informant completes the first 280-item instrument, which usually requires 25 to 30 minutes. However, if a longer critical item instrument is needed, a complete 430-item instrument for computer scoring is available. If a screening procedure is needed, a 131-item screening test is also available.

Unifactor Child and Adolescent Depressive Instruments

Instrument: **Reynolds Child Depression Scale (RCDS)**

Test author: William M. Reynolds

Purpose: The RCDS screens for depressive symptoms in children in schools and clinical settings. Written at a second-grade level, it contains 30 items and uses a 4-point rating scale. It is intended for children in grades three to six.

Administration: The RCDS can be administered to individuals or groups. It requires 10 minutes.

Scoring: The RCDS is hand-scorable for individual or group administration, but professional report service is also provided. Completed answer sheets will be scored and mailed within 24 hours of receipt (on the next business day). Form G for group screening generates a comprehensive survey report including group summary data, individual scores, and identification of individuals above critical cutoff scores. Reliability coefficients range from .87 to .91. Total sample alpha reliability is .90, and split-half reliability is .89. Validity has been consistently demonstrated since 1981.

Instrument: **Reynolds Adolescent Depression Scale (RADS)**

Test author: William M. Reynolds

Purpose: The RADS meets a vital need in the evaluation of adolescent mental health. It assesses depressive symptomatology in adolescents and is well suited for screening individuals or large groups of students in schools or clinical settings.

Scoring time: The RADS can be completed in 5 to 10 minutes.

Administration: The RADS consists of 30 items rated on a 4-point scale.

Purpose: The RADS can be used for large-scale intervention and prevention programs, for routine screening of individuals referred for behavior or conduct disorders and academic or substance-abuse problems, and for depression research. When used with the Suicidal Ideation Questionnaire (SIQ), which screens for adolescent suicidal ideation, the RADS and the SIQ form an efficient, low-cost mental health screening procedure for adolescents. Validity has been consistently demonstrated by research and clinical data from more than 12,000 adolescents over a 6-year period. Research has suggested that at least 10% of all adolescents experience significant depressive symptoms. Because the RADS can be administered quickly and easily, it is appropriate for large-group screening to help identify seriously depressed adolescents.

Scoring: The RADS may be handscored with a scoring key or by a professional computer scoring service providing a fast, cost-effective way to evaluate individual or group screenings. Completed answer sheets sent to Psychological Assessment Resource are scored and mailed within 24 hours of receipt (on next business day). Reliability coefficients by grade range from .91 to .94, with total sample alpha reliability of .92 and split-half reliability of .91. Six-week and three-month test-retest coefficients are .80 and .79, respectively. Validity has been consistently demonstrated by research and clinical data from more than 12,000 adolescents over 6 years.

Instrument: **Hamilton Depression Inventory (HDI)**

Test Authors: William M. Reynolds and Kenneth A. Kobak

Administration: Written at a fifth-grade reading level, the HDI can be administered in just 10 minutes to individuals or groups.

Scoring: The 23-item full-scale HDI provides a comprehensive evaluation. A 9-item short form is also available for use as a screening instrument when time constraints preclude using the full-scale HDI. A Major Depression Checklist allows for identification and evaluation of specific symptoms of Major Depression as delineated by the *DSM-IV.* It can be either hand-scored or scored rapidly and easily using the HDI Scoring Program.

TREATMENT CONSIDERATIONS

Sabatino and Altizer (1998) asked if a specific diagnosis of a mental disorder and a stated level of severity would make a difference in the prognosis or treatment outcomes. Little data is available on the efficacy of specific types of interventions as influenced by various presenting behaviors, at different ages, and in combination or in isolation from other interventions.

In reviewing the efficacy in children's mental health services, Henggeler (1994) noted that agreement exists that the current service delivery system does not meet the "needs of children" and is working "at tremendous human and financial cost . . . doing more harm than good" (p. 3). The United States frequently has the highest rates among the industrialized nations for child abuse, family abandonment, divorce, adolescent suicide, parental rejection and neglect, child and family drug problems, and domestic violence. Several recent studies (Bird, Gould, & Staghezza, 1993; Burns et al., 1995) concluded that only 40% of children ages 9 to 16 with mental disorders had access to mental health services.

Efficacy has improved as outpatient therapies designed for outpatient service delivery have appeared. Briefer therapies with a solution-oriented focus, and the evolution from analytical to client-centered, self-discovery therapies, to more behavioral and then cognitive-behavioral interventions, have revolutionized outpatient treatment.

Recent studies have demonstrated the effectiveness of outpatient psychotherapy with children (Kazdin, Bass, Ayers, & Rodgers, 1990; Weisz, & Weiss, & Donenberg, 1992). In terms of the types of psychotherapy, a meta-analysis of 150 outcome studies by Weisz, Weiss, Han, Grainger, and Morton (1995) found the effects of behavioral-oriented therapies more positive: cognitive, operant, modeling, social-skills training, parent training, and multimodal behavioral. Within the meta-analysis, neither the therapist's level of training nor type of training, including specialized treatment approaches, influenced treatment results with one very interesting exception: The professional providers produced the greatest treatment outcome gains in children with depression.

There is also strong evidence that the efficacy of a particular or specific psychotherapeutic approach is not as important as the conditions under which a treatment is offered. Saxe, Cross, and Silverman (1988) have shown that to obtain maximum benefits, a child's intervention/treatment program should be custom-tailored. Those factors to be considered in custom-tailoring include family (primary) support systems, agency (secondary) support systems, the developmental level of the child, comorbidity, past history of the child (abuse or neglect), and severity of the disorder. Clinicians are more likely to be in agreement on the form of treatment to be used when the presenting conditions are more severe (Kazdin, 1993). The degree of severity of specific clinical populations may be the most obvious factor to consider in designing a therapeutic intervention. Graham (1993) noted that agreement is higher among mental health clinicians on the form of treatment to be used when the presenting condition is more severe. In contrast there is less agreement with milder disorders about which therapy works best, and consequently about detailing treatment progress in terms of outcomes (Graham, 1993). A mental disorder's prognosis for improvement also influences substantiating the efficacy of one type of treatment against another. As a rule, pervasive developmental disorders such as autism have poor prognoses. Conduct disorders and ADHD obtain intermediate improvement, and anxiety and depressive disorders have good prognosis.

Demonstrating treatment effectiveness is more difficult in disorders where the child's growth or development would have produced desirable results unaided by psychotherapy. Because disorders such as anxiety and depression have a higher probability of abating without treatment, it is more difficult to substantiate whether improvement in course and condition of these mental disorders is related to a specific treatment or to other contributing conditions (Cheung & Zinn, 1991).

Children's treatment outcomes are more dependant upon conditions related to their security and well-being (freedom from threat) than are those of adults (Graham, 1993). The clinical behaviors and treatment outcomes are often related to the child's age, intelligence, and stability of primary social structure (Blanchard & Clarke, 1990). Other significant factors are the therapist, the treatment environment, and the motivation of the child and family to change (Hazelrigg, Cooper, & Borduin, 1987). Often, research data has not shown that one treatment seems better than another, according to Weissman and Markowitz (1994). This points out that when a child improves in mental health functioning, the skills of the therapist (the person) may influence treatment outcome more than the type of therapy (the art form) being used. Clients universally establish that therapists who are empathetic and patient, and who genuinely work to help the child and his or her family, are an asset to functionality (Gurman, Kniskern, & Pinsof, 1986).

Another factor affecting success in interventions with children is comorbidity (Bird, Gould, & Straghezza, 1993). Single conditions are easier to treat. To clinicians dealing with comorbidity, which condition should be treated in which order is frequently an issue (Blumberg, 1992). Since treatment is often limited to short time periods, the less prioritized comorbid disorder may not be treated, as evidenced by many care-givers' treatment plans. Intervention structures that are too broad in outcome goals, and too general in treatment, tend to scatter their effects in a broad manner, producing limited results.

There is little available research comparing service providers by discipline, level of training or degree, personality factors, or other features (Kazdin, 1993). In practically every research study completed in the 1990s, a final caveat always emerges: "more research is needed."

One difference between the interventions for children and adults is that children need to be treated within primary and secondary social groups (Costello, Burns, Angold, & Leaf, 1993). Frequently, the family must be reeducated and included in the therapeutic process. As the child grows stronger and becomes more functional, a carefully orchestrated transition from one treatment environment or system to another is essential. School-aged children cannot be offered a community-based service rich in support and acceptance and then return to a public school classroom where the teacher is punitive and inconsiderate. A total environment network of programs and services must be designed to form a safety net under the child and family. An intervention plan carefully matched to a child's and families presenting symptoms should produce better results more quickly.

WHICH THERAPEUTIC INTERVENTION WORKS WITH DEPRESSED CHILDREN?

Psychotherapy with children and families is the most frequent type of intervention (Tuma, 1989). Kazdin (1991) described psychotherapy as "an intervention which decreases distress, psychological symptoms and maladaptive behavior or which improves adaptive and pro-social functioning" (p. 785). Psychotherapy includes a number of traditional and new approaches, which are frequently grouped into at least five types: analytic or dynamic; client centered or self discovery; specialty children interventions using play, art, or drawing to facilitate communications; traditional behavioral modification; and behavioral and cognitive behavioral therapy, including a specific number of problem-solving and solution-oriented processes.

The major shift in therapeutic emphasis has been from the type of single intervention in a traditional sense toward the multimodal management of children across environments and in all their relationships (Grizenko, Papineau, & Sayegh, 1993). Depression has a tendency to threaten the very perception of having control over one's life. Therefore an extensive range of supportive efforts and activities that positively increase the functional skills or developmental status of a child are necessary. When children are confronted with behavioral problems that overwhelm them, they need additional support that helps them maintain positive outlooks and achievements (purpose) in their lives. Effective interventions increase the constructive coping capacity of the child, expanding available options while reducing risky and unwanted problematic behaviors. Interventions in any environment are designed to safeguard and promote the child's well-being, and to establish positive changes in attitudes and beliefs, to eliminate bad habits, and to teach socially acceptable behaviors many different ways. The depressed child must not be permitted to "drop-out" or become detached to decision making.

Certainly, one aspect of treatment is appropriate medical management. Depression and bipolar disorders result from or promote chemical disorders of the brain. These so-called chemical imbalances seem to respond best to a combination of psychopharmacology and psychotherapy. Medical management of psychopharmacology must be included in the treatment scheme. Other chapters in this volume will address psychopharmacology more completely, and therefore we will only note that it is an important consideration.

The therapeutic goal for most of those interventions reviewed briefly in this chapter will be management of thought in an effort to control feelings. Children isolated and blinded by feelings of abandonment and distrust find themselves disoriented emotionally and do not learn to trust their own judgement; hence they develop without a sense of trust for anyone, including themselves. Self-trust is taking the responsibility to direct the self in a responsible manner under someone else's rules. The development of self as an identity requires disciplined rule learning. The emergence of a usable value system also requires self-trust. There is a total emphasis on all aspects of the child's life, with the guided interactions being positive, rewarding, reassuring, and supportive, sharply reducing and maintaining that reduction on disturbing moods and emotions. Currently, the most frequently used form of psychotherapy to accomplish these goals is cognitive-behavioral therapy, which may occur individually, in groups, or in family structure (Wilkes, Belshwer, & Rush, 1994). It also overlaps into all aspects of the child's life, home, school, and community. The principle is that cognitive structuring and restructuring of thought involves awareness and dictates that thought overrules emotions.

COGNITIVE-BEHAVIORAL THERAPY

Kendall and Panichelli-Mendal (1995) reviewed studies where cognitive-behavioral forms of therapy (CBT) were the primary interventions with children and adolescents (ages 4 to 13 years). After the course of the CBT, the average treated child scored better on outcome measures than 71% of the nontreatment control peer group. Children ages 11 to 13 were more positively affected by CBT than were those in the 5- to 11-year age range. That finding is not surprising because early adolescents and preadolescent children have greater cognitive development than do their younger counterparts.

Reynolds and Coats (1986) reported one of the early studies on the effects of CBT combining behavioral therapy and relaxation training for the treatment of depression in adolescents. Their results demonstrated significant treatment results in contrast to other therapeutic approaches in combination. A year later, Stark, Reynolds, and Kaslow (1987) reported on their treatment efforts using CBT in clinical work with childhood depression. They used small groups, offering their program over a 3.5-month period (26 sessions) for one therapeutic hour. The content focused on affective education, social skills training, problem-solving training, self-instructional training, activities scheduling, relaxation training with positive imagery, and cognitive restructuring/cognitive modeling. They reported significant reductions in depressive symptoms in the treatment groups.

Another form of CBT that uses adjunct treatment techniques and a parent program is the Adolescent Coping with Depression Course (CWD/A; Clarke, Lewinsohn, & Hops, 1990). This program uses small groups of three to eight children. The program consists of 16 sessions lasting over 2 hours, with several joint parent-child sessions as well as individual parent sessions over an 8 week period. There are booster sessions at 4-month intervals over a 2-year period. The treatment content consists of mood monitoring, social skills training, relaxation training, positive/pleasant activities scheduling, instructive thinking/cognitive restructuring, communication skills training, negotiation, conflict resolution, and problem-solving training. In a controlled research study mixing parents and children and children alone, the authors reported a post-treatment reduction in diagnostic criteria for depression. The mixed group (parent and child) had a 47.6% reduction in diagnostic criteria, whereas the adolescent-only group had a 42.9% reduction, and the control group had a 5.3% reduction (Lewinsohn, Clarke, Rohde, Hops, & Seeley, 1996).

The studies on CBT (Kazdin & Marciano, 1998) using self-control training, relaxation training, and behavioral problem solving resulted in significant decreases in depressive symptoms compared to no-treatment control groups. In reviewing various applications in different environment with both adults and children suffering from depression, CBT has demonstrated significant clinical efficacy (Hallon, Shelton, & Davis, 1993). This appears to be true in a range of applications and conditions.

SCHOOL-BASED INTERVENTIONS

Clarke et al. (1995) studied 471 adolescents who self-reported depressive symptomatology and met criteria for current major depression or dysthymia. Experimental and control groups were established. A school psychologist and counselor conducted 15 45-minute group training sessions on coping with stress. Six months to a year later, 25% of the control nontreatment group and 14.5 percent of the experimental group reported sufficient depressive symptomatology.

This research (Clarke et al., 1995) shows the usefulness of group guidance in schools, at a significant cost savings over formal therapy. Further, the success rate from this early prevention program was clearly better than most recovery rates from therapy. Schools may be the ideal place for early prevention efforts such as this one. This study revealed that group therapy within the schools is clearly superior to treatment after the presence of a problem has been established. Stark, Brookman, and Frazier (1990) have also demonstrated the positive effects of school-based interventions when offered in group programs designed to prevent and reduce early symptoms of depression in children.

The richest of all the therapies could be education. Educators have a tremendous influence with children. They have the content requirements of curriculum, which they can use therapeutically to demonstrate accomplishment, growth, and development. Educators have access to a social interactive environment comprised of peers and adults and controlled by definitive rules.

FAMILY THERAPY

Family therapy receives good reviews throughout the helping professions, and research data substantiates its effectiveness (Markus, Lange, & Pettigrew, 1990) when used with children having conduct disorders. Gurman et al. (1986) obtained positive family therapy outcomes with younger children with Anorexia Nervosa and other psychosomatic complaints. Hazelrigg, Cooper, and Borduin (1987) conducted a meta-analysis on 10 family therapy studies and reported positive outcomes in family interaction and child ratings of behavior on children with conduct disorders.

Child and familial factors can influence how well family therapy might be suited to a child's treatment needs, according to Friesen and Koroloff (1990). Indicators for the use of family therapy include (a) when family conflict exists, especially unresolved parental conflict that cannot be resolved without external mediation; (b) when poor or rigid family organization curtails open family communications; and (c) when one of both parents are overly protective or possessive. Contraindicators for the use of familial therapy are when the problem resides mainly within the child and is not an outgrowth of the family network. However, even when the problem is mainly within the child, the family can still benefit from some supportive therapy that helps them cope with the child. A very significant therapy prohibitor is when one family member is dysfunctional (e.g., has a severe mental disorder, or other health factors).

A confusing issue is the differences among filial therapy, parent education, and parent support services. There is a common belief that parent education programs are as effective as family therapy. However, parent education programs have been poorly researched. Family support services are frequently defined as those broad-based services directed at providing social, emotional, and other basic needs of the family unit. The goal is to keep the family intact. This includes self help, support, and advocacy groups; information and referral sources; educational and training opportunities; respite care; and cash assistance or meeting the basic survival needs of the family unit.

Family support services have generally been evaluated as favorable. Parents who receive family support services are generally satisfied with these services and improve in outcomes, experiencing a significant reduction in stress and social isolation, displaying increased self-esteem, holding a more positive view of the children's behavior, and displaying increases in feelings of family decision-making competence and communication skills (Kazdin and Marciano, 1998).

Children may receive a range of family interventions: (a) collaborative family planning, (b) individual psychotherapy for family members, (c) the mother is hospitalized with the child and becomes active in the treatment program, and (d) inpatient parent training and support programs during hospitalization that continue after discharge (Dalton, Muller, & Forman, 1988).

INTERPERSONAL THERAPY (IPT)

Mufson et al. (1994) studied interpersonal therapy comprehensively and reported that it was one of the most promising types of psychotherapy. Interpersonal therapy is a short-term psychotherapy, normally consisting of 12 to 16 weekly sessions. It was developed specifically for the treatment of major depression and focuses on correcting current social dysfunction. It is solution oriented and focuses on "here and now" factors that directly interfere with social relationships, task achievement, and comfort in various environments.

Interpersonal therapy offers therapeutic intervention within the structure and boundaries of relationships. The aim of this intervention is to reduce depressive symptoms by promoting cognitive awareness of current problems within the context of personal relationships. Techniques often taught include self-monitoring of depressive feelings, exploratory questioning, problem clarification, identification of the link between affect and events, and communication skills. During therapy the client and therapist role-play real situations, and the therapist provides feedback regarding the patient's interpersonal style. IPT has been shown to be an effective means of reducing depressive symptoms in adolescents (Weissman & Markowitz, 1994).

PLAY THERAPY

The guidelines for play therapy have existed since 1872 (Axline, 1982). Carroll (1998) offered an excellent overview of the current rationale and procedures. The premise of play therapy is that preschool-aged children have not developed an awareness of their emotional needs and lack the language capabilities to express those feelings they are aware of. Play, not talk, is the natural medium of the child. Through play the child enhances sensory motor function, increases symbolic thought processes, imitates grownups, creates a world of make-believe, and expresses and acts out wishes and fantasies. The child creates play situations in which he can see the problem and develop what he needs to overcome it. The child enacts experiences that have been hurtful and threatening, creating a world of make believe and wishes and fantasies. Within the context of make-believe the child can act on the compulsion to repeat threatening experiences, identify with the aggressor, identify with the victim, master past events and behaviors, and prepare for the future.

Play therapy is an affective method of communicating with children. Axline's (1982) principles for play therapy for depressed children are:

1. Offer the child a warm, open relationship
2. Offer the child unconditional acceptance
3. Establish a permissive atmosphere
4. Observe and quickly recognize feelings the child is expressing and reflect those feeling back to him
5. Show respect for the child's feelings
6. Do not attempt to direct the child's play or feelings
7. Recognize that this is a gradual process that must not be hurried
8. Remove all limitations and restrictions except those necessary to establish reality

Individual play therapy is often accompanied by family therapy. Play sessions are 1/2 hour to 45 minutes in length once or twice a week. Family therapy is once a week for a full session period. The child is encouraged to do or say anything as long as it will not hurt him or the therapist. The child is reassured that what is said and done is between the child and the therapist. Play therapy assists the depressed child act out and express internal thoughts and fears (Kovacs & Gatsonis, 1994). Sand boxes with a range of toys, toy cars, trucks, houses, tools, doll houses with a wide range of character dolls, puppets, clay or playdough, drawing paper and easels, and Lego blocks and other toys that permit creative expression are all helpful tools. The therapeutic principle is to follow the child's lead and reflect his or her feelings, creating a path of self-expression through self-exploration and discovery.

DYNAMIC PSYCHOTHERAPY

Barber (1994) reported on the efficacy of short-term dynamic psychotherapy, offering the following standards of care: psychoanalytic therapy for childhood depression for those ages 7 to 12, related to the age-specific symptoms that occur and the intensification of the behaviors; suicidal intent; suicidal plan; social withdrawal from parents and peers; academic failure; guilt; shame; self-blame; and worthlessness. The developmental status of the child frequently results in a focus on oedipal conflicts: aggressive wishes and fantasies toward parents, intensification of defense mechanisms of repression, suppression, and denial. The depressed child often has underlying feelings of anger, isolation, and alienation from the parents that are displaced or transferred to the therapist. The therapist assists by differentiating the developmentally appropriate defense mechanisms of suppression, repression, denial, rationalization, and isolation of affect from the exaggerated and overwrought use of these same defenses. Defense mechanisms in the depressed child stand out because the child often overuses them until they are faulty. Reducing this dependence on the faulty defense structure with children requires the use of concrete examples based on the child's behavior as well as their judgement and insight as they formulate decision-making. The therapist offers suggestions and provides practice in the use of other defense structures, hoping to obtain more options and a greater range of flexibility.

If trust can be established in the therapeutic relationship with the depressed school-aged child, then receptiveness to the therapist's suggestions, clarifications, gentle confrontations, and occasional interpretations will be more easily received. Talking and the use of structured and unstructured games, more advanced and more creative play, and role-playing such as psychodrama will help the therapist share thoughts, feelings, and behaviors. However, when the depressed school-aged child is threatened and is resistant, or even defiant, then easy and relaxed games such as checkers, cards, tic-tac-toe, and hangman are useful ice-breakers and help reinstate more aggressive therapy. Recognizing the concrete preoperational stage of development for the younger children, a slow but steady effort should be made to help the child identify, categorize, separate, and isolate the affect and rationalization that are occurring in relationship problems with peers, parents, or others. The therapist should not even attempt to use abstract language or metaphors until the child is well past 12 years of age. Aggressive expression in therapy is considered a sign of progress. With older children therapists should also be aware of countertransference of feelings and should observe and modify their responses. It is not helpful to become overidentified with the adolescent, or to assume the parental role unconsciously, thus contributing to the adolescent's further rebellion and increasing resistance and bringing disruption to the therapeutic relationship.

As individual therapy progresses and the child becomes more expressive, family therapy can be initiated. It is not recommended that the therapist seeing the child individually and the family therapist be one in the same person. It does require that they have open communication and an excellent working relationship. The primary therapist also needs to initiate and maintain contact with the school system, social agencies, and other environments, including extended families across generational lines. The other consideration to the psychodynamic-oriented therapist is the insight and self-understanding of the child who is comorbid. Children with conduct disorders, ADHD, or learning disabilities will need coping skills for these problems as well as for the depression. They will need to understand the requirements made on them by these disorders in addition to the depression and what they can do about developing workable options. Psychotherapy must serve as a motivational platform helping the child see a future, set and realize goals, and feel that he has greater control of his life. Role-playing, videotaping and reviewing the videotapes are excellent therapies. Many depressed school-aged children enjoy videotherapy.

CASE STUDIES

In the following section two brief case studies are offered. The first provides a review of the diagnostic features and treatment plan for a 16-year-old adolescent female. This adolescent had a long history of multiple sexual abuses including incest. The emotional etiology was initial substantial episodic depression followed by residual dysthymia. An interesting aspect of the first case is that the school's response to the elevating agoraphobia and social phobias, including isolation, was to file charges against the mother for truancy. A juvenile judge saw the symptoms and ordered a psychological evaluation and corresponding treatment. It is appalling that the public school system, an assumed child-centered social institution, is less able to recognize psychological symptoms and respond than is our legal system. This one case, should it be common, makes one wonder who is pro-treatment and who is pro-punishment. It is also interesting that the family was more in denial of the abuse history than was the child. Family therapy seemed to relieve the situation. As the issue became more open in the home, the young woman showed increasing recovery from symptoms and (re)establishment of control over her own life.

The second case study presents a 9-year-old (age 7 when seen initially) male child who was a victim of sexual abuse by a stepfather and was forced to observe his biological mother and stepfather in primal activity. The family dynamics in response to him literally split the family (his grandmother and great-aunt) in two warring factions and participated legal action.

Both of the above cases responded well to treatment, not because of any great breakthrough in intervention strategies, but for the two most common reasons often associated with positive changes in thought, feelings, and behavior: a loving support system and available intrapersonal psychological resources. The therapist's job is to help the person unlearn old nonfunctional behaviors and replace these bad old habits with goal-oriented, positive, new, self-fulfilling feelings and self-directed thoughts, both of which produce positive functional behavioral outcomes.

Case Study in Adolescent Depression

M. S., now age 17, was referred by the court. She was unable to find the psychological resources to attend school on a regular basis. She had been in a regular high school the year before and had withdrawn from peers and the environment until she could no longer face going to school. The school's response was to cite the mother for the child's truancy. The juvenile court ordered that the child be seen psychologically.

M. S. is an attractive girl with dark black hair and eyes and olive-toned skin. She was neatly groomed and arrived for intake in a jogging suit. She was pleasant and cooperative but withdrawn. She was also only semialert and appeared fatigued with dark circles under her eyes. She sat with her neck rolled to one side in the chair as if she could not hold her head up straight. She acted dazed and exhausted. She reported that she was unable to sleep. Her mother reported that she stayed up most of the night roaming the house and then cat-napped during the day. M. S. reported being afraid. Her insight and judgment were good concerning issues other than those which focused on herself. She had a dry sense of humor and though socially oriented was guarded in social interaction. She offered a number of agoraphobic responses to school, shopping, and simply being out of the home.

Her history revealed that she had been sexually abused at age 7 by her father. She was sexually abused again at age 10 by her uncle, and then again at age 13 by a neighbor. She wanted an active social life but was very much afraid. Her thought was well organized, and she had relevant content. She was intelligent and had excellent social skills. There was no pattern of perceptual distortions. Her affect was positive, but she lacked a full range of emotions. She was dysthymic and had been so since age 13.

Her psychotherapy had a family orientation and included her mother and on occasion her brother. The mode was cognitive behavioral: replacing poorly understood feelings with thought and elevating awareness of feelings by verbal and written descriptions. Her mother served as a mirror, relating what she had observed in her behavior over the week, and pointing out if she was using thought control to restructure her perceptions. Progressive relaxation, in vivo visualization, thought stoppage, and thought blockage were used. One technique that greatly assisted her was role-playing situations as they occurred and then role-playing once she had refocused the problem aspect. She was particularly responsive to her mother's role-playing her observations of the client: "Oh, I didn't do that." The other helpful aspect was journaling and prioritizing goals and her responses to the barriers that might inhibit her from achieving them. Much of her feeling awareness came from the insight she gained in seeing her mother "play her." She enjoyed those sessions. Another helpful factor was in role-playing desired social interactions with selected people. Behaviorally, gradual desensitization was used to achieve movement toward entering various social relationships.

By the fifth session she had developed and prioritized a list of personal goals. She wanted to finish high school but was afraid of several of the students in the building that she had been attending. An arrangement was made at an optional high school, and the counselor assigned a peer mentor to be with her. She was able to fast-track her studies by concentrating her time on one course until it was completed and then going to a second course. She only needed to stay at the optional high school for 4 hours. She was able to find a job in the office of a supermarket with the help of a friend. She felt secure in the office and liked the people she was working with. The job went well. By summer she had begun dating a boy she had known all of her life and felt safe and secure with. They dated by going to his home. M. S. and his mother became best of friends. He taught her to drive, and she got her license shortly after school began.

She is still dating the same person, attending the optional high school, and working at the grocery store. She was able to develop feeling awareness and direct her anger (she had been highly agitated) at the source, her biological father. She and her mother have become very close in these sessions. She was placed on 50 mg four times a day of Zoloft, and has been taking 50 mg of Elavil before bedtime. She is now sleeping through the night, and is rapidly reclaiming her life in all aspects. She drives alone, shops with friends or her mother, and can remain in her home at night (someone is always there).

She still is not as active with peers as she would like. She is also still very fearful of strangers and strange situations. She is no longer fatigued in appearance, and she engages in social interactions with much more robustness and vitality. She has given herself a new goal recently. She wants a different job, where she meets the public, and she would like to attend a junior college. She is now being seen twice monthly.

Case Study in Juvenile Mood Disorder

C. W., age 7, was brought to the office by his aunt, who had been awarded temporary custody following allegations of emotional abuse by his biological mother. C. W.'s biological grandmother had been given the custody but had not followed court directives and had permitted the child to be seen by the biological mother and her husband (C. W.'s stepfather). In the process of having C. W. in his mother's home with the biological mother and stepfather, new instances of sexual abuse occurred. The family dynamics, especially among the two sisters, grandmother, and great aunt, could only be described as contempt for one another's behavior. The great aunt accused the grandmother of permitting physical and emotional harm to occur to the boy.

The child presented as a highly verbal 7-year-old. His verbality was random and merely a release, limited in content and meaning. His behaviors were also random, mimicking ADHD symptomology, which is often the case. He could not stay seated, and his behavior (like his verbal expression) was motor driven and hyperkinetic. The emotions underlying the child's behavior were characterized as racing thoughts, rapidly cycling moods, and disorganization in thought content. The child could not maintain focus; he had been fully toilet trained and was now having daytime encopresis and nocturnal enuresis. He had an irregular sleep pattern, was gaze avoidant, and clearly did not know whom to trust. He had many symptoms associated with a reactive attachment disorder; and, differentially, a dissociative disorder did seem highly likely. The two principal features of a dissociative disorder—psychogenic fugue (running away) and psychogenic amnesia (blank periods)—were not present. The child simply was unsafe, was insecure in the visitation environment, and felt emotionally unattached. In early human figure drawings he drew himself very small and would only draw his chief caretaker, his aunt, who wore her hair in a bouffant style. C. W. would not call any family member by a name or acknowledge the relationship factor. Later, he begin to call his maternal grandmother Mamaw and his great aunt Nanna. He called his primary caregiver "big hair" until very recently. When asked now who his mother is, he points to the care-giver but does not yet say the word "mother" or "mom." Human figure and kinetic family drawings were a major diagnostic tool and served to track his progress in family play therapy, the treatment mode which was utilized.

The first extended aspect of the treatment was to contact his care-giver's attorney and request a motion to the courts to stop all visitations with the grandmother in her home and to stop all visitations with the biological mother and stepfather. Two purposes were sought: One was protective in nature, but the other, just as important, was to provide him a much-needed sense of family identity. His drawing began to reflect this change. He now began to draw other members of his family in the background and off to the side of him, his primary care-giver, and her male friend. The other figures which he would not name but would respond with head shakes were his mother and stepfather. They were not drawn as people with humanoid characteristics. They were drawn as very dark and heavy circles from running the pencil in circles hundreds of times. Very rapidly, and very clearly, a new strong relationship began to emerge. He felt safe and protected with this dominant figure, and he drew the person as large and strong, occupying much of the page. He had made a definitive attachment with this care-giver's fiancee. This need for a secure giving male was very important to C. W. He preferred the direct support of the male care-giver and forced him to provide direct services to him, bathing, teeth brushing, and reading to him. In the process of supervising his baths, the adult male figure saw a flap of skin extending from the anal area in what appeared to be a prolapsed rectum.

In play therapy with C. W., he would not play with figures or dolls. He was too guarded in family relationships to enter into role play. He failed to respond to hearing repeatedly that it would help him if he could talk out or act out his feelings in the protection of the office without anyone else knowing. As he grew in secure relationship with the care-givers he began to talk to the adult male care-giver. He instructed him to get a pen and write down what he was going to say and his "mom" (big hair) was to take it to the doctor and read it. They filled up four pages of notes that C. W. dictated on a pattern of sexual and emotional abuse and what he had been made to witness between his mother and stepfather as supper, which was being prepared by his mother, burned on the stove. Once the material was on paper, I assumed that he would respond to direct questions as he usually did by nodding his head or looking at me. Instead, he talked freely in a nonstop fashion, this time with well-organized content, and he began to place emotions with his responses. Following this session his daytime encopresis stopped. His mood cycling fell into a normal range, and he began to express a full range of unguarded affect in behaviors though not in words. He still runs for his old behaviors when stressed; but the crucial mood rolls upon behavioral plot are half as frequent, and the duration has dropped by 60% or more.

The other interesting twist is that the once-squirming child who twisted himself in the chair and talked and moved randomly without self-directed response control has lost all of these ADHD symptoms. He is alert, fairly calm, socially well oriented and interactive, although he still is much more guarded in response to family dynamics.

An interesting parallel between the first and second case study is the adolescent girl presented as depressed with significant elevation in agitation. She was angry. Anger turned inward in children is often observed as depression. C. W., on the other hand, simply withdrew to a safety zone where he could survive. It would appear that he would have grown up unable to maintain relationships, presenting as a schizoaffective disorder. Further, it is highly probable that he would have recycled his abuse. While a number of symptoms were present on intake (ADHD, Reactive Detachment Disorder, Dissociative Disorder), C. W.'s diagnosis was Cyclothymic Disorder.

SUMMARY

In just over 20 years the mental health professions have altered beliefs and changed the focus on mood disorders in children. There are apparently two simultaneous occurrences. First, the professions slowly gained knowledge, some of which is data-based, on mental disorders in children. Childhood depression, like many other disorders affecting both adults and children, cannot be understood by simply boiling down what is known about adults. If that were not true enough, the absolute truth about treatment efficacy is that procedures used with children with mood disorders must address the developmental status of children, their cognitive level of functioning, and the uniqueness of their social learning experiences. One size does not fit all. At the moment, custom-tailored interventions appear to hold the greatest therapeutic efficacy. How they are applied and who applies them appears to be less important than the time at which they are brought to bear, and the therapeutic bond that exists facilitating communications between care-giver and patient. Children are not independent decision makers. Therefore, the augmentation of individual psychotherapy with family therapy also has produced excellent results.

The case for children with mood disorders has been summed up in these words: "Child mental health services are a prime example of the kind of service that can provide long-term benefits in exchange for relatively cheap early intervention" (Costello et al., Angold, & Leaf, 1993, p. 480). Why provide treatment to children when they may simply outgrow the problems? The answer is that by providing treatment to children, it may prevent a lifetime of distress (Kendall, 1994). The argument is not that treatment is supposed to eradicate all discomfort and illness, but treatment should help prepare a child for how to cope and compensate for the future. This seems to be particularly true as the levels of stress continue to mount in a complex society and the number of available support systems shrinks.

The standard of care provided for childhood mood disorders would be to identify symptoms early and offer preventative interventions; should symptoms, family, school, or other stress factors prevail in the face of genetic-family influences, then the state-of-the-art treatment is recommended. What that is will already have changed between the time of this writing and the time of the printing.

REFERENCES

American Psychiatric Association. (1980). *Diagnostic and statistical manual of mental disorders* (3rd ed.). Washington, DC: Author.

American Psychiatric Association. (1994). *Diagnostic and statistical manual of mental disorders* (4th ed.). Washington, DC: Author.

Andrus, J. K., Fleming, D. N., Neumann. M. A., Wassell, J. T. Hopkinds, D. D., & Gordon, J. (1991). Surveillance of attempted suicide among adolescents in Oregon. *American Journal of Public Health, 81,* 1067–1069.

Armbruster, P., & Schwab-Stone, M. E. (1994). Sociodemographic characteristics of dropouts from a child guidance clinic. *Hospital Community Psychiatry, 45,* 804–808.

Axline, V. (1982). Entering the child's world via the play experience. In G. L. Landreth (Ed.), *Play therapy: Dynamics of the process of counseling children* (pp. 47–57). Boston: Thomas.

Barber, J. P. (1994). Efficacy of short-term dynamic psychotherapy: Past, present, and future. *Journal of Psychotherapy Practice Research, 3,* 108–121.

Beck, A. T., Ward, C. H., Mendelson, M., Mock, J., & Erbaugh, J. (1961). An inventory for measuring depression. *Archives of General Psychiatry, 4,* 53–63.

Bird, H. R., Gould, M. S., & Staghezza, B. M. (1993). Patterns of diagnostic comorbidity in a community sample of children aged 9–16 years. *Journal of American Academic Child Adolescent Psychiatry, 32,* 361–368.

Blumberg, S. (1992). Initial behavior problems as predictors of outcome in a children's psychiatric hospital. In A. Algarin & R. Friedman (Eds.), *Fourth annual research conference proceedings for a system of care for children's mental health: Expanding the research base* (pp. 185–188). Tampa: University of South Florida, Research and Training Center for Children's Mental Health.

Bowlby, J. (1969). *Attachment* (Vol. 1). New York: Basic Books.

Brandenburg, N. A., Friedman, R. M., & Silver, S. E. (1989). *Epidemiology of childhood psychiatric disorders: Prevalence findings from recent studies.* Tampa, FL: Research and Training Center for Children's Mental Health.

Burchard, J., & Clarke, R. (1990). The role of individualized care in a service delivery system for children and adolescents with severely maladjusted behavior. *Journal of Mental Health Administration, 17,* 48–60.

Burns, B. J. (1994). The challenges of child mental health services research. *Journal of Emotional and Behavioral Disorders, 2,* 254–256.

Burns, B. J., Costello, E. J., Angold, A., Tweed, D., Stange, D., Farmer, E. M., & Erkanli, A. (1995). Children's mental health service use across service sectors. *Health Affairs, 14,* 147–159.

Butcher, J., Williams, C., Graham, J., Tellegen, A., Ben-Porath, Y., & Kaemmer, B. (1992). *Minnesota Multiphasic Personality Inventory–Adolescent (Manual for administration, scoring, and interpretation).* Minneapolis: University of Minnesota Press.

Cannon, T., Mednick, S., & Parnas, J. (1990). Two pathways to schizophrenia in children at risk. In L. Robins & M. Rutter (Eds.), *Straight and devious pathways from childhood to adulthood* (pp. 328–350). Cambridge, England: Cambridge University Press.

Carroll, J. (1998). *Introduction to therapeutic play.* Oxford, England: Blackwell Science.

Chess, S., & Thomas, A. (1977). *Origins and development of behavioral disorders.* New York: Brunner/Mazel.

Cheung, F., & Zinn, H. (1991). Mental health research issues of minority children and youth. In A. Algarin & R. M. Friedman (Eds.), *A system of care for children's mental health: Building a research base* (pp. 269–278). Tampa, FL: Research and Training Center for Children's Mental Health.

Clarke, G. M., Lewinsohn, P. M., & Hops, H. (1990). *Adolescent coping with depression course: Leaders manual for adolescent groups.* Eugene, OR: Castalia.

Clarke, G. M., Hawkins, W., Murphy, M., Sheeber, L. B., Lewinsohn, P. M., & Seeler, J. R. (1995). Targeted prevention of unipolar depressive disorder in an at-risk sample of high school adolescents: A randomized trial of a group cognitive intervention. *Journal of Academic Child and Adolescent Psychiatry, 34,* 312–321.

Cohen-Sandler, R., Berman, A., & King, R. (1982). A follow-up study of hospitalized suicidal children. *Journal of the American Academy of Child Psychiatry, 21,* 398–403.

Costello, E. J., Burns, B. J., Angold, A., & Leaf, P. J. (1993). How can epidemiology improve mental health services for children and adolescents? *Journal of American Academy of Child and Adolescent Psychiatry, 32,* 1106–1114.

Cytryn, L., & McKnew, D. H., Jr. (1996). *Childhood depression and its treatment.* New York: Norton.

Cytryn, L., McKnew, D. H., Zahn-Waxler, C., Radke-Yarrow, M., Gaensbauer, T. J., & Harmon, R. J. (1984). Affective disturbances in the offspring of affectively ill patients: A developmental view. *American Journal of Psychiatry, 141,* 219–222.

Dalton, R., Muller, B., & Forman, M. A. (1988). The psychiatric hospitalization of children: An overview. *Child Psychiatry and Human Development, 19,* 231–244.

Downey, G., & Coyne, J. C. (1990). Children of depressed parents: An integrative review. *Psychological Bulletin, 180,* 50–76.

Frank, R. G., & Dewa, C. S. (1992). Insurance, system structure, and the use of mental health services by children and adolescents. *Clinical Psychology Review, 12,* 829–840.

Friedman, R. (1990). Relating CASSP goals to a research design. In *Child and Adolescent Service System Program technical assistance research meeting: Summary of proceedings* (pp. 2–5). Washington, DC: National Institute of Mental Health.

Friesen, B. J., & Koroloff, N. M. (1990). Family centered services: Implications for mental health administration and research. *Journal of Mental Health Administration, 17,* 13–25.

Garfinkel, B., Froese, A., & Hood, J. (1982). Suicide attempts in children and adolescents. *American Journal of Psychiatry, 139,* 10.

Geller, B., Fox, L. W., & Clark, K. A. (1994). Rate and predictors of prepubertal bipolarity during follow-up of six to twelve year old depressed children. *Journal of the American Academy of Child and Adolescent Psychiatry, 33,* 461–468.

Glasser, K. (1968). Masked depression in children and adolescents. *Annual progress in child psychiatry and child development, 1,* 345–355.

Graham, P. J. (1993). Treatment of child mental disorders: Types, and evidence of effectiveness. *International Journal of Mental Health, 22,* 67–82.

Gould, R. E. (1965). Suicide problems in children and adolescents. *American Journal of Psychotherapy, 19,* 228–246.

Grizenko, N., Papineau, D., & Sayegh, L. (1993). Effectiveness of a multimodal day treatment program for children with disruptive behavior problems. *Journal of American Academic Child Adolescent Psychiatry, 32,* 127–134.

Gurman, A. S., Kniskern, D. P., & Pinsof, W. M. (1986). Research on the process and outcome in marital and family therapy. In S. L. Garafield & A. E. Bergin (Eds.), *Handbook of psychotherapy and behavior change* (p. 565). New York: Wiley.

Harrington, R. C., Fudge, H., Rutter, M. L., Pickles, A., & Hill, J. (1990). Adult outcomes of childhood and adolescent depression. *Archives of General Psychiatry, 47,* 465–473.

Hazelrigg, M. D., Cooper, H. M., & Borduin, C. M. (1987). Evaluating the effectiveness of families therapies: An integrative review and analysis. *Psychological Bulletin, 101,* 428–442.

Henggeler, S. W. (1994). A consensus: Conclusions of the APA Task Force Report on innovative models of mental health services for children, adolescents, and their families. *Journal of Clinical Child Psychology, 23,* 3–6.

Hoagwood, K., & Rupp, A. (1995). Mental health service needs, use and costs for children and adolescents with mental disorders and their families: Preliminary evidence. *Psychiatric Times* (March), 62–63.

Hallon, S. D., Shelton, R. C., & Davis, D. D. (1993). Cognitive therapy for depression: Conceptual issues and clinical efficacy. *Journal of Consulting and Clinical Psychology, 61,* 270–275.

Kagan, J. (1984). *The nature of the child.* New York: Basic Books.

Kalko, D. J. (1992). Short-term followup of child psychiatric hospitalization: Clinical description, predictors, and correlates. *Journal of the American Academy of Child and Adolescent Psychiatry, 31,* 719–727.

Kazdin, A. E. (1991). Effectiveness of psychotherapy with children and adolescents. *Journal of Consulting and Clinical Psychology, 59,* 785–798.

Kazdin, A. E. (1993). Adolescent mental health: Prevention and treatment programs. *American Psychologist, 48,* 127–141.

Kazdin, A. E., Bass, D., Ayers, W. A., & Rodgers, A. (1990). Empirical and clinical focus of child and adolescent psychotherapy research. *Journal of Consulting and Clinical Psychology, 58,* 644–657.

Kazdin, A. E., & Marciano, P. L. (1998). Childhood and adolescent depression. In E. J. Mash & R. A. Barkley (Eds.), *Treatment of childhood disorders* (pp. 321–340). New York: Guilford Press.

Kendall, P. C. (1994). Treating anxiety disorders in children: Results of a randomized clinical trial. *Journal of Consulting and Clinical Psychology, 62,* 100–110.

Kendall, P. C., & Panichelli-Mendel, S. M. (1995). Cognitive-behavioral treatments. *Journal of Abnormal Child Psychology, 22,* 107–121.

Knesper, O. J., Riba, M. B., & Schwenk, T. L. (1997). *Primary care psychiatry.* Philadelphia: W. B. Saunders.

Knitzer, J. (1993). Children's mental health policy: Challenging the future. *Journal of Emotional and Behavioral Disorders, 1,* 8–16.

Knitzer, J., Steinberg, Z., & Fleisch, B. (1990). *At the school house door: An examination of programs and policies for children with behavior and emotional problems.* New York: Bank Street College of Education.

Kovacs, M. (1981). Rating scales to assess depression in school aged children. *Acta Paedopsychiatrica, 46,* 305–315.

Kovacs, M. (1996). The course of childhood-onset depressive disorders. *Psychiatric Annuals, 26,* 326–330.

Kovacs, M., Akiskal, H. S., Gatsonis, C., & Parrone, P. L. (1994). Childhood-onset dysthymic disorder: Clinical features and prospective naturalistic outcome. *Archives of General Psychiatry, 51,* 365–374.

Kovacs, M., & Beck, A. T. (1977). An empirical-clinical approach toward a definition of childhood depression. In J. G. Schulterbrandt & A. Raskin (Eds.), *Depression in childhood: Diagnosis, treatment, and conceptual models* (pp. 112–120). New York: Raven.

Kovacs, M., & Gatsonis, C. (1994). Secular trends in age at onset of major depressive disorder in a clinical sample of children. *Journal of Psychiatric Res, 28,* 319–329.

Kovacs, M., Goldston, D., & Gatsonis, C. (1993). Suicidal behavior and childhood-onset depressive disorders: A longitudinal investigation. *Journal of the American Academy of Child and Adolescent Psychiatry, 32,* 8–20.

Kutash, K., & Rivera, V. R. (1995). Effectiveness of children's mental health services: A review of the literature. *Education and Treatment of Children, 18,* 443–477.

Lewinsohn, P. M., Clarke, G. N., & Rohde, P. (1994). Psychological approaches to the treatment of depression in adolescents. In W. M. Reynolds & H. F. Johnston (Eds.), *Handbook of depression in children and adolescents* (pp. 309–344). New York: Plenum Press.

Lewinsohn, P. M., Clarke, G. N., Rohde, P., Hops, H., & Seeley, J. R. (1996). A course in coping: A cognitive behavioral approach to the treatment of adolescent depression. In E. D. Hibbs & P. Jensen (Eds.), *Psychosocial treatments for child and adolescent disorders: Empirically based strategies for clinical practice* (pp. 109–135). Washington, DC: American Psychological Association.

Lewinsohn, P. M., Clarke, G. N., & Seeley, J. R. (1994). Major depression in community adolescents: Age of onset, episode duration, time to recurrence. *Journal of American Academy of Child and Adolescent Psychiatry, 33,* 809–818.

Lewinsohn, P. M., Klein, D. N., & Seeley, J. R. (1995). Bipolar disorders in a community sample of older adolescents: Prevalence, phenomenology, comorbidity, and course. *Journal of the American Academy of Child and Adolescent Psychiatry, 34,* 454–563.

Markus, E., Lange, A., & Pettigrew, T. F. (1990). Effectiveness of family therapy: A meta-analysis. *Journal of Family Therapy, 12,* 205.

Marttunen, M. J., Aro, H. M., Henriksson, M. M., & Lonnqvist, J. K. (1994). Antisocial behavior in adolescent suicide. *Acta Psychiatry Scandanivia, 89,* 167–173.

McMahon, R. J. (1994). Diagnosis, assessment, and treatment of externalizing problems in children: The role of longitudinal data. *Journal of Consulting and Clinical Psychology, 62,* 901–917.

Messer, S. C., & Gross, A. M. (1994). Childhood depression and aggression: A covariance structure analysis. *Behavior Research Theory, 32,* 663–677.

Mufson, L., Moreau, D., Weissman, M. M., Wickramaratne, P., Martin, J., & Samoilov, A. (1994). Modification of interpersonal psychotherapy with depressed adolescents (IPT-A): Phase I and II studies. *Journal of the American Academic of Child and Adolescent Psychiatry, 33,* 695–705.

National Center for Health Statistics Advance Report of Final Mortality Statistics, 1991. (1992). *Monthly Vital Statistics Report.* Hyattsville, MD: Public Health Service, 40(13).

National Mental Health Association. (1989). *Report of the invisible children project.* Alexandria, VA: Author.

Orbach, I., Gross, Y., & Glaubman, H. (1981). Some common characteristics of latency-age suicidal children: Tentative model based on case study analyses. *Suicide and Life Threatening Behavior, 11,* 3.

Patros, P. G., & Shamoo, T. K. (1989). *Depression and suicide in children and adolescents.* Boston: Allyn & Bacon.

Pecora, P. J., & Conroyd, M. K. (1982). Child and mental health services. In M. J. Austin & W. E. Hershey (Eds.), *Handbook on mental health administration* (pp. 556–577). San Francisco: Jossey-Bass.

Pfeffer, C. R. (1986). *The suicidal child.* New York: Guilford Press.

Pfeffer, C. R., Klerman, G. L., Hurt, S. W., Kakuma, T., Peskin, J. R., & Siefker, C. A., (1993). Suicidal children grow up: Rates and psychosocial risk factors for suicide attempts during follow-up. *Journal of American Academy of Child and Adolescent Psychiatry, 30,* 106–113.

Pfeiffer, S. I., & Strzelecki, S. (1990). Inpatient treatment of children and adolescents: A review of outcome studies. *Journal of the American Academy of Child and Adolescent Psychiatry, 29,* 847–853.

Poznanski, E. O., Grossman, J. A., Buchsbaum, Y., Banegas, M., Freeman, L., & Gibbons, R. (1984). Preliminary studies of the reliability and validity of children's depression rating scale. *Journal of American Academic of Child Psychiatry, 23,* 191–197.

Puig-Antich, J., Blau, S., Marx, N., Breengill, L., & Chambers, S. W. (1978). Prepubertal major depressive disorder: A pilot study. *Journal of the American Academy of Child Psychiatry, 21,* 545.

Rappley, M. (1999). Diagnosis and treatment of ADHD in children ages 3 years and younger. *Archives of Pediatric and Adolescent Medicine, 3,* 187–194.

Reynolds, W. M. (1988). Major depression. In M. Hersen & C. G. Last (Eds.), *Child behavior therapy case book* (pp. 85–100). New York: Plenum Press.

Reynolds, W. M. (1994). Assessment of depression in children and adolescence by self-report questionnaires. In W. M. Reynolds & H. F. Johnston (Eds.), *Handbook of depression in children and adolescents* (pp. 209–233). New York: Plenum Press.

Reynolds, W. M., & Coats, K. I. (1986). A comparison cognitive behavioral therapy and relaxation training for the treatment of depression in adolescence. *Journal of Consulting and Clinical Psychology, 54,* 653–666.

Reynolds, W. M., & Johnston, H. F. (Eds.). (1994). *Handbook of depression of children and adolescents.* New York: Plenum Press.

Reynolds, C., & Kamphaus, R. (1992). *Behavior assessment system for children–manual.* Circle Pines, MN: American Guidance Service.

Robins, L. N., & Regier, D. A. (1991). *Psychiatric disorders in America: The epidemiological catchment area study.* New York: Free Press.

Rohde, P., Lewinsohn, P. M., & Seeley, J. R. (1994). Are adolescents changed by an episode of major depression? *Journal of American Academic Child and Adolescent Psychiatry, 33,* 1289–1298.

Rutter, M. (1986). *The developmental psychopathology of depression: Issues and perspectives.* New York: Guilford Press.

Rutter, M. (1990). Commentary: Some focus on process consideration regarding effects of parental depression on children. *Developmental Psychology, 26,* 60–67.

Sabatino, D. A., & Altizer, E. A. (1998). Services and programs for children with E/BD. In D. A. Sabatino & B. L. Brooks (Eds.), *Contemporary interdisciplinary interventions for children with emotional/behavioral disorders.* (pp. 587–607). Durham, NC: Carolina Academic Press.

Sabatino, D. A., & Vance B. (1999). Comparison of BASC and MMPI-A. *International Journal of Special Education, 2,* 9–18.

Saxe, L., Cross, T., & Silverman, N. (1988). Children's mental health: The gap between what we know and what we do. *American Psychologist, 43,* 800–807.

Shaffer, D. (1974). Suicide in childhood and early adolescence. *Journal of Child Psychiatry, 15,* 275–291.

Sondheimer, D. L., Schoenwald, S. K., & Rowland, M. D. (1994). Alternatives to the hospitalization of youth with a serious emotional disturbance. *Journal of Clinical Child Psychology, 23,* 7–12.

Spitz, R. A., & Wolf, K. M. (1946). Anaclitic depression: An inquiry into the genesis of psychiatric conditions on early childhood. *Psychoanalytic Study of the child, 2,* 313–342.

Stark, K. D., Brookman, C. S., & Frazier, R. (1990). A comprehensive school based treatment program for depressed children. *School Psychology Quarterly, 5,* 111–140.

Stark, K. D., Reynolds, W. M., & Kaslow, N. (1987). A comparison of the relative efficacy of self control therapy and behavioral problem solving for depression in children. *Journal of Abnormal Child Psychology, 15,* 91–113.

Tuma, J. (1989). Mental health services for children: The state of the art. *American Psychologist, 44,* 188–199.

Turkington, C. (1983). Child suicide: An unspoken tragedy. *American Psychological Association Monitor, 14,* 15.

Wallerstein, J. S. (1991). The long-term effects of divorce on children: A review. *American Journal of Child and Adolescent Psychiatry, 30,* 346–360.

Watkins, J. T., Leber, W. R., Imber, S. D., Collins, J. F., Elkin, I., Pilkonis, P. A., Sotsky, S. M., Shea, M. T., & Glass, D. R. (1993). Temporal course of change in depression. *Journal of Consulting and Clinical Psychology, 61,* 858–864.

Weinberg, W. A., Rutman, J., Sullivan, L., Penick, E. C., & Dietz, S. G. (1973). Depression in children referred to an educational diagnostic center: Diagnosis and treatment. *Journal of Pediatrics, 83,* 1065.

Weissman, M. M., Leaf, P. J., & Tischler, K. J. (1988). Affective disorders in five United States communities. *Psychological Medicine, 18,* 141–153.

Weissman, M. M., Leckman, J. R., Merikangas, K. R., Jammon, G. D., & Prusoff, B. A. (1984). Depression and anxiety disorders in parents and children: Results from the Yale Family Study. *Archives of General Psychiatry, 41,* 845–852.

Weissman, M. M., & Markowitz, J. C. (1994). Interpersonal psychotherapy: Current status. *Archives of General Psychiatry, 51*(8), 599–606.

Weisz, J. R., Weiss, B., & Donenberg, G. R. (1992). The lab versus the clinic: Effects of child and adolescent psychotherapy. *American Psychologist, 47,* 1578–1585.

Weisz, J. R., Weiss, B., Han, S. S., Granger, D. A., & Morton, T. (1995). Effects of psychotherapy with children and adolescents revisited: A meta-analysis of treatment outcome studies. *Psychological Bulletin, 117,* 450–468.

Wilkes, T. C. R., Belshwer, G., & Rush, A. J. (1994). *Cognitive therapy for depressed adolescents.* New York: Guilford Press.

Wolk, S. I., & Weissman, M. M. (1996). Suicidal behavior in depressed children grown up: Preliminary results of a longitudinal study. *Psychiatric Annuals, 26,* 331–335.

Chapter 17

SOCIALLY AND EMOTIONALLY MALADJUSTED YOUTH

KENNETH M. ROGERS AND JASJEET K. MIGLANI

INTRODUCTION

Beginning with attempts by Kanner (1935) and later the American Psychiatric Association in its *Diagnostic and Statistical Manual of Mental Disorders,* researchers and clinicians who treat children and adolescents have attempted to label behaviors that cause problems in childhood. This is most often done to develop a treatment strategy or a prognosis based on current research findings. Although these labels do not always fully describe the problems with which youth suffer, they provide a common starting place for our discussion. For the purposes of this chapter, we will use *DSM-IV* terminology (American Psychiatric Association, 1994).

The United States is at a crossroads in determining what to do with children who suffer from emotional problems. During the early days of this country, children were viewed largely as the property of their parents, who were responsible for all aspects of the child's life. The majority of all of the child's waking hours were spent in the presence of his or her parents, usually on a farm. There was a great deal of room for the patient to be expressive without needing to constrain the child's behavior. The latitude in behavior that was allowed due to the open space and the lack of restraints served to benefit youth who had behavioral difficulties. As our society has progressed from being a largely agrarian society to being an industrial society, we have experienced a number of changes that have affected our children and our expectations. As we have begun living in smaller spaces in larger cities, youth who may have once been considered active may now be considered hyperactive. Further, the increased stress associated with adolescence has placed youth at greater risk for emotional difficulties.

A number of sociocultural issues have a direct effect on the development of emotional and behavioral problems. Among these are child maltreatment, poverty, and increased exposure to violence. It is estimated that 3 million children are the victims of maltreatment each year in the United States (National Committee to Prevent Child Abuse, 1995). Physical abuse has been linked to many psychiatric disorders, including posttraumatic stress disorder, depression, conduct disorder, attention-deficit/hyperactivity disorder, and poor social functioning (United States Public Health Service, 1999). Psychological maltreatment is believed to occur more often than physical maltreatment and is associated with depression, conduct disorder, and delinquency (United States Public Health Service, 1999). This type of treatment also impairs social and cognitive functioning.

The number of youth living in poverty has increased substantially in the past 10 years. Currently there are 13.2 million youth in this country who are living in poverty, and 4.9 of them are under age 6 (National Center for Children in Poverty, 1999). Ten percent of America's young children live in extreme poverty, in families with incomes of less than 50 percent of the poverty line. (In 1997, the extreme poverty line was $6,401 for a family of three.) The extreme poverty rate among young children is growing faster than the young child poverty rate. Research indicates that extreme poverty during the first five years of life has especially deleterious effects on children's future life chances compared to less extreme poverty experienced later in childhood. Extreme poverty leads to malnourishment at a time when the basic structure of the central nervous system is under development. Without adequate nutrition, these youth are at risk for neural underdevelopment, which leads to future learning difficulties, behavioral problems, and impaired development of cognitive skills.

The Surgeon General, as a result of the rapid increase that we have seen in violence in the past several years, declared violence a public health issue. Youth violence has been the area that has received the greatest increase, with a 60% increase in youth committing violent acts (OJJDP, 1996). Many of the victims of this violence are adolescents, with 20% of all violent crime victims being from this age group (Snyder and Sickmund, 1995). The late 1990s have seen a proliferation of cases that have spotlighted horrific violence directed at youth. It is not uncommon to hear youth describe feelings of being unsafe. In a recent study, 50% of youth reported having witnessed a violent act directed toward a friend or family member, and 29% of the youth in a juvenile corrections population had actually witnessed the murder of someone close to them (Vander Stoep, 2000). Witnessing such events place youth at risk for the development of anxiety disorders, such as posttraumatic stress disorder, and depressive disorders.

Approximately 20% of youths in the United States will suffer from an emotional/behavioral problem at some point during their childhood or adolescence. Unfortunately, treatment services for these youth are often unavailable because of lack of services or the inability to pay for such services. Despite the fact that children and adolescents are served by multiple systems (school, social services, health, etc.), these systems are not often equipped with the ability to recognize these problems. Once the problems are identified, there is no clear idea of what to do at that point; thus many teachers and parents may feel frustrated with identifying and accessing services for these youths. Consequently, the unmet needs in this population of youths is astounding. The lack of mental health treatment for these youths can have significant implications for their future development and mental health. Youths with unrecognized and untreated behavioral problems have higher levels of adult behavioral pathology and increased contact with the juvenile justice system.

HISTORICAL OVERVIEW AND CURRENT TRENDS

Our modern understanding of social and emotional adjustment in youths dates back to Josef Breuer's treatment of Anna O, who presented with a number of hysterical symptoms, related to the death of her father, in the 1880s. The treatment modality that was employed, psychoanalysis, was further developed by Sigmund Freud and served as the cornerstone for our understanding of mental illness from the time of its development until competing psychological and biological theories were developed in the early to mid-1900s. Although a better understanding of behavior was developed, psychiatric treatment was in its infancy and was available to only a few wealthy individuals in very confined areas of the world. Youth from families of modest means were afforded little opportunity even if very serious illness existed. There was a large reliance on community, religion, and state hospitalbased services, which offered more warehousing than actual treatment. Prior to the development of psychotropic drugs beginning with Thorazine in 1959, there was little useful treatment offered to psychiatric patients.

The development of the recognition of mental illness and the development of mental health treatment services for youths are a relatively recent advancement in American medicine. Prior to 1800, there was little recognition and understanding of mental illness. The United States was a new country and the health care system poorly developed. Beginning in the early 1800s, there was recognition that there were youths that suffered from emotional and behavioral problems. Problems that youths experienced were typically blamed on the family of origin, particularly the mother. The overriding issue at the time was how to conceptualize the behaviors of these youths. Many viewed behavioral problems as medical problems in need of treatment, whereas others viewed them as deviant behaviors in need of punishment. Treatment, as it existed, consisted mainly of warehousing youths in large institutional settings, which sometimes housed children and adults, criminals and noncriminals, and mentally ill and nonmentally ill individuals. Many youths were exploited for cheap labor and were commonly abused in these settings.

In New York in 1825, the "Houses of Refuge" were initially developed. These facilities, which had spread to 40 states by 1850, focused on treating and rehabilitating wayward youths. This was a step forward in that these facilities were for youths and not adults. Their size was also much smaller, with the average population being around 210 youths. The principles were based on benevolence and compassion and tended to focus on youths that were runaways or were incorrigible. Discipline was strict, and corporal punishment and meal deprivation were not uncommon. Although there was not a specific mental health component to the treatment program, school, church, and job training became standard portions of the treatment program. Unfortunately, families were forced to give up control of their children and were not allowed to participate in the rearing of their children.

By the mid-1800s there was a rudimentary appreciation for mental health principles in the American medical community. The American Psychiatric Association was founded in 1844. There was, for the first time, recognition that there were causal factors that affected behavior. Treatment in hospitals began to reflect the new appreciation for these causal factors, and treatment became more scientific. By the 1920s there was a greater understanding of the link between mental illness and emotional and behavioral problems. The emphasis on diagnosis and treatment of specific illnesses became more widespread. Treatment modalities such as group therapy and individual therapy became more common.

However, the development of treatment services for mentally ill youths lagged significantly behind that for mentally ill adults. There was no significant widespread integration of treatment services for youth prior to 1969, when the Joint Commission on Mental Health of Children (1969) issued its report *Crisis in Child Mental Health: Challenge for the 1970s.* The report asserted that there was probably no community in the country that provided an acceptable level of services for mentally ill children. The commission developed a comprehensive model for appropriate treatment services for this population. As a result of advocacy effort, the National Institute of Mental Health developed the Child and Adolescent Service System Program (CASSP) in 1983. The goal of the CASSP was to improve the system of service delivery to children and adolescents. The CASSP represented one of the first efforts to identify emotionally and behaviorally disturbed youths in a systematic and coordinated manner and to provide appropriate treatment services to these youths.

Although the psychological and biological underpinnings of many psychiatric disturbances had been identified, the 1980s ushered in the realization that many mentally ill youths continued to receive no psychiatric treatment. Many of these found themselves detained in the juvenile justice system. It has been estimated that as many as 60% of youths in the juvenile justice system suffer from an emotional disability (Otto, Greenstein, Johnson, & Friedman, 1992). Historically, these youths have posed a difficult problem for both the mental health and juvenile justice systems. These youths have been described as "mad" and "bad," both delinquent and mentally ill. Sadly, we know very little about this population, except that there is a great deal of unmet mental health care need in because most correctional facilities do not have adequate mental health services. Add in issues of race and ethnicity and the picture becomes even more dismal.

CLINICAL ASSESSMENT PROCESS: DIAGNOSIS AND TREATMENT

The clinical assessment of children and adolescents requires interviewing and gathering information from multiple sources, including the youths, parents, and the family, in order be comprehensive. Information on the youth's school performance, health status, and the result of standardized testing is essential. Because few clinician visits are initiated by the youth, it is important to ascertain the reason why the youth is being referred for evaluation and who is referring the youth for evaluation. The primary sources of information may vary based upon the age of the youth as well as his or her current living situation.

Parents

Parents are able to provide a developmental perspective on their children, including prenatal and perinatal history. Parents can provide the most comprehensive information on the child's prior medical and psychiatric history. The family's recollection of early developmental milestones and temperament provide insight into the temporal relation of current problems to the developmental course in the child. A parental and family psychiatric history will aid in assessing the youth's risk for psychiatric illness. The parents conceptualization of the child's problem and their expectations about treatment should be explored so that appropriate evaluation and treatment strategies can be developed that involve the child and the family.

School

Most school-aged children will spend an average of seven hours each weekday in an academic setting. During this time there is ample opportunity to observe many aspects of the child's behavior that may not be observed at home. These include interaction with other children, approaches to novel situations, frustration tolerance, and psychiatric symptoms that may be manifested more readily in a structured setting. Additionally, teachers are trained to teach children of a specific age and interact with children of this age on a daily basis; thus they are more likely to notice minor variations in children of the same age more quickly than parents, especially those who may have no older children. Although most teachers are burdened by the responsibility of educating many youths, most are willing to provide specific information on an individual child because it enables them to teach that child as well as other children more effectively because of the improvement to the classroom environment.

Child

The interview of a child or adolescent will vary depending on the developmental level of the youth. To conduct an interview effectively, the clinician must have an understanding of normal development and its associated milestones. For example, physically aggressive behaviors in a 3-year-old would be interpreted differently than the same behaviors in a 16-year-old.

Young children must often be interviewed along with their parents because they may feel very uncomfortable being away from their parents. This interview will focus more on the interaction between the parent and the child and will assess the parent-child relationship and the ability of the parent to provide a safe, loving environment for the child. The child's level of functioning can be assessed by observation of child behaviors as well as by using more standardized measures of behavior and development. Direct assessment of the infant during play can assist in determining the youth's ability to engage in imaginative or symbolic play.

School-aged children are usually able to engage in more direct conversation with the examiner. Some children may be unable to do so because of shyness, oppositional behavior, or communication difficulties. These youth will sometimes need to be approached in a manner similar to that for a young child. Because most school-aged children have been accustomed to spending 45 minutes to an hour in class daily, most are able to tolerate an interview of similar length if approached in an age-appropriate manner. The initial goal with children of this age is to establish good rapport and to make them feel comfortable in the interview setting. This may be accomplished by beginning with unstructured play and moving into a more focused interview as the hour progresses. The interview should begin with more open-ended questions and move to more multiple-choice and yes/no questions, as they become necessary. Activities that allow for more activity, such as drawing a house or family, may allow the child to remain more engaged for the evaluation period. Some games such as the *Thinking Feeling Doing*

Game may allow for a discussion of feelings in a manner that is nonthreatening for the child.

Because of their developmental level, the interview with the adolescent may provide as much or more information than other informants. As with all other youth, the initial goal of an evaluation with an adolescent is the establishment of rapport. The adolescent should be thanked for his or her participation, and ground rules for the evaluation should be clearly established. One of the primary concerns of most adolescents is confidentiality. The clinician should assure them that this would be the case unless they are ethically required to reveal specific information (suicidal or homicidal thoughts or dangerous behaviors). This will allow the adolescent to share information in a more honest manner. The clinician must be open to hearing what the adolescent is saying, even if it is contradictory to the thoughts of the clinician or the parents. Many adolescents may be angry or openly hostile because they may feel coerced into the evaluation by their parents or other adults. The interviewer must be able to diffuse this anger to complete the evaluation. As with all mental health evaluations, suicidal and homicidal ideation, dangerousness, substance use, sexual relationships, and psychosis must be explored.

Instruments

The assessment of children and adolescents is a complex task. Clinicians are often asked to determine a diagnosis, coping style, and strengths and weaknesses of a child in an hour to an hour and a half. This is an especially difficult task given that youths cannot often provide this information given the constraints of their developmental level or their emotional/behavioral disturbance. It is often difficult to assess the youth across multiple settings (i.e., school, home, community) in a meaningful way because it is often not feasible to have an extended evaluation with teachers or childcare providers. One method for obtaining a broader assessment of the child is the use of rating instruments and diagnostic interviews.

Rating scales are often a very useful means of obtaining objective data about a child's behavior from another individual. These rating scales may focus on an individual diagnostic category such as attention-deficit/hyperactivity disorder (ADHD) or may focus on broader measures of emotional or behavioral disturbance. At present, the most widely used broad measure is the Child Behavior Checklist (CBCL), which was developed by Achenbach and Edelbrock (1983). The CBCL provides scores on three domains: internalizing, externalizing, and total scores. Within each of these domains are several subscales. There are many advantages of the instrument. The first is that it was standardized on a very large population, which means that the frequency distribution for each symptom, as well as total symptom scores, is known. The instrument is highly reliable and resistant to informant bias. Second, the instrument can be used on a wide age range of individuals: ages 4 to 21. Third, there are multiple informant versions of the instrument so that information may be obtained from the youth, parent, or teacher. Finally, the length of the questionnaire is not unduly long given the amount of information obtained. In our experience, the informant can usually complete the form in 20 to 25 minutes.

Three other instruments that have similar uses include the Revised Behavior Problem Checklist (Quay, 1983; Quay and Peterson, 1983), the Conners' Parent Checklist, 1973), and the Global Assessment Scale (Spitzer, Gibson, & Endicott, 1973). A more recently developed instrument is the Scale for Assessing Emotional Disturbance (SAED; Epstein and Cullinan, 1998). Unlike the others, this scale was developed primarily for the identification of youths who qualify for the federal education category Emotional Disturbance and thus may be more limited in its generalizability to other settings.

The purpose of broad range instruments is to provide a screen for behavioral problems, but they give relatively little information on a specific diagnostic category or may be too long given the very focused information that may be desired by the clinician. For these types of situations, a diagnosis-specific instrument may be most useful. Some of the more widely used instruments for the most common childhood disorders are outlined in Table 17.1. The most widely used instrument in the Conners Parent Rating Scale. This is a 48-item scale that covers a wide range of symptoms associated with both ADHD and conduct disorder.

Many of the childhood rating scales have been adapted for use with children and adolescents from adult scales. The most notable examples of these are the Children's Depression Inventory (CDI) and the revised version of the Beck Depression Inventory, which were both based on the original Beck Depression Inventory. The Children's Depression Rating Scale was developed from the Hamilton Rating Scale for Depression (Hamilton, 1967). Unlike for depressive disorders, there have been relatively few scales developed for anxiety disorders. The most popular scale at present is the Children's Manifest Anxiety Scale, which was also developed from an adult scale.

The initial use of diagnostic instruments was for research purposes. The primary purpose was to allow information needed to make a diagnosis to be collected in a systematic manner without having to do exhaustive clinical interviews. These instruments increase the consistency of information gathered as well as reliability by removing the interpretation of clinicians that might interpret diagnostic information in different ways. Diagnostic instruments are of two types, structured and semistructured. Structured instruments are developed in a manner that does not allow for clinical judgment. The questions are worded in a particular manner on the interview form or on the computer screen and should be followed by the interviewer, who has little latitude to exercise clinical judgment. This offers the advantage of allowing the use of nonclinical interviewers who have been trained in the administration of the test. The disadvantage of these instruments is the assumption that they do not allow the interviewer to scrutinize or question an answer received, even if it is probable that the individual may not fully understand the question. The most widely used structured instruments are the Diagnostic Interview Schedule for Children (DISC; Costello, Edelbrock & Dulcan, 1984) and the Diagnostic Interview for Children and Adolescents (DICA, Herjanic & Campbell, 1977; Herjanic & Reich, 1982).

Semistructured instruments such as the Child Schedule for Affective Disorders and Schizophrenia (K-SADS; Ambrosini, Metz, Prabucki, & Lee, 1995; Chambers, Puig-Antich, & Hirsch, 1985) offer an alternative approach to the more structured interviews. In these instruments, phrasing is suggested, but the interviewer has the latitude to change the wording to increase patient understanding. Each individual criterion needed for the diagnosis can be scrutinized and evaluated. These instruments offer the

Table 17.1   Commonly Used Rating Scales for Most Prevalent Childhood Psychiatric Disorders

Attention-Deficit/Hyperactivity Disorder

Conners Parent Rating Scale	Goyette et al., 1978
New York Teachers Rating Scale	Miller at al., 1995
Eyeberg Child Behavior Inventory	Eyeberg and Ross, 1978
Self Control Rating Scale	Kendell and Wilcox, 1979

Depressive Disorders

Children's Depression Inventory	Kovacs and Beck, 1977
Beck Depression Inventory	Beck, 1978
Children's Depression Rating Scale	Pozanski et al., 1979, 1984

Anxiety Disorders

Children's Manifest Anxiety Scale	Castenada et al., 1956
Hamilton Anxiety Rating Scale	Clark and Donon, 1994
Yale-Brown Obsessive-Compulsive Scale	Goodman et al., 1989; Riddle et al., 1990
Leyton Obsessional Inventory	Cooper, 1970

advantage of obtaining more reliable information from individuals, but they have the disadvantage of requiring a trained clinician to administer, because a good understanding of the diagnostic system is required.

DIAGNOSIS AND FORMULATION

The source of psychiatric disturbances and behavioral difficulties in socially and emotionally maladjusted youths varies widely and encompasses several diagnostic categories, including substance use and disruptive mood, anxiety, and psychotic disorders. These disorders vary widely in their ages of onset and initial clinical manifestations. In many cases, these disorders may be antecedents to the adjustment, in other cases, the maladjustment may be a precipitant for the development of psychiatric conditions. This section will not attempt to cover all psychiatric disorders, as most are covered elsewhere in this volume in much greater detail, but we will focus on those disorders that are most related to social and emotional maladjustment.

Substance Abuse Disorders

The substance abuse disorders are among the most complex of all psychiatric disorders because of their relationship to other psychiatric symptoms, which they may induce or mask. For example, the abuse of substances can cause mood, anxiety, psychotic, or sleep disorders in individuals who do not otherwise have these disorders. Additionally, substance abuse can lead to cognitive and neurological impairments. On the other hand, many anxious individuals report that their symptoms are relieved as long as they are under the influence of their substance of choice.

Substance abuse disorders are divided into two categories: substance abuse and sub-

stance dependence. Substance abuse is characterized by the presence of at least one specific symptom that indicates that substance use has interfered with the individual's life
for at least a 12-month period. These symptoms include failure to fulfill major role
obligations, recurrent use in physically hazardous situations, recurrent legal problems,
and continued use despite social or interpersonal problems. Substance dependence is
the term that describes a much more severe substance use problem. Dependence is
characterized by the presence of at least three symptoms, which include physical symptoms such as tolerance and withdrawal experiences. The criteria also include behavioral
symptoms, such as increased use over time, inability to cut down on use, social and occupational impairment, and the continuation of use despite ongoing problems. Most
individuals who meet the criteria for dependence have a history of prior substance
abuse. Most children and adolescents have a relatively short history of substance abuse
and are less likely to have progressed to substance dependence.

Present data suggest that 21% of high school seniors had used alcohol in the last
month, and 8% had used marijuana (NIDA, 1996; SAMHSA, 1996). These estimates
do not include the high school dropout segment of this population, which is 15% to
20%; thus, the actual rate of use in this population is significantly higher. The impact of
adolescent substance abuse can be difficult to measure. Substance use has been found
to be related to an increased risk of human immunodeficiency virus/acquired immune
deficiency syndrome (HIV/AIDS) and other sexually transmitted diseases, such as gon-
orrhea, chlamydia, and human papilloma virus (HPV/genital warts). The increase in
sexual activity that is associated with adolescent substance abuse also places adolescents at risk for unwanted pregnancies. Approximately 20% of pregnant females who
abuse substances are adolescents who will often continue to abuse substances throughout their pregnancies (Pfefferbaum, 1997). This places the youth and the fetus at increased risk for prenatal and perinatal complications. Delivering a child during adolescence will have a significant impact on the social development of young females, who
often find themselves more socially isolated, and there is an increase in the number of
psychosocial stressors for the girls as compared with older women (Pfefferbaum, 1991).

Substance-abusing youths are also placed at increased risk for juvenile crime and
dangerous/self-injurious behavior. Furthermore, youths that abuse substances are less
likely to engage in academic pursuits and positive activities that will benefit them in
later life. The social contacts that are developed by adolescent substance abusers are
more likely to be other individuals who are engaged in similar behavior; therefore there
is an increased social benefit from continuing substance abuse and antisocial behaviors.
While youths are under the influence of substances, they are likely to commit acts that
they would have otherwise not engaged. Between 30% and 50% of youth in the juvenile
justice system were under the influence at the time that their offense was committed.

Mood Disorders

Perhaps more than all other psychiatric disorders, mood disorders have received increased attention over the past several years. It has only been 30 years since the existence of childhood depression was officially acknowledged, and it has been only in the
past 20 years that there have been significant advancements in the identification and as-

sessment of youths with bipolar disorder. Other mood disorders, including cyclothymia and dysthymia, have received little study in children.

The development of language skills and the ability to convey a mood state adequately has caused difficulty in recognizing mood disorders in young children. The ability to use language to relay information reliably to others is not present until a child is approximately 7 years of age. The ability to identify a mood state occurs later in many children, and many may not be able to describe a mood adequately until 10 years of age. This inability to acquire diagnostic information from the child has forced clinicians to depend on information from parents and rating scales, which may not provide a complete clinical picture.

Major depressive disorder is the most commonly described mood disorder in children. According to the *DSM-IV* (APA, 1994), individuals must have five out of nine symptoms for at least a two-week period. Necessary symptoms include (a) depressed or irritable mood and (b) a loss of interest or pleasure. The remaining criteria, of which four must be present, include disturbance in sleep, disturbance in appetite, feelings of worthlessness or inappropriate guilt, loss of energy, psychomotor agitation or retardation, decreased concentration, and recurrent thoughts of death. These symptoms must produce academic or social impairment.

The presentation of symptoms will vary depending on the age of the child. Young children are more likely to present with an irritable mood and somatic complaints as compared to a depressed mood, anhedonia, and feelings of hopelessness, which are seen in later adolescence and adulthood. These symptoms are likely to impact the child's desire and ability to engage in activities at both home and school. Because of the irritability and possible associated psychomotor agitation, many children may be identified more often as behavioral problems in school rather than as depressed individuals. Difficulty with concentration and impaired ability to follow through with academic tasks may place the youth at risk for falling behind on schoolwork. If symptoms persist over an extended time period, peer relations and social development may be negatively impacted. Thus many youth with primary affective difficulties may progress secondarily toward disruptive behavioral disorders.

The risk of suicide remains an issue in children and adolescents. There is little data on suicide in young children, although it is a problem that does occur. Because of a societal belief that children do not commit suicide, deaths of young children are often ruled as accidents even when they are the results of successful suicide attempts. In the case of older adolescents, suicide is the second leading cause of death behind accidents. Most youths who successfully commit suicide send a message to others of their feelings of wanting to die. It becomes incumbent upon mental health professionals to explore any thoughts of self-harm with youths and to take necessary steps to keep them safe.

Disruptive Disorders

No child psychiatric diagnosis has received as much attention and been as hotly debated in both the lay press and the psychiatric literature as much as ADHD and the other Disruptive Disorders, which include Oppositional Defiant Disorder (ODD) and Conduct Disorder (CD). ADHD continues to be one of the most common reasons for referral to child psychiatrists. Conservative estimates of the prevalence of ADHD are 3% to 5%, and boys have a greater incidence with a 3 : 1 to 5 : 1 ratio of boys to girls. Prevalence estimates of ODD and CD are less clear due to changes in diagnostic criteria in recent years. Most sources estimate the prevalence to be between 5% and 20%.

ADHD is characterized by an inappropriate attention span or by hyperactive/impulsive behaviors. The symptoms must be present for a six-month period and must begin by age 7. Many youth have only attention symptoms, which include (a) difficulty sustaining attention, (b) not seeming to listen when spoken to, (c) not following through on instructions, (d) having difficulty organizing tasks, (e) avoiding activities that require sustained mental effort, (f) often losing things necessary for tasks, (g) being easily distracted, and (h) being forgetful. In most situations, these youths receive relatively little attention because they cause few behavioral problems. Youths who have predominantly hyperactive/impulsive symptoms—fidgetiness, difficulty remaining seated, difficulty playing quietly, excessive motor movement, excessive talkativeness, intrusiveness, and difficulty awaiting turns—tend to garner more attention.

ADHD has no clear etiology. Several variables have an impact on the development of the disorder. No specific brain abnormalities have been associated with ADHD. There is speculation that there are subclinical brain insults that occur as a result of prenatal or perinatal insults, toxic exposures, or prematurity. The fact that children with hyperactive siblings or parents are more likely to have ADHD supports the assertion that there may be a genetic component to the disorder. The role of psychosocial factors is unclear. Youths who have prolonged emotional deprivation are more likely to display hyperactivity and poor attention spans. When placed in situations where there is more emotional nurturing, these symptoms tend to diminish. Ongoing stressors that produce anxiety are also likely to cause hyperactivity and inattention and may be a factor in perpetuating the symptoms. Some youths respond in this way to a situation that requires a very structured routine. There does not appear to be a relationship between socioeconomic status and ADHD.

ODD is a pattern of negativistic, hostile, and defiant behaviors that last at least 6 months. Symptoms include frequent loss of temper and arguments with adults, being frequently angry and spiteful, blaming other for mistakes, deliberately annoying people, and refusing to comply with adult requests. One of the difficulties with making a diagnosis of ODD is that many youths have symptoms consistent with the disorder, but because of the environment, the behaviors may be interpreted in a more positive manner than in other environments. Depending on the child's developmental level, these symptoms may be normal and adaptive and must be differentiated from more pathological situations in which the symptoms may produce more social and academic impairment. In about one quarter of youths, symptoms will spontaneously remit. In others, symptoms will remain stable, or the youths will begin to violate the rights of others, leading to a diagnosis of conduct disorder.

The essential feature of CD is a repetitive and persistent disorder in which the basic rights of others or other major age-appropriate societal norms or rules are violated. Symptoms do not occur spontaneously but evolve over time until there is a consistent pattern of aggression toward people and animals, destruction of property, deceitfulness, and violations of rules. Many of these youths fail to develop social attachments and tend to have poor peer relationships. This may lead to further withdrawal and self-isolation. The development of CD has been associated with negative parental attitudes and chaotic home environments. Parental psychopathology and criminality, as well as child abuse and neglect, have also been shown to have an association with the development of symptoms. There has been relatively little research on biological factors related to CD. There is some evidence that there may be an association with decreased noradrenergic functioning and decreased serotonin levels; however, this evidence is inconclusive at present.

Anxiety Disorders

For two reasons, the anxiety disorders are perhaps the most complex set of disorders facing clinicians who treat children and adolescents. First, all humans experience anxiety, which is a feeling of a diffuse, vague, unpleasant apprehension that is often accompanied by autonomic symptoms such as headache, palpitations, sweating, and stomach discomfort. Differentiating feelings of anxiety in an anxious individual from the symptoms of an anxiety disorder can be challenging even for an experienced clinician. There are eight anxiety disorders in *DSM-IV:* separation anxiety disorder, generalized anxiety disorder, specific phobia, social phobia, selective mutism, panic disorder, obsessive compulsive disorder, and posttraumatic stress disorder. We will consider the ones that are most important to child clinicians.

Separation anxiety disorder is the most common anxiety disorder in childhood. The disorder is characterized by developmentally inappropriate and excessive anxiety concerning separation from home or from those to whom the child is attached. Some degree of separation anxiety is part of normal development. For example, the child attending his first day of school is very reluctant to separate from his parents. The disorder occurs when the degree of anxiety is excessive for the child's developmental level and persists for at least a 4-week period. Periods of extreme terror and panic may ensue if the child is left in unfamiliar surroundings and if the primary caregiver is unavailable to provide support. The fear of being separated from the caregiver often leads to further fears and ruminations and an inability to separate from the caregiver. Other anxiety disorder may coexist with separation anxiety disorder.

Posttraumatic Stress Disorder (PTSD) and Acute Stress Disorder are less common in pediatric populations than many of the other anxiety disorders but are of great importance because of the level of morbidity and impairment associated with lack of treatment for the disorder. PTSD is a disorder that is characterized by exposure to a trauma that involved (a) actual or threatened death or serious injury and (b) a response of intense fear, hopelessness, or horror. Reexperiencing the trauma in ways such as dreams, flashbacks, and intrusive thoughts follows this exposure; avoidance of stimuli associated with the trauma and increased arousal are also hallmark features.

Many children in the United States are exposed to violence through communities in which they live or through physical and sexual abuse experienced in the home. Although there are many children at risk for the development of PTSD due to violent exposure, there are no epidemiological studies that examine the prevalence of PTSD in children. In studies where there is a clear trauma, 60% to 100% of children met criteria after 1 year (Pynoos et al., 1987). Traumas that have been previously studied as related to PTSD include criminal assault, combat, bone marrow transplantation, severe burns, and motor vehicle accidents. Violent, life-threatening events that occur in the lives of children may not be recognized as a risk factor in developing PTSD; hence PTSD may not be entertained as a diagnostic possibility for many children, the consequence of which may be sequelae including further behavioral acting out, depression, and future victimization.

CLINICAL CASE STUDY

Youths with emotional and behavioral problems usually do not fit into a single diagnostic category or have a simple mental health history. Often these are youths that have a long history of family dysfunction and have often been in multiple out-of-home placements (residential treatment centers, group homes, and foster care). Traumatic histories including physical and sexual abuse are not uncommon. In this section, we will present two cases that are representative of these youth: one of a child and the other of an adolescent.

Case 1

The patient is a 16-year-old girl who was admitted to a residential facility after setting fire to a bed mattress at her foster home. She stated that the reason for setting the fire was to "get away from those people who were smothering me," referring to her foster parents. The patient had been placed in foster care at age 10 due to sexual abuse at the hands of her father as well as maternal alcohol abuse. Since that time, she has been in six foster homes. These placements were usually disrupted by the patient's becoming physically aggressive toward the foster family or through sexual acting out behavior, usually directed toward older males. She also had four previous psychiatric hospital admissions, three admissions to residential treatment facilities, and has been placed at two group homes. Her prior psychiatric diagnoses have included bipolar disorder, conduct disorder, major depressive disorder, and alcohol abuse.

The patient described her symptoms as having begun around age 8, when she began feeling sad more days than not. She related this to her inability to do well academically in school and her inability to make friends. She was a self-described loner. Her home life was very chaotic. Her parents only loosely supervised her and her younger brother. Her mother was intoxicated most of the time, but in the patient's words "tried to be a good mother." Her father left home when she was 3 years old but returned when she was 8, and "life became a living hell." Her behavior became significantly worse in school, which ended with her threatening a peer with a knife. This led to her being arrested and sent to a juvenile detention facility at age 11.

During her time at the detention facility, her depressive symptoms worsened, because she "really missed my mom and my brother." She had a near-fatal suicide attempt in the detention center and was transferred to a psychiatric unit in a general hospital. She was started on an antidepressant and received both individual and group psychotherapy. During one of her therapy sessions, her history of sexual abuse was disclosed, and the allegations were reported to the department of social services. Following a social services investigation of the allegations, which found that the abuse had happened, the patient was removed from her parents custody. She was placed in a residential treatment center for approximately 6 months, followed by 8 months in a group home. Upon discharge she was admitted to her first foster care placement. Her depressive symptoms remitted, but the patient's behavioral symptoms and her abuse of alcohol, marijuana, and amphetamines appeared to escalate. She began working as a prostitute to pay for the substances. She was expelled from school in the eighth grade following a series of fights. After 6 months, the foster parents ended her placement after she ran away and could not be found for 4 days. She was located 300 miles away in another state.

Her mother became concerned about reuniting with her daughter and complied with the recommendation of substance abuse treatment and parenting classes. The patient was allowed to return home, where her behavior improved substantially. The period of stability for both mother and daughter lasted for approximately 6 months but then began to deteriorate when the parents divorced and the mother began dating another man who also attempted to assault the patient sexually in the home. Social services again intervened, and the patient was placed back in state custody.

The patient has been placed in several group homes, residential treatment facilities, and foster homes. Her behavior has been consistently problematic in each of these settings. Intermittently, she will have periods where there are few behavioral symptoms, mandatory drug screens will be negative, and sexual acting out is minimal. These usually occur during periods where her mother is doing well and she feels that there is a chance for reunification with her mother and brother.

Discussion

Behavioral disturbances in adolescence is usually not a spontaneous occurrence but is usually the result of years of problem behavior associated with family, school, and community problems. Problem behaviors are often maintained by ongoing problems within the family system. Additionally, many youths suffer from mental illnesses that impact on their functional ability. The behavioral problems cause individuals to view these youths through a punishment mode, which does not address the underlying issues that are impacting behavior. The lack of stable parenting figures and the unavailability of extended family leave the school as one of the only places that may have the opportunity to identify youths that are at risk for serious emotional and behavioral problems. It is not uncommon for many emotionally disturbed youths to spend a great deal of time in out-of-home placements. Even in the highest quality group homes and residential settings, the nurturing that developing children need to develop emotionally is often unavailable. The primary factor that determines a child's ability to develop good future relationships is the ability to form a close relationship with a primary caretaker.

Case 2

The patient is a 7-year-old male who was bought into the clinic by his foster mother and social services caseworker at the insistence of his first grade teacher. A note from the teacher indicated that the child had been spitting on other children, had intermittent periods of aggression toward the teacher, and was constantly running around the classroom. She also stated that he was behind academically and indicated that he would not pass the second grade.

The foster mother reported a history of problems that began at birth. The patient was born 6 weeks prematurely to a mother who abused alcohol and cocaine throughout her pregnancy. He spent the first month of his life in the neonatal intensive care unit prior to going home. He did not walk until about age 3 and did not begin speaking clearly until age 4. He was described as a relatively easy child who was rarely fussy. Behavioral symptoms first became prominent when he started in a nursery school at age 3. He was discharged from the nursery after 3 months due to physically aggressive behavior—biting and hitting—toward peers. He was placed in another nursery that was able to control his behavior until he began public kindergarten at age 4. His behavior continued at the same level of intensity until this referral. He has been diagnosed with fetal alcohol syndrome and ADHD in the past. He has been treated with stimulants and behavioral shaping strategies at the local mental health center.

The child has been in the custody of the current foster mother for 6 months. Prior to that time, he had been living with his grandmother, who was functioning as a foster mother. The patient's biological mother left the home when he was 6 months old and has not been in his life consistently since that time. The grandmother has significant medical problems and stated that she loves her grandson but will not be able to rear him due to her poor health. There are no other family members willing to care for the child, and it is likely that he will continue to live in a nonrelative foster care situation.

Discussion

Social and emotional adjustment in young children requires a stable environment and parenting figures in order to gain the sense of trust to be able to explore the environment. Successful individuation and self-development depend in large part on the child's feeling secure. Many youths do not have a stable biological parent, and more grandparents are becoming responsible for parenting their grandchildren. Unfortunately, in many cases these grandparents become elderly or ill or lack the resources and are unable to continue in this role. Thus, many of these children will end up in the foster care system. For youths who display problematic behaviors, multiple foster care placements are not unusual. For vulnerable youth these changes are very destabilizing, and many of these youths are never able to bond appropriately. This lack of attachment can lead to further alienation, social isolation, and problem behaviors.

SPECIFIC REMEDIAL AND TREATMENT APPROACHES

The modalities of treatment used with youths vary depending on the age of the child, diagnosis, severity of the problem, and functional level of the child. The therapist must have an understanding of the child's developmental level in order to treat a child effectively using psychotherapeutic modalities. Because it is often the guardian who has identified a problem and brought the child in for therapy, the child may not feel that a problem exists. The child may view the evaluation as punitive. Many youths with social and emotional problems have been in contact with a lot of "strangers," including social workers, court officers, physicians, and other therapists. The development of a therapeutic relationship under these circumstances may be difficult at best.

The role of the therapist is to provide treatment to the patient that will relieve his pain and suffering. There are many methods of accomplishing this task, and it depends a great deal on the training and experience level of the therapist but is also guided in large part by the needs of the youth. Many schools of psychotherapy promote a more passive approach, whereas others promote a more active approach. In either case, the development of a meaningful therapeutic relationship with the patient will determine the effectiveness of therapy. Although there are many approaches to nonbiological treatment of emotionally disturbed youth, we highlight four that we have found to be most effective with youths: individual, group, family, and multisystemic therapy.

Individual Psychotherapy

Individual psychotherapy is a term that identifies therapy that is done with an individual patient, with the focus being the alleviation of symptoms or personal growth. The types of therapy covered by these terms are numerous and varied in their approaches. They include supportive, psychodynamic, behavioral, and interpersonal approaches. Whatever approach is employed, the therapist must have a thorough understanding of a conceptual framework and its functioning in children. The theory of behavior, be it psychodynamic, behavioral, or developmental, drives the behavior of the therapist during sessions and provides a theoretical framework for interpreting information gleaned during the sessions. Each of these approaches uses specific skills to overcome deficits that youths may face. They may vary depending on the age of the child. For example, the themes of play therapy may drive the relationship between the therapist and a young child.

Group Therapy

Socialization is a major component of problems facing behaviorally disturbed youth. Whether it is impaired social skills or socialization with negative peers, socialization impacts the presentation and resolution of symptoms. The benefit of group therapy is having an adult figure as well as peers who can model behavior and help the youth problem-solve in a safe environment. Groups may be homogenous (specific disorders, gender, age) or may be more heterogeneous. Groups can be beneficial for most youths but must be chosen carefully so that the youth does not become overwhelmed and have a potentially negative experience.

Family Therapy

The problems of youth do not occur in a vacuum, but in the context of community and family. Most often, family therapy is used in combination with individual therapy, because as the youth begins to make positive changes, the family must be able to adapt in order not to sabotage the gains made by the youth. Families are sometimes resistant to therapy and identify the youth as having responsibility for all the problems occurring within the family system. It is only after establishing rapport with the family and approaching the case in a nonblaming manner that many families are able to engage in therapy. It is important to identify the members of the "family." In many cases these do not resemble the traditional family, but may consist of extended family members or even nonrelated individuals who must be invited if the therapy is to be successful.

Multisystemic Therapy

For many years severely behaviorally disturbed youth have been difficult to treat. The traditional treatments described above had short-term success, but this was usually not generalizable to other settings. Multisystemic therapy (MST) is a behavioral system that combines many treatment elements in a systematic manner. MST has been widely studied and researched and appears to be a very promising approach for the treatment of youth with serious behavioral and emotional disturbances (Henggeler et al., 1998).

PSYCHOPHARMACOLOGY

Pediatric psychopharmacology is a relatively young area of research and practice. The first pediatric psychopharmacological agents, the stimulants, were used in 1937. Many mental health professionals retain a strong bias toward using psychotherapy and behavioral therapies as their first line of treatment for most disorders and use psychopharmacological interventions only as their second line. The use of psychotropic medications with children and adolescents is further complicated by a variety of issues, including imprecise diagnostic classification schemes and normal changes in physical characteristics of children as they mature. Also, clinical trials of medications in children are far more expensive and draw from a much smaller subject population. Further, there are heightened concerns about the legal and ethical issues related to experimentation and informed consent in minors. It is the nature of child and adolescent psychopharmacology that the needs of the patients outrun the state of the art. In addition, clear answers to questions regarding long-term treatment for prevention of recurrence or relapse are lacking in the field of pediatric psychopharmacology. Until recently, the psychiatric treatment of children and adolescents has been almost exclusively an art, rather than a science. Unfortunately, once the clinician gets away from the best studied handful of child and adolescent disorders, there are very few if any acute studies. However, 50 or more years from the birth of psychopharmacology, the use of these drugs in children is becoming more popular. It is disconcerting that there is a lack of controlled data for child psychopharmacology. This is likely to improve over time as the American Psychiatric Association and the American Academy of Child and Adolescent Psychiatry are collaborating with clinicians in order to obtain a large database on clinical practice, which should provide more solutions to some unanswered questions.

The implementation of a treatment strategy in children and adolescents should always include detailed psychiatric and medical history and should target emotional and behavioral symptoms as well as the strengths and weaknesses of the patient and family. Careful attention should be paid to differential diagnosis, including medical/neurological and psychosocial factors contributing to clinical presentation and compliance issues. Nonpharmacologic interventions including psychotherapy and family and behavior therapy must always be considered as treatment options instead of, or in conjunction with, pharmacological treatments. Adolescents are usually more sensitive to issues regarding confidentiality than are children. Therefore, the guidelines for confidentiality and for sharing information between parent and child must be clearly stated. Finally, every effort should be made to minimize polypharmacy and resources and risks in the school, neighborhood and social support networks including religious group affiliation, which must be looked into as they influence the implementation and outcome of therapeutic interventions. A variety of psychopharmacological agents is being used to treat a wide range of psychiatric symptoms in youngsters. Psychostimulants (methylphenidate, dextroamphetamine, and magnesium permoline) are commonly prescribed for the treatment of ADHD to target symptoms of inattentiveness, impulsivity, and hyperactivity. The response rate for uncomplicated ADHD has been estimated to be about 70%. Tricyclic antidepressants (TCAs), clonidine, and guanfacine are being used as second-line agents for uncomplicated ADHD and for patients with ADHD and tics. Recently, bupropion has been used as a second-line agent for treatment-resistant cases and for children with ADHD and either major depression or dysthymia. Treatment with stimulants improves a wide variety of cognitive abilities (Bernstein, 1995) and improves performance in academic testing, personal communication, and school-based productivity. Concerns about treatment with stimulant medication in adolescents include the potential for abuse and dependence by the patient and friends, growth suppression, insomnia, and rebound effects consisting of increased excitability, activity, and irritability.

The antidepressant drugs are a heterogeneous group of compounds that have been found to be effective in the treatment of major depressive disorder, generalized anxiety disorder, panic disorder, and a variety of other conditions including PTSD. Controlled studies have failed to demonstrate that TCAs are superior to placebos in the treatment of childhood and adolescent depression. However, the selective serotonin reuptake inhibitors (SSRIs) fluoxetine, fluvoxamine, paroxetine, and sertraline have become popular and are the first drugs of choice, because of their lack of anticholinergic and cardiac side effects. A combination of antidepressants and antipsychotics is used in cases of depression with psychotic features. Some studies indicate that juvenile mood disorders may be more refractory to pharmacologic intervention than are adult mood disorders (Ryan, 1990). For treatment of refractory depression, the clinician should consider higher doses of partially effective antidepressants and augmentation strategies with mood stabilizers, other antidepressants, thyroid hormone (T3), and stimulants. Electroconvulsive therapy (ECT) has also been considered effective. Often the presenting problem in a depressed adolescent is an overt behavior problem, and the accompanying depression may not be detected. Poor school performance, change in grades, and irritability may be important markers of adolescent depression. Conduct disorder and substance abuse may further complicate treatment issues. Evaluation of treatment-refractory patients requires careful attention to diagnostic issues, particularly comorbidity. Appropriate monitoring of the drugs being used is a must to avoid toxicity and manage side effects—particularly sexual side effects in young adolescents.

Almost no studies have evaluated the treatment of juvenile mania. Based on the adult literature on bipolar disorders, mood stabilizers (lithium carbonate, valproic acid, and carbamazepine) may be useful in the acute management and prophylaxis of adolescent mania. In manic patients with psychotic symptoms, additional antipsychotic treatment is recommended. Lithium may be used in mentally retarded or autistic youths with severe aggression directed toward themselves or others. Patients with severe impulsive aggression with emotional lability and irritability who have an abnormal EEG may receive a trial of carbamazepine. Valproic acid is sometimes used in the treatment of adolescent mania, when other options have failed. Case reports suggest the use of valproate for mentally retarded children and adolescents with mood related behavioral symptoms that are resistant to lithium or carbamazepine (Geller & Luby, 1997). The initial laboratory workup is the same for carbamazepine and valproate acid, which includes hemoglobin, hematocrit, WBC, platelets, LFT, BUN, and creatinine measurement. Another recommendation for laboratory monitoring includes CBC and LFTs weekly for the first 4 weeks, monthly for 4 months, and every 3 months thereafter (Silverstein et al., 1983). Additional lab work for lithium treatment includes electrolytes, T3, TSH, and baseline EKG studies.

Antipsychotics are indicated for the treatment of childhood psychotic disorders. Positive symptoms show better improvement with treatment. However, atypical antipsychotics, clozapin, and risperdal appear to be more effective for negative symptoms. There are few reports of usefulness of high-potency benzodiazepines for treatment of acute agitation in acutely psychotic individuals therefore requiring lower doses of antipsychotics. Extrapyramidal reactions can be prevented in many cases by avoiding rapid neuroleptization or by using atypical antipsychotics. Propranolol (nonselective B adrenergic antagonist) has received considerable attention with regard to its potential use in patients with otherwise uncontrollable rage reactions and impulsive aggression or self-injurious behavior, especially those with evidence of organicity. Initial work-up should include a recent history and physical examination, with particular attention to medical contraindications: asthma, diabetes, bradycardia, heart block, cardiac failure, or hypothyroidism.

SPECIAL ISSUES

Suicide and Youth

The loss of young lives from any cause is always tragic, preventable deaths are doubly so. However, the high rate of youth suicide inspires added horror, pity, and concern. So many children abandon hopes in the future and despair of the possibility of sustaining relationships; this calls into question our own collective abilities as caring adults to protect our children and to convey a sense that life is worth living. Youth suicide also raises many important clinical and developmental questions. The rate of adolescent suicide has increased dramatically since 1960. Factors that may have contributed to this increase are the rise in depressive disorders among youths, the rise in the divorce rate, the dissolution of the nuclear family, and the availability of firearms (Pfeffer, 1988). Although there are environmental and sociocultural factors, the importance of psychopathology in youth suicide cannot be overestimated. Although the apparent prevalence of diagnosis and the degree of comorbidity vary across studies and gender, the most common diagnoses are depression, substance abuse, and conduct disorder, especially with antisocial behaviors. One common but problematic diagnosis often assigned to adolescents who attempt suicide is adjustment disorder. In practice, this area frequently means nothing more than that the suicide attempt has occurred in apparent reaction to an upsetting event, most often a fight, the breakup of a romance, or a parental separation.

The personality profiles of suicidal adolescents are also diverse, but borderline personality disorder appears to be the single most common personality disorder. However, there have been reports that young adolescents who complete suicide fall into four personality types: paranoid, impulsive, uncommunicative, and perfectionistic/self-critical. The relationship of alcohol and substance abuse to youth suicidal behavior is worth paying attention to. Adolescents with substance abuse have a 5 to 7-time greater risk of suicidal ideation or suicide attempts than adolescents without substance abuse disorders. A developmental perspective is essential in understanding the nature and cause of suicidal behavior, for example, hormonally mediated changes in the modulation of mood and aggression and amplification of preexisting ambivalence toward parents regarding separation/individuation. Teenagers' senses of identity are not fully consolidated. Clusters of contagious suicides in adolescents have been reported in apparent response to a suicide in the community. Suicidal behavior is associated with a family history of attempted or completed suicide. Postmortem and in vivo cerebrospinal fluid (CSF) and receptor studies of suicide attempters and completers suggest a possible risk between suicidality and abnormalities is serotonergic regulation.

The assessment, treatment, and prevention of the potentially suicidal youngster require a multifaceted approach that seeks primarily to reduce the severity and prevent the occurrence of a suicidal event and to decrease suicidal risk factors. Either misunderstanding or overestimating the patient's suicidal risk may have deleterious consequences for treatment planning. In evaluating the suicidal child, careful assessment of the dynamic and interpersonal context of symptoms and circumstances, the seriousness and persistence of suicidal intent, the fantasies and motivations for suicide, the psychiatric and personality risk factors, the access to weapons or lethal means, and the interpersonal resources are of extreme importance along with contingency planning and suitable disposition. In recent years, suicide prevention programs have been implemented as part of high school curricula and aim to foster awareness of warning signs of suicidal behavior and skills in appropriate response to suicidal tendencies encouraged in one's peers. However, suicide and nonfatal suicide behavior in children and adolescents are mental health problems that requires extensive research efforts with a special focus on early identification, prevention, and intervention. Aside from the risk of physical harm or death, a suicidal crisis offers an opportunity for therapeutic intervention that must be vigorously seized.

Violence and Youth

Mental health professionals are frequently called on to assess and treat youngsters with aggression. A number of studies indicate that approximately 10% of patients presenting to psychiatric hospitals have manifested violent behavior toward others just prior to being admitted to these hospitals. Persons under age 25 make up nearly 50% of all victims of a serious violent crime. According to FBI reports, 2,900 juveniles were arrested for murder in 1996. Nearly a million U.S. students took guns to school during 1998 (Parents Resource Institute for Drug Education), and gunshot wounds to children ages 16 and under have increased 300% in major urban areas since 1986. Experience with violence—whether as a witness or victim—is very common among youths and is associated with increased rates of psychiatric symptoms. The link is especially strong for externalizing symptoms such as antisocial behavior and combativeness. However, violence also increases the risk of internalizing symptoms, such as anxiety or depression. The link between violence and psychiatric symptoms is strong for both boys and girls and across racial and ethnic groups. The growing problem of violence in America is fueled by a sense of alienation and violence in the media, coupled with easy access to guns as a unique critical factor. According to recent studies, guns kill more American teenagers than all natural causes combined. Other research-identified risk factors for violent behavior include violence at home or in the neighborhood, alcohol abuse, drug trade, and association with older delinquent juveniles or adults. Juvenile delinquency has also been shown to develop along other paths, resulting from a lack of support and structure in the community, developmental problems, psychiatric disorders, and genetic predisposition. Juvenile delinquency is most often blamed on moral degeneration, however, extensive research supports the perspective that delinquency and violence are public health problems. Aside from the human cost, teen violence causes a heavy economic price as well. We can not violence-proof our children and adolescents. They are anxious, playful, and active. Such healthy traits, when mixed with exposure to aggression, can cause death. Therefore, a collaborative effort among child and adolescent psychiatrists, other professionals, parents, and community leaders is a must to stem the tide of juvenile violence. Also, understanding and implementing strategies to reduce violence are important not only for the safety of society and patients in treatment settings, but also for the safety of mental health professionals who themselves are at increased risk of being assaulted.

REFERENCES

Achenbach, T. M., & Edelbrock, C. (1983). *Manual for the Child Behavior Checklist and Revised Child Behavior Profile.* Burlington: University of Vermont, Department of Psychiatry.

Amborsini, P. (1987). Pharmacotherapy in child and adolescent major depressive disorder. In H. Y. Meltzer (Ed.), *Psychopharmacology: The third generation of progress* (pp. 1247–1254). New York: Raven.

Ambrosini, P. J., Metz, C., Prabucki, K., & Lee, J. (1989). Videotape reliability of the third revised edition of the K-SADS. *Journal of American Academy of Child and Adolescent Psychiatry, 28,* 723–728.

American Psychiatric Association. (1994). *Diagnostic and statistical manual of mental disorders* (4th ed.). Washington, DC: Author.

Beck, A. T. (1978). *Depression inventory.* Philadelphia:Philadelphia Center for Cognitive Therapy.

Campbell, M., & Spender, E. K. (1988). Psychopharmacology in child and adolescent psychiatry: A review of the past five years. *Journal of the American Academy of Child and Adolescent Psychiatry, 27,* 269–279.

Castenda, A., McCandless, B., & Palermo, D. (1956). The children's form of the Manifest Anxiety Scale. *Child Development, 27,* 317–326.

Chambers, W., Puig-Antich, J., & Hirsch, M. (1985). The assessment of affective disorders in children and adolescents by semi-structured interview. *Arch General Psychiatry, 42,* 696–702.

Clark, D. B., & Donon, J. E. (1994). Reliability and validity of the Hamilton Anxiety Rating Scale in an adolescent sample. *Journal of American Academy of Child and Adolescent Psychiatry, 33,* 354–360.

Cook, P. J. (1982). The role of firearms in violent crime. An interpretive review of the literature. In M. E. Wolfgang & N. A. Weinch (Eds.), *Criminal violence* (pp. 236–291). Beverly Hills, CA: Sage.

Cooper, J. (1970). The Leyton Obsessional Inventory. *Psychological Medicine, 1,* 48–64.

Costello, A. J., Edelbrock, C., & Dulcan, M. K. (1984). *The National Institute of Mental Health Diagnostic Interview Schedule for Children: Final Report.* Bethesda, MD: National Institute of Mental Health.

Duncan, N. K. (1996). Treatment of children and adolescents. *The American Psychiatric Press Synopsis of Psychiatry,* 1191–1208.

Epstein, M. H., & Cullinan, D. (1998). *Scale for assessing emotional disturbance.* Austin, TX: PRO-ED.

Eyberg, S. M., & Robinson, E. A. (1982). Parent-child interaction training. Effects on family functioning. *Journal of Clinical Child Psychology, 11,* 130–137.

Geller, B., & Luby, S. (1997). Child and adolescent bipolar disorders: A review of the past 10 years. *Journal of the American Academy of Child and Adolescent Psychiatry, 36,* 1168–1176.

Goodman, W. K., Price, L. H., Rasmussen, S. A., & Mazure, C. (1989a). The Yale-Brown Obsessive-Compulsive Scale: I. Development, use and reliability. *Arch General Psychiatry, 46,* 1006–1011.

Goodman, W. K., Price, L. H., Rasmussen, S. A., & Mazure, C. (1989b). The Yale-Brown Obsessive-Compulsive Scale: II. Validity. *Arch General Psychiatry, 46,* 1012–1016.

Goyette, C. H., Conners, C. K., & Ulrich, R. F. (1978). Normative data on Revised Conners Parent and Teacher Rating Scales. *Journal of Abnormal Child Psychology, 6,* 221–236.

Hamilton, M. A. (1967). Development of a rating scale for primary depressive illness. *British Journal of Social and Clinical Psychology, 6,* 278–296.

Henggeler, S. W., Schoenwold, S. K., Borduem, C. M., Rowland, M. D., & Cunningham, P. B. (1998). *Multisystemic treatment of antisocial behavior in children and adolescents.* New York: Guilford Press.

Herjanic, B., & Campbell, W. (1977). Differentiating psychiatrically disturbed children on the basis of a structured interview. *Journal of Abnormal Child Psychology, 5,* 127–134.

Herjanic, B., & Reich, W. (1982). Development of a structured psychiatric interview for children: Agreement between child and parent on individual symptoms. *Journal of Abnormal Child Psychology, 10,* 307–324.

Joint Commission on Mental Health of Children. (1969). *Crisis in child mental health: Challenge for the 1970's.* New York: Harper & Row.

Kanner, L. (1935). *Child psychiatry.* Springfield, IL: Thomas.

Kendall, P. C., & Wilcox, L. E. (1979). Self-control in children: Development of a rating scale. *Journal of Consulting Clinical Psychology, 47,* 1020–1029.

Kovacs, M., & Beck, A. T. (1977). An empirical clinical approach towards a definition of childhood depression. In J. G. Schulterbrandt & A. Raskin (Eds.), *Depression in children: Diagnosis, treatment and conceptual models* (p. 126). New York: Raven.

Lewis, D. D., Balla, D. A., & Shanok, S. (1979). Violent juvenile delinquents: Psychiatric, neurological, psychological and abuse factors. *Journal of the American Academy of Child Psychiatry, 18,* 307–319.

Miller, L. S., Klei, R. G., Piacentini, J., & Abikoff, H. (1995). The New York Teacher's Rating Scale for Disruptive and Antisocial Behavior. *Journal of the American Academy of Child and Adolescent Psychiatry, 34,* 359–370.

National Center for Children in Poverty. (1999). Young children in poverty fact sheet. [On-line] 99. Columbia University, New York.

National Committee to Prevent Child Abuse. (1995). *Current trends in child abuse reporting and fatalities. The results of the 1994 annual 50 state survey.* Chicago: Author.

National Institute of Mental Health. (1982). *Television and behavior: Ten years of scientific progress and implications for the eighties.* Rockville, MD: National Institute of Mental Health. DHHS Publ. No. [ADM] 821195.

Otto, R., Greenstein, J., Johnson, M., & Friedman, R. (1993). Prevalence of mental disorders among youth in the juvenile justice system. In *Responding to the mental health needs of youth in the juvenile justice system.* Seattle: National Coalition for the Mentally Ill in the Criminal Justice System.

Pfeffer, C. R. (1988). Suicidal behaviour among children and adolescent: Risk identification and intervention. *American Press Review of Psychiatry, 7,* 386–402.

Pfeffer, C. R. (1997). Suicide and suicidality. In J. M. Weiner (Ed.), *Textbook of child and adolescent psychiatry* (pp. 727–738). New York: Wiley.

Pfeffer, C. R., Klerman, G. L., Hurt, S. W., & Kakuma, T. (1993). Suicidal children grow up: Rates and psychosocial risk factors for suicide attempts during follow up. *Journal of the American Academy of Child and Adolescent Psychiatry, 32,* 106.

Pfefferbaum, B., & Overall, J. E. (1984). Decision about drug treatment in children. *Journal of the American Academy of Child Psychiatry, 23,* 209–214.

Pfefferbaum, B. (1997). Posttraumatic stress disorder in children: A review of the past 10 years. *Journal of the American Academy of Child and Adolescent Psychiatry, 36,* 1503–1511.

Poznanski, E. O., Cook, S. C., & Carroll, B. J. (1979). A depression rating scale for children. *Pediatrics, 64,* 442–450.

Poznanski, E. O., Grossman, J. A., & Buchsbaum, Y. (1984). Preliminary studies of the reliability and validity of the Children's Depression Rating Scale. *Journal of American Academy of Child Psychiatry, 23,* 191–197.

Pynoos, R. S., Frederick, C., & Nader, K. (1987). Life threats and posttraumatic stress in school age children. *Archives of General Psychiatry, 44,* 1057–1063.

Quay, H. C. (1983). A dimensional approach to behavior disorder: The Revised Behavior Problem Checklist. *School Psychology Review, 12,* 244–249.

Quay, H. C., & Peterson, D. R. (1983). *Manual for the Revised Behavior Problem Checklist.* Unpublished manuscript. Coral Gables, FL: University of Miami Press.

Riddle, M. A., Hardin, M. T., King, R., & Scahill, L. (1990). Fluoxentine treatment of children and adolescents with Tourette's and obsessive compulsive disorders: Preliminary clinical experience. *Journal of American Academy of Child and Adolescent Psychiatry, 29,* 45–48.

Ryan, N. (1990). Heterocyclic antidepressants in children and adolescents. *Journal of Child and Adolescent Psychopharmacology,* 1.21–31.

Shaffer, D., Erhardt, A. A., & Greenhill, L. L. E. (1985). *The clinical guide to child psychiatry.* New York: Free Press.

Shaffer, D., Garland, A., Gould, M., Fisher, P., & Trautman, P. (1988). Preventing teenage suicide: A critical review. *Journal of American Academy of Child and Adolescent Psychiatry, 27,* 675.

Snyder, H., & Sickmund, M. (1995). *Juvenile offenders and victims: A national report.* Washington, DC: Office of Juvenile Justice and Delinquent Prevention.

Spitzer, R. L., Gibson, M., & Endicott, J. (1973). *Global Assessment Scale.* New York: New York State Department of Mental Hygiene.

Tardiff, K. (1996). Violence. *The American Psychiatric Press Synopsis of Psychiatry,* 1191–1208.

United States Public Health Service. (1999). *Mental health: A report of the surgeon general.* Washington, DC: US Government Printing Office.

Vander Stoep, A. (2000). *Mental health and substance use of detained youth: An epidemiological study. A System of Care for Children's Mental Health.* Tampa: University of South Florida, Florida Mental Health Institute.

World Health Organization. (1987). *Drugs for children.* Denmark: Author.

SECTION III

Special Interventions with Children and Adolescents

Chapter 18

PSYCHOPHARMACOLOGICAL INTERVENTIONS FOR CHILDREN WITH CHALLENGING BEHAVIORS

AMOR S. DEL MUNDO, ANDRES J. PUMARIEGA, BOONEY VANCE, AND CURTIS KAUFFMAN

INTRODUCTION

The use of psychopharmacological agents in the treatment of childhood psychiatric disorders and behavioral disturbances presents significant fears. A more panic fear expressed both by parents and educators is that of children's being labeled and stigmatized. Fears also involve short-term side effects, long-term impacts on the growth and development of children, and the potential of addiction. An unspoken fear that often underlies such concerns is the "pathologizing" of childhood behavior, which results in empowerment of parents, teachers, and children themselves; the loss of input and control due to the technical nature of decision making process (Gadow, 1997). Mental illness affects at least 12% (7–12 million) of American children and adolescents. Depression occurs in about 3% to 5% of children and youth. Anxiety disorders affect approximately 10% to 15% of children, and ADHD affects 3% to 7% of school-aged children. Childhood-onset bipolar disorder (otherwise known as manic depressive illness) has a chronic course into adulthood and can have serious consequences. Schizophrenia is a chronic mental and cognitive disorder marked by characteristic psychotic symptoms, such as hallucinations and delusions, disturbances in aspect and form or thought, and markedly impaired cognitive function. Anorexia nervosa and bulimia affect a high percentage of adolescents—a total of 3% to 5% with significant psychological and medical morbidity, and even mortality. Mental health problems are considered barriers to learning. They can interfere with the child's overall functioning at home, at school, and in the community.

PAST AND PRESENT LEADERS

Pioneering child and adolescent psychiatrists began to recognize the potential benefits of pharmacological interventions in the treatment of children with serious mental and emotional disturbances. As far back as the late 1930s, Bradley (1937) identified that stimulants reduced school refusal and hyperactivity and improved the school performances of children identified as hyperactive. It was not until the 1960s that investigators proceeded to test the effectiveness of stimulants in treating children with ADHD using double-blind, placebo-controlled research methodology. These trials formally opened the era of psychopharmacology with children, not only by establishing the most commonly used pharmacological agents with children, but also by setting double-blind, placebo-controlled trials as standard for establishing efficacy (Barkley, 1977). Increasing numbers of well designed clinical trials of psychotropic agents with children and adolescents in recent years have led to more formal indications for the use of these agents (Campbell & Cueva, 1995). Comparative studies so far have shown pharmacological intervention to be superior to behavioral intervention in the treatment of ADHD (Rappaport, Denny, DuPaul, & Gardner, 1994), equal with such interventions in the treatment of anxiety and depressive disorders and equal in the treatment of eating disorders. However, source studies suggest that the combination of pharmacological and cognitive behavioral approaches is superior to the use of either of the above (Pfefferbaum, 1997; Kolko, Bukstein, & Barron, 1999).

PHARMACOLOGICAL INTERVENTION IN ASSESSMENT: ITS SIGNIFICANCE IN RELATION TO DIAGNOSIS, TREATMENT INTERVENTION, AND HABITATION

Depression

Childhood depression is now recognized as a widespread, debilitating, and often chronic illness affecting 3% to 4% of children and youth that interferes with mood, cognition, behavior, socialization, and development. In addition, this illness can result in significant numbers of lost school days, lost workdays for parents and other care-givers, and considerable treatment expense and distress for the family (Fleming & Offord, 1990).

Children and adults with depression were initially treated with tricyclic antidepressants (TCAs), such as amitriptyline (Elavil), imipramine (Tofranil), nortriptyline (Pamelor), amoxapine (Doxepin), and desipramine (Norpramine). Although they were effective with adults, they had mixed efficacy with children and adolescents. TCAs are known to produce high incidence of adverse effects, especially with children. Central side effects of TCAs include drowsiness, ataxia, anxiety, insomnia, nightmares, confusion, decreased cognition, and seizures. Dry mouth, blurred vision, and constipation commonly result from a blockade of muscarinic cholinergic receptors. In addition, TCAs can precipitate delusions and worsen psychoses in patients with schizophrenia. In overdose, TCAs are potentially life threatening. Seizures, coma, respiratory depression, hypotension, cardiac arrhythmia, and acute renal failure commonly occur in TCA overdoses in children, and death usually results from cardiac arrhythmics secondary effects on cardiac conduction. Children are more vulnerable than adults to the toxic effects of TCAs because they produce greater proportion of cardiotoxic metabolites (Pumariega, Muller, & Rivers-Buckeley, 1982; Ryan, 1990; DeVane & Salle, 1996).

The new class of selective serotonin reuptake inhibitors (SSRIs) such as fluoxetine

(Prozac), paroxetine (Paxil), sertraline (Zoloft), fluvoxamine (Luvox), and citalpram (Celexa) has been successful in effecting favorable therapeutic outcomes in adults with markedly better effect profiles. Though most of these agents have not undergone Food and Drug Administration trials for children and adolescents, preliminary clinical studies of SSRIs with children with depression have shown efficacy greater than placebo and equal or greater efficacy than TCAs (DeVane & Salle, 1996). The SSRIs have a relatively safe side-effects profile, very low lethality after overdose, and easy once-a-day administration, all of which favor this antidepressant as first-line medication. The most frequent adverse effects are nausea, headache, diarrhea or loose stools, insomnia, dry mouth, and sexual dysfunction (predominantly in males). Adverse effects appear to decrease in frequency and severity with chronic dosing (DeVane & Salle, 1996; Grimsley & Iann, 1992).

The SSRIs appear to be safer than TCAs in acute overdose. Doogan (1991) reports four cases of sertraline poisoning that resolved with no significant sequelae and without need for intensive monitoring. However, severe intoxication with sertraline in a child after accidental ingestion has been reported; prolonged tachycardia, hypertension, hallucinations, coma, and hyperthermia occurred in this patient (Kaminski, Robbins, & Weibley, 1994).

The use of TCAs is now reserved for children who do not respond to SSRIs. However, there are also new adrenergic agents such as bupropion (Wellbutrin), venlafaxine (Effexor), and mirtazapine (Remeron), which are increasingly used in treating depression as alternatives to the TCAs and which have much safer side-effects profiles. Lithium, valproic acid, or stimulant coadministration to augment the efficacy of antidepressants are also means of addressing treatment-resistant depression. When depression in a youngster is severe, it is often accompanied by psychotic features (such as hallucinations, problems with reality testing, or violent behavior); in fact, this occurs more frequently with children than with adults. The addition of antipsychotic medication in such circumstances can be beneficial, especially with the newer antipsychotic medications such as olanzepine and risperidal, which have fewer extrapyramidal side effects (Ryan, 1990; Gadow, 1997).

Anxiety Disorders

Anxiety disorders (panic disorder, obsessive-compulsive disorder, generalized anxiety disorders, social phobia, and posttraumatic stress disorder) are the most common psychiatric disorders in both children and adults, affecting approximately 10% to 15% of children. Although the majority of children with anxiety disorders do not experience serious impairment, a significant percentage of them go on to have significant disruption of their academic, social, and interpersonal function as a result of the severity of their illnesses. Some of these disorders, such as posttraumatic stress disorder and obsessive-compulsive disorder, used to be considered rare among children and adolescents but are now known to affect significant percentages within these age groups.

The SSRIs, benzodiazepines, beta adrenergic blockers, alpha adrenergic blockers, antihistamines, and buspirone have been used to provide antianxiety effects for adolescents and children suffering from anxiety disorders or anxiety symptoms associated with other conditions. Children with anxiety disorders respond very well to treatment with SSRIs. These medications not only contribute to the relief of the typical physiological symptoms of anxiety but are also quite effective in addressing the cognitive aspects of these disorders, such as worrying, initial insomnia, rumination, decreased concentration, and repetitive or intrusive thinking or behaviors (Murdoch & McTarish, 1992; Bernstein, Borchardt, & Perwien, 1996).

There are few reports on the use of benzodiazepines, such as alprazolam (Xanax) and clonazepam (Klonopin) in adolescents and children. Short-term use may be considered in cases of acute situational anxiety such as posttrauma or postsurgery, or in the short-term management of anxiety disorders prior to the onset of action of the SSRIs, which can be delayed by 2 to 3 weeks from initiation. Benzodiazepines have been found helpful as part of preoperative sedation to reduce anticipatory anxiety before surgery. These are safe and effective drugs, but there are clinical problems like risks for abuse and dependence, sedation, withdrawal symptoms, and disinhibition of impulsive or aggressive behaviors (Bernstein, Borchardt, & Perwien, 1996).

Beta blockers (propranolol) and alpha blockers (clonidine) are also helpful in controlling anxiety disorders, especially in children or adolescents with periodic range outburst. Propranolol and clonidine can improve affective, cognitive, and physiologic symptoms of PTSD. Antihistamines like diphenhydramine (Benadryl) and hydroxyzine (Atarax or Vistaril) are the two most commonly used in treating anxiety disorders in children. Antihistamines are quite safe to administer, with the risk of sedation and behavioral disinhibition being the most common side-effects. Behavioral disinhibition can be seen in an occasion patient, particularly in children with problems with impulsivity or motor tics (Bernstein, Borchardt, & Perwien, 1996).

Attention-Deficit/Hyperactivity Disorder

Attention-Deficit/Hyperactivity Disorder (ADHD) is one of the most prevalent and persistent psychiatric disorders in school-aged children, affecting 3% to 7% percent of this population. It is a psychiatric disorder characterized by serious and continuous difficulties in three specific areas attention span, impulse control, and extraneous motoric activity. ADHD is a chronic disorder that starts in early childhood and can extend through adulthood and that has negative effects on a child's life in the home, school, and the community (American Psychiatric Association, 1994). This is a disorder that has significant future consequences in terms of academic achievement or completion, especially due to the high level of comorbidity of learning disorders as well as its symptoms. It is also associated with other adverse psychiatric and social comorbidity in longitudinal studies, such as comorbid bipolar and conduct disorder, criminal activity or incarceration, unemployment and auto accidents (Barkley, Fischer, Edelbrock, & Smallish, 1990; Cantwell, 1996). Data from national surveys showed a 100% increase in diagnosis between 1900 and 1993, from approximately one million to two million cases. ADHD is probably over-diagnosed because of failure to consider psychiatric conditions that are either comorbid or have similar presenting symptoms. These include mood disorders (bipolar disorder or depressive disorder), anxiety disorders, intermittent explosive disorder, child abuse/neglect, substance abuse, or chaotic home environments (Cantwell, 1996).

Given the difficulties in distinguishing the symptomatology associated with this condition, careful evaluation of children suspected of having ADHD is essential. Unfortunately, too often children who are suspected of having ADHD are superficially evaluated by inexperienced medical and nonmedical professionals and are prematurely placed on medication trials. An initial diagnostic appointment should be directed by a doctoral-level mental health professional (psychologist or psychiatrist) who should collect developmental, educational, social, and family-history data. During the initial assessment, each child should be observed during an academic analog task. A series of parent and teacher rating forms should also be completed in order to ensure multi-informant observation of symptoms. A computerized continuous performance task test should be administered to obtain an objective baseline measure of attention, both for comparison with established age and gender norms and for later outcome measures after medication administration, useful both in determining efficacy and dose titration. A child psychiatrist should confirm that he or she met criteria for ADHD and that no primary mood, anxiety, adjustment, or pervasive developmental disorder better explains the child's presenting symptoms (Rosenberg, Holttum, & Gershon, 1994).

The nature of the findings should then be explained to parents, teachers, and the child. Informed consent should also be obtained for any medication trial. However, treatment should not consist solely of stimulant medication. There are significant impairments associated with ADHD that are best addressed through educational or psychosocial interventions, such as associated specific learning disorders or deficits in self-esteem. Additionally, children with ADHD can be taught to develop self-control and self-monitoring skills to enhance their attention span and reduce their impulsivity, thus reducing the need for medication. A number of highly effective cognitive-behavioral interventions should be coupled with pharmacotherapy for enhanced treatment efficacy (Pelham & Murphy, 1986; Barkley, Fischer, Edelbrock, & Smallish, 1990).

ADHD is highly responsive to behavioral and pharmacologic treatment. Stimulants remain the drug of first choice. Seventy percent of ADHD children respond to methylphenidate (Ritalin or Dexedrine), and the remaining 30% are selective responders. Pemoline (Cylert) and Adderall (a combination of various amphetamines), both of which are longer-acting types or preparations of stimulants, are also useful alternatives for nonresponders or those children who require more extensive symptom coverage. All forms of stimulants should be tried before moving to nonstimulants (Bernstein, 1995; Rosenberg, Holttum, & Gershon, 1994).

Although children differ significantly in age and body weight, contemporary studies generally do not index stimulant dosages by body weight according to Handen et al. (1999). Patient needs to be monitored for any adverse drug effects such as decreased appetite, dizziness, drowsiness, lack of sleep, stomachache, headache, tics, nervous movements, anxiety, disinterest in others, euphoria, nightmares, sadness, and staring into space. Most of these side effects are dose related and are subject to individual differences. Many of these diminish within 1 to 2 weeks of beginning the medication, and all except the possibility of tics disappear upon ceasing pharmacotherapy. These risks can be reduced by giving the patient small doses at the beginning of therapy and working up slowly to the smallest dose that achieves meaningful results. Earlier reports of growth retardation with the stimulants have not been proven in controlled studies, with any effect on growth being related to its effect on appetite (DuPaul, Barkley, & McMurray, 1994).

Clonidine (Catapres), an alpha adrenergic antagonist, can be used as an adjunctive medication along with a stimulant for children who have significant difficulties with impulsivity, aggression, or sleep. This medication needs to be carefully titrated to prevent hypotension or bradycardia as significant side effects. There are four cases of sudden death with the use of Clonidine and about 20 emergency room reports of significant cardiac side effects (Swanson et al., 1995). Response to the stimulants characterized by mood lability, crying spells, and irritability can be suggestive of either misdiagnosed or comorbid depression. In children where ADHD is accompanied by major depressive disorder or anxiety disorder, combination of stimulant and antidepressant medication like bupropion (Wellbutrin) or the SSRIs is beneficial. Major antipsychotic tranquilizers such as thioridazine (Mellaril) have been used to manage children with ADHD and high levels of aggression and impulsivity by older practitioners. Their significant short-term and long-term side effects make them unacceptable for this purpose (see the section on schizophrenia). New agents are being tested for ADHD, and in the future clinicians will probably have broader therapeutic options (DuPaul, Barkley, & McMurray, 1994; Elia, Boncherding, Rapoport, & Keyson, 1991).

Bipolar Disorder

Childhood-onset bipolar disorder (otherwise known as manic depressive illness) has a chronic course into adulthood and can have serious consequences. Children and adolescents with this disorder have a high rate of suicide. Violent behavior can occur during severe manic episodes. Children with rapid mood cycling show a poor response to treatment. The effective diagnosis of this disorder can often be life-saving and significantly change the short- and long-term outcome for children (Geller & Luby, 1997).

Although lithium carbonate has been considered the first-line agent for the treatment of bipolar disorder and is known to improve its course and prognosis, only 50% to 60% of individuals with bipolar disorder achieve significant control of their symptoms with lithium alone. With children and adolescents, it is imperative to have a choice of medications that can effectively and safely be given in chaotic environments because of their rapid cycling and the abrupt onset of suicidality. It is particularly important to have medication that is safer than lithium if taken in overdose. Mood-stabilizing agents such as valproate (Depakote), carbamazepine (Tegretol), or clonazepam are alternatives frequently used with children with bipolar disorder given the above parameters, especially due to their efficacy in rapid cycling mood states. Valporate and carbamazepine have the added beneficial feature that blood levels can be measured, with established norms for therapeutic ranges and toxic levels. Since bipolar disorder can be accompanied by psychotic symptoms such as hallucinations and delusional thinking, which can be additionally dangerous, the concomitant use of antipsychotic medication is often necessary (Geller & Luby, 1997; see also the next section).

Schizophrenia and Other Psychotic Disorders

Schizophrenia is a chronic mental and cognitive disorder marked by characteristic psychotic symptoms, such as hallucinations and delusions, disturbances in affect and form of thought, and markedly impaired cognitive function. Early onset of schizophrenia is often associated with negative symptoms (such as blunting of emotional expressiveness and lack of volition to pursue interests). It has a very poor prognosis associated with cognitive deterioration and even documented morphological brain changes (Remschmidt et al., 1994).

Antipsychotic medications have been clearly shown to be effective in treatment of psychotic symptoms. The older antipsychotics, such as chlorpromazine (Thorazine), thioridazine (Mellaril), haloperidol (Haldol), fluphenazine (Prolixin), and thiothixine (Navane), were proven efficacious in the treatment of psychotic symptoms in schizophrenia and other disorders with associated symptoms, such as mood disorder. However, these agents have significant short-term side effects, such as oversedation, Parkinsonian-like extrapyramidal symptoms (EPS), and anticholinergic-like side effects, and are not particularly efficacious in addressing negative symptoms in schizophrenia. Their chronic and high-dosage use is also associated with tardive dyskinesia, an involuntary movement disorder especially involving buccofacial and fine motor movement, which can become irreversible. Children and adolescents may be at particularly high risk for developing extra pyramidal side effects as well as tardive dyskinesia. They continue to have a role in the management of acute psychosis, especially in their injectable form, and as second-line agents (Groevich et al., 1996).

The newer atypical antipsychotics, such as risperidone, olanzeprine, quentepine, and clozapine, may prove more useful in the treatment of schizophrenia and psychotic symptoms in general given both their relatively lower side effects and their better efficacy in treating negative symptoms (Werry & Aman, 1993). Risperidone provides positive and negative symptom reduction as well as relatively low rates of EPS, especially when dosing is gradually titrated. Clozapine provides positive and negative symptom reduction, though hematological side effects (drops in platelet counts) are possible. There is limited data available on the use of olanzepine or quentepine in children and adolescents.

Eating Disorders

Anorexia nervosa and bulimia affect a high percentage of adolescents (a total of 3–5%), with significant psychosocial and medical morbidity and even mortality (both from starvation effects and suicide). Antidepressant medications have been shown to be an important component in the treatment of eating disorders, not only through their effects on comorbid depressive or anxiety disorders, but also directly through their effects on neurochemical mechanisms related to binge eating and satiety. SSRIs like fluoxetine (Prozac) can reuce binge eating and purging. TCAs such as imipramine (Tofranil), trazodone (Desyrel), and desipramine (Norpramine) have been helpful in the treatment of bulimia, while amitriptyline (Elavil) has been reported to be beneficial in the treatment of anorexia nervosa. Mood stabilizers like carbamazepine or lithium are effective in the presence of bipolar disorders comorbid with bulimia. Cyproheptadine (Periactin), a drug with antihistamine and antiserotonergic properties, is an effective adjunct in the treatment of patients with the restricting type of anorexia nervosa, either as an appetite stimulant or through reduction of gastrointestinal malaise (Steiner & Lock, 1998).

Tourette's Disorder and Other Tic Disorders

Children and adolescents with tic disorders, including Tourette's Disorder, suffer from spontaneous involuntary motor and verbal behaviors as well as associated hyperactivity and impulsivity problems. Some psychotropic medications have demonstrated efficacy in controlled studies of the treatment of tic disorders, including antipsychotics such as haloperidol and pimozide (Campbell, Rapoport, & Simpson, 1999) and desipramine (Singer et al., 1995) Clonidine has been suggested as another treatment and has support from uncontrolled studies but mixed results in controlled studies (Riddle et al., 1999).

Autism

The fourth edition of the *Diagnostic and Statistical Manual of Mental Disorders* (*DSM-IV:* APA, 1994) defines pervasive developmental disorders as severe, pervasive impairments in multiple areas of socioemotional and cognitive development, such as social interaction and communication or stereotyped behavior, interests, and activities. The impairments in these most severe childhood psychiatric disorders are significant when compared to a person's chronological and expected developmental level. The best known of these disorders is Autistic Disorder, although other forms such as Asperger's Disorder, Rett's Disorder, and Acute Disintegrative Disorder have been recently defined.

Pharmacotherapy is a valuable adjunct in comprehensive treatment and habilitation programs designed to improve a variety of associated symptoms and enhance developmental progression. The administration of risperidone has been used successfully to diminish hyperactivity, self-injurious behavior, and aggressive behavior (Perry et al., 1997). The SSRIs have been used to diminish obsessive-compulsive and stereotypical behaviors and to improve social reciprocity and learning (McDougle, 1998). The administration of major tranquilizers like haloperidol reduces behavioral symptoms and accelerates learning (Perry et al., 1997). Clinical studies of dipamine antagonists used to control self-injurious behavior in PDD populations yielded mixed results. Sedative hypnotics can be used for the management of agitation, but these can cause disinhibition and thus are not good treatment options in the presence of self-injurious behaviors (Werry & Aman, 1995). Naltrexone, an opiate antagonist, is currently being investigated to reduce autistic symptoms. Initial studies with Naloxone, an injectable opiate blocker, reported positive effects in eight of ten patients treated. Positive results were reported in studies with orally administered. Naltrexone in 38 of 45 autistic patients, including 24 of those 28 with self-injurious behavior (Sandman, 1991).

Symptomatic Management of Children with Serious Emotional Disturbances

In addition to the treatment of defined diagnostic entities, psychopharmacological treatment can be used for the management of behaviors seen in children with serious emotional disturbances that do not respond to behavioral or psychosocial interventions.

Aggression, Agitation, and Violent Behavior

The majority of children who present for psychiatric treatment are brought in by family members concerned about their aggressive behavior. Unpredictable rage or intermittent explosive behavior can be managed with the use of mood stabilizers like lithium, valmoric acid, or carbamazepin. The medications can also be effective in treating complex partial seizures, or psychomotor seizures, another condition that should be suspected in children with unprovoked aggression and no recall of the episodes. Clonidine, an apresynaptic alpha adrenergic blocking agent, is also effective. Beta blockers such as propranolol are also used to control aggression in children. In cases of severe aggression or agitation, short-acting benzodiazepines such as lorazepam (Ativan) can be beneficial. Aggressive children with comorbid affective disorders can benefit from a trial of SSRIs, which have also been shown to reduce impulsivity and aggression over long-term use. Rarely should antipsychotic medication be used to manage aggressive disorder, and only then in acute situations when other treatments have failed (Arredondo & Butler, 1994; Popper & Zimnitzky, 1996).

Enuresis

Enuresis consists of repeated urination into clothes or in bed twice weekly for at least 3 consecutive months. According to the *DSM-IV* (APA, 1994), the diagnosis is not made until the child is at least 5 years old. Children with enuresis are at higher risk for developmental delays. TCAs, particularly imipramine, can be effective in controlling enuresis on a short-term basis. However, tolerance often develops after 6 weeks of therapy. Desmopressin acetate (DDAVP), an antidiuretic administered intranasally, has been shown to be effective in reducing enuresis. Electrolyte levels should be checked early in treatment (Thompson & Rey, 1995).

Mood Lability, Compulsive Behaviors, and Self-Injurious Behaviors

Children and adolescents presenting with mood lability and self-injurious behaviors (SIBs) can benefit from SSRIs or mood stabilizers (lithium, depakote, tegretol). Naltrexone, an opiate blocker, appears to be the only treatment option for some children with SIBs. These include children with autism, children with serious emotional disturbance with a history of traumatization, or youth with incipient serious personality disorders, who fail to respond to other treatments. The opiate hypothesis maintains that patients engage in SIBs either because they are partially analgesic or because SIBs supply a "fix" for an additional endogenous opiate system. Learning, memory, and compliance are also improved with opiate blockers. Formal evaluation of chronic treatment and long-term effects have not been reported (Sandman, 1991).

Sleep Disturbance

Sleep disturbance can accompany a variety of emotional and psychiatric disorders in children. The type of sleep disturbance and the associated symptoms often dictate the type of pharmacological intervention to be used. Children with initial insomnia can be treated with mild antihistamines such as diphenhydramine (Benadryl) or hydroxyzine

(Vistaril), or with clonidine if significant problems with agitation or impulsivity interfere with sleep. They may require treatment with sedative hypnotics; although the concerns about tolerance dependence and addiction also apply for this application, so its use should only be for short durations. Trazodone, with its longer-acting profile, may be used as a sleep aid in children who have problems with both initial insomnia and intermittent insomnia. Adjunctive agents for disrupted sleep may be useful when a child's sleep needs to be regularized so that it provides sufficient rest to allow for normal function at school on the following day. They are typically not needed over the long term unless levels of stressors in the environment are not addressed, or the child suffers from one of the above disorders that may require more definitive treatment (Popper & Zimnitzky, 1996).

Other types of sleep disturbance require different interventions. The tricyclic antidepressants have a role in the treatment of somnambulism (sleepwalking) or pavor nocturnus (night terrors, a condition in which a child may appear as if they were having a nightmare but not have any recall). These conditions (along with some forms of enuresis) can be considered disturbances of initial stages of sleep—namely, when the child transitions from deep to shallower sleep—and can resolve themselves with nervous system maturation, usually by adolescence, but may cause nighttime safety concerns in the meantime (Balon, 1994). Narcolepsy, a rare sleep disorder that involves continual involuntary transition into sleep at all hours of the day, is another condition for which the stimulants is an efficacious agent and should be suspected when a child continually falls asleep during the day in the face of adequate nighttime sleep and no other emotional problems (Dahl, Holttum, & Trubnick, 1994).

FORMULATION AND DIAGNOSIS

Psychodynamic formulation has been described for child and adolescents to complement diagnosis and guide management. The developmental status of the child in his or her more or less dependent relationship within a family should be of interest to clinicians. Features of developmentally immature patients should be taken into consideration, such as the role of the child as an organism and a person with a disorder and as a symptom bearer in a family. The dynamic formulation should include a summary paragraph concerning the complaints of the patient, the diagnosis, and the precipitating events, such as genetics, social deprivations, traumatic, and other factors that might contribute to the presentation or symptoms. The explanation of central conflicts provides a preliminary interpretation of how the patient presents. The predictive responses concerning the therapeutic situation are based upon prior factors (Shapiro, 1989). Understanding the predisposing, precipitating, and sustaining factors in a patient's life will help tremendously in understanding the biological and genetic components and how they interact with the social and physical environments.

The emerging psychiatric diagnostic nosology, based on a more descriptive, nontheoretical approach, eventually led to the development of the *DSM-IV* (APA, 1994). This classification scheme has allowed for the specific testing of the efficacy of different treatment modalities, including medications, which in turn has led to advances in the development of such treatments (Gittleman-Klein, Spitzen, & Cantwell, 1978). However, it is important to note that this diagnostic system is far from flawless. It is in a constant state of evolution based on available epidemiological and mechanistic (biological or psychological) research findings. There are also problems with the reliability and validity of clinician-administered diagnoses, which often do not strictly adhere to the criteria set by the diagnostic nosology. Systematic diagnostic instruments, such as the Diagnostic Interview Schedule for Children (DISC; Shaffer et al., 1996) and the Diagnostic Interview for Children and Adolescents (DICA; Reich, Weiner, & Herjanic, 1994) based on the *DMS-IV,* have established reliability and validity and can be administered by either clinicians or trained lay interviewers to systematically evaluate the presence of diagnosed mental or emotional disorders as the presence of subdiagnostic symptomatology.

One of the main areas in which the diagnostic system lacks good research findings is the diagnosis of children and adolescents. Although many studies have shown that the criteria for many disorders can be equally applied to adults and children, the emergence of symptoms in children can often be gradual and incomplete, thus leading to inconclusive diagnostic findings. There are also developmental variations on how different symptoms are expressed. For example, anhedonia (the loss of interests or pleasure commonly seen in depression) in adults is quite different on the surface from complaints of boredom in children, but they are essentially the same symptom.

Additionally, the functional level or level of behavioral severity, and consequently the needed level of care or restrictiveness in children, may not correlate with seriousness of the associated diagnosis, especially given the problems caused by disruptive behavioral symptomatology (Caron & Rutter, 1991). Quite often, the severity of a child's condition is not necessary related to his or her diagnostic or formal clinical status. It may be more clearly expressed in the child's inability to meet the expectations and requisite adaptive behaviors necessary for him or her to successfully negotiate roles within the family, with peers, and in school or other organized settings. This has led at times to the exclusion of children with so-called behavioral disorders that have no immediately identified biological basis, often referred as having serious emotional disturbances, from treatment settings. Another reason for their exclusion is the fact that treating and caring for such children may actually be more difficult and taxing on school and mental health professionals than it is for children with readily identified biologically based disorders. Additionally, interventions may at times improve more formal clinical symptoms but may not address the children's function in the significant areas of their lives. This may in fact be explained by the focus on negative behaviors or symptoms in treatment and care planning, whereas the development of positive adaptive capacities receives secondary or incidental attention.

The efficacy of a pharmacological agent may not be predictive of diagnostic certainty for a given child. For example, stimulants and sedative-hypnotics have nonspecific effects on attention, activity level, or agitation. Response to these agents do not predict the diagnosis of either ADHD or anxiety disorders, and many children who do not have these conditions may respond nonspecifically to these agents and others, thus complicating the diagnostic picture.

ASSESSMENT AND MONITORING/REASSESSMENT

Assessment in child psychiatry or mental health in general requires information from multiple observers in the evaluation of symptomatology because of the unreliable nature of the report of any single observer involved (parents, teachers, friends, or the child). A number of instruments have been designed to collect multi-informant data and score in an integrative manner for diagnostic assessment and treatment-outcome monitoring. Empirically derived instruments that measure behavioral symptomatology and social function have been developed as a means of identifying children with significant emotional or behavioral disturbances and of assessing them across different settings and environments. They offer a complementary alternative to diagnostically driven identification. Additionally, these serve as efficient means of screening populations of children, because many are directly self-administered by key informants, such as the child, parent, and teacher, without needing significant interviewer assistance. The Child Behavior Checklist/Teacher Report Form/Youth Self Report (Achenbach, 1991) is the prime example of this type of instrument. Additionally, instruments that evaluate a child's level of function globally or across different life domains have been found to be invaluable in assessing the effectiveness of treatment modalities or an overall treatment plan. The Child and Adolescent Functional Assessment Schedule (Hodges & Wong, 1996) and the Children's Global Assessment of Function (Shaffer et al., 1983) are examples of such functional instruments.

Multi-informant information is also needed to evaluate specific types of behaviors or symptoms and their responses to pharmacological intervention across different settings and environments. The Conners' Scales (for ADHD; Conners, 1969; Conners & Wells, 1997), the Child Depression Inventory (Kovacs, 1981), the State-Trait Anxiety Scale (STAIC; Spielberger, 1973), and the Yale-Brown Obsessive Compulsive Scale for Children (Y-BOCS-C; Goodman & Price, 1992) are examples of instruments that measure specific areas of symptomatology. To determine efficacy and adjunct dosages, these rating scales should be obtained from parents, teachers, and youths. This information benefits the clinician, school personnel, and parents by organizing information about drug responsiveness in ways that are most directly usable by school personnel and parents. Functional data from the school environment is invaluable in making rational decisions about the efficacy of a given pharmacological agent or dose for a given child.

When using antidepressant or mood-stabilizing agents, the need for adequate time to allow for build-up of serum levels should be considered. It often takes 2 to 3 weeks, or even longer, before adequate responses can be seen. Stimulants and short-acting benzodiazepines are exceptions, with effects often seen in hours or days. Therefore, adequate treatment periods should be considered before discontinuation of medication. Another complicating factor is the differential time course and dosage in different agents for efficacy on different symptoms. For example, in ADHD a complicating phenomenon in evaluating medication-dose efficacy is the reported findings of a curvilinear relationship between dose and attentional improvement, resulting in a therapeutic window effect, as compared to a more linear relationship between dose and efficacy in reducing hyperactivity and impulsivity (Rosenberg et al., 1994). This latter finding may complicate the validity and reliability of different observers. For example, teachers may be torn between identifying the effects on attention and learning versus the effects on disruptive behaviors in the classroom. More research needs to be done in these areas.

SPECIFIC AND SPECIAL ISSUES

A number of specific and special issues need to be addressed in order to ensure the success and effectiveness of pharmacological interventions.

Integration with Other Treatment Modalities

Pharmacotherapy is never a sole modality in treating children and adolescents with serious emotional disorders or mental illnesses. A multimodal treatment approach guided by a multidisciplinary team is the most effective approach. Pharmacotherapy is often best used for rapid symptom relief and return to function. Cognitive, behavioral, and psychosocial therapies, however, have been shown to be most effective in relapse prevention and the development of long-term adaptive skills (Cantwell, 1996). A well integrated multimodal treatment approach requires education of and close communication among different clinicians, educators, and parents. Joint definition of intervention, treatment goals, tracking of target symptoms, evaluation of level of function, close monitoring of medication side effects, and fidelity/adherence to treatment modality techniques and dosage must be achieved for such an approach to be successful.

Ideally, such an integrated treatment plan should be coordinated across agencies or settings in which the child or adolescent is involved. Unfortunately, such integration is not encouraged due to fears by agencies of incurring significant portions of the total costs of treatment, including medical treatment. This is most often seen in the lack of coordination with school districts around behavioral and pharmacological management. Interagency systems of care with clear interagency agreements can set the stage for such treatment integration (Pumariega et al., 1997).

Cultural Competence in Psychopharmacotherapy

A common assumption about psychopharmacotherapy is that since this is an area of intervention that is biologically based, cultural competence principles are not important in its implementation. However, research is emerging that challenges this assumption and makes cultural competence a critical principle in psychopharmacotherapy as well as in other areas of mental health treatment and services. Significant cultural bias found in clinical psychiatric diagnostic assessment of children and adolescents can readily lead to inappropriate use or level of action of the cytochrome P450 enzymes, and core monitoring can determine the level of dosage needed to achieve therapeutic action as well as the emergence of side effects (Sramek & Pi, 1996; Rudorfer & Potter, 1999).

Role of Professionals in Pharmacotherapy

The close and effective collaboration among different professionals of different disciplines can ensure the success of pharmacotherapy within the context of school-based mental health services as well as that of the overall treatment program for children.

Case Managers

In different systems of care, the role of case manager may be defined as a separate role or may be integrated into the role of other professionals, such as therapists or even psychiatrists. Case managers have critical roles to play in the implementation of pharmacotherapy. They can provide objective assessment of the child's baseline symptoms/behaviors and function as well as assessment of his/her response and of side effects, at times also using observer rating versions of many of the instruments described above. They can also facilitate the communication of observations and concerns from the child and family relating to the use of medications. The maintenance of adherence with medication regiments can also become a major focus of their work, both by supporting the child and family in this endeavor as well as by providing valuable feedback to the psychiatrist or other medical professional about the practicality of the regimen prescribed.

Psychiatrists

Child and adolescent psychiatrists, or general psychiatrists in manpower shortage areas, have critical roles in the treatment of children with serious emotional and mental disturbances. They can provide effective diagnostic evaluation for children suspected of serious disorders and can serve as clinical consultants to other professionals in interdisciplinary treatment teams in the construction, implementation, and reevaluation of treatment plans. They can initiate pharmacotherapeutic treatment and, upon stabilizing the child's condition, transition care to other medical professionals. They can consult with other mental health professionals on the implementation of a wide range of therapeutic modalities, including psychotherapeutic, behavioral, group, and family interventions. Child and adolescent psychiatrists can be involved in program consultation and community education around emotional and psychiatric disorders, and can provide systems of care consultation. Child and adolescent psychiatrists, with their combined medical and mental health training, can serve as effective interphase liaisons between medical and nonmedical professionals. In these days of more systematic treatment approaches, child and adolescent psychiatrists can also help design protocols as well as policy and procedures for pharmacological treatment within school settings (Pumariega et al., 1997).

Other Medical Professionals

Pediatricians are actively involved in monitoring the physical and cognitive development of children. They can provide screening assessment and first-line treatment for children with uncomplicated emotional and behavioral disorders, as well as assume care for children with more serious disorders in consultation with child psychiatrists. They can also care for concomitant physical illness in children with behavioral and emotional disturbances. Family physicians can serve some of the roles defined above, but their more limited training in childhood development limits their involvement in assessment. However, they can work closely with families on their child's overall physical and emotional health. Nurse practitioners and school nurses can also play important roles in providing screening evaluation, monitoring the efficacy of pharmacotherapy in consultation with child psychiatrists, and in outreach to the home and the community involving education about emotional disorders and mental illness.

Teachers and Other Educational Professionals

Educational professionals can serve important roles in effective pharmacotherapy within a school context. They can readily provide objective observations on a child's behavior either naturalistically or with the aid of rating tools. This is due to their ready access to other children for comparative assessment, which can be invaluable in diagnosis and in monitoring medication efficacy/outcomes. They can help destigmatize emotional and psychiatric disorders and its treatment with pharmacotherapy among other students and their families. They are in excellent positions to observe and report side effects, especially those affecting learning or cognition. Educational professionals can also reassure children and parents as they face decisions about initiating pharmacotherapy.

School psychologists can serve important roles in psychopharmacological treatment through their performance of psychoeducational testing, which can help to refine the selection of target symptoms and evaluation of the efficacy of treatment on educational function. They can also develop behavioral interventions to complement pharmacological treatment and improve the child's overall functioning.

Parental and Child Education; Consent and Alliance

True informed consent is the cornerstone of decision making about pharmacological interventions. The parents and the child, where appropriate, need to be fully informed of the risk and benefits of any medication in an interactive discussion using appropriate language that is understandable and allows for questions and responses. Side effects of medications and what the parents and child can do when side effects occur should be carefully discussed. Parents should also understand the importance of regular follow-ups to monitor for responses to medication and side effects. Collaboration with parents is essential in making dose adjustments and in ensuring adherence with medication treatment. This involves helping parents feel empowered to make the ultimate decisions around medication and feeling an equalization of the power differential associated with dealing with medical professionals (Werry & Aman, 1993).

It is also extremely important to educate parents and teachers about emotional and psychiatric disorders and the use of pharmacological agents as a means of empowerment and of demystifying psychopharmacology, with a resultant increase in comfort with such treatment. In the age of consumerism, there is ready information access on the World Wide Web and through advocacy groups, lay-oriented books, and educational materials. Parents and educators should be suspicious of professionals who hide behind technical language and incomprehensible terminology.

An issue that often arises in pharmacological treatment is the reluctance on the part of parents to allow school personnel knowledge of whether a child is on a psychotropic medication. Parents in such situations often fear discrimination and stigma from the resultant labeling of their child if this information is disclosed. However, this lack of disclosure can result in serious problems if the child experiences adverse effects without the knowledge of someone in the school setting. The achievement of a stigma-free environment in schools needs to be a high priority among school professionals and mental health professionals. This should involve education of both school professionals and children, as well as the development of appropriate procedures for medication administration that do not single out children adversely.

The importance of addressing medication treatment directly with the child cannot be overlooked. The clinicians involved should evaluate and address the child's self-concept and self-esteem and perceived stigma due to taking medications. They should also address fears of side effects as well as the realities of such. Children and teens can at times shift the responsibility and locus of control for their symptoms or problems, and their active involvement and control need to be encouraged. Clinicians need to enlist treatment adherence by the child, including honest reporting of side effects and developmentally appropriate responsibility for taking and keeping track of medications (Werry & Aman, 1993).

REFERENCES

Achenbach, T. (1991). *Integrative Guide for the CBCL 4–18, YSR, and TRF Profiles.* Burlington: University of Vermont, Department of Psychiatry.

American Psychiatric Association. (1994). *Diagnostic and statistical manual of mental disorders* (4th ed.). Washington, DC: American Psychiatric Press.

Arredondo, D., & Butler, S. (1994). Affective co-morbidity in psychiatrically hospitalized adolescents with conduct disorder or oppositional defiant disorder: Should conduct disorder be treated with mood stabilizers? *Journal of Child and Adolescent Psychopharmacology, 4,* 151–158.

Balon, R. (1994). Sleep terror disorder and insomnia treated with trazodone: A case report. *Annals of Clinical Psychiatry, 6,* 161–163.

Barkley, R. (1977). A review of stimulant drug research with hyperactive children. *Journal of Child Psychology and Psychiatry, 18,* 137–165.

Barkley, R., Fischer, M., Edelbrock, C., & Smallish, L. (1990). The adolescent outcome of hyperactive children diagnosed by research criteria: An eight year prospective follow-up study. *Journal of the American Academy of Child and Adolescent Psychiatry, 29,* 546–555.

Bernstein, J. G. (1995). *Drug therapy in psychiatry.* St. Louis: Mosby.

Bernstein, G., Borchardt, C., & Perwien, A. (1996). Anxiety disorders: A review of the past 10 years. *Journal of the American Academy of Child and Adolescent Psychiatry, 35,* 1110–1119.

Bradley, C. (1937). The behavior of children receiving benzadrine. *American Journal of Psychiatry, 95,* 577–585.

Campbell, M., & Cueva, J. (1995). Psychopharmacology in child and adolescent psychiatry: A review of the past seven years. Part II. *Journal of the American Academy of Child and Adolescent Psychiatry, 34,* 1262–1272.

Campbell, M., Rapoport, J., & Simpson, G. (1999). Antipsychotics in children. *Journal of the American Academy of Child and Adolescent Psychiatry, 38,* 537–545.

Cantwell, D. (1996). Attention deficit disorder: A review of the past 10 years. *Journal of the American Academy of Child and Adolescent Psychiatry, 35,* 978–987.

Caron, C., & Rutter, M. (1991). Co-morbidity in child psychopathology: Concept, issues, and research strategies. *Journal of Child Psychology and Psychiatry, 32,* 1063–1080.

Conners, C. K. (1969). *Conners rating scales.* Toronto: Multi-Health Systems.

Conners, C., & Wells, K. (1997). *Conners-Wells Self-Report Scale.* North Tonawanda, NY: Multi-Health Systems.

Dahl, R., & Trubnick, L. (1994). A clinical picture of child and adolescent narcolepsy. *Journal of the American Academy of Child and Adolescent Psychiatry, 33,* 834–841.

DeVane, C., & Salle, F. (1996). Serotonin selective reuptake inhibitor in child and adolescent psychopharmacology: A review of published experience. *Journal of Clinical Psychiatry, 57,* 56–66.

Doogan, D. (1991). Toleration of safety of sertraline: Experience worldwide. *International Journal of Clinical Psychopharmacology, 6 (Suppl.),* 47–56.

DuPaul, G., Barkley, R., & McMurray, M. (1994). Response of children with ADHD to methylphenidate: Interaction with internalizing symptoms. *Journal of the American Academy of Child and Adolescent Psychiatry, 33,* 894–903.

Elia, S., Boncherding, B., Rapoport, J., & Keyson, C. (1991). Methylphenidate and dextroamphetamine treatments of hyperactivity: Are there true non-responders? *Psychiatric Research, 36,* 141–155.

Fleming, S., & Offord, D. (1990). Epidemiology of childhood depressive disorders: A critical review. *Journal of the American Academy of Child and Adolescent Psychiatry, 29,* 571–580.

Gadow, K. (1997). An overview of three decades of research in pediatric psychopharmacology. *Journal of Child and Adolescent Psychopharmacology, 7,* 219–236.

Geller, B., & Luby, S. (1997). Child and adolescent bipolar disorder: A review of the past 10 years. *Journal of the American Academy of Child and Adolescent Psychiatry, 36,* 1168–1176.

Gittleman-Klein, R., Spitzen, R., & Cantwell, D. (1978). Diagnostic classification and psychopharmacological indications. In J. Werry (Ed.), *Pediatric psychopharmacology: The use of behavior modifying drugs in children* (pp. 148–160). New York: Brunner/Mazel.

Goodman, W., & Price, L. (1992). Assessment of severity and change in obsessive-compulsive disorder. *Psychiatric Clinics of North America, 15,* 861–869.

Groevich, S., Findling, R., Rowane, W., Friedman, L., & Schilz, C. (1996). Risperidone in the treatment of children and adolescents with schizophrenia: A retrospective study. *Journal of Child and Adolescent Psychopharmacology, 6,* 251–257.

Grimsley, S., & Iann, M. (1992). Paroxetine, sertraline and fluvoxamine: New selective serotonin reuptake inhibitors. *Clinical Pharmacy, 11,* 930–957.

Henden, B. L., Feldman, H. M., Lurier, A., & Murray, P. J. H. (1999). Efficacy of methylphenidate among preschool children with DD and ADHD. *Journal of American Academy of Child and Adolescent Psychiatry, 38,* 805–819.

Hodges, K., & Wong, M. (1996). Psychometric characteristics of a multidimensional measure to assess impairment: The Child and Adolescent Functional Assessment Scale. *Journal of Child and Family Studies, 5,* 445–467.

Kaminski, C., Robbins, M., & Weibley, R. (1994). Sertraline intoxication in a child. *Annals of Emergency Medicine, 23,* 1371–1374.

Kolko, D., Bukstein, O., & Barron, J. (1999). Methylphenidate and behavior modification in children with ADHD and co-morbid ODD or CD: Main and incremental effects across settings. *Journal of the American Academy of Child and Adolescent Psychiatry, 38,* 578–586.

Kovacs, M. (1981). Rating scales to assess depression in school-aged children. *Acta Paedopsychiatrica, 46,* 305–315.

Murdoch, M., & McTarish, D. (1992). Sertraline: A review of its psychodynamic and pharmacokinetics properties, and therapeutic potential in depression and obsessive-compulsive disorders. *Drugs, 44,* 604–624.

Pelham, W., & Murphy, H. (1986). Attention deficit and conduct disorders. In M. Hersen (Ed.), *Pharmacological and behavioral treatment: An integrated approach* (pp. 180–184). New York: Wiley.

Pfefferbaum, B. (1997). Posttraumatic stress disorder in children: A review of the past 10 years. *Journal of the American Academy of Child and Adolescent Psychiatry, 36,* 1503–1511.

Popper, C., & Zimnistzky, B. (1995). Child and adolescent psychopharmacology update: January, 1994–December, 1994. *Journal of Child and Adolescent Psychopharmacology, 5,* 1–40.

Perry, R., Pataki, C., Munoz-Silva, D., Armenteros, J., & Silva, R. (1997). Risperidone in children and adolescents with pervasive developmental disorder: Pilot trial and follow-up. *Journal of Child and Adolescent Psychopharmacology, 7,* 167–179.

Pumariega, A., Muller, B., & Rivers-Buckeley, N. (1982). Acute renal failure secondary to amoxapine overdose. *Journal of the American Medical Association, 282,* 3141–3142.

Pumariega, A., Nace, D., England, M., Diamond, J., Mattson, A., Fallon, T., Hansen, G., Lourie, I., Marx, L., Thurber, D., Winters, N., Graham, M., & Weigand, D. (1997). Community-based systems approach to children's managed mental health services. *Journal of Child and Family Studies, 6,* 149–164.

Rapport, M., DuPaul, G., & Kelly, K. (1989). Attention deficit hyperactivity disorder and methylphenidate: The relationship between gross body weight and drug responses in children. *Psychopharmacology Bulletin, 25,* 285–290.

Reich, W., Weiner, Z., & Herjanic, B. (1994). *Diagnostic Interview for Children and Adolescents–Revised (for DSM-IV) Computer Program: Child/Adolescent Version and Parent Version.* North Tonawanda, NY: Multi-Health Systems.

Remschmidt, H., Schulz, E., Martin, M., Warnke, A., & Trott, G. (1994). Childhood onset schizophrenia: History of the concept and recent studies. *Psychopharmacology Bulletin, 20,* 713–725.

Riddle, M., Bernstein, G., Cook, E., Leonard, H., March, J., & Swanson, J. (1999). Anxiolytics, adrenergic agents, and naltrexone. *Journal of the American Academy of Child and Adolescent Psychiatry, 38,* 546–556.

Rosenberg, D., Holttum, S., & Gershon, S. (1994). *Psychostimulant textbook of pharmacotherapy for child and adolescent psychiatric disorders* (pp. 19–50). New York: Brunner/Mazel.

Rudorfer, M., & Potter, W. (1999). Metabolism of tricyclic antidepressants. *Cell and Molecular Biology, 19,* 373–409.

Ryan, N. (1990). Heterocyclic antidepressants in children and adolescents. *Journal of Child and Adolescent Psychopharmacology, 1,* 21–31.

Sandman, C. (1991). The opiate hypothesis in autism and self injury. *Journal of Child and Adolescent Psychopharmacology, 1,* 237–248.

Shaffer, D., Gould, M., Brasic, J., & Piven, J. (1983). A children's global assessment scale (CGAS). *Archives of General Psychiatry, 40,* 1228–1231.

Shaffer, D., Fisher, P., Dulcan, M., Davies, M., Piacentini, J., Schwab-Stone, M., Lahey, B., Bourdon, K., Jansen, P., Bird, H., Canino, G., & Regier, D. (1996). The NIMH Diagnostic Interview Schedule for Children Version 2.3 (DISC 2.3): Description, acceptability, prevalence rates, and performance in the MECA study. *Journal of the American Academy of Child and Adolescent Psychiatry, 35,* 865–877.

Shapiro, T. (1989). The psychodynamic formulation in child and adolescent psychiatry. *Journal of the American Academy of Child and Adolescent Psychiatry, 28*(5), 675–680.

Singer, H., Brown, J., Quaskey, S., Rosenberg, L., Mellits, E., & Denckla, M. (1995). The treatment of attention deficit disorder in Tourette's syndrome: A double-blind, placebo-controlled study with clonidine and desipramine. *Pediatrics, 95,* 74–81.

Spielberger, C. (1973). *Preliminary test manual for the State-Trait Anxiety Inventory for Children.* Palo Alto, CA: Consulting Psychologists Press.

Sramek, J., & Pi, E. (1996). Ethnicity and antidepressant response. *Mount Sinai Journal of Medicine, 63,* 320–325.

Steiner, H., & Lock, J. (1998). Anorexia nervosa and bulimia nervosa in children and adolescents: A review of the past 10 years. *Journal of the American Academy of Child and Adolescent Psychiatry, 37,* 352–359.

Swanson, J., Flockhart, D., Udea, D., Cantwell, D., Connor, D., & Williams, L. (1995). Clonidine in the treatment of ADHD: Questions about safety and efficacy. *Journal of Child and Adolescent Psychopharmacology, 5,* 301–304.

Thompson, S., & Rey, J. (1995). Functional enuresis: Is desmopressin the answer? *Journal of the American Academy of Child and Adolescent Psychiatry, 34,* 266–271.

Werry, J., & Aman, M. (1993). *Practitioners guide to psychoactive drugs for children and adolescents.* New York: Plenum Press.

Chapter 19

CULTURAL COMPETENCE IN TREATMENT INTERVENTIONS

ANDRES J. PUMARIEGA

RATIONALE FOR CULTURAL COMPETENCE IN CHILDREN'S MENTAL HEALTH

Child and adolescent mental health has a history of interest in cross-cultural issues impacting on children and families, as witnessed by the work of early pioneers such as Erickson (1963), Berlin (1978, 1983), Minuchin (1974), and Spurlock (Spurlock, 1985, Wilkinson & Spurlock, 1986). However, the focus on serving culturally diverse children and families has traditionally been narrowly defined toward certain segments of the population, such as children living in inner cities or immigrant children. The attitude of most individuals in the field, and in society in general, has at best neglected the importance of these issues. However, recent demographic changes in the United States have served to underscore the significance of these issues and place them in the forefront of service delivery and policy in child mental health. In the past 20 years, there has been remarkable growth in what were termed minority groups, at a much faster rate than the mainstream European-background population in America. In many areas of the United States, including most large cities and many states in the Southwest, there are no longer minority populations; rather, there is a plurality of different ethnic, racial, and cultural groups. This will be the case for America as a whole before the year 2050, and among the under-18-year-old population by the year 2030. These changes are happening most rapidly in areas not typically associated with multiple racial/ethnic groups, such as the South and Midwest. Most of the growth in culturally diverse populations has been in the under-18 age group, both as a result of higher birth rates and increased immigration by younger ethnically diverse individuals. Culturally diverse youth already constitute 30 percent of the population under the age of 18, and close to 40 percent by 2020 (U.S. Bureau of the Census, 1998).

It would be a mistake to assume that these growing culturally diverse populations are in any way monolithic or homogeneous. They compromise a wide array of national origins, ethnicities, and races, many of which are overlapping. For example, there are numerous nationalities of Hispanics/Latinos in the United States; Mexican-Americans comprise the majority (about 2/3), but Puerto Ricans, Dominicans, Cubans, different Central American nationalities, and different South American nationalities are also included. Hispanics/Latinos have a varied racial and cultural heritage, including a strong American Indian background in mainland Latinos, a strong African heritage among Caribbean Latinos, and a strong European backgrounds among South Americans. Their reasons for originally arriving in the United States include economic immigration, political exile and refuge, and relocation by multinational corporations; and many groups have been in the United States for decades, some even before the landing of the Mayflower. Hispanics/Latinos range linguistically from monolingual Spanish, monolingual English, bilingual, to speaking many local dialects. This same level of diversity is seen within the other three main ethnic/racial groups.

Although these populations are rapidly becoming the numerical majority in the United States, they unfortunately still suffer from inequities in socioeconomic status, education, and political influence, as well as access to health and human services. This is reflected in significantly lower mean household income and levels of education, higher mortality rates (including infant mortality), higher unemployment, and higher rates of physical health problems and morbidities. Studies, such as the Epidemiological Catchment Area Study, point to equivalent levels of mental health needs among these populations when controlled for socioeconomic status, although poverty does play a significant role in higher mental health morbidity among them (Cheung & Snowden, 1990).

Culturally diverse groups, and particularly those in the four underserved and underrepresented ethnic/racial groups (African Americans, Latinos/Hispanics, Asian Americans, and American Indians), are currently still being discriminated against in the U.S. mental health system. A number of barriers to mental health care access exist for these populations. These include the lack of minority practitioners, lack of culturally appropriate services, and the lack of knowledge and skill among majority practitioners around cross-cultural issues. The persistent lack of public child and adolescent mental health services has a disproportionate impact on these underserved groups. As a result of the lack both of appropriate services and practitioners who are appropriately prepared to serve these populations, they are either underrepresented in public mental health settings, are shunted to other service systems, or are placed in overly restrictive levels of care, such as in inpatient facilities or incarceration/juvenile detention (Pumariega, Glover, Holzer, & Nguyen, 1998, Pumariega, Johnson, & Sheridan, & Cuffe, 1995; Cuffe, Waller, Cuccaro, Pumariega, & Garrison, 1995; Pumariega, Atkins, Rogers, Montgomery, Nybro, Caesar & Millus, 1999). The morbidity and mortality resulting from such neglect is already resulting in high social and financial costs for our society at large as well as high personal costs for minority children and their families. Such problems as high homicide and suicide rates, substance abuse, homelessness, teenage pregnancy, and school drop-out and illiteracy are at least partial results of these barriers and the policies that created them.

CONCEPTS OF CULTURE AND IMPACT ON HUMAN BEHAVIOR

In order to begin to understand the special needs of minority individuals, a conceptual framework of the role of culture in human behavior and development is necessary. The work of Spiegel (1971) and Kluckhorn (1953) has contributed to the understanding of

UNIVERSE

CULTURE   SOMA

SOCIETY   PSYCHE

GROUP (FAMILY)

Figure 19.1   Transactional Field of Human Experience
Source: Adapted from Spiegel (1971, p. 42).

this linkage. They define culture as part of a transactional field that influences human behavior and is made up of a series of interdependent levels or foci. Culture is the focus of the interface between a society and the greater physical universe, where the meaning of social behavior and knowledge of the meaning and function of guidelines for the maintenance of the social system, linguistic systems, and systems of beliefs and values are found (see Figure 19.1). According to Spiegel and Kluckhorn, basic cultural values attempt to define humans' relationship to four basic domains: nature, time, activity, and relationships. Different cultures define these relationships in ways that are adaptive according to the group's environmental and relational context. Table 19.1 gives examples of the different value orientations generally found within these four domains. These value orientations can also be influenced by other contextual factors, such as educational and economic background, and cannot be stereotyped across individuals within cultural groups, though some commonalities can be found within certain cultures. For example, Eastern and Indian cultures have long oriented their relationship with nature toward one of harmony, whereas Western cultures have placed a premium on overcoming the forces of nature for the greater human good. Many non-Western cultures focus either on the here and now or on past traditions and customs in terms of time, and do not place much emphasis on punctuality, whereas Western cultures focus on the future and time efficiency. Most non-Western cultures place more emphasis on the individual's identity in terms of familial/tribal membership or familial roles, rather than in terms of occupation career roles. Relational lines also vary greatly, with some non-Western cultures emphasizing either hierarchical relations or kinship networks

Table 19.1   Cultural Value Domains and Orientations/Preferences

Domains		Orientations/Preferences	
Man-Nature	Subjugation	Harmony	Mastery
Time	Past	Present	Future
Activity	Being	Being-in-becoming	Doing
Relational	Lineal	Collateral	Individual

Source: Adapted from Spiegel (1971, p. 163).

rather than focusing on either the value of the individual or intimacy between individuals.

Value orientations, and the beliefs and practices that arise from them, have particular importance in clinical interaction with children and families from diverse cultural backgrounds. The definition of behavioral and emotional normality is largely culturally determined. Cultural values help define psychosocial developmental norms and expectations and childrearing patterns. For example, normative expectations for such widely varied developmental tasks as toilet training, leaving a child unsupervised, readiness and process for expression of sexuality and intimacy, and readiness to leave the parental home are all governed by culture. Expected role functioning in different contexts is also largely culturally governed. These include definitions of gender roles (female versus male characteristics), familial roles (expectations of fulfilling roles as mother, father, child, sibling, grandparent, uncle or aunt, cousin, etc.), and much influence on occupational roles (degree of deference to superiors, performance expectations, etc.). Acceptable patterns for interpersonal communication are also largely culturally governed. For example, even within different Hispanic/Latino groups there may be wide differences in the acceptability of affective expressiveness, with some groups expected to be reticent and reserved and others being very expressive and voluble. Norms around behaviors or behavioral patterns and adaptive cognitive or psychological strategies or mechanisms differ widely among cultures. For example, motoric hyperactivity in male children is not seen as abnormal by many different cultural groups (including Latinos and African Americans), whereas for other groups it may be seen as highly deviant (such as for Asian Americans). Some cultures value coping mechanisms for stress reduction such as reaction-formation and affective reversal or sublimation of anxiety into productivity, whereas others may value humor, abreaction, and symbolic representation of conflicts in rituals or artistic forms.

Human psychological development is a key process through which culture has significant impact on behavior and adaptation. A child responds to cultural expectations for role functioning, interpersonal relationships and communication patterns, and behavioral norms. However, for most culturally diverse children, this may involve being conversant with at least two cultural systems. A number of authors, including deAnda (1984), have already proposed that an optimal adaptation for minority children and particularly adolescents is the development of the capacity for biculturality or even multiculturality. Such adaptation implies the development of knowledge and skills in at least two cultural traditions; the youth retains his or her original cultural heritage but becomes adept at meeting the expectations of a different culture. It also implies the development of flexibility to operate in different cultural contexts, the development of a stable self-image and values based on selective adoption of the best values and beliefs of different cultures, and openness to different cultural viewpoints and perspectives. Inability to develop these adaptational characteristics results in a number of patterns with adverse psychological consequences. These include margination, reification, or mummification of the culture of origin, overacculturation to the mainstream culture, and resultant identity diffusion or negative identity formation as defined by Erikson (1968) and cultural conflict that is either internalized or externalized between generations in the family (Szapocznik, Scopetta, & Tillman, 1978).

It is important to view the lack of development of these cross-cultural skills in culturally diverse youngsters not as disorders, but as developmental tasks that they can achieve given the proper environmental support and opportunities, which are often lacking in the difficult socioeconomic and social circumstances in which they grow up. Remarkably, many do develop them despite very adverse circumstances, including poverty and discrimination. In fact, with an increasingly pluralistic society, these may also be critical (and equally difficult) tasks for children from the mainstream culture. Sue (1981) describes the process of racial identity formation and provides a developmental framework for understanding these particular mental health issues. Sue's work suggests that the identity formation process can be assessed and that therapeutic interventions can be designed to facilitate the development of a healthy bicultural adjustment. However, behaviors that may be offensive to the larger society are likely to be exhibited during identity development, causing many helpers to see a healthy but painful process as pathologic. Inappropriate responses may inhibit healthy outcomes and contribute to role confusion and identity diffusion.

Culture likewise has a major influence on how we experience, understand, express, and address emotional, behavioral, and mental distress and dysfunction. It greatly influences the type of symptomatology that is used to express distress and which may characterize different disorders. Somatization, for example, is often a frequent symptom associated with depression and anxiety disorders in Hispanics and Asian Americans. It is less stigmatizing and culturally sanctioned to deal with somatic expressions rather than emotions, and it leads to access to services through the general health system rather than mental health professionals. Differences in language and idiomatic expressions can determine how different symptoms are identified. Symptoms may also take on different meanings in different cultural contexts. For example, the term *blue* may have clinical significance to a psychiatrist, but to an African American it may reflect a state resulting from chronic oppression, and to a Hispanic it may not make any sense at all because it would be interpreted literally (feeling a color). Cultural values may also dictate who the reliable reporters and observers are as well as where it is appropriate to discuss different symptoms and problems. For some time it was assumed that Asians suffered more somatic symptoms than others, but recent research has demonstrated that they report somatic symptoms to physicians but are able to identify emotional responses and symptoms only to close friends and family. Different clustering of symptoms may also vary among different groups. For example, fewer Africans than Britons identified as depressed meet diagnostic criteria for major depression (Draguns, 1984).

Attributional beliefs about mental illness and emotional stress are largely culturally determined, and these influence an individual or family's attitudes and responses. For example, mental illness can be viewed through a Western biopsychosocial perspective, or through the perspective of religion (God's will), spirituality (spirit possession), or interpersonal/supernatural beliefs (caused by hexes or spells). Culture also defines the role and level of function that the "sick" individual is to fulfill within both the family and the greater society. For example, the mentally ill individual may be expected to behave in a fragile or invalid manner, or to carry on normal responsibilities despite their illness, or have a special spiritual role for the society. Finally, cultural values and beliefs also influence patterns of help-seeking behavior. Individuals of different cultures may seek different types of assistance, ranging from neighborhood wise ladies or *co-madres,* traditional healers (such as *curanderos, santeros, espiritas,* root doctors, medicine men/women, etc.), religious (ministers, priests, rabbis, mullahs), primary care physicians, to mental health professionals, with these usually being the last to be consulted. The orientation of healers and healing approaches is largely governed by attributional beliefs and may differ greatly from that of the professional establishment (ceremonies/rituals, incantations, prayers, herbal remedies, sweat lodges, spiritual counseling, psychotherapy, psychopharmacology; (Rogler & Cortes, 1993).

Various risk factors for psychopathology are influenced by cultural background and immigration status. Risks for certain forms of psychopathology or morbidity that are commonly seen in mainstream populations, such as substance abuse, eating disorders, and suicidality, increase with increased exposure to Western cultural values and practices (Swanson, Linskey, Quintero-Salinas, Pumariega, & Holzer, 1992, Pumariega, 1986, Pate, Pumariega, Hester, & Garner, 1995). This increase in risk may be a result of the loss of previously protective cultural values and beliefs (such as different attitudes about the use of substances, suicide, and body image, or family support) and exposure to risk-enhancing factors (such as media exposure and peer pressure with lesser family support, Pumariega, Swanson, Holzer, Linskey, & Quintero-Salinas, 1992, Pate, Pumariega, Hester, & Garner, 1992). Added stressors from the process of immigration and acculturation itself can lead to increased risk for emotional disturbance. These include previous traumatic exposure in their homelands (war, terrorism, famine), loss of extended family, difficult and traumatic journeys to the United States (crossing rivers, capsizing in rafts, witnessing deaths), margination, discrimination, and poverty.

CULTURAL COMPETENCE MODEL

Cross, Bazron, Dennis, and Isaacs (1989), in their monograph titled *Towards a Culturally Competent System of Care,* defined the prerequisites for culturally appropriate or competent services for minority children and their families. They defined the cultural competence model as a set of congruent behaviors, attitudes, and policies that are found in a system, agency, or a group of professionals that enables them to work effectively in a context of cultural difference. They identified a spectrum of cultural competence that has been demonstrated by society at large and by institutions in particular and that ranges across cultural destructiveness (genocide, lynching, ethnic cleansing), cultural incapacity (segregation, discrimination, immigration quotas, services that break up families), cultural blindness ("equal" treatment for all, but not making distinctions in services offered or differences in values or beliefs), cultural precompetency (realization of differences but insufficient provision of services), cultural competence, and cultural proficiency (provision of innovative services and research).

Cross et al. (1989) went on to define the particular qualities that culturally competent practitioners and agencies must embody and achieve. For the individual practitioner, they included qualities such as being aware and accepting of cultural differences, awareness of their own culture and the biases it may create, understanding the dynamics of working across cultures, acquisition of cultural knowledge, and acquiring and adapting practice skills to fit the cultural context of the client. They also drew on the work of Wilson (1982), who summarized a number of the qualities to be developed un-

Table 19.2 Personal Attributes/Attitudes Essential for Practitioner Cultural Competence

Personal qualities that reflect genuineness, accurate empathy, nonpossessive warmth, and a capacity to respond flexibly to a range of possible solutions.

Acceptance of ethnic difference between people.

A willingness to work with clients of different ethnic minority groups.

Articulation and clarification of the therapists' personal values, stereotypes, and biases about their own and others' ethnicity and social class, and ways these may accommodate or conflict with the needs of ethnic minority clients.

Personal commitment to change racism and poverty.

Resolution of feelings about one's professional image in fields that have systematically excluded people of color.

Source: Wilson (1982).

der areas of attitudes, knowledge, and skill (see Tables 19.2, 19.3, and 19.4). Many of these attributes do not differ from qualities found in good clinicians or mental health professionals, but others are specifically oriented to the needs of culturally diverse children and families.

Cross et al. (1989) also defined four main qualities to be demonstrated by culturally competent agencies or institutions. These include valuing and adapting to cultural diversity, ongoing organizational self-assessment; understanding and managing the dynamics of cultural difference, the institutionalization of cultural knowledge and skills through training, experience, and literature, and instituting service adaptations to serve culturally diverse clients and their families better. They go on to specify that such adaptations include addressing barriers to care (cultural, linguistic, geographic, or economic), levels of staffing that reflect the composition of the community being served, needs assessment and outreach, training in communication or interviewing skills, and modifications in actual assessment and treatment procedures and modalities.

Table 19.3 Areas of Knowledge Essential for Practitioner Cultural Competence

Knowledge of the culture (history, traditions, values, family systems, artistic expressions) of ethnic minority clients.

Knowledge of the impact of class and ethnicity on behavior, attitudes, and values.

Knowledge of the help-seeking behaviors of ethnic minority clients.

Knowledge of the role of language, speech patterns, and communication styles in ethnically distinct communities.

Knowledge of the impact of social service policies on ethnic minority clients.

Knowledge of the resources (agencies, persons, informal helping networks, research) that can be utilized on behalf of ethnic minority clients and communities.

Recognition of the ways that professional values may conflict with or accommodate the needs of ethnic minority clients.

Knowledge of power relationships within the community, agency, or institution and their impact on ethnic minority clients.

Source: Wilson (1982).

Table 19.4   Areas of Skill Essential for Practitioner Cultural Competence

Techniques for learning the cultures of ethnic minority client groups.

Ability to communicate accurate information on behalf of ethnic minority clients and their communities.

Ability to discuss openly racial and ethnic differences and issues and to respond to culturally-based cues.

Ability to assess the meaning ethnicity has for individual clients.

Ability to differentiate between the symptoms of intrapsychic stress and stress arising from the social structure.

Interviewing techniques reflective of the therapist's understanding of the role of language in the client's culture.

Ability to utilize the concepts of empowerment on behalf of ethnic minority clients and communities.

Capability of using resources on behalf of ethnic minority clients and their institutions.

Ability to recognize and combat racism, racial stereotypes, and myths in individuals and institutions.

Ability to evaluate new techniques, research, and knowledge as to their validity and applicability in working with ethnic minorities.

Source: Wilson (1982).

APPLICATION OF CULTURAL COMPETENCE PRINCIPLES IN CLINICAL INTERVENTIONS

Clinical Environment

The concept of cultural competence has direct applications in the clinical setting in the interface between the child and adolescent psychiatrist and the child and his or her family. We will present how these concepts are applied at different stages of clinical work. Even before the child and the family actually present for a clinical visit, the clinician must be aware of how cultural differences can impact access to the care desired. The clinic or facility may have inadvertently developed barriers such as how the telephone referral is handled over the phone (e.g., either too formal or impersonal or not sufficiently respectful), the geographic location of the clinic (away from accessible transportation or the neighborhood), and the appointment hours available (which may not match the work and activity hours of the family). The clinic setting and decor may not reflect the cultural values of the populations being served, such as having sufficient room for extended family or kin. In fact, some clinics may actively discourage attendance by such related individuals during initial visits, even though they may have information critical for the diagnostic process. Registration and financial procedures may also serve to enhance an atmosphere of impersonality and mistrust.

Engagement and Therapeutic Alliance

The establishment of a therapeutic alliance may be the most critical factor in treatment success with culturally diverse youth and families (Bernal, Bonilla, Padilla-Cotto, &

Perez-Prado, 1998). Once the child and family present for their initial appointments, the clinician must be attentive to how his or her nonverbal and verbal cues and those of the family are perceived within their cultural context and the impact these have on the establishment of a therapeutic alliance. For example, even the manner in which a handshake is approached can have vastly different meanings in different cultures. In many Native American tribes, a soft handshake is the appropriate sign of respect and trust with either gender. On the other hand, Hispanic males expect a firm handshake, whereas females expect a softer one. Avoidance of eye contact, which may be misperceived as a sign of dishonesty or even psychopathology by majority clinicians, is a sign of respect among Asians and a self-protective adaptational stance among African Americans. It may be important to establish quickly who the main spokesperson for the family is and to direct inquiries through that individual, at least initially. Gender-based differences in different cultures in interpersonal communication, communication of intimate information, and boundaries also need to be recognized and addressed (Bracero, 1998).

A number of factors may impinge on the minority family's motivation for clinical assistance. It is important to establish whether the motivation is primarily their own or is enforced by some outside agent or agency (e.g., school, welfare department, etc.), which may lead to resentment and disinterest. If the referral resulted from the failure of a cultural practitioner to address the problem, the family may be dealing with demoralization and frustration. Whether such care is sanctioned by the family elders/decision-makers, such as grandparents, is very important, and they should be involved as soon as possible. The clinician should ascertain the degree of stigma associated with mental illness and seeking psychiatric help in the culture and how this could affect the family's comfort with the consultation. The expectations and outcomes of the evaluation should be readily established so they may be dealt with openly and misconceptions or disappointments can be prevented (Cross et al., 1989).

Other important factors that can adversely impact the establishment of a therapeutic alliance with culturally diverse youth and families is that of clinicians' preexisting biases and stereotypes. Some studies have established how such biases can adversely affect the perception of minority clients from the outset of the clinical interaction (Abreu, 1999). Clinicians need to become aware of their previous-learned perceptions of diverse cultural and racial groups and should actively prevent these from entering into their interaction of their diverse clients.

Clinical Assessment

The principles of cultural competence can also be applied to the assessment of the psychosocial functioning of the individual child within his or her sociocultural context. The earlier points about cultural factors involved in the expression, reporting, and assessment of symptomatology need to be accounted for in clinical evaluations. Such differences in the interpretation of emotional experiences, the labelling and interpretation of symptomatology, and the degree of self-disclosure affect the cross-cultural and cross-ethnic validity of most of the diagnostic instruments used in clinical assessment, because the large majority of these were normed with primarily Anglo-American populations. Results from any such instruments require interpretation within the youngster's sociocultural context as well as support by careful clinical observation (Canino et al., 1994).

The cultural and family context of symptomatology must also be considered in the assessment of a minority child. Symptomatology may be occurring in the context of a culturally normative period of transition, such as a grief/mourning period or a maturational stage. One must also assess whether cross-cultural dynamics play a role in the symptomatology, such as intergenerational conflicts around acculturation, discrimination, and margination from the majority culture or the youth's own culture. The impact of experiences such as poverty and deprivation or traumatic immigration should also be considered (Koss-Chioino & Vargas, 1999).

In assessing the behavior and psychosocial development of minority children, one must consider that the expected norms for these may differ considerably among different cultural groups; different psychological and cognitive skills are reinforced according to different cultural values. Minority children are also exposed to different family structures, role expectations, and communication patterns than are majority children. When minority children are evaluated against the norms for the majority, Euro-American culture, they may be erroneously found to be deficient or abnormal. For example, African American children are frequently overrepresented in the disruptive behavior diagnoses, but the greater emphasis on motoric development in Afrocentric cultures is not taken into account in coming to such diagnostic conclusions (Fabrega, Ulrich, & Mezzich, 1993, Kilgus, Pumariega, & Cuffe, 1995). Another misconception, that African American children have lower levels of self-esteem than whites, was proven erroneous by a number of studies that found that they actually had higher levels of self-esteem and used each other as models for comparison. Native American children are often assessed as quiet or lacking in social skills due to being socialized to use longer pauses between turns at conversation. When the Native American child pauses for a polite silence of up to 30 seconds after the previous speaker, children or adults of other cultures usually break the silence, leaving the Native American child out of the conversation. In the diagnostic interview, this behavior is often misinterpreted. In fact, a particular source of stress for the culturally diverse child is the conflicting developmental expectations from within and outside their families and communities, with the risk of being labelled as dysfunctional by either (Powell et al., 1983, Gibbs & Huang, 1989, Philips, 1983).

In order to ascertain the roles of culture and cultural values in the functioning of the minority child more accurately, the clinician must become knowledgeable about the developmental norms and childrearing patterns of the populations that he or she serves. Although there are excellent resource materials for reference, the best source of such information is the family itself. Modifications to the traditional diagnostic interview are needed for this purpose. The techniques used are often termed ethnographic interviewing, with the best overall reference for them to be found in the article "Teaching Ethnographic Methods to Social Service Workers" by Green and Leigh (1989). Green and Leigh have adapted the work of Spradley (1979) to allow human service professionals a window on the reality experienced by their clients. In general, such techniques involve having the family member serve as the cultural guide for the clinician by making a series of open-ended inquiries about different cultural aspects of family life. For example, one might ask the parent or grandparent about the usual expectations for behavior or self-control by asking, "How are boys supposed to behave and mind in your community?" The clinician might need to mark a transition from the typical psychiatric interview and actively enlist the cooperation of the family member in this task. One might also incorporate some of these techniques in the interview with the child to evaluate his or her understanding of cultural expectations. In addition, consultants from the cultural group or community to which the family belongs can also provide much contextual information about normal development, behavioral norms, and role-functioning expectations. In interviewing the child, the clinician should as much as possible include in the interview or the interview area symbols significant to the child's culture in order to facilitate expression of their conflicts in culturally syntonic ways. This might include having dolls and figures of the appropriate racial group or reading materials that could elicit cultural themes.

It is not uncommon to serve children from families who do not speak English in clinical settings. Unfortunately, the importance of language and communication in obtaining accurate clinical information is totally overlooked in many mental health settings. Translation and interpretation is relegated as a menial or informal task rather than as one that is central to the clinical process. This is reflected in the use of disembodied telephonic translating services or untrained translators, such as housekeeping or lower-level care staff, and the use of family members without regard to the impact on family relations, particularly the use of siblings or the child him- or herself. This latter practice should be absolutely prohibited except in emergencies due to the adverse impact it can have on family relations. Interpreters should have proper training in both their skill and the content area of interpretation, in this case child mental health. They should understand the culture of the child and family and be ready to address verbal, nonverbal, and implicit communications (Altarriba & Santiago Rivera, 1994).

Care Planning and Selection of Interventions

The treatment planning and interpretive process are critical in the effective treatment of the minority child. The minority family may well feel a strong power differential between themselves and the professional, which is often the case when dealing with agents of the majority culture. They may often choose to acquiesce passively and later not follow recommendations. It is important to address this perception and empower the family in making treatment decisions for their child. One must ensure that a true consensus is developed with the family around the understanding of the child's problems and possible illness. This may involve using terminology and concepts acceptable in their cultural belief system. It is also important to present treatment options in a demystifying manner understandable to the family, but in a manner that is not condescending to them. Such options should include cultural or folk practitioners and consultants whenever indicated, as well as the option not to pursue treatment at all.

One of the most obvious care planning decisions in the mental health treatment of culturally diverse children and their families involves clinician assignment. The assignment of a therapist/clinician from the same or similar cultural, ethnic, or racial background would seem to be the most culturally competent approach to treatment. In fact, some studies suggest that such matching leads to better engagement in treatment and better outcomes (O'Sullivan & Lasso, 1992). However, there are some realities that mitigate this choice. First, the availability of such a matched clinician is likely to be low, especially in geographic areas where the child belongs to a marked numerical minority. Overall, minority mental health clinicians are far outnumbered by culturally diverse children and families seeking services. Minority clinicians are not necessarily culturally competent in terms of their clinical skills, and the acculturation process inherent in professional training may reduce their degree of cross-cultural effectiveness. Also, there are times when minority families deliberately do not want to see a clinician from their own community out of concern for confidentiality and potential stigma.

Modalities that focus on immediate needs and problems and interpersonal processes and have a present orientation are more acceptable and practical than those emphasizing insight and a future orientation. Explanatory models of illness or psychological distress also play a role in the family's acceptance of the care plan and therapeutic approaches being recommended (Callan & Littlewood, 1998). It is important, in selecting target behaviors for intervention or role function expectations for improvement goals, that cultural norms for these be taken into account. Additionally, for behavioral interventions, the selection of family interveners needs to be consonant with the normative family roles for the culture. For example, if grandparents have a greater role in discipline than parents, they need to be highly involved in developing and implementing any protocols for behavioral interventions for disruptive behaviors.

Pharmacotherapy

A common assumption about psychopharmacotherapy is that because this is an area of intervention that is biologically based, cultural competence principles are not important in its implementation. However, research is emerging that challenges this assumption and makes cultural competence a critical principle in psychopharmacotherapy as well as in other areas of mental health treatment and services. The interpretation, expression, measure, and threshold of behavioral and emotional symptoms can also vary across cultures, making the establishment of baselines and outcomes more challenging. Significant cultural bias found in clinical psychiatric diagnostic assessment of children and adolescents (Kilgus et al., 1995; Fabrega et al., 1993), which can readily lead to the inappropriate use or withholding of psychopharmacotherapy for culturally diverse children. For example, Zito, Safer, dosReis, Magder, and Riddle (1997) found that African American children were less likely to receive stimulant medications than were Caucasian children in treatment settings. The perception by ethnic and racial minorities of psychopharmacological agents as a means for social control adversely influences the acceptability of these agents among such populations. Cultural and ethnic norms around family medical decision-making and consent need to be considered in presenting the recommendations to use such agents and soliciting informed consent, where elders assume a greater role than in traditional White middle-class families. It is important to educate and obtain true informed consent from the true family decision-makers or elders in order to obtain optimal treatment compliance. This also involves demystifying the use of medications and addressing misperceptions based both on traditional cultural beliefs as well as on the perceived power differential with the clinician (e.g., the medication will "control his thinking"). Discussion of biological and genetic factors can also serve to alleviate feelings of guilt on the part of the family, who may often feel responsible for the child's illness or problems as a result of their socioeconomic limitations.

Additionally, there are cross-racial and cross-cultural biological considerations that need to be attended to in psychopharmacological treatment. A new science of ethnopsychopharmacology is developing its own body of literature pointing to genetic and nutritional factors that can contribute to differential pharmacological responses across ethnic and racial groups (Lin, Poland, & Nasaki, 1993). A case in point relates to the metabolism of most pharmacological agents, especially the selective serotonin reuptake inhibitor (SSRI) antidepressants. These agents are metabolized by a series of liver enzymes called cytochrome P450 enzymes, and various of these enzymes are responsible for the metabolism of different agents. Genetic polymorphisms have been described for many drug metabolizing enzymes in Caucasian, Asian, and African populations (Smith & Mendoza, 1996). Additionally, nutritional factors such as citrus and corn content in the diet, which vary in different ethnic groups, inhibit the action of some of these enzymes. The level of action of the cytochrome P450 enzymes can determine the level of dosage needed to achieve therapeutic action as well as the emergence of side effects (Rudorfer & Potter, 1999).

Psychosocial Therapies

In individual psychotherapy, the clinician must address the dynamics of cultural differences and power differentials with the child as clearly as with the family. The presence of identity or role confusion as a result of acculturation conflicts should also be addressed empathetically, but also empowering the child to make his or her own flexible choices around cultural values and identification. It is also important to address specific areas of cultural conflict, such as role pressures on children to serve as a cultural broker with their family, pressures not to betray their culture, and negative identification against their culture of origin. A value-neutral approach, where the clinician models openness to the diverse cultural influences that the child is exposed to, is quite effective in achieving these goals. The therapist can also use judicious self-disclosure with the child when he or she has personally experienced any of these conflicts. It is also important to address issues of confidentiality in psychotherapy so the clinician is neither perceived as driving a wedge between the patient and his or her family nor used by the patient as a means of resisting dealing with family issues (Gibbs & Huang, 1989; Baker, 1999).

Culturally diverse population of children and families have been shown to be more accepting and responsive to psychotherapeutic approaches that have a practical here-and-now focus. Cognitive-behavioral approaches, which are inherently oriented towards these principles, are most frequently used, with results from studies and case reports suggesting good response by culturally diverse clients (Elligan, 1997; Williams, Chambless, & Steketee, 1998; Longshore, Grills, & Annon, 1999). Interpersonal approaches, which focus on an important attributional issue in emotional/behavioral problems for non-Western cultures, show promise in their use with diverse populations (Mufson, Weissman, Moreau, & Garfinkel, 1999; Rosello & Bernal, 1999; Brown, Schulberg, Sacco, Perel, & Houck, 1999). Psychoanalytically, insight-oriented interventions are not contraindicated, and no stereotypes should be drawn about the ability and capacity of culturally diverse children and families to respond to these approaches. However, psychoanalytically oriented approaches have tended to include inherent cultural biases, such as encouraging separation-individuation and challenge of traditional parental authority and roles, which can be counterproductive in engaging families from more traditional cultures (Cabaniss, Oquendo, & Singer, 1994). When cultural values and beliefs are effectively addressed, culturally diverse clients also benefit from these approaches (Aslami, 1997). Some therapists have developed interventions that are specific for particular ethnic and racial groups and have been evaluated for efficacy (Malgady, Rogler, & Costantino, 1990; Constantino, Malgady, & Rogler, 1994; De Rios, 1997). Group psychotherapy, particularly group approaches that integrate cultural and ethnic identity themes as well as a psychoeducational approach addressing culturally consonant coping approaches, have also been reported as both well accepted and successful (Guanipa, Talley, & Rapagna, 1997; Yancey, 1998, Salvendy, 1999).

All treatment of minority children must have a contextual orientation in order to address cultural issues effectively. This means that the therapist must evaluate the familial, neighborhood, community, and cultural contexts of the child's dysfunctional behaviors, address the environmental factors that contribute to the problem behaviors, and also enhance strengths that the child and family bring to the efforts at problem-solving (Koss-Chioino & Vargas, 1999). The therapist should help parents develop effective behavioral management skills that are consonant with their values and beliefs. They must respect culturally established means of communication and family role functioning, but at the same time fostering flexibility on the part of the family to accommodate differing points of view that might be espoused by their more bicultural offspring. This involves addressing intergenerational acculturation conflicts, which may stem from parental fears of abandonment by their acculturating child, while also facilitating the family in their role of transmission of traditional cultural values and beliefs in a nonconflicting fashion. The family can also accept greater acculturation by the child if empowered in dealing with the majority culture more effectively (Montalvo & Gutierrez, 1983; Szapocznik & Kurtines, 1989; Koss-Chioino & Vargas, 1999).

In a contextual approach, the therapist should also engage the family in using community resources that can facilitate both the enhancement of their traditional strengths as well as the introduction into new cultural viewpoints. This includes the use of school settings, churches, community organizations, and informal kinship networks, from which the family is often cut off or marginated (Spurlock, 1985; Gutierrez-Mayka & Contreras-Neira, 1998; Garrison, Roy, Azar, 1999; Koss-Chioino & Vargas, 1999). Using a cultural consultant in therapy, with the family's consent, can also be useful in dealing with issues around the interpretation of traditional beliefs and values as well as potential distortions of these for dysfunctional purposes.

CHALLENGES TO THE CULTURAL COMPETENCE OF SYSTEMS OF CARE

In recent years, managed behavioral health models and technology in health and mental health systems have had particular impact on culturally diverse populations, particularly on children and their families. Many are covered under Medicaid for health and mental health benefits, and states increasingly pursue managed behavioral health approaches for their Medicaid programs. Public managed behavioral health, combined with the privatization of many of these services, tends to be oriented toward middle-income populations that do not deal with the multiple stressors that culturally diverse children and families face and uses different types of services, particularly fewer social support services. It also has relocated many mental health services away from traditional ethnic community and neighborhood settings and towards unfamiliar and uncomfortable suburban settings. The exclusive provider panels developed for such managed care plans also tend to exclude culturally diverse practitioners due to their having fewer formal credentials as well as their serving higher risk and higher utilizing (and higher cost) clients.

The response to these challenges has been to operationalize further the definition of culturally competent mental health services, at both the provider and systems level. This has led to the development of standards for culturally competent mental health services for mental health practitioners, provider organizations, health plans, and organized systems of care. Examples of such standards include the Guidelines for Culturally Competent Managed Mental Health Services by the National Latino Behavioral Workgroup, sponsored by the Western Interstate Commission on Higher Education (Pumariega et al., 1997), and the Standards for Cultural Competence in Managed Care Mental Health by the Center for Mental Health Services (Four Racial/Ethnic Panels, 1999). These outline specific best practice standards for significant aspects of mental health systems (including governance, benefit design, quality assurance/improvement, information systems, and staff training and support) and clinical practice (access portals, triage and assessment, care planning, case management, treatment services, case management, and linguistic support). They also set out a process for cultural competence planning for systems of care that is based on a needs assessment of the diverse populations being served and that involves the leadership and front line providers. The Surgeon General's Report on Mental Health (U.S. Office of the Surgeon General, 1999) also outlines significant issues in ethnic/racial mental health disparities and will be followed by a focused report in this area. Research in epidemiology and services research examining mental health disparities for minority and underserved youth is also pointing the way toward the system of care reforms needed to improve the cultural competence of child mental health services (Pumariega, 1996; Glover & Pumariega, 1998).

REFERENCES

Abreu, J. (1999). Conscious and nonconscious African-American stereotypes: Impact on first impression and diagnostic ratings by therapists. *Journal of Consulting and Clinical Psychology, 67*(3), 387–393.

Altarriba, J., & Santiago Rivera, A. (1994). Current perspectives on using linguistic and cultural factors in counseling the hispanic client. *Professional Psychology. Research and Practice, 25*(4), 388–397.

Aslami, B. (1997). Interracial psychotherapy: A report of the treatment of an inner-city adolescent. *Journal of the American Academy of Psychoanalysis, 25*(3), 347–356.

Baker, A. (1999). Acculturation and reacculturation influence: Multilayer contexts in therapy. *Clinical Psychology Review, 19*(8), 951–967.

Berlin, I. N. (1978). Anglo adoptions of Native Americans: Repercussions in adolescence. *Journal of the American Academy of Child and Adolescent Psychiatry, 17,* 387–388.

Berlin, I. N. (1983). Prevention of emotional problems among Native American children: Overview of developmental issues. In S. Chess & A. Thomas (Eds.), *Annual progress in child psychiatry and development* (pp. 320–333). New York: Brunner/Mazel.

Bernal, G., Bonilla, J., Padilla-Cotto, L., & Perez-Prado, E. (1998). Factors associated to outcome in psychotherapy: An effectiveness study in Puerto Rico. *Journal of Clinical Psychology, 54*(3), 329–342.

Brown, C., Schulberg, H., Sacco, D., Perel, J., & Houck, P. (1999). Effectiveness of treatments for major depression in primary care practice: A post-hoc analysis of outcomes for African-American and white patients. *Journal of Affective Disorders, 53*(2), 185–192.

Bracero, W. (1998). Intimidades: Confianza, gender, and hierarchy in the construction of Latino-Latina therapeutic relationships. *Cultural Diversity and Mental Health, 4*(4), 264–277.

Cabaniss, D., Oquendo, M., & Singer, M. (1994). The impact of psychoanalytic values on transference and countertransference: A study in transcultural psychotherapy. *Journal of the American Academy of Psychoanalysis, 22*(4), 609–621.

Callan, A., & Littlewood, R. (1998). Patient satisfaction: Ethnic origin or explanatory model? *International Journal of Social Psychiatry, 44*(1), 1–11.

Canino, G., Bird, H., Rubio-Stipec, M., Woodbury, M., Ribera, J., Huertas, S., & Seeman, M. (1987). Reliability of child diagnosis in a hispanic sample. *Journal of the American Academy of Child and Adolescent Psychiatry, 26*(4), 560–565.

Cheung, F. K., & Snowden, L. (1990). Community mental health and ethnic minority populations. *Community Mental Health Journal, 26*(3), 277–291.

Constantino, G., Malgady, R. G., & Rogler, L. H. (1994). Storytelling through pictures culturally sensitive psychotherapy for hispanic children and adolescents. *Journal of Clinical Child Psychology, 23*(1), 13–20.

Cross, T. L., Bazron, B. J., Dennis, K. W., & Isaacs, M. R. (1989). *Towards a culturally competent system of care.* Washington, DC: CASSP Technical Assistance Center, Georgetown University Child Development Center.

Cuffe, S., Waller, J., Cuccaro, M., Pumariega, A. J., & Garrison, C. Z. (1995). Race and gender differences in the treatment of psychiatric disorders in young adolescents. *Journal of the American Academy of Child & Adolescent Psychiatry, 34*(11), 1536–1543.

DeAnda, D. (1984). Bicultural socialization: Factors affecting the minority experience. *Social Work, 29,* 101–107.

De Rios, M. (1997). Magical realism: A cultural intervention for traumatized Hispanic children. *Cultural Diversity and Mental Health, 3*(3), 159–170.

Draguns, J. G. (1984). Assessing mental health and disorder across cultures. In P. B. Petersen, N. Sartorius, & A. J. Marsella, *The cross-cultural context (Vol. 7). Cross-cultural research and methodology series* (pp. 31–58). Beverly Hills, CA: Sage.

Elligan, D. (1997). Culturally sensitive integration of supportive and cognitive-behavioral therapy in the treatment of a bicultural dysthymic patient. *Cultural Diversity and Mental Health, 3*(3), 207–213.

Erikson, E. H. (1963). *Childhood and society.* New York: Norton.

Erikson, E. H. (1968). *Identity, youth, and crisis.* New York: Norton.

Fabrega, H., Ulrich, R., & Mezzich, J. (1993). Do Caucasian and Black adolescents differ at psychiatric intake? *Journal of the Academy of Child and Adolescent Psychiatry, 32,* 407–413.

Four Racial/Ethnic Panels. (1999). *Cultural competence standards for managed care mental health for four racial/ethnic underserved/underrepresented populations.* Rockville, MD: Center for

Mental Health Services, Substance Abuse and Mental Health Administration, U.S. Department of Health and Human Services.

Garrison, E., Roy, I., & Azar, V. (1999). Responding to the mental health needs of Latino children and families through school-based services. *Clinical Psychology Review, 19*(2), 199–219.

Gibbs, J. T., and Huang, L. N. (1989). A conceptual framework for assessing and treating minority youth. In J. T. Gibbs & L. N. Huang (Eds.), *Children of color: Psychological interventions with minority youth* (pp. 1–29). San Francisco: Jossey-Bass.

Glover, S., & Pumariega, A. J. (1998). The importance of children's mental health epidemiological research with culturally diverse populations. In M. Hernandez & M. Isaacs (Eds.), *Promoting cultural competence in children's mental health services.* Baltimore: Brookes.

Green, J. W., and Leigh, J. W. (1989). Teaching ethnographic methods to social service workers. *Practicing Anthropology, 11,* 8–10.

Guanipa, C., Talley, W., Rapagna, S. (1997). Enhancing Latin American women's self-concept: A group intervention. *International Journal of Group Psychotherapy, 47*(3), 355–372.

Gutierrez-Mayka, M., & Contreras-Neira, R. (1998). A culturally receptive approach to community participation in system reform. In M. Hernandez & M. Isaacs (Eds.), *Promoting cultural competence in children's mental health services.* Baltimore: Brookes.

Kilgus, M., Pumariega, A. J., & Cuffe, S. (1995). Race and diagnosis in adolescent psychiatric inpatients. *Journal of the American Academy of Child and Adolescent Psychiatry, 34*(1), 67–72.

Kluckhorn, F. R. (1953). Dominant and variant value orientations. In C. Kluckhorn & H. A. Murray (Eds.), *Personality in nature, society, and culture.* New York: Knopf.

Knight, G. P., Virdin, L. M., Ocampo, K. A., & Roosa, M. (1994). An examination of the cross-ethnic equivalence of measures of negative life events and mental health among hispanic and anglo-american children. *American Journal of Community Psychology, 22*(6), 767–783.

Koss-Chioino, J., & Vargas, L. (1999). *Working with Latino youth: Culture, development and context.* San Francisco: Jossey-Bass.

Lin, K., Poland, R., & Nasaki, G. (1993). *Psychopharmacology and psychobiology of ethnicity.* In D. Spiegel (Series ed.), *Progress in psychiatry: Vol. 39.* Washington, DC: American Psychiatric Press.

Longshore, D., Grills, C., & Annon, K. (1999). Effects of a culturally congruent intervention on cognitive factors related to drug-use recovery. *Substance Use and Misuse, 34*(9), 1223–1241.

Malgady, R. G., Rogler, L. H., & Constantino, G. (1990). Hero/heroine modeling for Puerto Rican adolescents: A preventive MH intervention. *Journal of Consulting and Clinical Psychology, 58*(4), 469–474.

Minuchin, S. (1974). *Families and family therapy.* Cambridge, MA: Harvard University Press.

Montalvo, B., & Gutierrez, M. (1983). A perspective for the use of the cultural dimension in family therapy. In C. J. Fallicov, *Cultural perspectives in family therapy.* Gaithersburg, MD: Aspen.

Mufson, L., Weissman, M., Moreau, D., & Garfinkel, R. (1999). Efficacy of interpersonal psychotherapy for depressed adolescents. *Archives of General Psychiatry, 56*(6), 573–579.

O'Sullivan, M., & Lasso, B. (1992). Community mental health services for hispanics: A test of the culture compatibility hypothesis. *Hispanic Journal of Behavioral Sciences, 14*(4), 455–468.

Pate, J., Pumariega, A., Hester, C., & Garner, D. (1992). Cross cultural patterns in eating disorders. *Journal of the American Academy of Child and Adolescent Psychiatry, 31*(5), 802–809.

Philips, S. U. (1983). *The invisible culture.* New York: Longman.

Powell, G. J., Yamamoto, J., Romero, A., & Morales, A. (Eds.), (1983). *The psychosocial development of minority group children.* New York: Brunner/Mazel.

Pumariega, A. J. (1986). Acculturation and eating attitudes in adolescent girls. *Journal of the American Academy of Child and Adolescent Psychiatry, 25*(2), 276–279.

Pumariega, A. J., Swanson, J., Holzer, C. E., Linskey, A., & Quintero-Salinas, R. (1992). Cultural context and substance abuse in Hispanic adolescents. *Journal of Child and Family Studies, 1*(1), 75–92.

Pumariega, A. J., Johnson, P., Sheridan, D., & Cuffe, S. (1995). Race, gender, age, depressive symptomatology, and substance abuse in high-risk adolescents. *Cultural Diversity and Mental Health, 2*(2), 115–123.

Pumariega, A. J. (1996). Culturally competent program evaluation in systems of care for children's mental health. *Journal of Child and Family Studies, 5*(4), 389–397.

Pumariega, A. J., Balderrama, H., Garduno, R., Hernandez, M., Hernandez, P., Martinez, F., Romero, J., Saenz, J., Torres, J., Sanchez, M., & Keller, A. (1997). *Cultural competence guidelines in managed care mental health services for Latino populations.* Boulder, CO: Western Interstate Commission for Higher Education.

Pumariega, A. J., Glover, S., Holzer, C. E., & Nguyen, N. (1998). Utilization of mental health services in a tri-ethnic sample of adolescents. *Community Mental Health Journal, 34*(2), 145–156.

Pumariega, A. J., Atkins, D. L., Rogers, K., Montgomery, L., Nybro, C., Caesar, R., & Millus, D. (1999). Mental health and incarcerated youth: II. Service utilization in incarcerated youth. *Journal of Child and Family Studies, 8*(2), 205–215.

Rogler, L. H., & Cortes, D. E. (1993). Help-seeking pathways: A unifying concept in mental health care. *American Journal of Psychiatry, 150*(4), 554–561.

Rosello, J., & Bernal, G. (1999). The efficacy of cognitive-behavioral and interpersonal treatments for depression in Puerto Rican adolescents. *Journal of Consulting and Clinical Psychology, 67*(5), 734–745.

Rudorfer, M., & Potter, W. (1999). Metabolism of tricyclic antidepressants. *Cell and Molecular Biology, 19,* 373–409.

Salvendy, J. (1999). Ethnocultural considerations in group psychotherapy. *International Journal of Group Psychotherapy, 49*(4), 429–464.

Smith, M., & Mendoza, R. (1996). Ethnicity and pharmacogenetics. *The Mount Sinai Journal of Medicine, 63,* 285–290.

Spiegel, J. (1971). *Transactions: The interplay between individual, family, and society.* J. Papajohn, (Ed.). New York: Science House.

Spradley, J. (1979). *The ethnographic interview.* New York: Holt, Reinhart, & Winston.

Spurlock, J. (1985). Assessment and therapeutic interventions of Black children. *Journal of the American Academy of Child and Adolescent Psychiatry, 24,* 168–174.

Sue, D. W. (1981). *Counseling the culturally different.* New York: Wiley.

Swanson, J., Linskey, A., Quintero-Salinas, R., Pumariega, A. J., & Holzer, C. E. (1992). Depressive symptoms, drug use and suicidal ideation among youth in the Rio Grande Valley: A bi-national school survey. *Journal of the American Academy of Child and Adolescent Psychiatry, 31*(4), 669–678.

Szapocznik, J., Scopetta, M. A., & Tillman, W. (1978). What changes, what remains the same, and what affects acculturation in Cuban immigrant families. In J. Szapocznik & M. C. Herrera (Eds.), *Cuban Americans: Acculturation, adjustment, and the family.* Washington, DC: COSSMHO.

Szapocznik, J., & Kurtines, W. (1989). *Breakthroughs in family therapy with drug abusing and problem youth.* New York: Springer.

U.S. Bureau of the Census. (1998). *Resident population of the United States: Estimates by sex, race, and hispanic origin.* Washington, DC: U.S. Department of Commerce.

U.S. Office of the Surgeon General. (1999). *Mental health: A report of the surgeon general.* Rockville, MD: U.S. Department of Health and Human Services, Substance Abuse and

Mental Health Services Administration, Center for Mental Health Services, National Institutes of Health, National Institute of Mental Health.

Valle, R. (1986). Cross-cultural competence in minority communities: A curriculum implementation strategy. In M. R. Miranda & H. H. L. Kitano (Eds.), *Mental health research and practice in minority communities: Development of culturally sensitive training programs.* Rockville, MD: National Institute of Mental Health, ADAMHA.

Wilkinson, C., & Spurlock, J. (1986). *The mental health of Black Americans: Psychiatric diagnosis and treatment.* New York: Plenum Press.

Williams, K., Chambless, D., & Steketee, G. (1998). Behavioral treatment of obsessive-compulsive disorder in African-Americans: Clinical issues. *Journal of Behavioral Therapy and Experimental Psychiatry, 29*(2), 163–170.

Wilson, L. (1982). *The skills of ethnic competence.* Unpublished manuscript. Seattle: University of Washington.

Yancey, A. (1998). Building positive self-image in adolescents in foster care: The use of role models in an interactive group approach. *Adolescence, 33*(130), 253–267.

Zito, J., Safer, D., dosReis, S., Magder, L., & Riddle, M. (1997). Methylphenidate patterns among Medicaid youths. *Psychopharmacological Bulletin, 33,* 143–147.

Chapter 20

SYSTEMS OF CARE FOR CHILDREN AND ADOLESCENTS WITH SERIOUS EMOTIONAL DISTURBANCE

NANCY C. WINTERS AND ANDRES J. PUMARIEGA

INTRODUCTION: THE CHILD WITH SERIOUS EMOTIONAL DISTURBANCE

Children and adolescents with serious emotional disturbance (SED) present a significant challenge to the agencies responsible for their care, including education, health, child welfare, mental health, juvenile justice, and developmental disabilities. The term SED itself can be confusing, because definitions of SED vary across agencies serving children. SED in the educational system has been used to describe children eligible for special education services based on emotional or behavioral problems. This concept responded to the mandate by the Education for All Handicapped Children act (PL 94-142) passed in 1975. The more recent Individuals with Disabilities Education Act (IDEA) of 1990 (PL 101-476) maintains the requirement that the emotional or behavioral disturbance adversely affect school performance.

In mental health, SED generally refers to the presence of a psychiatric disorder accompanied by significant functional impairment. The Center for Mental Health Services (CMHS) within the Substance Abuse and Mental Health Services Administration (SAMHSA) defines children with a serious emotional disturbance as:

> persons from birth up to age 18, who currently or at any time during the past year have a diagnosable mental, behavioral or emotional disorder of sufficient duration to meet diagnostic criteria specified within the *DSM-III-R*, that resulted in functional impairment which substantially interferes with or limits the child's role or functioning in family, school, or community activities. (U.S. Government, 1993)

There are definitions of SED used in child welfare, juvenile justice, and developmental disabilities. These definitions have different aims; the educational definition is used for determining eligibility for special education services, and the mental health definition is intended for use as a basis for mental health service system planning.

Epidemiological studies that have examined the prevalence of mental disorders in youth have assigned SED status to those with the highest severity of problems. Recent epidemiological studies of youth have demonstrated that a significant percentage of children and adolescents, ranging from 14% to 20%, have mental health disorders, and that about 7% of all children have a serious disorder (Brandenburg, Friedman, & Silver, 1990; Costello, Burns, Angold, & Leaf, 1993). More recent estimates appear to be higher, a recent CMHS-sponsored report on the prevalence of serious emotional disturbance in children and adolescents (Friedman et al., 1996) reviewed the epidemiological data on SED in children and adolescents 9 to 17 years old. The report recommended a range of 5% to 9% for the prevalence of serious emotional disturbance and extreme functional impairment, and 9% to 13% for serious emotional disturbance with substantial functional impairment.

Despite recognition of the high prevalence of serious emotional disturbance among children and adolescents, there is a critical shortage of services for this vulnerable population. At any one time, less than 1% of children in the United States receive mental health treatment in hospital or residential settings, and another 5% are served in out-patient or community-based settings. The majority of children with SED receive insufficient or no mental health services whatsoever (Tuma, 1989; Inouye, 1988), despite the fact that budgets dedicated to financing both public and private mental health services for children have grown exponentially since the 1970s. Total expenditures for children's mental health services have grown to 4.8 billion, comprising approximately 7% of the total national mental health budget (Burns, Taube, & Taube, 1990).

A broad array of morbidities associated with emotional disturbance and mental illness in children is increasing at an alarming rate. These include suicide, homicide, substance abuse, child abuse, teenage pregnancy, school drop-out, youth crime, and associated institutionalization and incarceration. In addition to mental health, many other health and human service agencies (schools, welfare, child protection, juvenile justice, and public health) have experienced the increasing impact of these psychosocial morbidities associated with emotional disturbance in children. Often, each of these agencies functions as an isolated piece of the service system puzzle, addressing part of the youth's needs with little or no coordination with other agencies serving the same youth (Knitzer, 1982).

Access to mental health services is also an unmet need for increasing numbers of culturally diverse populations of children. In the United States and Western Europe, such populations are increasing both in overall numbers and in proportion to the rest of the population. This is a result of both higher birth rates and accelerating immigration in populations of non-European background. Children from these populations experience higher levels of stressors, such as poverty, discrimination, acculturation stress, and exposure to violence and trauma. These stressors are associated with their minority status in society as well as the difficulties involved in immigration. These culturally diverse child populations have traditionally been underserved by mental health, health, and human services, both in terms of overall access to services and the cultural competence of the services available to them. The increasing cost of serving these populations of children and adolescents needs to be balanced against their high risk for psychosocial morbidity, including potential long-term outcomes of loss of productivity as citizens and the costs of welfare dependency and institutionalization (Cross, Bazron, Dennis, & Isaacs, 1988; Pumariega & Cross, 1997).

Even as there is a growing recognition of the needs of children with emotional disorders, there are increasingly limited resources available to fund child mental health and human services. Because of the public's increasing disenchantment with governmental programs and its resistance to increased taxation as a solution to social problems, policy makers are looking for ways of limiting or even cutting the public budgets dedicated to health and human services. Private funding for such services has experienced similar constraints. Business and industry have also expressed increasing concerns about the rising costs of health and mental health care, especially the growing percentage of such spending on child and adolescent mental health.

Reconciling the need for increased access to services for these youth with the need to control ever-growing health care costs presents a major challenge to the continued development of organized systems of care for children and adolescents. In order not to experience restriction or curtailment of services, child mental health providers are facing increased pressures to demonstrate both improved clinical- and cost-effectiveness of their services. These trends highlight the progressively important role of health services research as a source of information for providers, policy makers, and payors (Hoagwood, Jensen, Petti, & Burns, 1996).

HISTORY OF TREATMENT FOR SED CHILDREN

The history of mental health services for children differs significantly from the history of services for adults. Mental health services for adults were originally located in large state-operated institutions, based on the work of such pioneers as Dorothea Dix in Massachusetts. The orientation of this work was toward providing sanctuary, or asylum, to those dealing with mental illness, and sheltering them from the demands of the outside world. From its earliest origins, however, mental health services for children have emphasized a community and interdisciplinary orientation. In the United States, these services began in response to a perceived need for counseling of juvenile offenders rather than incarcerating them with adult offenders.

In the 1890s and 1900s, America, much as today, was undergoing rapid cultural changes due to immigration and economic changes due to industrialization and urbanization. These social pressures led to marked increases in a number of new social problems, such as child abuse and neglect, child industrial labor, and decreased school attendance and behavior problems, as well as crime committed by juveniles. The first state compulsory education laws were enacted in the 1860s and the first child abuse laws were fashioned after the animal cruelty laws in the 1880s. In the next two to three decades, the first child welfare, juvenile justice, and public health services in the nation followed these developments.

The first mental health clinic for children was founded at the University of Pennsylvania in 1896 and focused on school problems. The juvenile court clinics in Chicago and Boston were founded in the early 1900s, giving rise to the first interdisciplinary child mental health services in the nation, staffed by physicians, social workers, and psychologists. The success of these clinics led the Commonwealth Foundation to commission a study, which, in 1922, recommended and funded the development of child guidance clinics throughout the United States. These clinics were to be staffed with interdisciplinary teams of professionals to serve the child and the family. At first, these clinics were staffed primarily by social workers, but in time they attracted pediatricians, psychologists, psychoanalysts, and psychiatrists, and later served as the basis for the first child psychiatry programs in the nation.

These child guidance clinics were quite different and were removed from the specialty-driven medical system that was evolving in tertiary medical centers; further, they did not encourage the practice of hospital-bound care. They provided low-cost services oriented to the needs of the child and the family, with treatment modalities evolving to include individual psychodynamic psychotherapy, family therapy, crisis intervention, and even day treatment programs. Many of these clinics have survived to this day. They served as models for the community mental health centers developed in the 1960s under federal legislation that sought to decrease the large populations of institutionalized adults in state mental hospitals (Berlin, 1991).

Advances in psychopharmacotherapy facilitated the deinstitutionalization of adults to the community under the care of the new mental health centers. The medicalization of psychiatry starting in the 1970s, however, served paradoxically to move psychiatric services toward a more hospital-based, tertiary care model. This left the child guidance clinics and the community mental health centers without significant psychiatric participation. Community-based services were neglected, leaving these clinics generally understaffed, underfunded, and with narrow choices of interventions that included medication, counseling, or multiple hospitalizations.

The United States also experienced a rapid increase in the population of poor and minority children and adults with higher levels of need for mental health services. Many of these children were placed in the custody of child welfare agencies or placed in out-of-home residential care and juvenile detention facilities, whereas children with insurance coverage were placed in the new medically oriented psychiatric facilities, thus overtaxing the resource capacity of many agencies and funders. The lack of integrated services under this approach led to a marked increase in homelessness among seriously mentally ill adults as well as children and families in the late 1970s and 1980s (England & Cole, 1992).

The findings of the Joint Commission on the Mental Health of Children (1969) led to a growing recognition that youngsters with mental health disorders were either not receiving mental health services or were served in overly restrictive settings. A study published by the Children's Defense Fund, *Unclaimed Children* (Knitzer, 1982), further documented that two thirds of the children with serious emotional disorders were not receiving services. Those who were receiving services were receiving uncoordinated and largely ineffective care. This led to the establishment in 1984 of the Child and Adolescent Service System Program (CASSP), under the auspices of the National Institute of Mental Health and later CMHS.

CASSP had as its goal the development of systems of care for youth with SED. These systems were intended to address the need for family-centered, culturally competent care that would involve interagency coordination and access to a full continuum of services. A monograph entitled *A System of Care for Children and Youth with Serious Emotional Disturbances* (Stroul & Friedman, 1986) outlined the system of care concept. The CASSP core values and guiding principles that were articulated in this monograph provided a framework for the system of care concept and have guided subsequent system of care reform efforts. CASSP principles emphasize that care should be child-centered and family-focused, children and their families should have access to individualized, community-based services provided in the most normative environment that is clinically appropriate. Individualization of care is central to the system of care concept, emphasizing services that fit the individual child and family's needs, rather than placing the child in existing categorical services that may meet needs of the agency, but not be optimal for the individual child.

The CASSP principles also specify that services should be culturally competent, as well as coordinated and integrated among the different child-serving agencies. Family involvement is central to the system of care concept; it is sought at multiple levels, including treatment, decision-making, and system policy-making. An increased understanding of the enormous burden that youth with SED pose for their families has led to recognition of the importance of providing support to families and strengthening their natural support systems, along with providing mental health services targeted to children.

CASSP led to other system of care initiatives, including the Fort Bragg project in North Carolina and the Ventura County project in California. The Robert Wood Johnson Mental Health Services Program for Youth (RWJ-MHSPY) funded seven national systems of care projects from 1990 to 1995. In 1993, CMHS launched the Comprehensive Community Mental Health Services for Children and Their Families Program (also known as the Children's Services Program), a grant program that currently supports 62 system of care projects across the United States.

Although different system of care projects may serve different target populations of children with SED, they have in common an organized delivery system of mental health and other human services to children with SED, delivered in a coordinated manner using the values and philosophy embodied in the CASSP principles.

CHARACTERISTICS OF THE SED CHILD

Despite definitional variations, it is recognized across agencies that children and adolescents with SED have serious problems in developmentally important areas of functioning, including family and peer relationships, school behavior and performance, self-care, and emotional/behavioral functioning. They tend to receive services in multiple service sectors, including mental health, child welfare, education, developmental disabilities, juvenile justice, health, and substance abuse.

In addition to significant problems in functioning, youth with SED have multiple psychiatric diagnoses, including both internalizing and externalizing disorders. Costello et al., (1998) found the prevalence of SED to be highest in association with conduct and/or oppositional disorders, followed by anxiety disorders and attention-deficit/hyperactivity disorder (ADHD). In the CMHS Report to Congress on 22 system of care demonstration projects (Macro International, 1997), *DSM-IV* psychiatric diagnoses were obtained in a sample of 9,682 children. In this sample, 30% of the children had two distinct diagnoses. Thirty-five percent of the children were diagnosed with conduct-related disorder; 16% with other diagnoses such as substance abuse, eating disorders, somatic disorders, speech disorders, enuresis, and phobia, and psychotic disorder was diagnosed in 2% of the sample. Of children with conduct disorder, 22%

had a secondary diagnosis of substance abuse, whereas children with depressive disorder were most likely to have secondary diagnoses of conduct disorder (23%) or substance use disorder (20%).

Children with SED often come to the attention of child-serving agencies not due to symptoms of their psychiatric disorders (e.g., depressed mood, inattentiveness, thought disorder), but due to associated behavioral problems, including truancy, aggression, legal referrals, and severe socially maladaptive behaviors, including sexual offending. These impairments put youths at higher risk for out-of-home placements in foster care, residential treatment centers, incarceration, or repeated psychiatric hospitalizations. Although these out-of-home placements generally provide needed respite for stressed and burdened families, they are often not as effective as community-based approaches in addressing the problems the child has in the family environment that will need to be dealt with again when the child returns home.

In general, the prevalence of SED has been found to be higher in males than in females. The sample described in the CMHS Report to Congress (Macro International, 1997) consisted of 62% males and 38% females. This may underrate the number of females with SED who have severe internalizing problems and are not disruptive enough to come to the attention of child-serving agencies. The prevalence of SED has been found to be twice as high in low socioeconomic groups as in with high socioeconomic groups (Costello and Messer, 1995). SED and associated disorders also appear to have high rates of stability and chronicity (Costello et al., 1999), supporting the view that SED in children is analogous to chronic mental illness (Looney, 1988). When seen in this context, it is clear that many children with SED will need ongoing rather than time-limited services, where the goal may be maintenance at a best-possible level of functioning rather than complete resolution of symptoms.

ASSESSMENT OF THE SED CHILD

Assessment of SED children must be comprehensive in scope due to the nature of their multiple psychiatric diagnoses and problems in functioning. Children with SED, especially those who are culturally different, have a high prevalence of conduct symptoms and externalizing behaviors, with the result that underlying internalizing diagnoses may be missed (Caron & Rutter, 1991; Kilgus, Pumariega, & Cuffe, 1995). Thus, the psychological and emotional difficulties of children with SED need to be kept in focus along with their behavioral problems. In order to make sense of maladaptive behaviors and to provide opportunities for positive change, one must understand problems in thinking, self-image disturbances, psychological conflicts, and problems in affective regulation. This requires the availability of an experienced clinician to interview the child or adolescent in a setting that facilitates communication.

In a comprehensive assessment, all domains of the child or adolescent's functioning are relevant, including family life, behavior and achievement in school, peer relationships, self-care ability, adaptive behavior in the community, and the presence of unsafe or self-harm behaviors, including alcohol and drug use. A developmental perspective is important in identifying which developmental tasks have or have not been achieved by the child and how this affects his ability to cope with the demands of his age. Given the developmental and evolving nature of serious mental and emotional disorders in children, the full symptom picture of a disorder such as bipolar disorder, for example, is often not seen until late adolescence or adulthood. This highlights the importance of frequent reevaluations and an ongoing diagnostic process. To this end, youths with SED benefit from having access to sophisticated diagnostic settings and diagnosticians at nodal points in their treatment.

In the assessment process, multiple informants are needed to obtain an accurate picture of the youth's behaviors in different contexts. Because SED children so often perform poorly in educational settings, it is important to ascertain their level of intellectual functioning and the presence of learning disabilities. Identifying strengths and problems in the youngster's ability to learn and process information can be important in developing successful treatment interventions as opposed to continued exercises in frustration and failure.

As the system of care model has evolved, strength-based assessment and treatment planning have become increasingly important. Feedback from family members who want strengths to receive more attention has been influential in this trend. Assessment of the child and family's strengths along with weaknesses and problems makes good sense clinically in that change is most easily accomplished in a climate of motivation and experiences of success.

With the growing influence of families and other stakeholders on the care of children, outcomes that involve improvement in functioning in addition to symptom reduction have assumed increased importance. Systematic assessment of functioning is very useful in identifying target areas for intervention as well as in measuring response to treatment. Naturalistic functional indicators such as school attendance, the ability to stay out of legal trouble, making friends, and getting along with family members (often the measures that are most meaningful to families) should be coupled with standardized assessments that quantify the level of functioning in different functional domains. Such assessments can be helpful for establishing appropriate levels of care as well as for tracking and monitoring outcomes.

There are a number of validated and reliable instruments for use in assessment of child and adolescent functioning. The Child Behavior Checklist (CBCL; Achenbach and Edelbrock, 1983) has been used frequently as a screening tool to identify children at risk of having significant emotional/behavioral problems. Those children scoring above the 90th percentile for age and sex are at risk for SED. The CBCL can also be used to yield scores on social competence in three areas: at school, with peers and family, and in social activities. There is also a Teacher's Report Form (TRF) and Youth Self-Report (YSR) form (Achenbach, 1991). The Children's Global Assessment Scale (CGAS; Shaffer et al., 1983), a child-oriented version of the Global Assessment of Functioning, can also be used to rate functional impairment. It assigns a global score of impairment from 0 to 100. Children scoring 60 or below are usually found to show significant impairment (Bird et al., 1990). A more recent instrument now in wide use is the Child and Adolescent Functional Assessment Scale (CAFAS; Hodges, 1990). The CAFAS has the advantage of separately rating different domains of functioning (e.g., home, community, school, thinking, substance use) using specific criteria. These instruments have demonstrated acceptable validity and reliability.

THE CLINICAL MODEL IN SYSTEMS OF CARE

The wraparound approach has become central to the system of care concept. Wraparound is a philosophy and approach, rather than a set of services. Central to this approach is the requirement that services be designed to fit the unique and specific needs of children and families. The wraparound process as described by VanDenBerg and Grealish (1996) includes the following elements: (a) Wraparound efforts are based in the community; (b) services and supports are individualized to meet the needs of the children and families, rather than being driven by priorities of categorical services; (c) parents are included in every level of the planning process; (d) the process is culturally competent and is based on unique values, strengths, and the social or racial composition of the child and family; (e) the process must have access to flexible, noncategorical funding; (f) the process must be implemented on an interagency basis and owned by the larger community; (g) the services must be unconditional, so that when needs change, the services are modified rather than the child or family being rejected; and (h) outcomes must be measured so that the process is developed on an empirical scientific basis.

The wraparound model, with its emphasis on individualized, strength-based services, lends itself to nontraditional services. Examples of these services include home-based therapies, therapeutic foster care in lieu of residential treatment, therapeutic mentoring, parent and child skills training and "coaching," use of respite services as a part of mental health treatment, and family advocates as service team members. Results of service effectiveness studies suggest that nontraditional services (especially case management, home-based services, and therapeutic foster care) are effective in altering service-level outcomes, such as change in placements and service intensity (Jensen et al., 1996).

The role of case manager is also critical to the wraparound process. Other terms have been used for the case management function in systems of care, depending on the specific functions. These include care management, care coordination, and service coordination. In general, case management implies a client-level role with more direct contact and service to the family. Friesen and Poertner (1995) use the term *case management* when discussing activities aimed at improving circumstances of specific children and families and *service coordination* for activities that have implications for a broader set of children and families or for the service system. Because SED children have such complex needs typically involving multiple service systems, the case manager serves to ensure that children and families receive appropriate, timely, and coordinated services. The case manager has been described as the "glue" of treatment planning, playing a critical role in needs assessment, service planning, service implementation, service coordination, monitoring and evaluation, and advocacy (Stroul, 1996). The Child Mental Health Service Initiative of CMHS views case management as occupying a critical role and requires case management for all youngsters offered access to services in a system of care.

Family-centered models of case management are particularly compatible with the system of care and wraparound philosophies. These models emphasize the child's and family's strengths as well as needs, and seek to provide the family with the skills and resources needed to care for a child with SED. The family-centered intensive case management model is a team case management approach described by Evans et al., (1996). It uses parent advocates and flexible service funds to purchase economic and social supports, along with in-home respite care. The family-centered case manager's aim is to support the skills of family members in functioning as the natural case managers for their children. Developing and maintaining positive working alliances with parents is the cornerstone of effective case management in work with SED children. The effective case manager also needs to build cohesive service teams that develop a shared understanding of the problems being addressed and agree on appropriate desired outcomes that are meaningful to the child and family.

Service planning within systems of care lends itself to using an ecological conceptual framework that maintains a systemic overview. In this framework, the child is understood in the context of the family as well as the school, neighborhood, and larger community environments in which he or she lives. This model also takes into account the different service systems that can impact the child and family, including mental health, social services, education, health, substance abuse, vocational services, and recreational services. In the child's ecological system, factors such as the parents' untreated medical problems or changes in their work environment can be understood as significant influences on the child's functioning, and therefore appropriate targets for service interventions.

Quality psychiatric diagnostic assessment and clinically appropriate treatment interventions are central components in the system of care model. No amount of wrapping services around a youngster can substitute for a missed or inaccurate diagnosis. A diagnosis of major depression, ADHD, or psychosis, for example, can point to effective pharmacologic interventions. Increasingly, medications are showing effectiveness for childhood psychiatric disorders. Some examples of demonstrated benefits of pharmacologic agents include the following: (a) Psychostimulants have well-demonstrated efficacy for ADHD; (b) serotonergic antidepressants have now been shown to be effective for child and adolescent major depression (Emslie et al., 1997); (c) mood stabilizing medications are useful for bipolar disorder and aggression; and (d) the atypical antipsychotics now have clinical indications for bipolar disorder, aggression, psychosis and Tourette's disorder (Del Mundo, Pumariega, & Vance, 1999).

With increasing recognition of the biological underpinnings of psychiatric disorders, it is appropriate to use medications for children with serious emotional disturbance who are likely to suffer the greatest developmental impact. Without appropriate medications, many of these seriously disturbed youngsters are likely to be maintained in restrictive levels of care for longer periods of time. It is thus important that youngsters with SED are triaged early for psychiatric assessment and pharmacotherapy and that the psychiatrist works closely with the child, family, and other service providers. This may necessitate a higher frequency of psychiatric appointments for symptomatic children. As stated above, diagnostic assessment in children also generally needs to be ongoing and repeated due to the evolving nature of childhood mental health disorders (Del Mundo, Pumariega, & Vance, 1999).

CLINICAL VIGNETTES ILLUSTRATING THE WRAPAROUND APPROACH

The following clinical vignettes, adapted from case management services in a system of care program, illustrate some of the principles of the wraparound process, including family-centered case management, strength-based treatment planning and the use of nontraditional services.

Vignette 1

A. L. was a 15-year-old Caucasian male when he entered the case management program. A. L. had been diagnosed with ADHD and oppositional defiant disorder. He also had a history of physical abuse and witnessing domestic violence between his parents, leading to posttraumatic stress disorder. He had particular problems with female authority figures. A. L. had been in multiple alternative school settings, including the most structured schools, all of which were unable to manage his noncompliant and aggressive behavior. Previous attempts at counseling and pharmacotherapy for A. L. had been unsuccessful due to his family's lack of transportation to appointments and their antimedication attitudes.

Initial planning meetings with the youth and family led the case manager to implement a different treatment strategy. First, an individual therapist and a family therapist, both of whom met with family members in their home or an office close to their home, were engaged. A mentor for the youth was brought in who initially provided social experiences that were more positive than the negative peer influences in the youth's neighborhood. Later, the mentor's role was reoriented toward skills training around anger management, to reduce anger outbursts between the youth and his mother.

In the next phase, the youth transitioned to a family-owned business that offered a mentored job experience. In this setting, A. L. performed supervised work under the supervision of a female boss. When problems arose, they were processed with the help of a son with counseling experience. A. L. progressed well with his social skills in this work setting; initially he questioned whenever he was asked to perform a task, and said inappropriate things to customers under his breath. Eventually, he was able to take more initiative on the job and blended into the culture of the business. This mentored job experience allowed for a break from individual therapy, which restarted when the youth was ready to work on family relationship issues. The youth's mother developed a trusting relationship with the home-based family therapist and agreed to a medication evaluation for A. L. by a physician who was willing to meet with them in their home. In this wraparound plan, the goal was to create the least restrictive learning environment where the youth was likely to be successful. The job experience lasted 8 months and led to the youth's seeking out other work opportunities. Sensitivity to the family's attitudes and preferences, as well as changing interventions that matched the child's developmental needs and strengths, were the elements of successful wraparound planning.

Vignette 2

J. T. was a 14-year-old Hispanic female who entered case management following state hospitalization for a serious suicide attempt. She had had two prior hospitalizations for suicidal behavior that were complicated by use of drugs and alcohol. J. T. lived with her mother, a single parent whose primary language was Spanish. J. T. had had previous trials of outpatient counseling that had not been successful. She and her mother had a highly conflictual relationship; J. T.'s mother was very concerned about her but was unable to enforce any rules or limits. After an initial needs assessment, the first service put into place by the case manager was a Spanish-speaking home-based therapist who was able to develop a collaborative relationship with J. T.'s mother, helping her identify which behaviors were acceptable and unacceptable for J. T. J. T.'s mother was then encouraged to seek out voluntary services from the child welfare agency in order to access more support in her parenting role.

Over time, the child welfare caseworker, the case manager, and the mother developed a highly collaborative relationship in which the caseworker played the limit-setting role, informing J. T. that she had to comply with drug and alcohol treatment and school attendance in order to remain in her home. This allowed J. T.'s mother to maintain a more positive and more comfortable relationship with her. J. T.'s mother was able to alert the team when she saw signals of impending mental health crises so that additional supports could be put into place for J. T. Several individual therapists were tried, and J. T. eventually made a good connection with an experienced child and adolescent psychiatrist who did psychotherapy with J. T. and kept her on minimal medications. J. T. was helped to attend school and earn her high school diploma by an incentive plan that provided her with periodic funds to purchase new outfits contingent on regular school attendance. Culturally competent services, cooperative relationships among the team and the family, and access to flexible funds were the elements of successful wraparound planning for J. T.

MODELS OF INTERAGENCY COLLABORATION IN SYSTEMS OF CARE

Interagency collaboration within systems of care is another critically important element necessary to ensure access to comprehensive and coordinated treatment for children with SED. Interagency collaboration is facilitated by a number of organizational and structural characteristics. Formal interagency agreements, for example, have increasingly been implemented to improve services coordination either to overlapping populations or to targeted high-risk populations. Other structural mechanisms short of formal interagency agreements have also been used to facilitate interagency collaboration, one example is colocation of staff or services, which allows multiple agencies to provide services to overlapping consumers at common sites. In this model, one agency may provide services at another agency's site or at neutral community-based sites such as schools, churches, or community centers where consumers feel a greater sense of comfort and less stigma.

Interagency plans constructed by interagency teams and families formally outline the accountability for different services by different agencies and how the services will be coordinated. These plans usually designate a lead agency that takes responsibility for the coordination of the service plan. Blended funding agreements have also been used to facilitate the purchase of flexible services from the budgets of multiple participating agencies for common clients. Such blended funding allows for the purchase of wraparound services that fall outside of (but generally complement) the categorical services delivered by different agencies, such as the purchase of tutoring services or a "shadow" for a child or home repair service for a family (Friesen & Poertner, 1995). Another funding model involves "braiding" of funds, in which agencies develop formal or informal agreements about combining their funds into integrated treatment plans for individual children or groups of children.

The fiscal and organizational elements that support interagency collaboration have been challenged by the competing trends of escalating needs and limited funding. In an effort to gain efficiencies and stem rising costs, state and federal governments have adopted new approaches to downsizing, streamlining, and privatizing of governmental services. State governmental agencies have also progressively engaged in devolution of responsibility and funding of services to more local levels.

With these developments, agencies are increasingly turning to managed care approaches to finance and organize mental health and social services. Managed care approaches are relatively new in mental health and human services, and those that have existed were developed with adult and private sector populations in mind. These approaches have relied on a priori benefit restrictions based on actuarial analyses. This often leads to the selecting out of poorer populations that are high users of services, with a benefit package aimed instead at large pools of relatively healthy, minimally impaired populations from higher socioeconomic backgrounds that typically use fewer services.

When applied to child mental health services, the benefits restriction approach used in traditional behavioral managed care risks depriving poor, underserved, and more impaired children of timely and effective intervention and prevention services. This results in fragmentation of care and a shifting of the burden of services and costs to the other child-serving agencies and systems. The shifting of costs to other systems can seriously limit the potential for interagency collaboration, as well as raise the likelihood of increased morbidity in these populations due to their receiving inadequate mental health services. Managed care models for children's mental health need to emphasize community-based treatment and prevention of morbidity through enhancing family and community resources as well as providing clinical services for the child (Pumariega et al., 1997).

Although there are common challenges and pressures faced by human service agencies interfacing with the mental health needs of children and families, some challenges are unique to the scope of responsibility of different agencies. Challenges unique to different child-serving agencies follow.

Welfare/Social Services

The populations of children in state custody are well known to be at high risk for serious emotional and behavioral disturbances (Pumariega, Johnson, & Sheridan, 1995). The child welfare system has traditionally been a high consumer of mental health services, both directly for its wards as well as for the treatment of parents and other family members in the service of family reunification. Rising rates of SED and serious mental illness (SMI) in this population have had a significant impact at a number of levels.

These include increased numbers of traumatized children recovering from serious abuse and neglect, the task of reunifying families after abuse, and the difficulties for families on the welfare rolls of caring for children with SED/SMI.

Given the cutbacks in public child mental health services associated with downsizing and managed behavioral health, increasing numbers of families have returned to the practice of giving up children to state custody due to their inability to care for them. This aggravates the already critical shortage of out-of-home residential placements available for children in state custody, particularly therapeutic and nontherapeutic foster homes. The high prevalence of serious mental illness and substance abuse among the adult homeless population also presents a major challenge for social service agencies and often requires the assistance of volunteer and religious entities to provide support services (Culhane, Averyt, & Hadley, 1998). Another recent trend has been the increasingly important role that access to adequate levels of mental health services plays in aiding families on welfare to return to work under state welfare reform initiatives. The goal of facilitating former welfare recipients' participation in the workforce has placed a greater premium on improved family functioning (Bazelon Center for Mental Health Law, 1996).

Different initiatives have been developed to address the integrated mental health and social service needs of these large at-risk populations. Some states have moved into managed welfare services under capitated or case-rate mechanisms, with providers credentialed to provide the whole array of social service, residential, and mental health services, along with built-in incentives to "step down" to the least restrictive levels of care and family reunification. The colocation of mental health services within the offices of governmental welfare agencies, volunteer welfare programs, and shelter programs is now becoming widely accepted and greatly facilitates integrated service delivery. Another promising modality for integrated service delivery is that of family preservation services with strong case management components. These approaches attempt to prevent out-of-home placements or to transition children with SED back to families with multiple needs. Initial results of these family preservation approaches have been promising (Rivera & Kutash, 1994).

Education

The educational system faces the impact of increased educational demands for average students due to the increased technological and informational demands in our society. In addition, the increasing needs of children with learning disorders and SEDs are placing added burdens on schools. This occurs in the context of underfunding of school districts due to downward pressures on property taxes and other means of funding education. This lack of funding is especially felt in the area of special education services. Many school districts actively avoid the mandates of federal laws such as the Individualized Disability Education Act (IDEA) and Section 504 (which outlines services for mentally ill or emotionally disturbed children), often underidentifying children with covered disabilities and temporizing by addressing their needs informally through the services of regular classroom teachers to prevent added service commitments.

A recent salutary development in the area of interagency systems of care is the renewed interest in school-based services. These go beyond traditional school mental health consultation services and involve the colocation of health and mental health professionals within schools to provide a wide array of direct and indirect/preventive health and mental health services. School-based mental health services serve as an ideal core service for a children's system of care and provide an excellent accessible portal of entry that is nonstigmatizing and is a naturalistic setting to observe behavior and integrate interventions into the child's environment. These services are often funded through blended Medicaid fee-for-service and managed care funding, serving to augment limited school funding. A number of these models have been implemented in Baltimore, Maryland, rural South Carolina; Charlotte, North Carolina; Portland, Oregon; and other locations. They have had documented success in reducing psychosocial morbidity and increasing access to needed services (Flaherty & Weist, 1999; Motes, Melton, Pumariega, & Simmons, 1999; Casat, Rigsby, Sobelewski, & Gordon, 1999). Innovative legislative approaches ensuring interagency collaboration in IDEA-mandated services have been promoted in California through a law that mandates interagency collaboration in the development and implementation of individualized educational plans when these involve areas outside formal education services (Schacht & Hansen, 1999).

Juvenile Justice

A number of studies have documented high rates of SEDs among youth in the juvenile justice system (Atkins et al., 1999). These youth are typically diverted into this agency due to their propensity to display aggressive or disruptive behaviors, following successive disciplinary interventions in the schools, as well as out-of-home placements. Youths entering the juvenile justice system have typically underutilized mental health services when compared to cohorts who remain in the mental health system (Pumariega et al., 1999). There is also greater racial disparity in the population of youths that are served by juvenile justice. This may be due to the poverty and adversity these youths face, as well as the lack of culturally competent services in mental health and other agencies and systems.

Despite the similarities in their populations, the juvenile justice and mental health systems have significant differences in their service orientations and philosophies. The juvenile justice system has faced a recent split in its orientation between those who still promote the rehabilitation of its consumers versus those who promote a more purely punitive and containment or public safety approach. This often clashes with the treatment mentality and orientation of the mental health system, although the latter suffers due to the lack of focus on behavioral containment and long-term follow-up.

Areas of natural collaboration between these systems are the prevention of youths' entry into the juvenile justice system (particularly into detention/incarceration) and the treatment of youths with SEDs within the juvenile justice system. Multisystemic therapy (MST), a therapeutic approach combining home-based and wraparound approaches within a systemic context, has been tested with youth at risk of detention and incarceration. It has resulted in significant reductions in out-of-home placements, externalizing criminal behaviors, rates of arrest and incarceration, and treatment costs (Henggeler, Schoenwald, Borduin, Rowland, & Cunningham, 1998).

Public Health/Primary Care

Children and adults served in primary care settings, particularly in public settings, have been known to have a higher risk for mental illness and emotional disorders (Costello, 1986). The integration of mental health services into primary care has long held the promise of providing greater access due to lower stigmatization and regular contact with covered individuals in the primary care setting. The benefits of such integration include the potential to provide earlier, more preventive services and to screen for risk for emotional disturbance or mental illness as a part of routine maintenance health care. Such integration has the potential to reduce costs of higher-end services and to improve the population's mental health (Shandle & Christianson, 1988). In support of these efforts, a special version of the *Diagnostic and Statistical Manual of Mental Disorders* of the American Psychiatric Association (1994) was developed for the recognition of sub-threshold mental disorders by primary care practitioners (Jellinek, 1997). The collaboration between community mental health agencies and public health departments has been minimal over time, however, especially because the latter have a diminishing role in the service system (Polivka, Kennedy, & Chaudry, 1997).

In some publicly funded health plans, mental health services are being integrated into general health services, with primary care practitioners having a greater role as direct mental health providers and psychiatrists and other mental health professionals serving in consulting or supporting roles. This has been especially attractive in rural communities, which have suffered from chronic shortages of mental health services and professionals (Bird et al., 1998). There are limitations in this model due to the lack of training for primary care practitioners in detecting, diagnosing, and treating mental disorders. Additionally, the limited contact time that primary care physicians and practitioners have with clients compromises their abilities to screen and diagnose mental health problems effectively (Glied, 1998).

ACCOMPLISHMENTS OF SYSTEMS OF CARE PROJECTS

With the growing interest in community-based services for children, research on child mental health services has increasingly focused on evaluation of interagency community-based interventions and systems of care. Evaluations have included community-based residential approaches, nonresidential intensive community-based approaches, and clinical, functional, and cost outcomes of interagency systems of care (Rivera & Kutash, 1994; Kupermine & Cohen, 1995; Pumariega & Glover, 1997).

A number of innovative community-based models for children that provide intensive and individualized services are undergoing initial evaluation studies. These include different types of day treatment programs, school-based interventions, wilderness programs, crisis mobile outreach teams, therapeutic in-home emergency services, time-limited hospitalization with coordinated community services, intensive case management, and family support services. Studies involving these modalities have demonstrated significantly better outcomes than have traditional outpatient or residential services. These include reduced levels of externalizing and internalizing symptoms, improved family functioning, and reduced use of more restrictive services (Pumariega & Glover, 1997; U.S. Surgeon General, 1999).

The wraparound model of care embodies the child- and family-centered, community-based approach that is central to the system of care model. A number of studies of wraparound programs have reported positive outcomes, such as reduction of externalizing behavioral problems and out-of-home placements, improved levels of child and family functioning, and increased consumer/family satisfaction (Pumariega & Glover, 1997; U.S. Surgeon General, 1999).

Studies of community-based service systems for children that utilize innovative interventions along with interagency coordination and family empowerment are being undertaken. Initial outcome data on overall service system functions in community-based systems of care in Vermont, New York, and Ventura County, California, have demonstrated reduced hospitalization rates and days, decreased out-of-home placements and less restrictive placements, significantly lower incidence of negative behaviors severe enough to put children at risk of out-of-home placement, and lower rates of overall problem behaviors (Jordan & Hernandez, 1990; Bruns, Burchard, & Yoe, 1995, Evans, Armstrong, & Kuppinger, 1996).

Several recent evaluation projects of system of care programs have sparked considerable debate. Evaluation of the Fort Bragg Project in North Carolina involved a controlled study in which traditional military (CHAMPUS) benefits were compared with an expanded continuum of care in which a wide array of individualized and family-centered services was delivered. The evaluation by Bickman and colleagues (1996a) found that in the demonstration site, there was increased access to services; families were more satisfied with services; care was provided in less restrictive environments; and children stayed in treatment longer. No differences between the two groups were shown in either clinical outcomes or costs in the Fort Bragg project. Another study in Stark County, Ohio (Bickman et al., 1997, 1999), also found no difference in clinical or functional status between a system of care group and a usual care group.

Preliminary evidence from uncontrolled evaluations in the CMHS Children's Services Program indicates some improvement in outcomes, including better academic performance and attendance, a decrease in contacts with law enforcement, diversion of some children from restrictive placements, and improvements in CAFAS scores in several domains of functioning (MACRO International, 1997).

There has been considerable debate and little consensus about how to interpret these results. One recommendation made as a result of these findings is to focus on the nature and efficacy of the treatments and service components provided within systems of care (Jensen et al., 1996; Weisz et al., 1997; Hoagwood, 1997). An important question that has been raised is how to evaluate the systems changes that have been created. The improved family satisfaction, increased interagency collaboration, and less restrictive levels of care that are being demonstrated suggest that system-level and family-level outcome indicators may be important along with clinical and functional outcomes. A multidomain model of outcomes for mental health care that includes symptoms, functioning, consumer perspectives, environments, and systems has been proposed (Hoagwood et al., 1996); this model broadens the view of outcomes that are relevant to assessing effectiveness of services.

Another benefit of system of care demonstration projects has been the implementation of innovations in service delivery, including blended funding, managed care/ system of care hybrids, and colocation of different agency workers, as in the CMHS-funded sites located in Santa Barbara County, California and Charleston, South Carolina, as well as in emerging nonprofit managed care entities such as Community Behavioral Health (owned by the City of Philadelphia) and Aurora Behavioral Health in eastern Wisconsin. These programs have used system of care approaches to develop case management and community-based, integrated, interagency services to reduce duplication and improve the efficiency and effectiveness of mental health and human services to high-need populations of children and families.

SUMMARY

Children and adolescents with SEDs represent approximately 9% to 13% of the child and adolescent population. These children generally have multiple psychiatric diagnoses coupled with significant functional impairment in several domains of functioning. Children and adolescents with SED also tend to be involved with multiple child-serving agencies, creating the risk of uncoordinated and fragmented services. The past two decades have seen broad national initiatives aimed at developing systems of care guided by the CASSP principles. These principles specify that services within a system of care should be coordinated, integrated across systems, community-based, culturally competent, and individualized to the needs of children and families.

Children with SED benefit greatly from comprehensive diagnostic assessment and structured functional assessments. They should have early access to both psychosocial therapies and pharmacotherapy. Case management services and the wraparound approach are central to the systems of care approach. The wraparound approach for SED children and their families attempts to strengthen their natural support systems, increase adaptive skills, and provide supports to minimize the burden of caring for an SED child. Services delivered in a family-centered approach, using an ecological conceptual framework, are most compatible with the system of care concept. Nontraditional service elements show promise in improving outcomes for children with SED. Judgements on the overall success of system of care initiatives await more controlled studies.

REFERENCES

Achenbach, T. M., & Edelbrock C. (1983). *Manual for the Child Behavior Checklist and Child Behavior Profile.* Burlington: University of Vermont, Department of Psychiatry.

Achenbach, T. M. (1991a). *Manual for the Teacher's Report Form and 1991 Profile.* Burlington: University of Vermont, Department of Psychiatry.

Achenbach, T. M. (1991b). *Manual for the Youth Self-Report and 1991 Profile.* Burlington: University of Vermont, Department of Psychiatry.

Atkins, D., Pumariega, A. J., Rogers, K., Montgomery, L., Nybro, C., Jeffers, G., & Sease, F. (1999). Mental health and incarcerated youth: II. Prevalence and nature of psychopathology. *Journal of Child and Family Studies, 8*(2), 193–204.

Bazelon Center for Mental Health Law. (1996). *An uncertain future: How the new welfare law affects children with serious emotional disturbance and their families.* Washington, DC: National Technical Assistance Center for Children's Mental Health.

Berlin, I. (1991). Development of the subspecialty of child and adolescent psychiatry. In J. Weiner (Ed.), *Textbook of child and adolescent psychiatry* (pp. 8–15). Washington, DC: American Psychiatric Press.

Bickman, L. (1996). Implications of a children's mental health managed care demonstration project. *Journal of Mental Health Administration, 23,* 137–145.

Bird, H. R., Yager, T. J., Steghezza, B., Gould, M. S., Canino, G., & Rubio-Stipec, M. (1990). Impairment in the epidemiological measurement of childhood psychopathology in the community. *Journal of the American Academy of Child and Adolescent Psychiatry, 29,* 796–803.

Bird, D., Lambert, D., Hartley, D., Beeson, P., & Coburn, A. (1998). Rural models for integrating primary care and mental health services. *Administration and Policy in Mental Health, 25,* 287–308.

Brandenburg, N., Friedman, R., & Silver, S. (1990). The epidemiology of childhood psychiatric disorders. Prevalence findings from recent studies. *Journal of the American Academy of Child and Adolescent Psychiatry, 29,* 76–83.

Bruns, E., Burchard, J., & Yoe, J. (1995). Evaluating the Vermont system of care. Outcomes associated with community-based wrap-around services. *Journal of Child and Family Studies, 4,* 321–339.

Burns, B., & Taube, C. (1990). Mental health services for adolescents. Contract paper prepared by the Office of Technology Assessment, U.S. Congress Cited in U.S. Congress Office of Technology Assessment (November, 1991). *Adolescent health: volume II. Background and effectiveness of selected prevention and treatment services* (OTA-H-466). Washington, DC: U.S. Government Printing Office.

Caron, C., & Rutter, M. (1991). Co-morbidity in child psychopathology: Concepts, issues, and research strategies. *Journal of Child Psychology and Psychiatry, 32,* 1063–1080.

Casat, C., Rigsby, M., Sobelewski, J., & Gordon, J. (1999). School-based mental health services: A pragmatic view of a program. *Psychology in the Schools, 36*(5), 403–414.

Costello, E. J. (1986). Primary care pediatrics and child psychopathology. *Pediatrics, 78,* 1044–1051.

Costello, E. J., Angold, A., & Keeler, G. (1999). Adolescent outcomes of childhood disorders: The consequences of severity and impairment. *Journal of the American Academy of Child and Adolescent Psychiatry, 38*(2), 121–128.

Costello, E., Burns, B., Angold, A., & Leaf, P. (1993). How can epidemiology improve mental health services for children and adolescents? *Journal of the American Academy of Child and Adolescent Psychiatry, 32*(6), 106–117.

Costello, E. J., & Messer, S. C. (1995). *Rates and correlates of serious emotional disturbance: Secondary analysis of epidemiologic data sets.* Paper prepared for Center for Mental Health Services, Rockville, MD.

Costello, E. J., Messer, S. C., Bird, H. R., Cohen, P., & Reinherz, H. Z. (1998). The prevalence of serious emotional disturbance: A re-analysis of community studies. *Journal of Child and Family Studies, 7*(4), 411–432.

Cross, T., Bazron, B., Dennis, K., & Isaac, M. (1989). *Towards a culturally competent system of care for children with serious emotional disorders.* Washington, DC: Georgetown Technical Assistance Center for Children's Mental Health.

Culhane, D., Avery, J., & Hadley, T. (1998). Prevalence of treated behavioral disorders among adult shelter users: A longitudinal study. *American Journal of Orthopsychiatry, 68,* 63–72.

Del Mundo, A., Pumariega, A., & Vance, H. (1999). Psychopharmacology in school-based mental health services. *Psychology in the Schools, 36*(5), 437–450.

Emslie, G. J., Weinberg, W. A., Kowatch, R. A., Hughes, C. W., Carmlody, T. J., & Rush, A. J. (1997). Fluoxetine treatment of depressed children and adolescents. *Archives of General Psychiatry, 54,* 1031–1037.

England, M. J., & Coles, R. (1992). Building systems of care for youth with serious mental illness. *Hospital and Community Psychiatry, 4,* 630–633.

Evans, M. E., Armstrong, M. I., & Kuppinger, A. D. (1996). Family-centered intensive case management: A step toward understanding individualized care. *Journal of Child and Family Studies, 5*(1), 55–65.

Flaherty, L., & Weist, M. (1999). School-based mental health services: The Baltimore models. *Psychology in the Schools, 36*(5), 379–390.

Friedman, R. M., Katz-Leavy, J. W., Manderscheid, R. W., & Sondheimer, D. L. (1996). Prevalence of serious emotional disturbance in children and adolescents. In R. W. Manderscheid & M. A. Sonnenschein (Eds.), *Center for Mental Health Services Mental Health, United States, 196* (71–89). Washington, DC: U.S. Government Printing Office.

Friesen, B. J., & Poertner, J. (Eds.). (1995). *From case management to service coordination for children with emotional, behavioral, or mental disorders.* Baltimore, MD: Brookes.

Glied, S. (1998). Too little time? The recognition and treatment of mental health problems in primary care. *Health Services Research, 33,* 891–910.

Henggeler, S. W., Schoenwald, S. K., Borduin, C. M., Rowland, M. D., & Cunningham, P. B. (1998). *Multisystemic treatment of antisocial behavior in children and adolescents.* New York: Guilford Press.

Hoagwood, K. (1997). Interpreting nullity. The Fort Bragg experiment—A comparative success or failure? *American Psychologist, 52,* 546–550.

Hoagwood, K., Jensen, P. S., Petti, T., & Burns, B. J. (1996). Outcomes of mental health care for children and adolescents: I. A comprehensive conceptual model. *Journal of the American Academy of Child and Adolescent Psychiatry, 35*(8), 1055–1063.

Hodges, K. (1990). *Manual for the child and adolescent functional assessment scale.* Unpublished manuscript. Eastern Michigan University.

Inouye, D. (1988). Children's mental health issues. *American Psychologist, 43,* 813–816.

Jellinek, M. (1997). DSM-PC: Bridging primary care and mental health. *Journal of Developmental and Behavioral Pediatrics, 18,* 173–174.

Jensen, P. S., Hoagwood, K., & Petti, T. (1996). Outcomes of mental health care for children and adolescents: II. Literature review and application of a comprehensive model. *Journal of the American Academy of Child and Adolescent Psychiatry, 35*(8), 1064–1076.

Jordan, D., & Hernandez, M. (1990). The Ventura Planning Model: A proposal for mental health reform. *Journal of Mental Health Administration, 17,* 26–47.

Kilgus, M., Pumariega, A. J., & Cuffe, S. (1995). Influence of race on diagnosis in adolescent psychiatric inpatients. *Journal of the American Academy of Child and Adolescent Psychiatry, 35,* 67–72.

Knitzer, J. (1982). *Unclaimed children.* Washington, DC: Children's Defense Fund.

Kupermine, G., & Cohen, R. (1995). Building a research base for community services for children and families: What we know and what we need to learn. *Journal of Child and Family Studies, 4,* 147–175.

Looney, J. C. (Ed.). (1988). *Chronic mental illness in children and adolescents.* Washington, DC: American Psychiatric Press.

Motes, P., Melton, G., Pumariega, A., & Simmons, W. (1999). Ecologically-oriented school-based mental health services: Implications for service system reform. *Psychology in the Schools, 36*(5), 391–402.

Macro International, Inc. (1997). *Annual report to congress on the evaluation of the comprehensive community mental health services for children and their families program.* Atlanta, Georgia.

Polivka, B., Kennedy, C., & Chaudry, R. (1997). Collaboration between local public health and community mental health agencies. *Research in Nursing Health, 20,* 153–160.

Pumariega, A. J., Johnson, P., & Sheridan, D. (1995). Emotional disturbance and substance abuse in residential group homes. *Journal of Mental Health Administration, 22,* 426–431.

Pumariega, A. J., & Cross, T. (1997). Cultural competence in child psychiatry. In J. Noshpitz & N. Alessi (Eds.), *Handbook of child and adolescent psychiatry,* vol. 4 (pp. 473–484). New York: Wiley.

Pumariega, A. J., & Glover, S. (1998). New developments in services delivery research for children, adolescents, and their families. In T. Ollendick & R. Prinz (Eds.), *Advances in clinical child psychology* (Vol. 20). New York: Plenum Press.

Pumariega, A. J., Nace, D., England, M. J., Diamond, J., Mattson, A., Fallon, T., Hanson, G., Lourie, I., Marx., L., Thurber, D., Winters, N., Graham, M., & Wiegand, D. (1997). Community-based systems approach to children's managed mental health services. *Journal of Child and Family Studies, 6*(2), 149–164.

Pumariega, A. J., Atkins, D., Rogers, K., Montgomery, L., Nybro, C., Caesar, R., & Millus, D. (1999). Mental health and incarcerated youth: II. Service utilization. *Journal of Child and Family Studies, 8*(2), 205–215.

Rivera, V. R., & Kutash, K. (1994). *Components of a system of care. What does the research say?* Tampa: University of South Florida, Research and Training Center for Children's Mental Health.

Schacht, T., & Hanson, G. (1999). Evolving legal climate for school-based mental health services under the Individuals with Disabilities Education Act. *Psychology in the Schools, 36*(5), 415–426.

Shaffer, D., Gould, M. S., Brasic, J., Ambrosini, P., Fisher, P., & Bird, H. (1983). A Children's Global Assessment Scale (CGAS). *Archives of General Psychiatry, 40,* 1228–1231.

Shandle, M., & Christianson, J. (1988). Mental health care for children and adolescents in health maintenance organizations. In National Center for Education in Maternal and Child Health, *The Financing of Mental Health Services for Children and Adolescents.* Washington, DC: National Maternal and Child Health Clearinghouse.

Stroul, B. A. (1996). Service coordination in systems of care. In B. A. Stroul (Ed.), *Children's mental health: Creating systems of care in a changing society.* Baltimore, MD: Brookes.

Stroul, B. A., & Friedman, R. M. (1986). *A system of care for children and youth with severe emotional disturbance* (rev. ed.). Washington, DC: Georgetown University, CASSP Technical Assistance Center.

Tuma, J. (1989). Mental health services for children: The state of the art. *American Psychologist, 44,* 188–199.

U.S. Surgeon General. (1999). Children and mental health. *Mental health: A report of the Surgeon General.* Chap. 3, 123–220.

U.S. Government. (1993). *Federal Register* 58, 29425.

VanDenBerg, J. E., & Grealish, E. M. (1996). Individualized services and supports through the wraparound process: Philosophy and procedures. *Journal of Child and Family Studies, 5,* 7–22.

Weisz, J. R., Han, S. S., & Valeri, S. M. (1997). More of what? Issues raised by the Fort Bragg study. *American Psychologist, 52,* 541–545.

Author Index

Abikoff, H., 235, 270, 457
Abrantes, A. M., 285
Abreu, J., 502
Achenbach, T. M., 25, 57, 65, 93,
    101, 242, 245, 274, 339, 361,
    455, 486, 519
Ackerman, L., 210
Ackerman, P. T., 265
Adair, M., 338, 339, 340, 342
Addalli, K. A., 283, 296
Addy, C. L., 333
Adler, R. J. M., 237
Adson, D. E., 322
Agras, W., 323
Ainsworth, M. D. S., 388
Akiskal, H. S., 417
Alario, A. J., 335
Albach, F., 338
Albano, A. M., 400, 401, 402
Albert, A., 92
Albin, R. W., 63
Alderdice, F., 158
Algozzine, B., 139, 140, 144
Allan, J., 346
Allen, A. J., 286, 402
Allen, S. N., 340
Almond, P., 195, 206, 208
Altarriba, J., 504
Altizer, E. A., 431
Aman, M. G., 93, 481, 482, 489,
    490
Amaya-Jackson, L., 339, 341, 343,
    403
Ambrosini, P. J., 456, 519
American Academy of Child and
    Adolescent Psychiatry, 361,
    362, 364, 366, 367, 370, 389,
    396
American Academy of Child and
    Adolescent Psychiatry
    Work Group on Quality Is-
    sues, 272, 279
American Academy of Psychiatry
    and the Law, 102, 116n. 1
American College of Medical Ge-
    netics, 200, 201
American Council on Education,
    275
American Psychiatric Association,
    4, 5, 36, 45, 52, 61, 62, 63,
    66, 67, 77, 141, 144, 145,
    155, 189, 193, 196, 197, 198,
    199, 231, 232, 233, 234, 240,
    264, 265, 271, 276, 308, 313,
    314, 315, 316, 317, 322, 323,

334, 336, 341, 369, 390, 399,
    417, 418, 419, 424, 450, 459,
    478, 482, 483, 484
American Psychological Associa-
    tion, 102, 103, 116n. 1
Amess, P. N., 158
Anastasi, A., 56, 57, 58, 62, 63, 64,
    65, 66
Anastopoulos, A. D., 275
Andenor, L. T., 217
Andersen, A. E., 322, 323
Anderson, C. A., 233
Anderson, J. C., 157, 237, 390, 398
Anderson, M., 92
Ando, H., 270
Andrasick, F., 37, 58
Andreski, P., 333
Andrews, D. W., 251, 255
Andrus, J. K., 420
Angell, R. H., 338, 340
Anglin, R., 340
Angold, A., 270, 398, 431, 432, 443
Annon, K., 506
Appelbaum, P. S., 98
Applegate, B., 236, 237, 265
Archer, L., 209
Archer, R. P., 23
Ardali, C., 406
Arena, J. G., 37, 58
Arick, J., 195, 206, 208
Armbruster, P., 423
Armenteros, J., 482
Armstrong, M. I., 521, 528
Arndt, S. V., 286
Arnold, L. E., 267
Arnold, V., 338, 339, 340, 342
Arnsten, A. F. T., 287
Aro, H. M., 423
Arredondo, D., 483
Arrons, M., 192
Arroyo, W., 331, 334, 335, 340, 341,
    342, 343
Arvidson, J., 159
Asarnow, J. R., 269, 340
Asarnow, R., 209
Asbell, M. D., 287
Aschen, J., 286
Asher, S. R., 157
Aslami, B., 507
Asperger, H. C., 192, 193
Atkins, D. L., 495, 526
Atkins, M. S., 335, 341, 343
Attwood, A., 194
August, G. J., 267, 270
Ault, M. H., 38, 55

Avery, J., 525
Awadh, A. M., 16, 190, 194, 197,
    198, 199, 216
Axline, V., 437
Ayd, F. J., 383, 384, 387, 390
Ayers, S., 309
Ayers, W. A., 431
Ayllon, T., 37, 38
Aytaclar, S., 270
Azar, V., 507
Azrin, N. H., 38, 74
Azzam, P. N., 270

Bachrach, L. K., 322
Baer, D. M., 32, 38, 39, 40, 41, 42,
    43, 44, 47, 49, 55, 58, 78
Bagby, R. M., 100, 101
Bailey, J. N., 269
Bakan, D., 330
Baker, A., 506
Baker, L., 271, 315, 404
Balderrama, H., 508
Baldessarini, R., 285
Ball, J., 204, 208
Balla, D., 93, 184
Ballenger, J. C., 406
Balon, R., 484
Bandura, A., 41, 69
Banegas, M., 428
Banken, J. A., 190
Barber, J. P., 437
Barber-Foss, K. D., 131
Barclay, L., 126
Barkley, R. A., 36, 47, 56, 57, 62,
    65, 66, 263, 265, 267, 271,
    275, 476, 478, 479, 480
Barlow, D. H., 58, 72, 389
Barnard, K., 379
Baron, L., 331
Barone, D. F., 131
Barraclough, B., 307
Barrash, D. P., 39
Barrett, C. L., 65
Barrett, P. M., 389, 405
Barrickman, L. L., 286
Barrios, B. A., 45
Barron, J., 476
Bartolucci, G., 209
Bass, D., 252, 254, 431
Bates, E., 183
Bates, J. E., 239, 253
Bauman, K. E., 42
Baumgaertel, A., 287
Bayley, N., 21, 127, 130
Baysinger, C. M., 386

Bazelon Center for Mental Health Law, 525
Bazron, B. J., 499, 500, 502, 514
Beard, C. M., 309
Beaumont, J. G., 120
Beck, A. T., 41, 246, 437, 457
Beck, J. G., 37, 58
Becker, A. E., 309
Becker, D. F., 340
Bedi, G., 161
Beebe, D. W., 276
Beebe, S., 346
Beeson, P., 527
Begleiter, H., 269
Beidel, D. C., 386, 387
Beile, E. E., 125
Beitchman, J. H., 338, 339, 340, 342
Beitchman, M. D., 140, 145, 146, 155, 156, 157, 163
Bekken, K., 269
Bell, R. M., 308
Bellack, A. S., 6, 45, 62
Belshwer, G., 434
Belsky, J., 333, 334
Bemporad, J. R., 308, 309
Bender, L., 191
Bender, M. E., 283
Bender, P. K., 157
Bender, W. N., 142, 143, 155, 156, 162, 163
Benedek, E. P., 98, 342
Benevidez, D. A., 194
Benham, A. L., 91, 364
Bennetto, L., 250
Ben-Porath, Y. S., 23, 428
Benson, R. S., 338, 339, 340, 342
Bentzen, F. A., 142
Bergen, D., 365, 366, 367, 369
Bergh, C., 308
Bergland, M. M., 120
Berlin, I. N., 494, 516
Berman, A., 421
Bern, D. L., 387
Bernal, G., 501, 506
Bernet, W., 338, 339, 340, 342
Bernstein, G. A., 384, 390, 396, 398, 400, 401, 406, 478, 482
Bernstein, J. G., 479
Bernthal, J. E., 171
Berry, P. S., 156
Bessler, M. A., 296
Best, C. L., 333
Bettelheim, B., 215
Beutler, L. E., 28
Bhatara, V. S., 284
Biafora, F., 307
Bialik, R. J., 334
Bickman, L., 528
Biederman, J., 233, 263, 265, 267, 269, 270, 271, 282, 283, 285, 286, 385, 386, 390, 406, 407
Bierman, K. L., 238
Bigler, E. D., 125, 126
Bijou, S. W., 38, 55
Bingham, R., 369
Binkoff, J. A., 42, 43
Birch, H. G., 265, 385
Bird, A., 171
Bird, H. R., 236, 270, 389, 390, 431, 432, 485, 503, 517, 519, 526

Birmaher, B., 339
Black, B., 399
Black, M. M., 63
Black, S. A., 46, 47, 48, 68, 70, 71
Blake, D. D., 339
Blaskey, J., 132
Blass, J. P., 126
Blau, S., 63, 423
Blehar, M. D., 388
Bleiberg, J., 131
Bloom, M., 182
Blumberg, S., 432
Blumstein, A., 236
Bockian, N., 23
Boetsch, E., 155
Bolduc, E. A., 386
Boles, M., 284, 379
Boliek, C. A., 24
Boncherding, B., 480
Bongura, N., 283, 296
Bonilla, J., 501
Bonuagura, N., 235
Booth, S., 283
Bopp, M., 346
Borchardt, C. M., 384, 390, 396, 398, 400, 401, 406, 478
Borcherding, B., 282, 284
Borden, M. C., 194
Borduin, C. M., 432, 435, 526
Boretos, J. W., 125
Bourdon, K., 485
Bourgeois, B. F., 159
Bowen, M., 191
Bowen, R. C., 389
Bower, G. H., 33
Bowers, W. A., 322, 323
Bowlby, J., Jr., 360, 387, 388, 416
Bowring, M. A., 271
Boyle, M. H., 237
Bracero, W., 502
Bradley, C., 191, 282, 475
Brady, J. P., 37
Brady, M., 174
Brammer, M., 269
Brandenburg, N. A., 413, 514
Brannon, J. M., 237
Brasic, J., 486, 519
Braswell, L., 66, 267
Braun, D. L., 318
Braverman, C., 47, 48, 49, 55, 75
Breaux, A. M., 285
Breengill, L., 423
Bregman, J. D., 213, 214
Breier, J. I., 269
Bremmer, R., 209
Brendgen, M., 236, 239
Brent, D., 339, 340, 341
Breslau, N., 270, 333
Brestan, E. V., 247
Briggs-Gown, M. J., 373
Brinthaupt, V. P., 235
Britner, P. A., 111
Broadhurst, D. D., 332, 333
Broden, M., 53
Brodsky, A., 99, 115
Brodsky, S. L., 237
Brookman, C. S., 435
Brosig, C., 108
Bross, D. C., 343
Brown, C., 506

Brown, J., 482
Brown, M. M., 238
Brown, R. T., 159
Bruch, H., 309, 311, 315
Bruck, M., 108, 155
Bruininks, R. H., 127
Bruns, E., 528
Brust, J. D., 131
Bryan, T., 157
Bryson, S., 206
Bucher, B., 36
Bucholz, K. K., 269
Buchsbaum, Y., 428, 457
Buckley, N. K., 55
Bukstein, O. G., 338, 339, 340, 341, 342, 476
Bulik, C., 316
Bullmore, E. T., 269
Bunnell, D. W., 312
Burch, P. R., 241
Burchard, J., 432, 528
Burke, L. B., 284
Burns, B. J., 398, 424, 431, 432, 443, 514, 515, 528
Burt, D. B., 92
Bussey, K., 101
Butcher, J. N., 23, 428
Butler, S., 483
Butter, H. J., 334

Cabaniss, D., 507
Caddell, J., 283
Caesar, R., 495, 526
Caffey, J., 330
Calhoun, S. L., 275
Callaghan, C., 335, 341
Callan, A., 505
Camargo, C. A., 310
Camp, C. M. V., 58, 77
Campbell, D., 174
Campbell, M. C., 209, 215, 217, 476, 482
Campbell, W., 456
Canales, D. N., 130
Canino, G., 236, 270, 389, 390, 485, 503, 519
Cannon, T., 428
Canobbio, R., 340, 341
Canterbury, R., 340
Cantwell, D. P., 263, 269, 271, 275, 286, 404, 478, 480, 485, 487
Caplan, M. Z., 250
Capriotti, R. M., 47, 48, 49, 55, 75
Caputo, A. A., 237
Carey, D. J., 406
Carey, W. B., 386
Carlat, D. J., 310
Carlson, C. L., 267, 270
Carmlody, T. J., 521
Caron, C., 485, 518
Carpenter, R. L., 182
Carr, E. G., 42, 43
Carrey, N. J., 334
Carroll, B. J., 457
Carroll, J., 437
Carter, A. S., 203, 373
Casat, C. D., 270, 275, 286, 526
Casey, J. J., 269
Caspi, A., 387
Castellanos, D., 406

Castellanos, F. X., 267, 269, 285
Casteneda, A., 457
Cataldo, M. F., 42, 48
Catania, A. C., 33, 34, 35, 36, 37, 43, 77
Cautela, J. R., 6, 41
Ceci, S. J., 108
Celano, M. P., 159
Center for Disease Control, 119
Chalfant, J. C., 143
Chaloner, D., 318
Chambers, S. W., 423
Chambers, W., 25, 63, 339, 456
Chambless, D. L., 279, 506
Chandran, K. S. K., 286
Chaplin, D., 129
Chapman, R., 175, 182, 184
Charlton, A., 159
Chaudry, R., 527
Chen, L., 270
Chen, W. J., 270
Chen, Y. W., 92
Cherrick, I., 159
Cheryl, M. L., 235
Chess, J., 419
Chess, S., 385, 386
Cheung, F. K., 424, 432, 495
Cheung, K., 130
Chilappagari, S., 333
Chilcoat, H. D., 270
Chorpita, A. B., 400, 401, 402
Christ, M. A. G., 231, 233, 236
Christensen, C. P., 345
Christian, R. E., 237
Christianson, J., 527
Chrousos, G. P., 341
Chu, M. P., 269
Cicchetti, D., 93, 184, 206, 207
Clark, C., 174
Clark, D. B., 341, 457
Clark, K. A., 417
Clark, R., 362, 365, 367
Clarke, G. M., 413, 422, 434, 435
Clarke, G. N., 417, 435
Clarke, R., 432
Clarkin, J., 7
Cleckly, H., 237
Cleveland, L., 92, 270
Cleves, M., 269
Coats, K. I., 434
Coburn, A., 527
Coburn, T. H., 126
Coe, D., 205, 207
Coen-Kettenis, P., 275
Coggins, T. E., 182
Cohen, C., 92
Cohen, D. J., 203, 206, 207, 238, 270, 283, 285, 286
Cohen, E., 333
Cohen, J. A., 338, 339, 340, 342, 343, 344, 402, 403, 406
Cohen, M. J., 276
Cohen, P., 405, 517
Cohen, R., 527
Cohen, S. B., 217
Cohen-Sandler, R., 421
Coie, J. D., 233, 234, 235, 238, 239
Colder, C. R., 238, 239, 243
Cole, D., 194
Cole, R., 516

Coles, G. S., 141
Comas-Diaz, L., 79
Comings, B. G., 270
Comings, D. E., 269, 270
Conduct Problems Prevention Research Group, 232, 234, 249, 253
Conerly, S., 331
Conlin, S., 362, 365, 367
Conner, D. F., 286
Conners, C., 341
Conners, C. K., 7, 65, 93, 265, 274, 286, 457, 486
Conners, C. R., 25
Conners, K., 341
Connor, D. F., 286, 480
Connors, M., 312, 316, 317
Conroyd, M. K., 424
Constable, R. T., 271
Constantino, G., 507
Constantinou, J. E. C., 269
Conte, P. M., 159
Contreras-Neira, R., 507
Cook, E. H., Jr., 269, 482
Cook, S. C., 457
Cool, V. A., 159
Cooper, H. M., 432, 435
Cooper, J., 457
Cooper, P., 312
Copeland, D. R., 159
Corbett, J., 193
Corkum, P. V., 276
Cormier, C. A., 114
Cortes, D. E., 499
Cosgrave, M. P., 92
Costello, A. J., 25, 62, 66, 387, 456
Costello, E. J., 242, 270, 389, 390, 398, 431, 432, 443, 517, 518, 527
Coulter, M. L., 344
Courtney, M., 270
Cowdery, G. E., 42
Cowell, J. M., 158
Coyne, J. C., 417
Craske, M. G., 386, 387, 389
Craven, S. V., 239
Crawford, S. G., 160
Creak, M., 195
Crichton, P., 309
Crick, N. R., 237
Crisp, A. H., 311, 321
Cronbach, L. J., 3
Crook, W. G., 287
Crosby, C. A., 111
Crosby, R., 270
Cross, T. L., 431, 499, 500, 502, 514
Crowell, E. W., 275
Crowley, T. J., 235
Cruickshank, W. M., 142
Cuccaro, M., 495
Cuellar, I., 79
Cueva, J. E., 215, 476
Cuffe, S. P., 333, 335, 341, 495, 503, 505, 518
Culbertson, J. L., 26, 27
Culhane, D., 525
Cullinan, D., 270, 456
Culpepper, L., 402
Cummings, E., 92
Cunningham, P. B., 526

Curry, J. E., 241
Curry, J. F., 254
Curtis, S., 267, 270
Cytryn, L., 414, 418, 423

Dadds, M. R., 389, 405
Dahl, R., 484
Dalby, P. R., 131
Dale, P., 183
Dalton, R., 436
Daly, G., 269
D'Amato, G., 406
Damon, L., 331
Dana, R. H., 79
Dane, H., 254
Daneman, D., 319
Daniel, J. C., 131
Daniels, S. R., 309
Dansky, B. S., 333
Darrah, J., 127
Das, J. P., 270
Davalos, M., 360
Davenport, M. G., 159
Davidson, L. A., 126
Davies, M., 485
Davis, D. D., 435
Davis, G. C., 333
Davis, R. D., 23
Dawson, S., 214
DeAnda, D., 497
DeBellis, M. D., 341
Deblinger, E., 335, 341
DeGroot, J., 319
Deitz, J., 129
Del'Homme, M. A., 269
Delizio, R. D., 386
Del Mundo, A. S., 163, 217, 218, 521
DeMaise, L., 359
Denckla, M., 482
Denhoff, E., 265
Dennis, K. W., 499, 500, 502, 514
DePaul, G., 479, 480
De Rios, M., 507
Detlor, J., 285
Detries, J. C., 156
DeVane, C., 476, 477
DeVaugh-Geiss, J., 407
Devenny, D. A., 92
Dewa, C. S., 420
Diamond, J., 487, 488, 524
Dichtemiller, M., 377
Dickens, S. E., 100
Dickstein, D. P., 269
Dietz, S. G., 414, 418
Dignon, A., 318
Dinkmeyer, D., 280
Dinkmeyer, D., Jr., 281
Dinkmeyer, D. C., 281
Dinkmeyer, J. S., 281
Dishion, T. J., 234, 247, 251, 255, 280
Dodge, K. A., 238, 239, 253
Dogin, J. W., 286, 287
Dolan, B., 309
Donenberg, G. R., 431
Donnelly, M., 285
Donon, J. E., 457
Donovan, J. E., 341

Doogan, D., 477
Dorn, L. D., 341
Dorsey, M. F., 42
dosReis, S., 284, 379, 505
Downey, G., 417
Draguns, J. G., 498
Dratman, M., 204, 208
Drell, M. J., 342, 403
Droegemueller, W., 331
Dubey, D. R., 251
Duffy, J. H., 406
Dulcan, M. K., 236, 242, 272, 279,
     389, 397, 456, 485
Dumas, L. S., 345
Duncan, D., 162
Duncan, J. W., 79
Dunitz, M., 369, 370, 372
Dunn, S. E., 238, 243, 248
DuPaul, G. J., 271, 272, 275, 476
Durand, V. M., 42, 77
Durfee, M., 331
Dykens, E., 206, 207
Dykman, R. A., 265

Eaves, D. M., 194
Eaves, L., 307
Eaves, R. C., 190, 194, 197, 198,
     199, 208
Ecton, R. B., 251
Edelbrock, C. S., 25, 57, 62, 65, 66,
     242, 339, 455, 456, 478, 479,
     519
Edelsohn, G. A., 344
Edgell, D., 124
Edwards, P., 309
Egolf, B. P., 335
Ehoroco, M. C., 217
Eichelberger, M. R., 119
Eisenberg, H. M., 128
Eisenberger, J. G., 63
Elber, H. W., 9
Elder, G. M., 387
Elia, J. L., 282, 284, 285
Elia, S., 480
Elligan, D., 506
Elliot, A. N., 343
Elliot, S. N., 246
Ellis, A., 41
Ellis, M., 254
Emde, R. N., 369
Emslie, G. J., 286, 521
Endicott, J., 456
Engel, A. J., 212
England, M. J., 487, 488, 516, 524
Epstein, M. H., 270, 456
Erbaugh, J., 428
Erhardt, D., 341
Erikson, E. H., 494, 497
Erkanli, A., 431
Ernst, M., 284, 286
Ersahin, Y., 130
Esveldt-Dawson, K., 254
Eth, S., 331, 334, 335, 340, 341, 342,
     343
Evans, C., 396
Evans, I. M., 204
Evans, K. K., 322, 323
Evans, M. E., 521, 528
Everaerd, W., 338
Everson, M. D., 344

Ewing-Cobbs, L., 128, 130
Exner, J. E., 10, 22
Eyberg, S. M., 247
Eysenck, H. J., 387

Fabrega, H., 503, 505
Faherty, S. L., 348
Fairbanks, L. A., 331, 334, 340, 342
Fairburn, C. G., 323
Fallon, T., 487, 488, 524
Famularo, R., 343
Fantuzzo, J., 343
Faraone, S. V., 233, 263, 265, 267,
     269, 270, 271, 283, 386,
     390
Farel, A. M., 159
Faria, L. P., 270
Farmer, E. M., 431
Farrington, D. P., 236
Farwell, E. C., 270
Favell, J., 61
Fay, C. G., 128
Fay, G. C., 128
Fear, J., 316
Fedoroff, I. C., 310
Fee, V., 205, 207
Feehan, M., 237, 390
Feil, M., 284
Feindler, E. A., 251
Feldman, H. M., 285, 479
Fenson, L., 183
Fenton, T., 343
Ferguson, H. B., 406
Ferguson, R. J., 131
Ferster, C. B., 33, 34, 35, 37
Field, C. J., 93
Field, L. L., 160
Field, T., 360
Filipek, P., 269
Finch, A. J., 343
Finch, A. J., Jr., 343
Findling, R. L., 286, 287, 481
Finkelhor, D., 331, 334, 335
Finkelstein, R., 390
Finney, J. C., 9
Finney, J. W., 48
Fischer, M., 478, 479
Fisher, D., 28
Fisher, P., 245, 389, 397, 485
Fitzgerald, D. P., 241, 243, 244, 247,
     253, 254
Fitzgerald, G. A., 269
Fitzgerald, H. E., 368
Fitzgerald, M., 269
Flaherty, L., 526
Fleisch, B., 422, 424
Fleming, D. N., 420
Fleming, S., 476
Fletcher, J. M., 66, 128, 130, 159,
     271, 272
Fletcher, K. E., 286, 339
Flockhart, D., 480
Flynn, C., 339
Flynn, J. M., 141
Foa, E. B., 335, 340, 341
Folstein, M. F., 91
Folstein, S. E., 91
Fonagy, P., 368
Forehand, R., 79, 239
Forget, R., 128, 129

Forman, M. A., 436
Foster, O., 158
Four Racial/Ethnic Panels, 508
Fowler, M. G., 159
Fowler, R. D., 9
Fox, L. H., 65
Fox, L. W., 417
Fox, M., 386
Foxx, R. M., 74
Fraiberg, S., 360
Fraknoi, J., 204, 208
Francis, G., 398
Franco, N., 404, 405
Frank, R. G., 420
Frankel, K. A., 360
Frazer, D. R., 237
Frazier, J., 269
Frazier, R., 435
Frederick, C. J., 331, 334, 339, 340,
     342
Freeman, B. J., 190, 195, 204, 206,
     208
Freeman, L., 428
Freilinger, J. J., 171
French, J. L., 19, 20
French, N. H., 254
Freud, S., 384
Frick, P. J., 231, 232, 233, 234, 235,
     236, 237, 240, 241, 242, 243,
     253, 396
Friedman, D., 128, 129
Friedman, L., 481
Friedman, R. M., 413, 422, 453,
     514, 516
Friesen, B. J., 435, 520, 524
Froese, A., 421
Frost, A. K., 333
Fudge, H., 414
Fulbright, R. K., 271
Fuller, G. B., 216
Fuller, P. R., 37

Gable, R., 112
Gadow, K. D., 270, 271, 284, 285,
     475, 477
Gaensbauer, T. J., 342
Gagnon, I., 128, 129
Gajewski, N., 348
Galatzer-Levy, R., 106
Garber, J., 236
Garbin, M. G., 246
Gardner, J. F., 284, 379
Gardner, R., 107
Garduno, R., 508
Garfinkel, B. D., 406, 421
Garfinkel, P. E., 309, 311, 324
Garfinkel, R., 506
Garg, R., 159
Garner, D. M., 309, 311, 319, 321,
     323, 324, 499
Garrison, C. Z., 333, 495
Garrison, E., 507
Garvia, I. G., 343
Gatenby, C., 271
Gatsonis, C., 417, 420, 437
Gaub, M., 267, 270
Geist, D. E., 285
Geller, B., 285, 417, 480
Geller, R. J., 159, 239
Gemmer, T. C., 247

Gene Care, 201
Gentile, C., 340
Gerdtz, J., 213, 214
Gershon, S., 479, 486
Gersten, J., 63
Gersten, M., 386
Ghuabi, M., 340
Giaconia, R. M., 333
Giampino, T. L., 235, 283, 296
Giarretto, H., 345
Gibbons, R., 428
Gibbs, J. T., 503, 506
Gibson, M., 456
Giedd, J. N., 269, 285
Gilgen, J. W., 156
Gill, M., 4, 92, 269
Gillberg, C., 283
Gilliam, W., 362, 366, 367
Gill-Weiss, M. J., 93
Gittelman, R., 235
Gittens, T., 192
Gittleman-Klein, R., 485
Glasser, K., 416
Glaubman, H., 421
Glied, S., 527
Glod, C. A., 341
Glover, S., 495, 508, 527, 528
Glutting, J., 19, 24
Glynn, E. I., 53
Goenjian, A. K., 340
Golden, C. J., 57, 127
Golden, G. S., 284
Goldman, J., 63, 64, 65, 66
Goldstein, G., 6, 45, 62
Goldston, D., 420
Goncalves, A., 23
Gonzalez, A., 286
Goode, S., 208
Goodman, R., 269
Goodman, S. H., 270
Goodman, W. K., 457, 486
Goodrich, G., 28
Goodwin, J., 338
Goodwin, M. B., 235
Gordon, J., 420, 526
Gordon, M., 276
Gore, J. C., 271
Goskin, K. A., 360
Gosling, A., 285
Gottesman, R. L., 160
Gottfredson, M., 114
Gould, J., 193
Gould, M. S., 431, 432, 486, 519
Gould, R. E., 421
Gouze, K. R., 238
Goyette, C. H., 265, 457
Graff, R. B., 77
Graham, J. R., 23, 428
Graham, M., 487, 488, 524
Graham, P. J., 63, 158, 159, 432
Grandison, C., 360
Granger, D. A., 431
Gray, J. A., 386
Grealish, E. M., 520
Green, A. H., 107, 338, 340, 344
Green, B. F., 56, 57, 58
Green, J. W., 503
Green, P. A., 155
Green, S. M., 235, 237
Green, W., 209

Greenberg, M. T., 234
Greenberg, S. A., 99
Greenblatt, E., 158
Greenblatt, R. M., 158
Greene, E. L., 63
Greenhill, L. H., 265, 282, 284
Greenhill, L. I., 63
Greenspan, S., 361
Greenstein, J., 453
Gregg, J., 190
Gresham, R. M., 246
Greshman, F. M., 242
Griffin, S., 282
Grills, C., 506
Grimley, P., 340, 341
Grimm, J., 235
Grimsley, S., 477
Grisso, T., 100, 110, 111, 114
Grizenko, N., 433
Groevich, S., 481
Gross, Y., 421
Grossman, J. A., 428, 457
Grotpeter, J. K., 237
Gualtieri, C. T., 284, 286
Guanipa, C., 507
Guerry, S., 63, 64, 65, 66
Guevremont, D. C., 275
Guite, J., 270
Gulek, C., 19, 24
Gurlanick, M. J., 213
Gurley, D., 405
Gurman, A. S., 432, 435
Gustavson, C. R., 309
Gustavson, J. C., 309
Gutheil, T. G., 98, 99, 115
Guthrie, D., 204, 208
Guthrie, J. F., 310
Gutierrez, M., 507
Gutierrez-Mayka, M., 507

Hadley, T., 525
Hagen, E. P., 21
Haines, D. E., 120, 130
Hale, R. L., 19, 20
Hall, C., 159
Hall, J., 265, 276
Hall, R. V., 38, 53, 55, 58, 59
Hallahan, D. P., 142, 161
Hallin, A., 215
Hallon, S. D., 435
Halmi, K. A., 318
Hamburg, P., 309
Hamburger, S. D., 267, 269, 285
Hamilton, J., 398
Hamilton, M. A., 77, 456
Hammer, D., 93
Hammill, D. D., 140, 143, 161, 180
Hammond, M., 250, 252
Hammond, S., 56, 57
Hampe, E., 65
Han, S. S., 431, 528
Hand, L., 171
Handen, B. L., 285, 479
Handler, L., 22
Hansen, C., 404, 405
Hansen, G., 487, 488
Hanson, G., 104, 524, 526
Hanson, K., 231, 233
Hanson, R. K., 22
Hardesty, A., 209

Hardin, M. T., 286, 457
Harding, M., 282, 283
Hardy, J., 235
Hare, R. D., 237
Haring, T. G., 55
Harmatz, J., 285
Harmon, K. G., 131
Harmon, R. J., 360, 369
Harnish, J. D., 253
Harrington, R. C., 414
Harris, E., 307
Harris, G. T., 114
Harris, R., 193
Harris, S. R., 247
Harrison, P. L., 21
Harrist, A. W., 239
Harrop, J. W., 239
Hart, B., 47
Hart, E. A., 231, 233
Hart, E. L. E., 235, 236, 237
Hartley, D., 527
Hartman, S., 340
Hartmann, D. P., 45
Hartsung, J., 183
Harvey, M., 23
Hatcher, N. M., 26
Hathaway, S. R., 23
Hawi, Z., 269
Hawkins, R. C., 309
Hawkins, W., 422, 435
Hayes, S. C., 7
Hazel-Fernandez, L. A., 271
Hazelrigg, M. D., 432, 435
Health, A. C., 269
Heath, A., 307
Hechtman, L., 296
Hedges, D., 286
Hedrick, D., 183
Heemsbergen, J., 208
Helfer, R. E., 330
Hemyari, P., 119
Henggeler, S. W., 431, 526
Henriksson, M. M., 423
Henry, B., 387
Henry, D., 335, 341
Henry, M. M., 159
Hensen, M., 6
Henshaw, S. P., 155
Hentges, B. A., 270
Herjanic, B., 63, 456, 485
Herman, J. B., 386
Hernandez, M., 508, 528
Hernandez, P., 508
Herringkohl, E. C., 335
Herringkohl, R. C., 335
Herrmann, K. J., 286
Hersen, M., 6, 19, 24, 26, 45, 58, 62, 72, 390, 398, 404
Herson, J. H., 63
Hertzig, M. E., 198, 384, 385, 388
Herzog, D. B., 310
Hesselbrock, V., 269
Hester, C., 309, 319, 499
Heston, J., 340
Higgitt, A., 368
Hilgard, E. R., 33
Hill, J., 414
Hill, N. L., 237
Hinshaw, S. P., 233, 235, 236, 275, 283

Hirsch, M., 456
Hirschi, T., 114
Hirshfeld, D. R., 386
Ho, H. H., 194
Hoagwood, K., 284, 413, 515, 520, 528
Hoaz, J., 284
Hobbs, S. A., 160
Hock, M., 389
Hodges, K., 486, 519
Hodges, V. K., 242
Hogan, A., 157
Hogan, K., 208
Holahan, J. M., 271
Holborow, P. L., 156
Holburn, A. H. S., 125
Holcomb, P. J., 265
Holdgrafer, M., 204, 208
Hollon, S. D., 279
Holttum, S., 479, 486
Holzer, C. E., 495, 499
Honaker, L. M., 9
Hood, J., 421
Hooper, S. R., 159
Hopkinds, D. D., 420
Hopkins, J., 175
Hoppe, C., 235
Hops, H., 413, 434, 435
Horder, P., 389
Horner, R. H., 63
Houck, P., 506
Howard, W. T., 322
Howell, C. T., 101
Howells, K., 318
Huang, L. N., 503, 506
Huang, R. J., 175
Hubbard, J., 340
Hudson, J. I., 310, 318
Hudziak, J. J., 269
Huertas, S., 503
Hughes, C. W., 521
Hughes, J., 242
Hunsley, J., 22
Hunt, R. D., 270, 286, 287
Hunter, T., 406
Hunter, W. M., 344
Huntington, D. D., 156
Hurst, H., 112
Hurt, S. W., 420
Hyman, C., 233, 235, 238
Hynd, G. W., 146, 265

Iann, M., 477
Inouye, D., 514
Insel, T. R., 402
Isaac, M., 514
Isaacs, M. R., 499, 500, 502
Ismond, D., 286
Iwata, B. A., 42, 77, 251

Jackson, C., 160
Jackson, D., 38, 55, 58, 59
Jackson, K. L., 333
Jackson, L. J., 309
Jacob, T., 65
Jacobsen, J., 210
Jacobson, M. S., 312
Jaffe, K. M., 128, 129
James, B., 346
Jameson, J. D., 63

Jammon, G. D., 420
Jansen, P,. 485
Jaycox, L. H., 340
Jeffers, G., 526
Jellinek, M., 527
Jenkins, W. M., 161
Jennett, B., 126
Jennings, M. C., 132
Jensen, P. S., 236, 265, 284, 515, 520, 528
Jetton, J. G., 267, 270
Jodl, K. M., 111
Johnson, A., 158
Johnson, C., 284, 312, 316, 317, 319
Johnson, J. G., 270
Johnson, J. H., 9
Johnson, K. M., 340, 346
Johnson, M., 453
Johnson, P., 161, 495, 524
Johnson, R., 339
Johnston, H. F., 414, 428
Joint Commission on Mental Health of Children, 453
Jones, G. V., 389
Jones, J. G., 319, 335
Jordan, D., 528
Jordan, H., 208
Jung, C. J., 385

Kaczynski, N. A., 341
Kadin, A. E., 390
Kaemmer, B., 23, 428
Kagan, J., 66, 68, 386, 419
Kahng, S. W., 77
Kakuma, T., 420
Kalas, R., 242
Kalesnik, J., 364
Kalichman, S., 108
Kalish, B., 205
Kalmanson, B., 365
Kalsher, M. K., 42
Kaminski, C., 477
Kamphaus, R. W., 5, 25, 141, 236, 240, 241, 242, 243, 245, 274, 428
Kandel, D. B., 270
Kanfer, F. H., 6, 41
Kanner, L., 190, 192, 193, 450
Kaplan, B. J., 160
Kaplan, H., 190
Kaplan, S. J., 332, 333, 334, 335
Karayan, I., 340
Karl, S., 267
Kashani, J. H., 389, 390, 398, 399, 401, 403
Kaslow, N., 434
Katz, D. I., 126
Katz, M. M., 3, 6, 7
Katz-Leavy, J. W., 514
Katzman, D. K., 322
Kauffman, J. M., 142, 161
Kauffmann, A. S., 5, 6, 21
Kaufman, J., 339
Kaufman, N. L., 21
Kaye, W. H., 318
Kaysen, D. K., 269
Kazdin, A. E., 32, 37, 39, 46, 53, 58, 62, 213, 214, 233, 234, 252, 254, 280, 390, 431, 432, 433, 435, 436

Kearney, A. J., 41
Keenan, K., 233, 237, 239, 390
Keilutz, L., 157
Keith, T., 269
Keller, A., 508
Keller, F. S., 78
Keller, M. B., 405
Kelley, S. J., 346
Kelly, K. S., 100, 476
Kelly, M. S., 160
Kemp, S., 127
Kempe, C. H., 330, 331
Kemphaus, R. W., 21, 26
Kendall, P. C., 66, 389, 405, 434, 443, 457
Kendall-Tackett, K. A., 331, 334, 335
Kendler, K., 307, 319
Kennedy, C. H., 55, 527
Kessler, R., 307
Ketelaar, M., 127
Keyson, C., 282, 480
Keysor, B. G., 284
Khayrallah, M., 286
Kiessling, L. S., 402
Kihlgren, M., 159
Kilgus, M., 503, 505, 518
Kill, A. L., 92
Kilpatrick, D. G., 333
King, N. J., 389, 400, 405, 406
King, R. A., 407, 421, 457
Kingsley, D. P. E., 158, 251
Kinlan, J., 338, 339, 340, 342
Kinscherff, R., 343
Kinzie, J. D., 338, 340
Kirisci, L., 270
Kirk, S. A., 140, 142, 143
Kirk, U., 127
Kirkbride, V., 158
Kirt, W. D., 143
Kiser, L. J., 340
Klaric, S., 242
Klass, C. S., 360
Klee, T., 182
Klei, R. G., 457
Klein, D. F., 396, 399
Klein, G., 235
Klein, R. G., 235, 283, 296
Kleinman, C. S., 407
Klerman, G. L., 420
Klimes-Dougan, B., 248
Klin, A., 192, 193, 203
Klorman, R., 271
Kluckhorn, F. R., 495
Knee, D., 285
Kniskern, D. P., 432, 435
Knitzer, J., 413, 422, 424, 514, 516
Knott, V., 406
Knutson, J. F., 335
Koegel, L. K., 194
Koegel, R. L., 194
Kogan, N., 373
Kolko, D. J., 345, 476
Konig, P. H., 235
Koplowicz, H. S., 270
Korkman, M., 127
Koroloff, N. M., 435
Koss-Chioino, J., 503, 507
Kotchick, B. A., 79
Kovacs, M., 9, 25, 63, 271, 341, 414, 417, 420, 428, 437, 457, 486

Kowatch, R. A., 521
Kraemer, G. W., 386
Kraft, I. A., 406
Krain, A. L., 269
Kramer, L., 130
Krantz, P. J., 78
Krasner, L., 37
Krasowski, M. D., 269
Kraus, I., 270
Kraus, J. F., 119
Kraus, L., 106
Kraybill, E. N., 159
Kremenitzer, M. W., 285
Krener, P. G., 159
Kriegler, J. S., 339
Krohne, H. W., 389
Kronenberg, W. G., 240, 241
Krug, D., 195, 206, 208
Krug, S. E., 10
Kuhn, T. S., 32, 39, 42, 49, 58
Kuhne, M., 270
Kuiler, F., 340, 341
Kulp, S., 52
Kuperman, S., 269, 286
Kupermine, G., 527
Kuppinger, A. D., 521, 528
Kurland, L. T., 309
Kurtines, W., 507
Kutash, K., 422, 525, 527
Kutcher, S. P., 406
Kvas, E., 369, 370, 372
Kviz, F. J., 383

Labruna, V., 333, 334, 335
Lacadie, C., 271
Lacey, J. H., 308, 309
Lachar, D., 23, 27, 270, 274
Lahey, B. B., 231, 233, 235, 236, 237, 265, 270, 485
Lahey, P., 182
Lambert, D., 527
Lampron, L. B., 238, 241, 243, 247
Landry, S. H., 130
Lange, A., 435
Langer, L., 307
Langer, W., 359
Langner, T., 63
Lann, I. S., 58
LaPadula, M., 296
Larcombe, I. J., 159
Larrieu, J. A., 342, 403
Larsen, S., 143, 161
Larson, K. A., 157
Lasso, B., 504
Last, C. G., 390, 398, 404, 405
Lauer, S. J., 159
Laufer, M., 265
Lauterbach, D., 333
Lavori, P. W., 405
Law, S. F., 284, 285
Lawlor, B. A., 92
Lawson, L., 335
Lazarus, A. A., 5
Leaf, P. J., 414, 419, 432, 443
Leavitt, L., 173
Leckman, J. F., 206, 207, 267, 286, 402
Leckman, J. R., 420
Lecours, A. R., 124
LeCouteur, A., 204, 208

Leddy, M., 173
Lee, J., 456
Lehman, B. K., 270
Lehr, E., 131
Leigh, J. W., 503
Lelon, E., 263, 270
Lenane, M. C., 407
Lengua, L. J., 234
Lenhart, L. A., 239
Leonard, B., 131
Leonard, H. L., 285, 402, 407, 482
Leonhardt, T., 358, 365, 370,
Lesser, J., 92
Levers, C. E., 159
Levin, H. S., 128
Lewinsohn, P. M., 413, 417, 422, 434, 435
Lewis, J. F., 127
Lewis, K. R., 92
Lewis, M., 86, 96, 101
Lewis, S. W., 158
Liao, S., 128
Liaw, F., 377
Libby, M. E., 77
Liberman, A. M., 271
Liebenauer, L. L., 269
Lieberman, A., 360, 378
Light, J. G., 156
Lilienfeld, A. M., 265
Lilienfeld, S. O., 236
Lin, K., 506
Linch, N. S., 217
Lind, D. L., 37
Lindberg, J. S., 77
Lindgreen, S., 287
Linnoila, M., 286
Linskey, A., 499
Liotta, W., 268, 269
Liotus, L., 340, 341
Lipovsky, J. S., 347
Little, C., 373
Little, S. N., 242
Littlewood, R., 505
Livingston, R., 335, 383, 384
Lloyd, C. W., 61
Locasreco, J. J., 217
Lochman, J. E., 231, 233, 234, 235, 238, 239, 241, 243, 244, 247, 248, 249, 252, 253, 254
Lock, J., 481
Locke, B. J., 190
Loeber, R., 231, 233, 234, 235, 236, 237, 239, 240
Logan, G. D., 283
Logan, W. T., 146
Loney, J., 265
Long, K., 370
Long, N., 239
Long, S., 331
Longshore, D., 506
Lonigan, C. J., 343
Lonnerholm, G., 159
Lonnqvist, J. K., 423
Looff, D., 340, 341
Looney, J. C., 518
Lord, C., 204, 206, 208
Louis, P. T., 130
Lourie, I., 487, 488, 524
Lovaas, O. I., 36, 215
Love, R. S., 194

Loveland, K. A., 92, 270
Lowe, T. L., 285, 339
Lu, S., 270
Luby, J. L., 360
Luby, S., 480
Lucas, A. R., 191, 309
Lund, D., 37, 55, 58, 59
Lurier, A., 479
Luscomb, R., 275
Lynam, D. R., 235, 236
Lynch, F., 284, 379

Maag, J. W., 7
Macari, S., 369, 370, 372
Macaulay, B. D., 37
MacDonald, A. W., 270
MacDuff, G. S., 78
Macfarlane, A., 158
MacFarlene, K., 331
MacKenzie, S., 406
MacLean, C., 307
MacLellan, J., 204, 208
Macro International, 517, 518, 528
Madan-Swain, A., 159
Madden, P. A. F., 269
Magder, L., 505
Magee, T. N., 231
Maggio, W. W., 269
Maheay, L., 191
Mahone, C. H., 190
Malgady, R. G., 507
Malloy, P., 283, 296
Malmquist, C. P., 338, 342
Maloney, M. J., 309
Malphus, J., 360
Mangweth, B., 310
Mannarino, A. P., 343, 344
Mannuza, S., 235, 283, 296
Manoukian, G., 340
Manson, S., 340
Marans, W. D., 203
March, J. S., 335, 339, 340, 341, 343, 403, 482
Marchione, K. E., 271
Marciano, P. L., 435, 436
Marcotte, A. C., 402
Margolis, R. L., 269
Maris, A., 270
Markowitz, J. C., 424, 432, 436
Markus, E., 435
Marriott, S. A., 251
Marsh, W. L., 267, 269, 285
Martin, A., 340, 341
Martin, J., 436
Martin, K. M., 128
Martin, M., 389, 481
Martindale, A., 52
Martinez, F., 508
Martini, D. R., 399, 401
Marttunen, M. J., 423
Maruish, M. E., 26, 28
Marx, L., 487, 488, 524
Marx, N., 63, 423
Mash, E. J., 45, 62, 66
Masse, L. C., 250
Masten, A. S., 158, 340
Masters, J., 379
Matson, J., 205, 208
Matson, J. J., 77
Matson, J. L., 194

Matthews, W. S., 346
Matthews, Z., 343
Matthey, G., 345
Mattis, G., 400
Mattson, A., 487, 488, 524
Matula, K., 63
Maumary-Gremaud, A., 238, 239
Mawhood, L., 208
Mayer, G. R., 36, 49, 53, 55
Mayes, L., 360, 366
Mayes, S. D., 275
Mayo, N. E., 127
Mayo, P., 348
Mazure, C., 457
McBurnett, K., 236, 265
McCandless, B., 457
McCarron, M., 92
McCarthy, D. A., 21, 127, 130
McCarthy, E. D., 63
McCarthy, J. J., 143
McClannahan, L. E., 78
McClaskey, C. L., 238
McClellan, J., 338, 339, 340, 342, 407
McConaughy, S. H., 101, 361
McCordie, W. R., 128
McCullough, E. L., 335, 341
McDevitt, S. C., 386
McDougle, C. J., 217, 218, 219
McDuff, P., 239
McFarlane, A. C., 340
McGee, R. O., 157, 237, 387, 390, 398
McGill, P., 78
McGlashan, T. H., 340
McGough, J. J., 269
McGuire, J., 309
McHorney, C., 335
McHugh, P. R., 91
McInnis, M. G., 269
McIntosh, J., 107
McKay, G. D., 280, 281
McKay, J. L., 281
McKeown, R. E., 333
McKinley, J. C., 23
McKnew, D. H., Jr., 414, 418, 423
McLeer, S. V., 335, 339, 341
McMahon, R. J., 416, 423
McMurray, M., 479, 480
McNally, R. J., 340
McTarish, D., 478
Meador, A. E., 61, 62, 65, 66
Meagher, S. E., 23
Mealer, C., 275
Medicine Net, 200
Mednick, S., 428
Meesters, C., 401
Meheady, L., 162
Meichenbaum, D. H., 161
Meier, S. T., 22, 27
Meisels, S., 377
Melander, H., 283
Mellits, E., 482
Melnyk, L., 270
Melton, G. B., 115, 526
Mencl, W. E., 271
Mendelson, M., 428
Mendoza, R., 506
Meninger, S. R., 386
Mennin, D., 270, 271

Mercer, C. D., 141, 143
Mercer, J. R., 127
Merikangas, K. R., 267, 420
Merkelbach, H., 401
Merrell, A. W., 175
Merrill, K. W., 157
Merzenick, M. M., 161
Mesibou, G. B., 194
Messer, S. C., 517, 518
Metevia, L., 275
Metz, C., 456
Meyer, B. L., 238
Meyer, G. J., 22
Meyer, R. G., 240, 241
Mezzich, A. C., 341
Mezzich, J., 503, 505
Michael, J., 37, 78
Mick, E., 263, 267, 270
Mickalide, A. D., 310
Middle, C., 158
Mikulich, S. K., 235
Milberger, S., 270
Miler, D. H., 158
Miller, B., 309
Miller, J., 172, 173, 175, 181, 182, 184
Miller, L. C., 65, 66
Miller, L. S., 457
Miller, M. N., 309
Miller, S. L., 161
Miller-Johnson, S., 235, 238, 239
Millon, T., 23
Millus, D., 495, 526
Milroy, T., 296
Milsap, P. A., 340
Miltenberger, R. G., 36, 45, 55, 61, 62, 63, 77, 78
Minde, K., 360
Minde, R., 360
Minderaa, R. B., 286
Miner, M. E., 128
Minuchin, S., 315, 494
Mirzai, H., 130
Mishkind, M. E., 310
Mitchell, C. B., 309
Mitchell, J. E., 322
Mittenberg, W., 131
Mitts, B., 53
Mock, J., 428
Moes, D., 215
Moffitt, T. E., 114, 157, 234, 235, 236, 237, 387
Moitra, S., 236
Montalvo, B., 507
Montgomery, I., 112
Montgomery, L., 495, 526
Moore, P., 270
Morales, A., 503
Moreau, D., 436, 506
Morgan, A. E., 265
Morgan, C., 22
Morgan, K., 360
Morgan, S., 205, 275
Morisset, C., 379
Moritz, G., 340, 341
Moroz, G., 407
Morrer, S. H., 283
Morris, R., 203
Morrison, J. R., 269
Morton, T., 431

Mosley, I. F., 158
Mosley-Howard, S., 365
Motes, P. S., 309, 526
Motese, M. J., 194
Moveci, P., 339
MTA Cooperative Group, 283, 288
Mufson, L., 436, 506
Muller, B., 436, 476
Mundy, E., 271
Munoz-Silva, D., 482
Murdoch, M., 478
Muris, P., 401
Murphy, D. L., 286
Murphy, H., 479
Murphy, J., 270
Murphy, M., 422, 435
Murray, H. A., 22
Murray, P. J. H., 479
Murray, R. M., 158
Mutluer, S., 130
Myles, B. S., 217, 219

Nace, D., 487, 488, 524
Nader, K. O., 331, 334, 339, 340, 342
Najarian, L. M., 340
Nakamura, C. Y., 61
Nasaki, G., 506
Nassar, M., 309
National Center for Children in Poverty, 451
National Center for Health Statistics Advance Report of Final Mortality Statistics, 413, 420
National Committee to Prevent Child Abuse, 450
National Joint Committee on Learning Disabilities, 140
National Mental Health Association, 423
Neale, M., 307
Nelson, D. S., 219
Nelson, F., 269
Nelson, J. C., 407
Nelson, N. W., 171, 175
Nelson, R. O., 7
Neuman, R. J., 269
Neumann, M. A., 420
New, E., 198
Newcomer, P., 180
Newcorn, J., 265, 270
Newland, T. E., 21
Newman, K. L., 310
Newsom, C. D., 42, 43
Newton, J. S., 63
Nezu, A. M., 93
Nezu, C. M., 93
Nguyen, N., 495
Nichols, M., 379
Nippold, M., 175
Nobel, H., 65
Nolan, E. E., 284, 285
Noll, M-B., 275
Norman, D., 270
Norris, F. H., 333
Northwood, A. K., 340
Norton, A. M., 270
Norton, H. J., 275
Noyes, R., 286
Nugent, S. M., 270

Nunez, F., 331, 334, 340, 342
Nurcombe, B., 115
Nussbaum, M. P., 312
Nuttall, E., 364
Nybro, C., 495, 526
Nylander, J., 309

Oakland, T., 19, 24
Oates, R. K., 343
Oberkloid, F., 155, 156
O'Brien, W., 33, 36, 45, 58, 62, 67, 76, 77
Obrzut, J. E., 24, 131
O'Donnell, D., 282, 283
O'Donohue , W. T., 343
O'Fallon, W. M., 309
Offord, D. R., 237, 389, 476
Oldershaw, L., 101
O'Leary, K. D., 33, 36, 37, 38, 41, 42, 47, 62
Olesniewicz, M. H., 131
Olivardia, R., 310
Ollendick, T. H., 19, 24, 26, 61, 62, 65, 66, 194, 389, 400, 405, 406
Olley, J. G., 211
Olswang, L. B., 182
Ommaya, A. K., 125
O'Neill, R. E., 63
Oppenheimer, R., 318
Oquendo, M., 507
Orbach, I., 421
Orenchuk-Tomiuk, N., 345
Ornitz, E. M., 193
Ort, S. I., 286
Orvaschel, H., 339, 389, 390, 398, 399, 401, 403
Osnes, P. G., 204
Osofsky, J. D., 368
O'Sullivan, M., 504
Otto, R., 453
Ouellette, C., 270
Overmeyer, S., 269
Owens, R. E., 170, 171

Pace, G. M., 42
Padian, N., 339
Padilla-Cotto, L., 501
Pagani, L., 239, 250
Pakiz, B., 333
Palali, I., 130
Palermo, D., 457
Palmer, C. G., 269
Palmer, R., 318
Panak, W. F., 236
Paniagua, F. A., 32, 38, 39, 41, 42, 43, 44, 45, 46, 47, 48, 49, 52, 55, 59, 60, 61, 68, 69, 70, 71, 72, 73, 74, 75, 76, 77, 78, 79
Panichelli-Mendel, S. M., 434
Papanicolaou, A. C., 269
Papineau, D., 433
Pardini, D., 231
Parent, A. D., 120, 130
Park, K. S., 265, 271
Parker, J. D. A., 335, 341
Parker, J. G., 157
Parker, K. C. H., 22
Parks, S., 205, 206
Parnas, J., 428

Parrone, P. L., 417
Parrott, M. C., 33, 35
Partlett, D. F., 115
Pasamanack, B., 265
Pataki, C., 482
Pate, J. E., 309, 319, 499
Paterson, R. F., 38, 55
Patros, P. G., 421, 422
Patterson, D. R., 284
Patterson, G. R., 234, 239, 247, 250, 280
Paul, R., 170, 171, 172, 173, 175, 176, 182
Paulson, A., 362, 365, 367
Pawl, J., 378
Pearson, D. A., 270
Pearson, P., 92
Pecora, P. J., 424
Pekarsky, J., 360
Pelcovitz, D., 333, 334, 335
Pelham, W., 479
Pelham, W. E., 284
Pelham, W. E., Jr., 270, 283
Pena, E., 182
Penick, E. C., 414, 418
Pennington, B. F., 155, 156
Perel, J., 506
Perez-Prado, E., 501
Perlman, T., 296
Perper, J. A., 340, 341
Perrin, J., 270
Perrin, S., 390, 398, 404
Perrine, J., 270
Perry, D. G., 238
Perry, L. C., 238
Perry, N. W., 108
Perry, P. J., 286
Perry, R., 482
Persky, V. W., 383
Personger, M. A., 334
Perwien, A., 478
Perwien, B. A., 384, 390, 396, 398, 400, 401, 406
Peskin, J. R., 420
Peterson, B. S., 283
Peterson, D. R., 25, 456
Peterson, E., 333
Pethick, S., 183
Petrila, J., 115
Petti, T., 515, 520, 528
Pettigrew, T. F., 435
Pettit, G. S., 238, 239, 253
Petty, T., 158
Pfeffer, C. R., 420, 422, 423, 468
Pfefferbaum, B., 476
Pfeiffer, S. I., 414, 422
Pfister, K., 267, 270
Phil, D., 312
Philips, S. U., 503
Phillips, J. S., 41
Pi, E., 487
Piacentini, J., 245, 457, 485
Pickels, A., 206
Pickering, A., 316
Pickles, A., 414
Pike, K. M., 61, 65, 323
Pinderhughes, E. E., 234
Pine, D. S., 405
Pinsof, W. M., 432, 435
Piodrowski, A. Z., 9

Piper, M. C., 127
Piven, J., 486
Plante, E., 175
Pliszka, S. R., 283, 286
Poertner, J., 520, 524
Poland, R., 506
Poling, A. G., 22, 271
Polissar, N. L., 128
Polivka, B., 527
Pomeroy, C., 322
Pope, H. G., 318
Pope, H. G., Jr., 310
Popper, C., 483, 484
Porjesz, B., 269
Portwood, S. G., 111
Potter, H., 191
Potter, W., 487, 506
Povlishock, J. T., 126
Powell, G. C., 331, 336
Powell, G. J., 503
Powell, J. W., 52, 131
Powell, L., 348
Power, T. J., 275
Powers, M. D., 202, 203, 204
Powers, P., 319
Poythress, N. G., 115
Poznanski, E. O., 428, 457
Prabucki, K., 456
Prasad, M., 130
Prather, E., 183
Price, L. H., 457, 486
Primeaux, S., 92
Prinz, R., 107
Prior, M., 155, 156
Prizant, B., 182
Pruitt, D. B., 340
Prusoff, B. A., 420
Pryzbeck, T., 236
Pudenz, R. H., 125
Pugh, K. R., 271
Puig-Antich, J., 25, 63, 339, 423, 456
Pumariega, A. J., 5, 47, 48, 163, 217, 218, 309, 319, 335, 341, 476, 487, 488, 495, 499, 503, 505, 508, 514, 518, 521, 524, 526, 527, 528
Pursell, J., 319
Purvis, K. L., 271
Pynoos, R. S., 331, 334, 339, 340, 341, 342, 343, 403

Quaskey, S., 482
Quay, H. C., 19, 25, 190, 193, 235, 236, 237, 387, 456
Quik, K., 212
Quinsey, V. L., 114
Quintero-Howard, C. V., 322
Quintero-Salinas, R., 499

Rabiner, D. L., 238
Racine, Y. A., 237
Radbill, S. X., 329, 330
Raeusim, G., 203
Rajapakse, J. C., 269
Ralphe, D. L., 335, 341
Ramsey, C., 269
Rank, B., 193
Rao, U., 339
Rapagna, S., 507

Rapee, R. M., 389, 405
Rapoport, C. S., 284
Rapoport, D., 4
Rapoport, J. L., 259, 282, 285, 286, 480, 482
Rapoport, M., 476
Rappley, M., 422
Rasmussen, S. A., 457
Rater, M., 265, 271
Rath, B., 338, 340
Rauch-Elnekave, H., 160
Readen, M., 286
Realmuto, G. M., 270, 340
Reeve, C., 211
Reeves, D. L., 131
Regier, D. A., 270, 413, 417, 485
Rehbar, M. H., 141
Reich, T., 269
Reich, W., 63, 269, 456, 485
Reichler, R. J., 195, 204, 208, 215
Reid, J. B., 234, 247
Reid, R., 263, 275
Reilly, J., 183
Reimherr, F. W., 286
Reinecke, M. A., 276
Reinherz, H. Z., 333, 517
Reising, D., 285
Reiss, A., 286
Reiss, S., 93
Reitan, R. M., 126
Remschmidt, H., 481
Renner, B., 195, 204, 208
Renshaw, P. P., 269
Resnick, H. S., 333
Rey, J., 483
Reynolds, C. R., 25, 26, 141, 242, 245, 274
Reynolds, R., 237
Reynolds, W. M., 414, 428, 434
Reznick, J. S., 386
Reznick, S., 183
Ribera, J., 503
Riccio, C. A., 265, 275, 276
Rice, M. E., 114
Rich, W. D., 157
Richardson, D., 340, 341
Richert, W., 126
Richman, G. S., 42
Richman, N., 63
Riddle, M. A., 285, 286, 407, 457, 482, 505
Rifkin, L., 158
Riggs, S., 335
Rigsby, M., 526
Rimland, B., 193, 195, 204, 208
Rimm, D., 379
Rios, P., 204, 208
Risley, T. R., 38, 40, 43, 47, 55, 58
Rispens, J., 275
Risser, A., 124
Ritchie, G. F., 267, 285
Ritvo, A., 204, 208
Ritvo, E., 204, 208
Ritvo, F., 193
Ritvo, R., 190, 195
Rivara, J. B., 128
Rivera, V. R., 422, 525, 527
Rivers-Buckeley, N., 476
Rizzuto, M., 312, 313, 315
Roache, J. D., 270

Robbins, D. R., 399
Robbins, J. P., 340
Robbins, M., 477
Roberts, W. O., 131
Robertson, J., 360
Robertson, S. B., 160, 204, 208
Robins, L. N., 235, 236, 413, 417
Robinson, E., 322
Rock, A., 119
Rodger, R., 206
Rodgers, A., 431
Rodin, G., 319
Rodin, J., 310
Rodriquez, N., 340
Roebuck, T. M., 270
Rogers, A., 286
Rogers, K., 495, 526
Rogers, M., 265
Rogers, R., 16, 100
Rogers-Adkinson, D., 275
Rogers-Warren, A., 47, 78
Rogler, L. H., 499, 507
Rohde, P., 417, 435
Rojahn, J., 93
Rolls, B. F., 310
Romero, A., 503
Romero, I., 364
Romero, J., 508
Romm, S., 23
Rorschach, H., 22
Rorty, M., 316, 318
Rosello, J., 506
Rosenbaum, J. F., 386
Rosenberg, D., 479, 486
Rosenberg, L., 482
Rosenberg, M. B., 191
Rosenblatt, A., 269
Rosman, B., 315
Ross, C. A., 269
Ross, C. M., 276
Rossotto, E., 316, 318
Rotter, K. F., 144
Rotzberg, R. H., 142
Rouse, T. M., 119
Rowane, W., 481
Rowe, K. J., 272, 287
Rowe, K. S., 272, 287
Rowland, M. D., 414, 526
Roy, I., 507
Rubia, K., 269
Rubin, J., 365
Rubin, K. H., 346
Rubio-Stipec, M., 389, 390, 503, 519
Rudorfer, M., 487, 506
Rue, D., 338, 339, 340, 342
Rumer, R., 254
Runyon, D. K., 344
Rupp, A., 413
Rush, A. J., 434, 521
Russell, G. F. M., 308, 309, 310, 311
Russell, R. L., 265, 271
Russell, W. R., 125
Russo, D. C., 48
Russo, M. F., 237
Russo, M. J., 335
Rutman, J., 414, 418
Ruttenberg, B., 204, 205, 208
Rutter, M. L., 58, 196, 197, 204, 206, 208, 265, 368, 414, 417, 424, 485, 518

Ryan, N., 339, 476, 477

Sabatino, D. A., 429, 431
Sacco, D., 506
Sack, W. H., 338, 340
Sadock, R., 190
Saeed, M. A., 46, 61, 75, 76
Saenz, J., 508
Safer, D. J., 284, 379, 505
Saigh, P., 340
Sainato, D., 162
Sakai, J., 269
Salazar, A., 131
Salle, F., 476, 477
Sallec, F. R., 343
Saltz, P., 66
Salvendy, J., 507
Samoilov, A., 436
Sampen, S. E., 55
Samuel-Aikerman, M., 146
Sanchez, M., 508
Sandman, C., 482, 483
Sandra, F., 209
Sanson, A., 155, 156
Santiago Rivera, A., 504
Santos, C. W., 270
Sarfatti, S. E., 269
Saslow, G., 6
Satterfield, J. H., 235
Sattler, J. C., 202
Sattler, J. M., 4, 5, 20, 21, 25, 26, 27, 88, 145, 146
Saunders, B. E., 333
Saxe, L., 431
Sayegh, L., 433
Scahill, L., 267, 402, 407, 457
Schachar, R. J., 270, 283, 284, 285
Schacht, T. E., 104
Schafer, R., 4
Schaffer, D., 389, 397
Schanberg, S., 360
Scheer, P., 369, 370, 372
Scheeringa, M. S., 342, 403
Schell, A., 235
Scherer, W. M., 61
Schetky, D. H., 98
Schilz, C., 481
Schlacht, T., 526
Schlinger, H. D., 22
Schneider, B., 131
Schoenfeld, W. N., 78
Schoenwald, S. K., 414, 526
Schopler, E., 194, 195, 204, 205, 208, 211, 215
Schreiner, C., 161
Schroth, P., 204, 206, 208
Schubert, A. B., 269
Schulberg, H., 506
Schulz, E., 481
Schumacher, E., 286
Schumacher, S., 61
Schupak-Neuberg, K., 309
Schwab-Stone, M. E., 245, 267, 270, 423, 485
Schwartz, D., 309
Scopetta, M. A., 497
Scott, J., 174
Sease, F., 526
Sechrest, L., 56, 57

Secord, W. A., 180
Sedlack, A. J., 332, 333
Seeley, J. R., 417, 422, 435
Seeman, M., 503
Seidman, L. J., 270
Selzak, J. A., 383
Semel, E., 180
Semrud-Clikeman, M., 269
Sevin, B., 205, 207
Sevin, J. A., 194, 205, 207
Sexson, S. B., 160
Sgroi, S. M., 345
Shaffer, D., 236, 245, 421, 485, 486, 519
Shamoo, T. K., 421, 422
Shandle, M., 527
Shankweiler, D. P., 271
Shannon, M. P., 343
Shapiro, T., 198, 384, 388, 484
Share, D. L., 157
Sharp, W. S., 267
Shaw, C. R., 191
Shaw, D., 237
Shaw, H. E., 309
Shaywitz, B. A., 271, 272, 285
Shaywitz, S. E., 271, 272
Shee, S. M., 53
Sheeber, L. B., 422, 435
Sheldon, C. H., 125
Shelton, R. C., 435
Shelton, T. L., 275
Shenker, I. R., 312
Shenker, R., 235
Sheridan, D., 495, 524
Shuman, D. W., 99
Shunfield, L., 340, 341
Shurtleff, H. A., 128
Siassi, I., 63, 67
Sickmund, M., 451
Siefker, C. A., 420
Siegel, C. H., 342
Siegel, L. S., 276
Siegel, T. C., 252, 254
Siegel, Z., 198
Silberstein, L. R., 310
Silva, P. A., 157, 387, 390, 398
Silva, R., 482
Silver, H. K., 331
Silver, S., 514
Silver, S. E., 413
Silverman, A. B., 333
Silverman, F. M., 331
Silverman, J. A., 310
Silverman, N., 431
Silverman, W. P., 92
Silverthorn, P., 237, 396
Simeon, J. G., 406
Simmons, A., 269
Simmons, W., 526
Simon, R. I., 98
Simos, P. D., 269
Simpson, G., 482
Simpson, R. L., 217, 219
Sindelar, P. J., 191
Singer, H., 482
Singer, M. I., 340, 507
Singh, N. N., 93
Siqueland, L., 389
Skinner, B. F., 33, 34, 35, 36, 37, 38, 42, 43, 44

Skudlarski, P., 271
Sleator, E. K., 282
Slifer, K. J., 42
Sloane, H. N., 37, 55
Slobogin, C., 115
Sloper, T., 159
Small, A. M., 217
Smalley, S. L., 269
Smallish, L., 478, 479
Smart, D., 155, 156
Smit, A. B., 171
Smith, B., 56
Smith, M. G., 341, 506
Smith, S. M., 328, 329, 330
Snell, J. W., 269
Snidman, N., 386
Snow, M. E., 198
Snowden, L., 495
Snyder, H., 451
Sobelewski, J., 526
Sodersten, P., 308
Solomons, G., 265
Sondheimer, D. L., 414
Song, L., 340
Sontag, S., 308
Soriano, J., 267, 270
Spaccarelli, S., 335
Sparrow, S. S., 93, 184, 203, 206, 207
Spear, R., 161
Specker, B., 309
Spence, D. P., 100
Spencer, T. J., 269, 270, 281, 282, 283, 285, 286
Spiegel, J., 495, 496
Spieker, S., 379
Spielberger, C., 486
Spitz, R. A., 387, 388, 416
Spitzen, R., 485
Spitzer, R. L., 198, 456
Spock, A., 319
Spradley, J., 503
Sprafkin, J., 284, 285
Sprague, J. R., 63
Sprague, R. L., 265, 282, 285
Spreen, O., 124
Sprich, S., 270
Spurlock, J., 494, 507
Sramek, J., 487
Staghezza, B. M., 431, 432, 519
Stallings, P., 341
Stange, D., 431
Stark, K. D., 434, 435
Steele, B. F., 331
Steele, J. J., 406
Steer, R. A., 246
Stein, C. L., 63, 64, 65, 66
Stein, M. A., 269, 276
Stein, R. I., 309
Steinberg, A. M., 331, 334, 340, 341, 342
Steinberg, L., 389
Steinberg, Z., 422, 424
Steiner, H., 343, 481
Steingard, R. J., 269, 285, 286, 390
Steketee, G., 506
Sterges, J., 284
Sterling, J., 214
Sternberg, R. J., 161
Stevenson, J., 269, 286

Stewart, A. L., 158
Stewart, A. W., 93
Stewart, M. A., 269
Stice, E., 309
Still, G. F., 264
Stoel-Gammon, C., 182
Stokes, T. T., 204
Stone, W., 208
Stoner, G., 271, 272
Storey, K., 63
Storoschuck, S., 206
Stouthamer-Loeber, M., 233, 239, 240
Strasburger, L. H., 99, 115
Strauss, C. C., 390, 398
Strauss, M. A., 239
Strauss, R. S., 158
Straw, M., 53
Strayer, J., 238
Streiner, D., 209
Striegel-Moore, R. H., 310
Strong, R., 286
Stroul, B. A., 516, 520
Strzelecki, S., 414, 422
Stuebing, K. K., 271
Stumbo, P., 287
Sue, D. W., 498
Sullivan, J. M., 341
Sullivan, J. S., 128, 129
Sullivan, K., 335, 341
Sullivan, L., 414, 418
Sullivan, P., 307, 316
Sulzer-Azaroff, B., 36, 49, 53, 55
Summit, R. C., 331
Sunday, S. R., 318
Suomi, S. J., 386
Sutton-Smith, B., 343
Sverd, J., 284, 285
Swaab, H., 275
Swanson, H. L., 161
Swanson, J. M., 286, 480, 482, 499
Swedo, S. E., 402, 407
Sweeney, J. A., 7
Swerling, L., 161
Swettenham, J., 217
Szapocznik, J., 497, 507
Szatmari, P., 209
Szczepanski, R. G., 233, 234
Szymanski, L., 112

Tabriz, M. A., 339
Tager-Flusberg, H., 174
Tallal, P., 161
Talley, W., 507
Tam, D., 131
Tamm, L., 270
Tanguay, P., 209
Tannenbaum, L. E., 231, 233
Tannhouser, M. T., 142
Tannock, R., 263, 270, 271, 283
Tantam, D., 193
Tarter, R. E., 270
Tasse, M. J., 93
Taube, C., 514
Tavosian, A., 340
Taylor, C. B., 6
Taylor, C. M., 343
Taylor, E., 193, 269
Taylor, H. G., 66
Teal, M., 205, 207

Teicher, M. H., 341
Tellegen, A., 23, 428
Temple, E. P., 275
Tennenbaum, D. L., 65
Teplin, S. W., 159
Terdal, L. G., 45, 62, 66
Terr, L. C., 328, 331, 334, 336, 341, 343, 344, 346
Terry, R., 233, 234, 235, 238, 239
Thal, D., 183
Thatcher, R., 131
Thomas, A., 365, 385, 386, 419
Thomas, D., 112
Thomas, J. D., 53
Thomas, J. M., 360
Thomas, K. R., 131
Thompson, M., 309
Thompson, S., 483
Thorndike, R. L., 21
Thornell, A., 267, 270
Thuras, P., 267
Thurber, D., 487, 488, 524
Tibbs, R. E., 120, 130
Tidmarsh, L., 360
Tillman, W., 497
Timko, C., 310
Tipp, J., 236
Tischler, K. J., 414, 419
Tobin, A., 183
Todd, R. D., 269
Torbet, P., 112
Torres, J., 508
Townsend, J. P., 158
Tremblay, R. E., 236, 239, 250
Tremble, M., 193
Trott, G., 481
Troyer, R., 237
Trubnick, L., 484
Tsuang, M. T., 233, 270, 390
Tucker, D. M., 402
Tuma, A. H., 58
Tuma, J., 433, 514
Tuokko, H., 124
Tupper, D., 124
Turbolt, S. H., 93
Turell, S., 309
Turkington, C., 421
Turner, S. M., 386, 387
Tweed, D., 431
Twitchell, T. E., 124
Tyler, L., 237
Tyriell, J., 92

Udea, D., 480
Udwin, O., 340
Ullmann, L. P., 37
Ulrich, R. F., 265, 457, 503, 505
Unis, A. S., 254
U.S. Advisory Board on Child Abuse and Neglect, 332
U.S. Bureau of the Census, 494
U.S. Department of Education, 141
U.S. Department of Health and Human Services, 332, 333
U.S. Government, 513
U.S. Office of the Surgeon General, 508
U.S. Public Health Service, 450, 451
U.S. Surgeon General, 528

Vaituzis, A. C., 269
Valenti-Hein, D., 93
Valeri, S. M., 528
Vance, H. B., 5, 16, 163, 216, 217, 218, 429, 521
VanDenBerg, J. E., 520
van den Oord, E. J. C. G., 275
Vander Stoep, A., 451
van Engeland, H., 275
VanHorn, P., 360
Van Horn, Y., 231, 233
Vargas, L., 503, 507
Varley, C. K., 407
Vaughn, S., 157
Vauss, Y. C., 269
Vega, R., 159
Verda, M., 286
Verhegge, R., 309
Verhulst, F. C., 24, 405
Vermeer, A., 127
Versluis-den Bieman, H., 405
Vinson, B. P., 176
Vissing, Y. M., 239
Vitaro, F., 236, 239, 250
Vitiello, B., 284
Vitousek, K., 323
Vojvoda, D., 340
Volkmar, F. R., 192, 193, 203, 206, 207, 219
Vollero, H., 130
Vollmer, T. R., 58, 77
von Knorring, A., 283
Vrana, S., 333

Wadden, N., 206
Wagner, E. E., 248
Walco, G. A., 159
Waldman, I., 236
Walker, H. M., 55
Walkup, J. T., 286
Wallen, J., 335, 341
Waller, G., 318
Waller, J. L., 333, 495
Wallerstein, J. S., 417
Walsh, B. T., 285, 310
Walter, J. M., 267
Walters, E., 307, 319
Ward, C. H., 428
Wargo, J. B., 238
Warheit, G., 307
Warnke, A., 481
Warshaw, M., 310
Wassell, J. T., 420
Waterman, J., 331
Waters, E., 388
Watkins, J., 209
Watkins, R., 173
Wayland, K. K., 234, 238
Weaver, A., 269
Weber, W., 265, 267, 270, 271
Webster-Stratton, C., 250, 252
Wechsler, D., 21, 275, 276
Wechsler, R. D., 246
Weibley, R., 477
Weiffenbach, B., 269, 270
Weigand, D., 487, 488
Weinberg, W. A., 414, 418, 521
Weine, S., 340
Weiner, I. B., 4, 22
Weiner, Z., 485

Weiss, B., 431
Weiss, G., 296
Weissberg, R. P., 250
Weissbourd, B., 379
Weissman, M. M., 339, 414, 419, 420, 424, 432, 436, 506
Weist, M., 526
Weisz, J. R., 280, 431, 528
Wellage, L. C., 159
Wellen, E., 286
Wellen, R. A., 286
Wells, K. C., 239, 248, 249, 486
Weltzin, T. E., 318
Wenar, C., 204, 205, 208
Wender, E., 287
Wendon, P. H., 286
Werry, J. S., 19, 190, 191, 193, 265, 285, 390, 481, 482, 489, 490
Wetherby, A., 182
Wetzler, S., 3, 6, 7
Wheless, J. W., 269
Whidby, J. M., 241, 243, 244, 247, 253, 254
White, K. J., 238, 254
White, K. K., 238
Wickramaratne, P., 436
Wicks, J., 245
Wiebe, M., 205, 207
Wiegand, D., 524
Wiig, E. H., 180
Wilcox, L. E., 457
Wilens, T. E., 267, 269, 270, 281, 282, 283, 285, 286
Wilkes, T. C. R., 434
Wilkinson, C., 494
Williams, C., 428
Williams, C. D., 37
Williams, C. L., 23
Williams, K., 506
Williams, L. M., 331, 334, 335, 480
Williams, O. B., 28
Williams, S. C., 157, 237, 269, 390, 398
Williams, T. A., 9
Williamson, D., 339
Williard, J. C., 238
Willis, D. J., 26, 27
Willmore, L. J., 269
Wilson, F., 209
Wilson, G. T., 33, 36, 37, 38, 41, 42, 47, 61, 62, 65, 323
Wilson, L., 499, 500, 501
Wilson, R., 191
Wing, L., 193, 194
Winn, H. R., 128
Winsberg, B. G., 269
Winters, N., 487, 488, 524
Wisniewski, K. E., 92
Wolf, E., 205
Wolf, K. M., 416
Wolf, M. M., 38, 40, 43, 55, 56, 58
Wolfe, D. A., 340
Wolfe, V. V., 340
Wolff, P. L., 386
Wolpe, J., 41
Wolraich, M., 287
Wong, M., 486
Woodbury, M., 503
Woodward, J. A., 269
Woodward, M., 23

Woodworth, R. S., 22
Wozniak, J., 271
Wraith, R., 341
Wright, H., 358, 365, 370
Wright, M. O., 158
Wright, V., 285
Wrightsman, L. S., 108
Wunder, J., 405
Wyatt, G. C., 331, 336

Yager, J., 316, 318
Yager, T. J., 519
Yakolev, P. E., 124
Yamamoto, J., 503
Yancey, A., 507
Yates, A., 319, 335
Yehuda, R., 340

Yoder, D., 181
Yoe, J., 528
Yokota, A., 204, 208
Yoshimura, I., 270
Young, A. R., 140, 145, 146, 155, 156, 157, 163
Young, J. Z., 120
Young, S. E., 235
Yperen, T., 275
Ysseldyke, J. E., 139, 140, 143, 144
Yule, W., 27, 340
Yunginger, J. W., 383

Zakriski, A., 234
Zametkin, A. J., 268, 269, 284, 285, 286
Zeanah, C. H., 342, 403

Zelberger, J., 55
Zemcov, A., 126
Zero to Three, 364, 369
Zhang, H., 267
Zhang, Q., 233, 237, 239
Zimmerman, J., 157
Zimmerman, M., 307
Zimnitzky, B., 483, 484
Zinkin, B., 65
Zinn, H., 424, 432
Zito, J. M., 284, 379, 505
Zoccolillo, M. S., 233, 235
Zouridakis, G., 269
Zupan, B. A., 66

Subject Index

ABC. *See* Autism Behavior Checklist
ABC model, 38
  textbooks on, 41–42
Aberrant Behavior Checklist, 93
ABS. *See* Adaptive Behavior Scale, case study
Abuse:
  assessment of, 338–341
  case study, 348–349, 350
  causes of, 333–334
  definitional issues of, 331–332
  diagnostic interviews and, 339–340
  epidemiology of, 332–333
  by gender, 333
  impact of, 334–338
  by race, 332
  sexual, case study, 440
  symptom checklists for, 339–340
  treatment phases of, 344–348
ACTRS. *See* Conners Rating Scales
Acute Disintegrative Disorder, psychopharmacology and, 482
Acute lymphocytic leukemia (ALL), 158–159
Acute Stress Disorder, 461–462
Adaptive Behavior Scale, case study, 222
Adderall:
  Attention-Deficit/Hyperactivity Disorder and, 479
  See also Pemoline
ADHD. *See* Attention-Deficit/Hyperactivity Disorder
ADI. *See* Autism Diagnostic Interview
Adjustment Disorder, infant mental health and, 372
Adolescent Transitions Program, 251
ADOS. *See* Autism Diagnostic Observation Schedule
Affect, defined, 416
Affective disorder, defined, 416
Agoraphobia, 393
Alberta Infant Motor Scale, motor functioning and, 127
Alcohol Dependence, mood disorders and, 417–418
Alpha, defined, 58

Alprazolam, anxiety disorders and, 478
American Academy of Child and Adolescent Psychiatrists, 6
American Association of Mental Deficiency, 77
  Adaptive Behavior Scale, description of, 64
American Psychological Association Ethics Committee, 106
Amitriptyline:
  case study, 440
  depression and, 476
  eating disorders and, 481
Amoxapine, depression and, 476
Anafranil, eating disorders and, 322–323
Anger Control Training, 250–251
Anger Coping Program, 247–248, 253–255
Anorexia Nervosa:
  behavioral assessment of, 61
  case study, 319–320
  diagnosis and formulation of, 314–316
  historical perspectives on, 308
l'anorexie hystérique, 310
Antidepressants:
  eating disorders and, 322–323
  nontricyclic
    Attention-Deficit/Hyperactivity Disorder and, 286
  serotonergic, 521
  tricyclic (TCAs)
    anxiety disorders and, 405–406
    Attention-Deficit/Hyperactivity Disorder and, 285
    depression and, 476
    eating disorders and, 322–323, 481
    side effects of, 476–477
    sleep disturbance and, 484
    social/emotional maladjustment and, 467
Antisocial Personality Disorder (APD), 234, 241
  Attention-Deficit/Hyperactivity Disorder and, 270, 296
  callous-unemotional traits and, 237
Anxiety Disorders:
  behavioral treatment of, 405–406
  case study, 403–404

  comorbidity, 390
  course and outcome of, 404–405
  definition of, 383–384
  epidemiology of, 389–390
  ethological development of, 387–388
  genetic field theory and, 388
  historical perspectives of, 384–385
  indirect behavioral assessment of, 66
  infant mental health and, 372
  pharmacological treatment of, 406–407
  psychoanalytic perspectives of, 384–385
  psychological factors and, 389
  psychopharmacology and, 477–478
  social/emotional maladjustment and, 461–462
  temperament and, 385–386
Anxiety Disorders Interview Schedule for Children, 397
Anxiety Rating for Children (revised), 397
AOBC model, 38–39
  textbooks on, 41–42
Applied Behavior Analysis, 37
Arachnoid layer, defined, 123
Art therapy, abuse/trauma and, 346
ASIEP-2. *See* Autism Screening Instrument for Educational Planning (2nd edition)
Asperger's Disorder:
  vs. Autistic Disorder, 208–209
  characteristics of, 192–193, 200–201
  Pervasive Developmental Disorders and, 198
  psychopharmacology and, 482
Assessment:
  behavioral approaches to, 24–26
  computer-assisted, 9–10
  historical review of, 20–26
  intellectual, 20–22
  objective personality, 22–24
  parameters of, 3–4
  projective personality, 22
  psychological, current and future status of, 26–28
  recent developments in, 6–7
  traditional vs. new approaches to, 4–6
Atarax. *See* Hydroxyzine

Attention-Deficit/Hyperactivity
    Disorder:
  anxiety disorders and, 387
  assessment of, 6, 338–339
  behavioral assessment of, 45,
      46–47
  behavioral clinical case formula-
      tion and, 67
  with Behavioral Disturbance and
      Learning Disability, case
      study, 290–293
  case study, 68–71, 148–154,
      441–442, 522
  clinical assessment of, 272–275
  combined multimodal treatment
      of, 287–288
  comorbidity, 270–272
  Cruickshank's work on, 142
  current concepts of, 266–270
  depression and, 422–423
  diagnostic criteria for, 266
  Disruptive Behavior Disorders
      and, 235
  dynamic psychotherapy and,
      438–439
  gender-related differences in,
      263, 267
  genetic studies of, 269–270
  history of the diagnosis of,
      264–265
  indirect behavioral assessment of,
      66
  indirect measures using the Ab-
      breviated Conners Teacher
      Rating Scale of, 73–75
  infant mental health and, 372
  learning disabilities and, 145,
      156, 422–423
  with Mental Retardation, case
      study, 293–295
  Mental Status Exam and, 94–96
  neuropsychological tests and,
      275–276
  with Oppositional Defiant Disor-
      der, case example, 288–290
  outcomes in adolescence, 296
  outcomes in adulthood, 296
  Posttraumatic Stress Disorder
      and, 341
  psychopharmacology and,
      281–287, 478–480
  psychosocial treatment for,
      279–281
  rating scales and, 274–275, 277
  serious emotional disturbances
      and, 517
  social/emotional maladjustment
      and, 455
  Specific Learning Disabilities
      and, 271–272
  Student Behavior Survey and, 24
  systems of care and, 521
  target behavior and, 47
  treatment considerations in
      school settings, 278–279
  treatment planning of, 276–281
Atypical Pervasive Developmental
    Disorder, 197–198
Australian Temperament Project,
    155

Autism, as a term, 192
Autism Behavior Checklist,
    206–207
  case study, 223
Autism Diagnostic Interview, 206
Autism Diagnostic Observation
    Schedule, 205–206
Autism Screening Instrument for
    Educational Planning (2nd
    edition), 205
  case study, 222–223
Autism Society of America,
    195–196
Autistic Disorder, 189–192
  active-but-odd group, 195
  aloof group, 194
  vs. Asperger's Disorder, 208–
      209
  communication profiles of chil-
      dren with, 175
  communicative disorders and,
      173–174
  conceptual considerations of,
      193–195
  current definitions of, 195–199
  history of, 190–192
  vs. Mental Retardation, 210
  Mental Status Exam and, 92
  passive group, 194
  prevalence of, 190
  psychopharmacology and, 482
  vs. schizophrenia, 209–210
  specific scales for, 204–208
  teaching students with, 212–
      213
Autistic Research Institute, 218
Automatic reinforcer, defined, 36
Avoidance, defined, 35
Avoidant Disorder, 396
Axon, defined, 120

Basal ganglia, defined, 122
BASC. See Behavior Assessment
    System for Children
Baseline behaviors, defined, 202
Basic Achievement Skills Included,
    learning disorder and, 147
Battered Child Syndrome, 331
Bayley Motor Scale, closed head in-
    jury and, 128
Bayley Scales of Infant Develop-
    ment, 21
  child abuse and, 130
  communicative disorders and,
      177
  description of, 63
  limits of diagnosis based on, 77
  motor functioning and, 127
  purpose of, 367
Beck Depression Inventory, 7
  social/emotional maladjustment
      and, 456
Behavioral assessment:
  comprehensive, 45–61
    indirect vs. direct measure-
      ments of, 55–58
  defined, 32–33
  vs. functional analysis, 42–43
  history of, 43–45
  indirect, 61

Behavioral Assessment System for
    Children:
  Attention-Deficit/Hyperactivity
      Disorder and, 274
  case study, 245–246
  mood disorders and, 428–429
  Parent Rating Scale, case study,
      288–289, 291
  Teacher Rating Scale, case study,
      288–289, 291
Behavioral clinical case formula-
    tion, components of, 67–68
Behavioral disorders, treatment of,
    3–4
Behavioral inhibition, 386–387
Behavioral psychologists, defined, 32
Behavioral Screening Question-
    naire, description of, 63
Behavior analysis, applied, dimen-
    sions of, 39–40
Behavior analysts, defined, 32
Behavior assessment, current trends
    in, 76–78
Behavior Assessment System for
    Children, 25
  Disruptive Behavior Disorders
      and, 242
Behavior Disorders Identification
    Scale (home version),
    151–152
Behavior Modification, 37
Behavior Observation Scale, 206
Behavior Problem Checklist (re-
    vised), 57
  revised, 25
  social/emotional maladjustment
      and, 455–456
Behavior Rating Instrument for
    Autistic and Other Atypical
    Children (2nd edition), 205
Behavior Ruling Profile, learning
    disorder and, 147
Behavior therapists, defined, 32
Benadryl. See Diphenhydramine
Bender Visual Motor Gestalt Test, 4
  learning disorder and, 147
Benton Facial Recognition Test,
    learning disorder and, 147
Benton Judgment of Line Orienta-
    tion, learning disorder and,
    147
Benzedrine, Attention-Deficit/
    Hyperactivity Disorder
    and, 282
Benzodiazepine, anxiety disorders
    and, 406–407, 477–478
Berry Test of Visual Motor Integra-
    tion, learning disorder and,
    147
Binet, Alfred, 20
Binet-Simon Scale, 20–21
Bipolar Disorder:
  assessment of, 338–339
  Attention-Deficit/Hyperactivity
      Disorder and, 270, 271
  diagnosis of, 425–426
  psychopharmacology and, 480
Blind Learning Aptitude Test, 21
BOS. See Behavior Observation
    Scale

BOTMP. *See* Bruininks-Oseretsky Test of Motor Proficiency
Brain injury:
case study, 132–133
child abuse, 130–131
mechanisms of, 125–126
methods of intervention in, 132
motor impairments associated with, 127–129
psychological consequences of, 131–132
sports injuries and, 131
BRIAAC-2. *See* Behavior Rating Instrument for Autistic and Other Atypical Children (2nd edition)
British Working Party, 195
Brown Attention-Deficit Disorder Scale, learning disorder and, 147
Brown v. Board of Education, 104
Bruch, Hilda, 310–311
Bruininks-Oseretsky Test of Motor Proficiency:
brain injury and, 129
motor functioning and, 127
Bulimia Nervosa:
behavioral assessment of, 61
case study, 320
chronic, case study, 320
diagnosis and formulation of, 316–317
historical perspectives on, 308–309
Bupropion:
Attention-Deficit/Hyperactivity Disorder and, 286, 480
depression and, 477
social/emotional maladjustment and, 467
Buspirone, anxiety disorders and, 407, 477–478

CAFAS. *See* Child and Adolescent Functional Assessment Scale
California Psychological Inventory, 9
Callous-unemotional (CU) traits, 236–237
CAPA. *See* Child and Adolescent Psychiatric Assessment
CAPS-C. *See* Clinician-Administered PTSD Scale (child and adolescent version)
Carbamazepine:
Bipolar Disorder and, 480
eating disorders and, 481
Posttraumatic Stress Disorder and, 345
self-injurious behaviors and, 483
social/emotional maladjustment and, 467–468
CARS. *See* Childhood Autism Rating Scale
Catapres. *See* Clonidine
Cattell, James M., 20
Cattell Culture Fair Intelligence Tests, description of, 63

Caudate nucleus:
Attention-Deficit/Hyperactivity Disorder and, 269
defined, 122
CBCL. *See* Child Behavior Checklist
CDI. *See* Children's Depression Inventory; Communicative Development Inventory
Celexa, depression and, 477
Cell body, defined, 120
Center for Mental Health Services, 508, 513
Cerebellum, defined, 123
CGAS. *See* Children's Global Assessment Scale
Child Abuse, Prevention, Adoption, and Family Services Act (1988), 332
Child and Adolescent Functional Assessment Scale:
case study, 288–289, 291
psychopharmacology and, 486
serious emotional disturbances and, 519–520
Child and Adolescent Psychiatric Assessment:
Infant-Toddler Social and Emotional Assessment, 373
Child and Adolescent Service System Program (CASSP), 516–517
social/emotional maladjustment and, 453
Child and Adolescent Symptom Inventory, learning disorder and, 147
Child Assessment Schedule, Disruptive Behavior Disorders and, 242
Child Behavior Checklist, 25, 56–58, 93
anxiety disorders and, 397
Attention-Deficit/Hyperactivity Disorder and, 274
behavioral assessment and, 45
case study, 222, 245–246, 294–295, 403
description of, 65
Disruptive Behavior Disorders and, 242
learning disorder and, 147
Posttraumatic Stress Disorder and, 339
psychopharmacology and, 486
purpose of, 367
serious emotional disturbances and, 519
social/emotional maladjustment and, 455
Child custody, 106–108
Child Development Project, 360
Childhood Abuse Prevention and Treatment Act (1974), 359
Childhood Autism Rating Scale, 204–205
Childhood Depression Inventory, 9
Childhood Disintegrated Disorder, 198, 200
Childhood Onset Pervasive Devel-

opmental Disorder (COPDD), 196–198
Childhood PTSD Interview (child form), 339
Childhood PTSD Reaction Index, 340
Childhood schizophrenia, 209
Child PTSD Symptom Scale, 340
Children Apperception Test, 4
Children's Depression Inventory:
description of, 65
functional assessment and, 68
Posttraumatic Stress Disorder and, 341
psychopharmacology and, 486
social/emotional maladjustment and, 456
Children's Depression Rating Scale, social/emotional maladjustment and, 456
Children's Global Assessment Scale
psychopharmacology and, 486
serious emotional disturbances and, 519
Children's Impact of Event Scale, Posttraumatic Stress Disorder and, 340
Children's Manifest Anxiety Scale:
anxiety disorders and, 397
social/emotional maladjustment and, 456
Children's Memory Scale, learning disorder and, 147
Children's PTSD Inventory, 340
Children's Services Program. *See* Comprehensive Community Mental Health Services for Children and Their Families Program
Child Schedule for Affective Disorders and Schizophrenia, social/emotional maladjustment and, 456
Child Screening Inventory, description of, 63
Chlorpromazine:
Attention-Deficit/Hyperactivity Disorder and, 286
schizophrenia and, 481
Chronic lung disease (CLD), 158–159
Citalpram, depression and, 477
Clinical Evaluation of Language Fundamentals (3rd edition), 179, 180
Clinician-Administered PTSD Scale (child and adolescent version):
Posttraumatic Stress Disorder and, 339
Clomipramine, anxiety disorders and, 407
Clonazepam:
anxiety disorders and, 478
Bipolar Disorder and, 480
Clonidine:
Attention-Deficit/Hyperactivity Disorder and, 286–287, 480

Clonidine (*continued*)
  Posttraumatic Stress Disorder
    and, 345
  social/emotional maladjustment
    and, 467
  Tourette's Disorder and, 482
Closed head injury (CHI), 128
Clozapine, schizophrenia and, 481
Cocaine Dependence, mood disorders and, 417
Cognitive-behavioral therapy:
  abuse/trauma and, 347
  anxiety disorders and, 405–406
  cultural competence and,
    506–507
  eating disorders and, 323
  mood disorders and, 434–435
  Posttraumatic Stress Disorder
    and, 343–344
Columbia University, 20
Communication and Symbolic Behavior Scale, communicative
  disorders and, 177
Communicative Development Inventory:
  case study, 181, 182–186
  communicative disorders and, 177
Communicative disorders:
  assessment of, 174–180
  case study, 180–181
  leaders in the field of, 181–182
Comorbidity, defined, 155–156
Comprehensive Community Mental Health Services for Children and Their Families Program, 517
Comprehensive System for
  Rorschach, 22
CompuPsych, 9
Computerized tomography (CT),
  Attention-Deficit/Hyper-
  activity Disorder and,
  268–269
Concurrent validity, defined, 367
Conduct Disorder:
  assessment of, 239–243
  Attention-Deficit/Hyperactivity
    Disorder and, 270
  behavioral assessment of, 46
  behavioral clinical case formula-
    tion and, 67
  callous-unemotional traits and,
    236–237
  comorbidity, 235–236
  defined, 232
  Disruptive Disorders and,
    459–461
  dynamic psychotherapy and,
    438–439
  effects of stimulants on, 283
  factors associated with, 234–239
  family factors in, 239
  gender differences in, 237
  indirect behavioral assessment of,
    66
  learning disorder and, 145
  onset of, 236
  peer factors in, 238–239
  Posttraumatic Stress Disorder
    and, 341, 343

serious emotional disturbances
  and, 517–518
social cognitive processes and,
  237–238
Student Behavior Survey and, 24
symptoms of, 240
target behavior and, 47
Conners Rating Scales:
  behavioral assessment and, 56–58
  description of 7, 9, 65
  functional assessment and, 68
  learning disorder and, 147
  Parent Rating Scales, 93
    Attention-Deficit/Hyper-
      activity Disorder and,
      275
    case study, 294–295
    Posttraumatic Stress Disorder
      and, 341
    social/emotional maladjust-
      ment and, 456
  psychopharmacology and, 486
  revised, 25
  Teacher Rating Scales, 69, 71
    Attention-Deficit/Hyper-
      activity Disorder and, 275
    case study, 152, 294–295
    Posttraumatic Stress Disorder
      and, 341
Content validity, defined, 367
Continuous Performance Test:
  Attention-Deficit/Hyperactivity
    Disorder and, 276
  description of, 66
  learning disorder and, 147
Coping Power Program, 249
Cortex, defined, 120
Covert conditioning, defined, 41
CPT. *See* Continuous Performance
  Test
CPTSRI. *See* Childhood PTSD Re-
  action Index
Criminal court, 108–109
Cruickshank, William, 142
Cultural competence:
  application of, 501–507
  challenges to, 507–508
  clinical assessment and, 502–504
  conceptual framework for,
    495–499
  intervention and, 504–505
  model of, 499–501
  psychopharmacology and,
    505–506
  psychosocial therapies and,
    506–507
  rationale for, 494–495
  therapeutic alliance and, 501–502
Cyclothymic Disorder:
  case study, 442
  characteristics of, 426–427
Cylert. *See* Pemoline
Cyproheptadine, eating disorders
  and, 481

Datheus, Arch Priest of Milan, 329
*Daubert v. Merrell-Dow Pharmaceu-
  ticals,* 102
Delinquency, 108–109
Dementia pralcocissina, 190–191

Dendrite, defined, 120
Depakote. *See* Valporic acid
Depression:
  acute, chronic, and masked,
    418–419
  aggressive behaviors and, 423
  Attention-Deficit/Hyperactivity
    Disorder and, 422–423
  case study, 439–441
  degrees of, 419
  diagnosis of, 423–424
  factors and changes within,
    417–418
  learning disabilities and, 422–423
  psychopharmacology and,
    476–477
  suicide and, 420–422
  See also Mood disorders
Desipramine:
  Attention-Deficit/Hyperactivity
    Disorder and, 285
  depression and, 476
  eating disorders and, 481
Desmopressin acetate, enuresis and,
  483
Desyrel. *See* Trazodone
Developmental delay, 173
Developmental Disorders:
  Mental Status Exam and, 91–93
  See also Pervasive Developmen-
    tal Disorders
Development Sentence Scoring,
  communicative disorders
  and, 177, 178, 179
Devereux Behavior Rating Scale
  (School), learning disorder
  and, 147
Deviation IQ method, 21
Dexedrine. *See* Methylphenidate
Dextroamphetamine, Attention-
  Deficit/Hyperactivity Dis-
  order and, 282–283
Dextrostat, Attention-Deficit/
  Hyperactivity Disorder
  and, 282–283
Diagnostic Checklist for Behavior-
  Disturbed Children (Form
  E-2), 207
Diagnostic Interview for Children
  and Adolescents:
  anxiety disorders and, 397
  behavioral assessment and, 62
  description of, 63
  psychopharmacology and, 485
  social/emotional maladjustment
    and, 456
Diagnostic Interview Schedule for
  Children:
  behavioral assessment and, 58
  case study, 9, 245–246
  Disruptive Behavior Disorders
    and, 242
  Infant-Toddler Social and Emo-
    tional Assessment, 373
  psychopharmacology and, 485
  social/emotional maladjustment
    and, 456
DICA. *See* Diagnostic Interview
  for Children and Adolescents

Differential Ability Scales, learning disorder and, 147
Differential reinforcement, defined, 34
Differential reinforcement of other behavior, 47
    case study, 74–75
Dimethylglycine (DMG), 220
Dinosaur School, 250
Diphenhydramine:
    anxiety disorders and, 478
    sleep disturbance and, 483–484
DISC. See Diagnostic Interview Schedule for Children
Discriminative stimuli, defined, 34
Disintegrative psychosis, 193
Disruptive Behavior Disorders, 459–461
    assessment issues in, 251–252
    assessment of, 239–243
    case study, 243–246
    clinical issues in, 252–255
    cognitive-behavioral interventions in, 247–251
    defined, 231–234
    infant mental health and, 372
    interventions in, 247
    See also Conduct Disorder; Oppositional Defiant Disorder
Dissociative Disorder, case study, 442
Divorce, 106–108
Dix, Dorothea, 515
Down syndrome:
    communication profiles of children with, 174
    communicative disorders and, 173
    Mental Status Exam and, 92
Doxepin, depression and, 476
Draw-a-Person, 4
DRO. See Differential reinforcement of other behavior
DTLA-4, learning disorder and, 147
DuPaul Rating Scales:
    Attention-Deficit/Hyperactivity Disorder and, 275
    Parent Rating Scale, case study, 288–289
    Teacher Rating Scale, case study, 288–289
Dura, defined, 123
Dynamic psychotherapy, mood disorders and, 437–439
Dyslexia. See Specific Reading Disorder
Dysthymic Disorder:
    characteristics of, 426
    learning disorder and, 145
    Posttraumatic Stress Disorder and, 340, 343

Eating Attitudes Test, 324
Eating Disorder Inventory, description of, 65
Eating disorders:
    assessment of, 311–314
    atypical forms of, 317
    comorbidity, 318

current status of, 309–310
detection and prevention of, 323–324
differential diagnosis of, 317
interventions and rehabilitation, 321–323
leaders in the field of, 310–311
medical evaluation of, 313–314
populations, 318–319
psychological/psychiatric assessment of, 312–313
psychopharmacology and, 322–323, 481
risk factors, 318–319
serious emotional disturbances and, 517
See also Anorexia Nervosa; Bulimia Nervosa
Education for All Handicapped Children Act (1975), 104, 513
Effexor. See Venlafaxine
Elavil. See Amitriptyline
Elective Mutism:
    behavioral assessment of, 46
    case study, 75–76
    ethnic issues, 79
Electroconvulsive therapy (ECT), social/emotional maladjustment and, 467
Ellen, Mary, 330
Emotional disorders. See Serious emotional disturbances
Encopresis, measurement of target behavior and, 49, 52
Enuresis:
    measurement of target behavior and, 49, 52
    psychopharmacology and, 483
    serious emotional disturbances and, 517
Escaping, defined, 35
E-2. See Diagnostic Checklist for Behavior-Disturbed Children (Form E-2)
Exhibition, behavioral assessment of, 61
Expansion mutations, Attention-Deficit/Hyperactivity Disorder and, 269–270
Experimental Analysis of Behavior (EAB), 33, 43
Eysenck Personality Questionnaire, 57

Facilitated communication (FC), 219
Fast Track Program, 231, 249–250
Fear Survey Schedule for Children:
    anxiety disorders and, 397
    behavioral assessment and, 61
    description of, 65
Feeding Disorder of Infancy or Childhood, 52
    infant mental health and, 372
Feingold diet, 287
Fenfluramine, Attention-Deficit/Hyperactivity Disorder and, 286
Fernald, Grace, 143

Fetishism, behavioral assessment of, 61
Finger Tapping Test, 126
    brain injury and, 128
Fluoxetine, 218
    anxiety disorders and, 407
    Attention-Deficit/Hyperactivity Disorder and, 286
    depression and, 476–477
    eating disorders and, 323, 481
    Posttraumatic Stress Disorder and, 345
    social/emotional maladjustment and, 467
Fluphenazine, schizophrenia and, 481
Fluvoxamine:
    depression and, 477
    eating disorders and, 323
    social/emotional maladjustment and, 467
Focal assessment, 4–6
    example of, 7–9
    instruments of, 8
Folstein Mini-Mental State Exam, 91
Forebrain, defined, 122
Forensic evaluation, 103–104
    therapeutic vs. legal practice contexts in, 98–103
Foundling Family Hospital, 329
Fragile X Syndrome:
    Mental Status Exam and, 92
    symptoms of, 201
Fraiberg, Selma, 360
Freedom from Distractibility (FFD), 275–276
Frontal lobe, defined, 120
Functional analysis:
    vs. behavioral assessment, 42–43
    current trends in, 76–78
    defined, 32, 202
    expansion of, 38–42
    history of, 33–38
Functional assessment:
    of behavioral changes, 58–61
    defined, 33
Functional Assessment Interview, description of, 63
Functional magnetic resonance imaging (fMRI), Attention-Deficit/Hyperactivity Disorder and, 268–269

Galton, Sir Francis, 20
Gault, in re, 109, 110
Generalized Anxiety Disorder:
    Attention-Deficit/Hyperactivity Disorder and, 270
    characteristics of, 399–400
    clinical vignette, 399–400
    criteria for, 391–392
    Posttraumatic Stress Disorder and, 340, 343
    psychopharmacology and, 407
Genetic field theory, 388
GFTA. See Goldman-Fristoe Test of Articulation
Gilliam Autism Scale, case study, 222

Glial cells, defined, 120
Global Assessment Scale, social/emotional maladjustment and, 456
Globus pallidus:
  Attention-Deficit/Hyperactivity Disorder and, 269
  defined, 122
Golden Cage, The, 311–314
Goldman-Fristoe Test of Articulation:
  communicative disorders and, 178, 179
Goldstein, Kirk, 142
Greenspan, Stanley, 360
Grip Strength Test, 126
Guanfacine:
  Attention-Deficit/Hyperactivity Disorder and, 286–287
  social/emotional maladjustment and, 467
Guidelines for Culturally Competent Managed Mental Health Services, 508
Guide to Assessment of Test Session Behavior (GATSB), 24
Gull, Sir William, 310
Guthrie, R. E., 33
Gyri, defined, 120

Haldol. *See* Haloperidol
Halo errors, defined, 274
Haloperidol:
  Attention-Deficit/Hyperactivity Disorder and, 286
  Autistic Disorder and, 482
  schizophrenia and, 481
  Tourette's Disorder and, 482
Halstead-Reitan Neuropsychological Test Battery for Children, motor functioning and, 126
Hamilton:
  Anxiety Rating Scale, 397, 398
  Depression Inventory, mood disorders and, 430–431
  Rating Scale for Depression, social/emotional maladjustment and, 456
Harvard Infant Study Laboratory, 386
HDI. *See* Hamilton, Depression Inventory, mood disorders and
Heller's syndrome, 193
Hindbrain, defined, 123
Hiskey-Nebraska Test of Learning Aptitude, description of, 63
Home Situations Questionnaire, description of, 66
Hydroxyzine:
  anxiety disorders and, 478
  sleep disturbance and, 483–484
Hyperkinetic impulse disorder, 265. *See also* Attention-Deficit/Hyperactivity Disorder
Hyperkinetic Reaction of Childhood Disorder, 265. *See also* Attention-Deficit/Hyperactivity Disorder

Hypothalamus, defined, 122

Illinois Test of Psycholinguistic Abilities, 143
  description of, 65
Imipramine:
  Attention-Deficit/Hyperactivity Disorder and, 285
  depression and, 476
  eating disorders and, 322–323, 481
  enuresis and, 483
Individual Education Plan (IEP), 105–106, 278
Individuals with Disabilities Education Act (IDEA; 1991):
  Attention-Deficit/Hyperactivity Disorder and, 273–274, 278–279
  characteristics of, 104
  serious emotional disturbances and, 513, 525
  special education and, 199
Individual Treatment Plans (ITP), 4
Infant and Toddler Mental Status Exam, 367–368
Infanticide, 328–329
  legal protection against, 330
Infantile Autism, 198
Infant mental health:
  assessment of, 361–368
  developmental, 362–366
  measures of, 366–367
  at-risk populations, 368
  case study, 373–377
  diagnosis of, 369–377
  disciplines involved in, 362
  historical overview of, 359–361
  interventions and rehabilitation, 377–380
Infant-Toddler Social and Emotional Assessment, 373
Institutional Review Boards (IRBs), 33
Instrumentally proximal event, defined, 44
Instruments for Assessing Understanding and Appreciation of Miranda Rights, 100, 111
Internal consistency reliability, defined, 58
International Congress of the World Association of Infant Mental Health, 359
Interpersonal therapy (IPT), mood disorders and, 436
Interrater errors, defined, 274
Interrater reliability, defined, 366–367
Interviews:
  child, Attention-Deficit/Hyperactivity Disorder and, 273
  parent, Attention-Deficit/Hyperactivity Disorder and, 272
Interview Schedule for Children, 25
  description of, 63
Intrasubject replication designs, defined, 37

IOWA Conners Rating Scale, Attention-Deficit/Hyperactivity Disorder and, 275
ITMSE. *See* Infant and Toddler Mental Status Exam
ITSEA. *See* Infant-Toddler Social and Emotional Assessment

Journal of Applied Behavior Analysis, 37
Journal of Child and Adolescent Psychiatry, 6
Journal of the Experimental Analysis of Behavior, 37

K-ABC. *See* Kaufman Assessment Battery for Children
KAIT. *See* Kaufman Adolescent and Adult Intelligence Test
Kaufman Adolescent and Adult Intelligence Test:
  description of, 21
  learning disorder and, 147
Kaufman Assessment Battery for Children:
  description of, 4, 21, 63
  learning disorder and, 147
Kent v. United States, 110
Kiddie-SADS. *See* Schedule for Affective Disorders and Schizophrenia in School Age Children
Kirk, Samuel, 143
Klonopin. *See* Clonazepam
Koop, C. Everett, 119
K-SADS. *See* Schedule for Affective Disorders and Schizophrenia in School-Age Children

Lasègue, Charles, 310
Law. *See* Forensic evaluation
Learning disorder:
  assessment of, 143–147
  Attention-Deficit/Hyperactivity Disorder and, 156, 422–423
  case study, 148–154
  cognitive behavioral approaches and, 161
  comorbidity, 155–156
  defined, 140–141
  depression and, 422–423
  dynamic psychotherapy and, 438–439
  externalizing disorders and, 156–157
  history of, 141–143
  indirect behavioral assessment of, 66
  internalizing disorders and, 156
  medical factors in, 158–160
  medication and, 163
  remediation, 161–163
  social skills and, 157
  treatment of, 161
Legal system:
  protection of children, history of, 330–331
  See also Forensic evaluation

Leiter Informal Piagetian Assessment, communicative disorders and, 178
Leniency errors, defined, 274
Limbic system, defined, 122
Lithium carbonate:
    Attention-Deficit/Hyperactivity Disorder and, 286
    Bipolar Disorder and, 480
    eating disorders and, 323, 481
    self-injurious behaviors and, 483
    social/emotional maladjustment and, 467–468
Louisville Behavior Checklist, description of, 66
Luria-Nebraska Neuropsychological Battery (children's revision), motor functioning and, 127
Luvox. See Fluvoxamine

MacArthur Communication Development Inventory, 183–184
MACI. See Millon Adolescent Clinical Inventory
Magnetic source imaging (MSI), Attention-Deficit/Hyperactivity Disorder and, 269
Major Depressive Disorder:
    Attention-Deficit/Hyperactivity Disorder and, 270
    behavioral clinical case formulation and, 67
    diagnosis of, 521
    episodes of, 417–418
    ethnic issues, 79
    indirect behavioral assessment of, 66
    Posttraumatic Stress Disorder and, 340, 341, 343
    Recurrent, 425
    Single Episode, 425
Maladjustment, social/emotional:
    assessment of, 453–457
    case study, 462–464
    current trends in, 451–453
    diagnosis and formulation of, 457–462
    historical overview of, 451–453
    instruments, 455–457
    psychopharmacology, 466–468
    treatment approaches, 464–466
Marching Test, 126
MASC. See Multidimensional Anxiety Scale for Children
Master treatment plan (MTP), 278
Matching Familiar Figures Test, 68
    Attention-Deficit/Hyperactivity Disorder and, 275
    description of, 66
    learning disorder and, 147
Mayo Clinic, 9
McCarthy Scales of Children's Abilities, 21
    child abuse and, 130
    description of, 63
    motor functioning and, 127
    Motor Scale, closed head injury and, 128

MECA. See Methods for the Epidemiology of Children and Adolescent Mental Disorders
Medulla, defined, 123
Mellaril. See Thioridazine
Mental Measurements Yearbook, 367
Mental Retardation:
    assessment of, 6
    Attention-Deficit/Hyperactivity Disorder and, 270
    vs. Autistic Disorder, 210
    indirect behavioral assessment of, 66
    Mental Status Exam and, 91–93, 95–96
    methylphenidate and, 285
    perceptual motor theory and, 142
Mental Status Exam:
    age-related modification of, 90–91
    case study, 94–96
    content of, 89–90
    defined, 86–87
    in diagnosis and treatment planning, 96
    focal assessment and, 7
    Infant-Toddler, 91
    process of, 88
    purposes of, 86–87
    recording of, 93–95
    use with special populations, 91–93
Methods for the Epidemiology of Children and Adolescent Mental Disorders, 389–390
Methylphenidate:
    Attention-Deficit/Hyperactivity Disorder and, 282–283, 286, 479
    Autistic Disorder and, 218
    case study, 290, 293
    Mental Retardation and, 285
Metropolitan Achievement Tests, description of, 65
Midbrain, defined, 122–123
Millon Adolescent Clinical Inventory, 23
Millon Adolescent Personality Inventory, 23
Minimal brain damage, 265. See also Attention-Deficit/Hyperactivity Disorder
Minimal brain dysfunction, 265. See also Attention-Deficit/Hyperactivity Disorder
Minnesota Multiphasic Personality Inventory:
    computer-assisted assessment and, 9
    description of, 23
    mood disorders and, 428–429
Minnesota Perception Diagnostic Test (revised):
    case study, 151
    learning disorder and, 147
Miranda v. Arizona, 109–111

Mirtazapine, depression and, 477
Momentary time sampling recording system, defined, 53
Monoamine oxidase inhibitors, Attention-Deficit/Hyperactivity Disorder and, 286
Montreal Delinquency Prevention Program, 250
Mood, defined, 416
Mood disorders:
    case study, 441–442
    cognitive-behavioral therapy and, 434–435
    description of, 458–459
    diagnosis of, 424–428
    dynamic psychotherapy and, 437–439
    family therapy, 435–436
    historical perspectives on, 415–417
    infant mental health and, 372
    interpersonal therapy and, 436
    intervention in, 433–435
    play therapy and, 437
    school-based interventions, 435
    treatment of, 431–433
    Weinberg criteria for, 414–415
Morton, Richard, 310
Motor-Free Visual Perception Test, learning disorder and, 147
Motor functioning:
    evaluation of, 126–127
    neuroanatomy of, 123–125
    See also Brain injury
MSE. See Mental Status Exam
Multidimensional Anxiety Scale for Children, 397
    Posttraumatic Stress Disorder and, 340
Multimodal Treatment of ADHD (MTA), 283
Multiple-baseline designs (MBDs), 59–61
    format of, 60
Multisystemic therapy (MST):
    serious emotional disturbances and, 526
    social/emotional maladjustment and, 466
Myelin, defined, 120
Myklebust, Helmer, 143

Naglieri Nonverbal Ability Test, learning disorder and, 147
Naloxone, Autistic Disorder and, 482
Naltrexone, Autistic Disorder and, 482
National Institute of Mental Health, 453, 516
National Latino Behavioral Workgroup, 508
National Society for Autistic Children, 194
National Society for the Prevention of Cruelty to Children, 330
Navane, schizophrenia and, 481

Nefazodone, Attention-Deficit/
Hyperactivity Disorder and,
286
Negative reinforcement, defined, 35
NEPSY, motor functioning and,
127
Neuron, defined, 120
New York Longitudinal Study of
Child Development, 385
New York State Institute Adapted
Mental Status Exam, 92
Nisonger Child Behavior Rating
Form, 93
NMH Diagnostic Interview Sched-
ule for Children, anxiety dis-
orders and, 397
Norepinephrine, anxiety disorders
and, 405–406
Norpramine. See Desipramine
Nortriptyline:
Attention-Deficit/Hyperactivity
Disorder and, 285
depression and, 476

Obsessive-Compulsive Disorder:
behavioral assessment of, 45
characteristics of, 394–395,
401–402
clinical vignette, 402
cognitive-behavioral therapy and,
405–406
psychopharmacology and, 407
Olanzeprine, schizophrenia and,
481
Open head injury (OHI), 129–130
Operant conditioning, defined, 33
Oppositional Defiant Disorder:
assessment of, 239–243
Attention-Deficit/Hyperactivity
Disorder and, 270
behavioral clinical case formulation and, 67
callous-unemotional traits and,
236–237
case study, 522
comorbidity, 235–236
defined, 232
Disruptive Disorders and,
459–461
effects of stimulants on, 283
factors associated with, 234–239
family factors in, 239
gender differences in, 237
indirect behavioral assessment of,
66
learning disorder and, 145
Mental Status Exam and, 94–95
onset of, 236
peer factors in, 238–239
Posttraumatic Stress Disorder
and, 341, 343
social cognitive processes and,
237–238
Student Behavior Survey and, 24
symptoms of, 240
target behavior and, 47
Oregon Social Learning Center, 250
Orton, Samuel, 142–143
Osgood, Charles, 143
Other Health Impaired (OHI), In-

dividuals with Disabilities
Education Act and, 278
Owen, Robert, 330

Paired Associate Learning Test,
Attention-Deficit/
Hyperactivity Disorder
and, 275
Pamelor. See Nortriptyline
Panic Attack, 392
Panic Disorder:
characteristics of, 392–393, 400
clinical vignette, 400
cognitive-behavioral therapy and,
405–406
Separation Anxiety Disorder
and, 398–399
PAPA. See Preschool Age Psychi-
atric Assessment
Parallel forms reliability, defined, 58
Parent-Adolescent Communication
Scale, description of, 65
Parenting Stress Index, purpose of,
367
Parent Interview for Autism, 207
Parent Management Training
(PMT), 280
Parietal lobes, defined, 121
Paroxetine:
depression and, 477
Posttraumatic Stress Disorder
and, 345
social/emotional maladjustment
and, 467
Partial interval time sampling, de-
fined, 52–53
Paxil. See Paroxetine
PDDRS. See Pervasive Develop-
mental Disorders Rating
Scale
Peabody Picture Vocabulary Test,
description of, 65
Pedophilia, behavioral assessment
of, 61
Peel, Sir Robert, 330
Pemoline:
Attention-Deficit/Hyperactivity
Disorder and, 282, 479
case study, 293
Perceptual motor (PM) theory, 142
Periactin, eating disorders and, 481
Permanent product recording system, defined, 52
Personality Inventory for Children,
24
anxiety disorders and, 397
Attention-Deficit/Hyperactivity
Disorder and, 274
learning disorder and, 147
Personality Inventory for Youth, 24
mood disorders and, 429
Pervasive Developmental Disorders:
assessment of, 6, 201–204
behavioral assessment of,
203–204
behavioral clinical case formulation and, 67–68
behavioral interventions in, 47,
213

case study, 220–224
defined, 189
development-based assessment
of, 203
differential diagnosis for,
208–210
educational intervention in,
215–216
family treatment with, 213
indirect behavioral assessment of,
66
infant mental health and, 372
informal observation of, 202–203
interventions in, 210–219
language intervention in,
216–217
Mental Status Exam and, 92
psychopharmacology and,
217–219
special education and, 199
Pervasive Developmental Disorders
Rating Scale, 207–208
PES. See Preschool Evaluation
Scale
Pharmacology. See Psychopharmacology
Phenelzine, Attention-Deficit/
Hyperactivity Disorder
and, 286
Phobias, serious emotional distur-
bances and, 517
PIA. See Parent Interview for
Autism
Pia mater, defined, 123
PIC. See Personality Inventory for
Children
Pimozide, Tourette's Disorder and,
482
PIY. See Personality Inventory for
Youth
Play therapy:
abuse/trauma and, 346
mood disorders and, 437
Pons, defined, 123
Porteus Mazes, Attention-Deficit/
Hyperactivity Disorder and,
275
Positive reinforcement, defined, 35
Positron emission tomography
(PET), Attention-Deficit/
Hyperactivity Disorder and,
268–269
Posttraumatic Stress Disorder:
anxiety disorders and, 461–462
assessment of, 338–339
characteristics of, 402–403
clinical vignette, 403
comorbidity, 340–341
diagnosis of, 341–343, 395–396
diagnostic interviews and symptom checklists for, 339–340
events and, 334
sexual abuse and, 335–336
Precentral gyrus, defined, 121
Predictive validity, defined, 367
Prefrontal cortex, Attention-
Deficit/Hyperactivity Disorder and, 269
Premature Ejaculation, behavioral
assessment of, 61

Preschool Age Psychiatric Assessment:
Infant-Toddler Social and Emotional Assessment, 373
Preschool Evaluation Scale:
case study, 221
Preschool Language Scale:
case study, 222
communicative disorders and, 178
Primary motor area, defined, 121
Problem-Solving Skills Training (PSST), 280
Programming, defined, 34
Prolixin, schizophrenia and, 481
Promoting Alternative Thinking Strategies (PATHS), 249
Protriptyline, Attention-Deficit/ Hyperactivity Disorder and, 285
Providence, Sally, 360
Prozac. See Fluoxetine
Psychological Assessment Resources (PAR), 9–10
Psychopharmacology:
assessment and, 486
case study, 522
cultural competence and, 487, 505–506
formulation and diagnosis and, 484–485
infant mental health and, 379
leaders in the field, 475–476
role of professionals in, 487–490
special issues in, 487–490
Psychotic Disorder, serious emotional disturbances and, 517
PTSD Reaction Index, 339
Putamen, defined, 122

Quentepine, schizophrenia and, 481

Racemine amphetamine, Attention-Deficit/Hyperactivity Disorder and, 282
RADS. See Reynolds Adolescent Depression Scale
Rate of responding, defined, 44
Raven's Progressive Matrices:
description of, 63
learning disorder and, 147
RCDS. See Reynolds Child Depression Scale
Reactive Detachment Disorder:
case study, 442
infant mental health and, 372
Reading Disorder, behavioral clinical case formulation and, 67
Real-Life Rating Scale, 207
Recency errors, defined, 274
Rehabilitation Act (1973), 104
Attention-Deficit/Hyperactivity Disorder and, 278
Reinforcement of Corresponding Reports, defined, 69
Reinforcement of Do-Report Correspondence, defined, 69
Reinforcement Set-Up on Promises, defined, 73

Reiss Scales for Children's Dual Diagnosis, 93
Reitan-Indiana Test Battery for Children, motor functioning and, 126
Remeron, depression and, 477
Rett's Disorder, 198, 200
Mental Status Exam and, 92
psychopharmacology and, 482
Reversal design, defined, 58–59
Reynolds Adolescent Depression Scale:
mood disorders and, 430
Reynolds Child Depression Scale:
mood disorders and, 429–430
Risperidone, 218
Autistic Disorder and, 482
schizophrenia and, 481
Ritalin. See Methylphenidate
RLRS. See Real-Life Rating Scale
Robert Wood Johnson Mental Health Services Program for Youth (RWJ-MHSPY), 517
Rorschach Inkblot Technique, 22
Rorschach Prognostic Rating Scale, 22
Rossetti Infant-Toddler Scale, communicative disorders and, 177

SAED. See Scale for Assessing Emotional Disturbance
SALT. See Systematic Analysis of Language Transcripts
Sanctis, Sante de, 190–191
S-B-IV, learning disorder and, 147
SBS. See Student Behavior Survey
Scale for Assessing Emotional Disturbance:
social/emotional maladjustment and, 456
Schedule for Affective Disorders and Schizophrenia in School-Age Children, 25, 58
anxiety disorders and, 397
behavioral assessment and, 62
description of, 63
epidemiological version, Posttraumatic Stress Disorder and, 339
present and lifetime version, Posttraumatic Stress Disorder and, 339
Schizophrenia:
vs. Autistic Disorder, 209–210
psychopharmacology and, 480
as a term, 191
School Behavior Checklist:
description of, 66
learning disorder and, 147
School Situations Questionnaire, description of, 66
Science and Human Behavior, 35
Secretin, 218
Selective Mutism, indirect behavioral assessment of, 66
Selective serotonin reuptake inhibitors:
aggression and violent behavior and, 483

anxiety disorders and, 405–406, 477–478
assessment and, 7
Attention-Deficit/Hyperactivity Disorder and, 286, 480
Autistic Disorder and, 482
depression and, 476–477
eating disorders and, 323, 481
Posttraumatic Stress Disorder and, 345
self-injurious behaviors and, 483
side-effects of, 477
social/emotional maladjustment and, 467
use of, with autism, 218–219
Self-Control Rating Scale:
description of, 66
learning disorder and, 147
Self-injurious behavior:
functional analysis of behavior and, 36
psychopharmacology and, 483
Separation Anxiety Disorder:
assessment of, 391
behavioral assessment of, 61
characteristics of, 398–399
clinical vignette, 399
cognitive-behavioral therapy and, 405–406
epidemiology of, 389
genetic field theory and, 388
Posttraumatic Stress Disorder and, 340, 343
Sequenced Inventory of Communicative Developments:
case study, 180, 183
communicative disorders and, 177, 178
Serious emotional disturbances:
accomplishment of systems of care projects, 527–529
assessment of, 518–520
case study, 522–523
characteristics of, 517–518
clinical model in systems of care and, 520–521
defined, 513–515
education and, 525–526
history of treatment, 515–517
Individuals with Disabilities Education Act and, 278
juvenile justice and, 526
models of interagency collaboration in systems of care and, 523–527
public health/primary care and, 527
symptomatic management of, 482–484
treatment of, 3–4
welfare/social services and, 524–525
Sertraline:
Attention-Deficit/Hyperactivity Disorder and, 286
case study, 440
depression and, 477
eating disorders and, 323
Posttraumatic Stress Disorder and, 345

Sertraline (*continued*)
  social/emotional maladjustment
    and, 467
Severity errors, defined, 274
Sexual Aversion Disorder, behavioral assessment of, 61
S-FRIT, learning disorder and, 147
SICD. *See* Sequenced Inventory of Communicative Developments
Simon, Theodore, 20
Single positron emission tomography (SPECT), Attention-Deficit/Hyperactivity Disorder and, 268–269
Single-subject designs, defined, 37
Skinner, B. F., 33–38
Skinnerian paradigm, 43–45
Skull fractures, 129–130
Sleep Disorder, infant mental health and, 372
Slosson Visual-Motor Performance Test, learning disorder and, 147
Smith, Bob, 9
SNAP, Attention-Deficit/Hyperactivity Disorder and, 275
Social Anxiety Scale for Children (revised), 397
Social Phobia:
  characteristics of, 393–394, 396
  cognitive-behavioral therapy and, 405–406
Social Skills Rating System, case study, 246
Society for the Prevention of Cruelty to Animals, 330
Specific Arithmetic Disorder, Attention-Deficit/Hyperactivity Disorder and, 271
Specific language impairment (SLI), 172–173
Specific language impairment–expressive (SLI-E), 172–173
Specific Learning Disabilities:
  Attention-Deficit/Hyperactivity Disorder and, 270–272
  Individuals with Disabilities Education Act and, 278
Specific Phobias:
  characteristics of, 393–394, 400–401
  clinical vignette, 401
Specific Reading Disorder:
  Attention-Deficit/Hyperactivity Disorder and, 271–272
  magnetic resonance imaging and, 271–272
Specific Writing Disorder, Attention-Deficit/Hyperactivity Disorder and, 271
Speech disorders, serious emotional disturbances and, 517
SSRIs. *See* Selective serotonin reuptake inhibitors
STAIC. *See* State-Trait Anxiety Inventory for Children
Standards for Cultural Competence

in Managed Care Mental Health, 508
Stanford-Binet Intelligence Scale:
  case study, 294–295
  description of, 20–21, 63
Stanford v. Kentucky, 103
State-Trait Anxiety Inventory for Children:
  anxiety disorders and, 397
  psychopharmacology and, 486
Statistical guess, defined, 44
Stimulants:
  Attention-Deficit/Hyperactivity Disorder and, 282–284, 479
  side effects of, 283–284
  social/emotional maladjustment and, 467
  Tourette's syndrome and, 285
Strange Situation Test, anxiety disorders and, 388
Strauss, Alfred, 142
Stroop Test, Attention-Deficit/Hyperactivity Disorder and, 275
Structural magnetic resonance imaging (sMRI), Attention-Deficit/Hyperactivity Disorder and, 268–269
Structured diary, defined, 202
Structured Interview of Reported Symptoms, 100
Student Accommodation Plan, 278–279
Student Behavior Survey, 24
Subcortex, defined, 122
Substance Abuse and Mental Health Services Administration (SAMHSA), 513
Substance Abuse Disorders:
  diagnosis and formulation of, 457–458
  mood disorders and, 417
  Posttraumatic Stress Disorder and, 340
  serious emotional disturbances and, 517
Suicide, 468–469
  depression and, 420–422
Sulci, defined, 120
Symbolic psychosis, 193
Systematic Analysis of Language Transcripts:
  communicative disorders and, 177, 178, 179
Systematic Training for Effective Parenting (STEP), 280–281
System of Multicultural Pluralistic Assessment, motor functioning and, 127

Tact, defined, 43
Tally frequency count, defined, 202
Target behavior:
  behavioral definition of, 47–48
  defined, 202
  measurement of, 49–55
Teacher Report Form:
  Attention-Deficit/Hyperactivity Disorder and, 274
  case study, 294–295

Tegretol. *See* Carbamazepine
Temporal lobes, defined, 121–122
Test for Severe Impairment, 91–92
Test of Language Development, communicative disorders and, 178, 179, 180
Test of Memory and Learning, learning disorder and, 147
Test of Nonverbal Abilities, learning disorder and, 147
Test of Nonverbal Intelligence, description of, 64
Test-retest errors, defined, 274
Test-retest reliability, defined, 58, 366
Thalamus, defined, 122
Thematic Apperception Test, 22
Therapeutic alliance, cultural competence and, 501–502
Thioridazine:
  Attention-Deficit/Hyperactivity Disorder and, 286, 480
  schizophrenia and, 481
Thiothixine, schizophrenia and, 481
Thompson v. Oklahoma, 103
Thorazine. *See* Chlorpromazine
Tofranil. *See* Imipramine
Tourette's Disorder:
  Attention-Deficit/Hyperactivity Disorder and, 270
  psychopharmacology and, 482
  stimulants and, 285
  systems of care and, 521
TOVA, Attention-Deficit/Hyperactivity Disorder and, 275
Tower of Hanoi, Attention-Deficit/Hyperactivity Disorder and, 275
Tranylcypromine, Attention-Deficit/Hyperactivity Disorder and, 286
Trauma:
  assessment of, 338–341
  case study, 348–349
  causes of, 333–334
  diagnostic interviews and, 339–340
  epidemiology of, 332–333
  history of, 328–330
  impact of, 334–338
  by race, 332
  symptom checklists for, 339–340
  treatment interventions for, 343–348
  treatment phases of, 344–348
Trazodone:
  eating disorders and, 481
  sleep disturbance and, 484
Treatment and Education of Autistic and Related Communication Handicapped Children (TEACCH), 211
TRF. *See* Teacher Report Form
Tricyclic acid, Attention-Deficit/Hyperactivity Disorder and, 285

Unmarried Mother in German Literature, The, 329

U.S. Senate Committee on Labor and Human Resources, 119

Valporic acid:
Bipolar Disorder and, 480
eating disorders and, 323
Posttraumatic Stress Disorder and, 345
self-injurious behaviors and, 483
social/emotional maladjustment and, 467–468
Venlafaxine:
Attention-Deficit/Hyperactivity Disorder and, 286
depression and, 477
Vineland Adaptive Behavior Scales, 57, 93
case study, 181, 184, 292, 294–295
purpose of, 367
Vineland Social Maturity Scale, description of, 64
Vistaril. See Hydroxyzine
Visual Analogue Scale for Anxiety (revised), 397

Watson, J., 33
Wechsler, David, 21
Wechsler Individual Achievement Test, case study, 292
Wechsler Intelligence Scale for Children:
Attention-Deficit/Hyperactivity Disorder and, 275–276
case study, 149–150, 246, 292
characteristics of, 21, 64

communicative disorders and, 179
focal assessment and, 4–6, 57
indexes on, 11
learning disorder and, 147
limits of diagnosis based on, 77
psychological interpretive report, 10–15
psychometric summary, 12
Wechsler Memory Scale, learning disorder and, 147
Wechsler Preschool and Primary Scale of Intelligence:
characteristics of, 21, 64
communicative disorders and, 178
Wellbutrin. See Bupropion
Werner, Hing, 142
Werry-Weiss-Peters Activity Rating Scale, 57, 66
Western Interstate Commission on Higher Education, 508
Whole-interval recording system, defined, 52
Wide Range Achievement Test:
case study, 151, 294–295
description of, 65
Wide-Range Assessment of Memory and Learning, learning disorder and, 147
Wide-Range Assessment of Visual Motor Abilities, learning disorder and, 147
Williams syndrome, Mental Status Exam and, 92
WISC. See Wechsler Intelligence Scale for Children

Wisconsin Card Sort Test, Attention-Deficit/Hyperactivity Disorder and, 275
Woodcock-Johnson Reading Mastery Tests (revised), learning disorder and, 147
Woodcock-Johnson Scale of Independent Behavior:
brain injury and, 128
case study, 295
World Association of Infant Mental Health (WAIMH), 358
World Association of Infant Psychiatry. See International Congress of the World Association of Infant Mental Health
Wundt, William, 20

Xanax. See Alprazolam

Yale-Brown Obsessive Compulsive Scale for Children:
case study, 404
psychopharmacology and, 486
Yale–New Haven Middle School Social Problem Solving Program, 250
Y-BOCS-C. See Yale-Brown Obsessive Compulsive Scale for Children

Zero to Three/National Center for Infants, Toddlers, and Families (ZTT), 358
Zoloft. See Sertraline